Natural Toxins

Proceedings of the 6th International Symposium on Animal, Plant and Microbial Toxins, Uppsala, August 1979

Editors

D. EAKER and T. WADSTRÖM

Institute of Biochemistry, Uppsala, Sweden

PERGAMON PRESS

OXFORD · NEW YORK · TORONTO · SYDNEY · PARIS · FRANKFURT

U.K.	Pergamon Press Ltd., Headington Hill Hall, Oxford OX3 0BW, England
U.S.A.	Pergamon Press Inc., Maxwell House, Fairview Park, Elmsford, New York 10523, U.S.A.
CANADA	Pergamon of Canada, Suite 104, 150 Consumers Road, Willowdale, Ontario M2J 1P9, Canada
AUSTRALIA	Pergamon Press (Aust.) Pty. Ltd., P.O. Box 544, Potts Point, N.S.W. 2011, Australia
FRANCE	Pergamon Press SARL, 24 rue des Ecoles, 75240 Paris, Cedex 05, France
FEDERAL REPUBLIC OF GERMANY	Pergamon Press GmbH, 6242 Kronberg-Taunus, Hammerweg 6, Federal Republic of Germany

First edition 1980

British Library Cataloguing in Publication Data

International Symposium on Animal, Plant and Microbial Toxins, *6th, Uppsala, 1979*
Natural toxins.
1. Toxins - Congresses
I. Title II. Eaker, D
III. Wadström, T
615.9'5 QP631 80-40898

ISBN 0-08-024952-3

Supplement No 2 1980 to the journal *Toxicon.*

In order to make this volume available as economically and as rapidly as possible the authors' typescripts have been reproduced in their original forms. This method has its typographical limitations but it is hoped that they in no way distract the reader.

Printed in Great Britain by A. Wheaton & Co., Ltd., Exeter

Contents

CYTOLYTIC TOXINS

PHOSPHOLIPASES AND CELL MEMBRANES

ENTEROTOXINS

LIPID A AND ENDOTOXIN

Preface

Poisons produced by living organisms have fascinated man for many centuries, and various of them have been exploited for good and devious ends from ancient times down to the present. Unlike most of the man-made environmental poisons that pervade the industrialized world today, most of the natural poisons produced by living things are unstable in nature, and nearly all cases of accidental poisoning by such toxins involve direct contact with the organisms that produce them. In most of the industrialized nations of the world, natural toxins are not serious problems because, owing to climatic conditions and urbanization, poisonous insects and animals are rare, and in the case of microorganisms, because contacts have been minimized by better hygiene and controls on the production and distribution of foodstuffs and water or because the unpleasant consequences of such contacts have been largely eliminated by immunization. However, the tropical climates of most developing countries favor proliferation of all forms of life. Serious and even fatal diseases in man and livestock caused by toxins of various microorganisms are often endemic, and more than 100 000 human deaths occur each year as a consequence of bites or stings by poisonous snakes, insects and spiders. Diarrhea diseases caused by various microorganisms are the major cause of infant mortality in the world. Furthermore, the mycotoxins produced by certain molds render a very large fraction of the cereal and peanut production of many developing countries unfit for consumption by man or beast. The latter toxins are especially dangerous owing to the insidious nature of their effects.

For two reasons, natural toxins have received steadily increasing attention during the last two decades: firstly, because we realize that better methods for their detection and the diagnosis, treatment and prevention of the diseases that they cause are among the prerequisites for social and economic progress in many of the developing nations of the world. The second reason is the realisation that the often awesome potency of the most powerful natural toxins is due to very specific interference with vital molecular processes involved in the maintenance of cell integrity and in the communication among different cells. Natural toxins are thus emerging in their own right as extremely valuable tools for the study of some of the most fundamental mechanisms of life.

The concensus among the participants was that the 6th International Symposium on Animal, Plant and Microbial Toxins held in Uppsala in August 1979 under the co-sponsorship of the International Society on Toxinology and the University of Uppsala was a great success both scientifically and socially. The scientific success relects in no small part the high relevance of the subject matter and the competence of the chairmen who put together the 16 different sessions. The meeting was attended by 319 registered participants, and including non-registered locals attendance exceeded 400 on most days. The next international meeting of the International Society on Toxinology will be held in Brisbane, Australia, during July 1982.

Of the 235 abstracts submitted for the meeting, 209 arrived in time for publication in the special issue of TOXICON (volume 17, supplement 1, 1979). 207 papers were actually presented at the meeting: 78 orally and 129 in poster form. Although nearly all of the papers presented were worthy of publication, it did not seem feasible to publish the entire proceedings, which might have run to well over 2000 pages. Working within a page limit of 800 - 1000 pages, we therefore decided to invite submission of manuscripts of only the invited oral papers, which were mainly of review character, and the special workshop presentations, which were tightly organized and also contained considerable amounts of review material. We felt that the remaining free communications, which mainly represented new, original research on a broad range of topics would inevitably be published elsewhere anyway. In any case, the publication of the abstracts meant that all participants had the opportunity to record their participation in print.

Of the 124 manuscripts thus requested for these proceedings, 83 were received and appear here under the authorship of 228 authors. Although we had correctly estimated the time required for the editorial work at two full months, most of the manuscripts arrived late in October 1979, toward the end of the period that we had reserved for the job, and owing to teaching and other committments we were unable to return in earnest to the task until mid-Spring of this year. A delay of somewhat more than one month in the submission of the manuscripts has thus delayed completion of the book by about half a year. We hope that you readers will find the volume worth waiting for.

Uppsala, June 1, 1980

David Eaker Torkel Wadström

Plenary Lectures

VENOM GLANDS, VENOM SYNTHESIS, VENOM SECRETION AND EVOLUTION

E. Kochva, U. Oron, M. Ovadia, T. Simon and A. Bdolah

*Dept. of Zoology, George S. Wise Faculty of Life Sciences,
Tel Aviv Univ., Ramat Aviv, Israel*

ABSTRACT

This paper reviews the embryonic development, structure and function of the compound oral glands of non-venomous and venomous snakes in comparison with other exocrine glands, mainly the pancreas. It discusses the phylogenesis of the snake venom glands and proposes a hypothesis for the co-evolution of the two-component, phospholipase-containing toxin and the anti-toxic factor(s) found in the blood serum of snakes.

KEYWORDS

Venom; snake; evolution; phospholipase A; toxin; embryonic development; exocrine glands; anti-toxin; enzyme inhibitor; Viperidae.

INTRODUCTION

In his paper on the evolution of enterosecretory proteins, Adelson (1971) states that "genetic changes in the time and location of expression of the functionally different, related genes led to the evolution of functionally specialized regions of the gut" and that "the ability to secrete related proteins remained constant among the gut-derived glands." He sees as a special case "the ability of several specialized non-entodermal tissues to secrete proteins related to entodermal proteins", which could evolve by "a change in the pattern of gene-activation...... allowing expression of a formerly repressed entodermal gene in a non-entodermal tissue". Extensive evidence in support of these suggestions has since been accumulated (Dayhoff and co-workers, 1975), and hypotheses on the evolution of toxins from certain pancreatic enzymes have been proposed (Eaker, 1975; Heinrikson, Krueger and Keim, 1977; Ivanov and Ivanov, 1979; Strydom, 1977). Given these hypotheses one might expect to find similarities also in the morphology of the glands secreting these compounds, i.e. the pancreas and the compound oral glands of snakes; these similarities should then be more evident in the more primitive glands of the non-venomous species.

EMBRYOLOGY AND MORPHOLOGY

Snakes have developed a variety of exocrine glands in the mouth. The two major types are found in the supra-labial region and are represented by Duvernoy's glands in the colubrid snakes and by the venom glands in the Viperidae and Elapidae *sensu lato* (Kochva, 1978b).

We shall start this comparison with the embryonic development of Duvernoy's glands and the venom glands of Viperidae. In all species thus far examined the gland develops from a common, ectodermal primordium, together with the dental lamina of the maxilla (Fig. 1a). At later stages, the primordium of Duvernoy's gland branches in a symmetrical pattern, while in the Viperidae branching is restricted to the posterior region of the gland (Figs. 1b-d). From what meager evidence is available, the development of the venom glands of the Elapidae and the Atractaspidinae seem to resemble the pattern of Duvernoy's glands rather than the viperid venom glands.

In general terms, the embryonic development already provides some clues suggesting that the venom glands of the Viperidae are the more specialized and should be expected to differ from other glands also in the adult. The similarities with other exocrine glands such as the pancreas, should be looked for among Duvernoy's glands of the non-venomous snakes. The great variability of these glands should facilitate the search and make it possible to find glands with a general pattern not dissimilar to that of the pancreas. An example of such a gland is given in Fig. 2. The venomous snakes, and mainly the vipers, show a different morphology

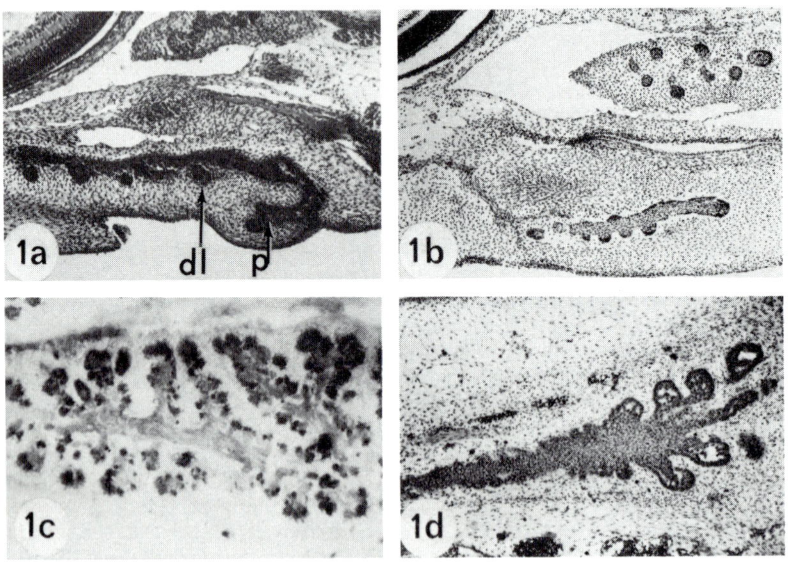

Fig. 1. Embryonic development of oral glands. a) Early stage of dental lamina with gland primordium in *Natrix tesselata*; approx. 80x. b) First branching of gland primordium in *Spalerosophis cliffordi*; approx. 50x. c) Later branching of gland in *Spalerosophis*; approx. 40x. d) Branching of venom gland primordium in *Vipera palaestinae*; approx. 60x. dl - dental lamina; p - primordium of Duvernoy's gland.

that can be clearly seen even at lower magnifications of the light microscope (Figs. 3a-c). At the ultrastructural level the differences are more evident: In all glands examined, including the Elapidae, the cells are filled with secretory granules; only the Viperidae and Crotalidae show a very small number of granules, compensated for by the wide lumina that store large amounts of venom (Figs. 4a-c). *Vipera palaestinae* and the other Viperidae and Crotalidae thus show a gland that is well adapted for having a large amount of venom in store to use effectively even in several consecutive strikes, in connection with a simple and efficient way of replenishing the dose(s) injected (Kochva, 1978a).

Looking at the amounts of venom found in the gland lumina and the small number of secretory granules in the cells, the question was asked whether these secretory granules are the only avenue of venom secretion or whether there was an alternative, direct route of secretion, e.g. from the cisternae of the rough endoplasmic reticulum into the lumen. The latter pathway was suggested for other exocrine glands (cf. Isenman and Rothman, 1979).

In order to answer this question, some histochemical and immunohistochemical techniques were applied, at the level of the light and electron microscopes (Figs. 5a-d). The results show that all secretory cells contain the venom components examined, some of which could be identified in the same secretory granules. Admittedly, not all our evidence is direct and overlapping, but it appears nevertheless that the venom is secreted through these granules, despite their scarcity.

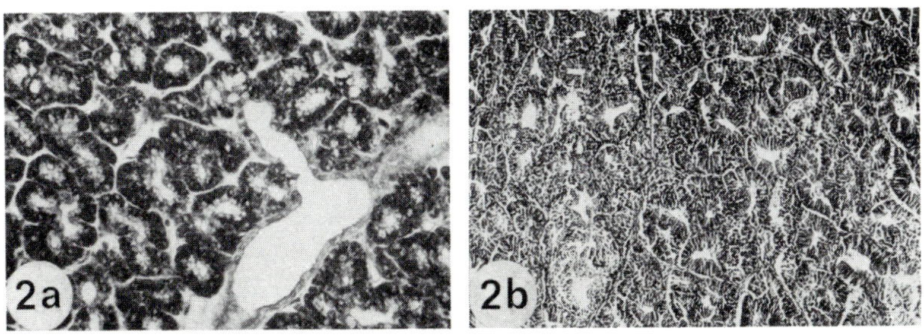

Fig. 2. Comparison of pancreas and Duvernoy's gland. a) Pancreas of *Vipera palaestinae*; approx. 200x. b) Duvernoy's gland of *Aparallactus modestus*; approx. 200x.

PHYSIOLOGY

Quantitative evidence on the synthesis and secretion of venom is now available from work done on the Cascavel, *Crotalus durissus terrificus* at Riberão Preto by Marchi, Haddad and De Lucca (1978), on the Tsefa, *Vipera palaestinae*, by Oron and Bdolah (1978b) in Tel Aviv and on the sea snake *Laticauda semifasciata* by Takeda, Yoshida and Tamiya (1974). Radioautographic and morphometric calculations (Fig. 6) support the assumption that the intracellular transport of venom proteins in both *Crotalus* and *Vipera* follows the conventional pattern of exocrine glands, as documented by Palade (1975) for the mammalian pancreas. In *Crotalus* there is a variable number of intracisternal granules (Brasileiro, 1976) that follows a different labelling pattern.

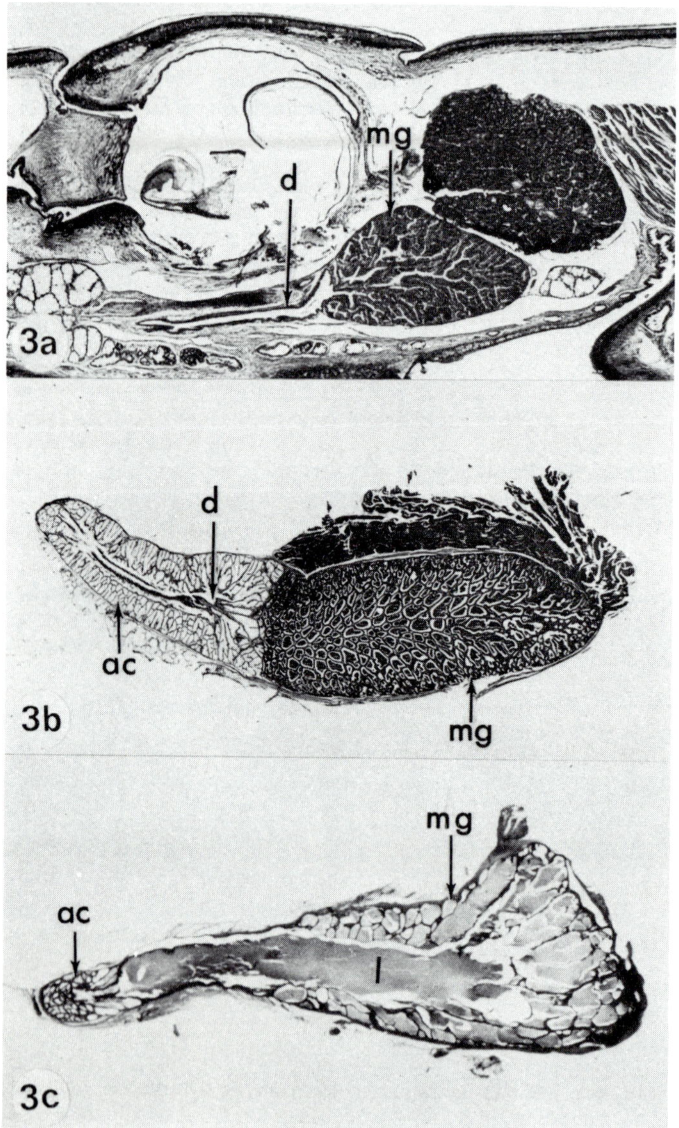

Fig. 3. Adult morphology of oral glands. a) Duvernoy's gland of *Chilorinophis*; approx. 40x. b) Venom gland of *Walterinnesia aegyptia*; approx. 12x. c) Venom gland of *Vipera palaestinae*; approx. 20x. ac - accessory gland; d - duct; l - lumen; mg - main gland.

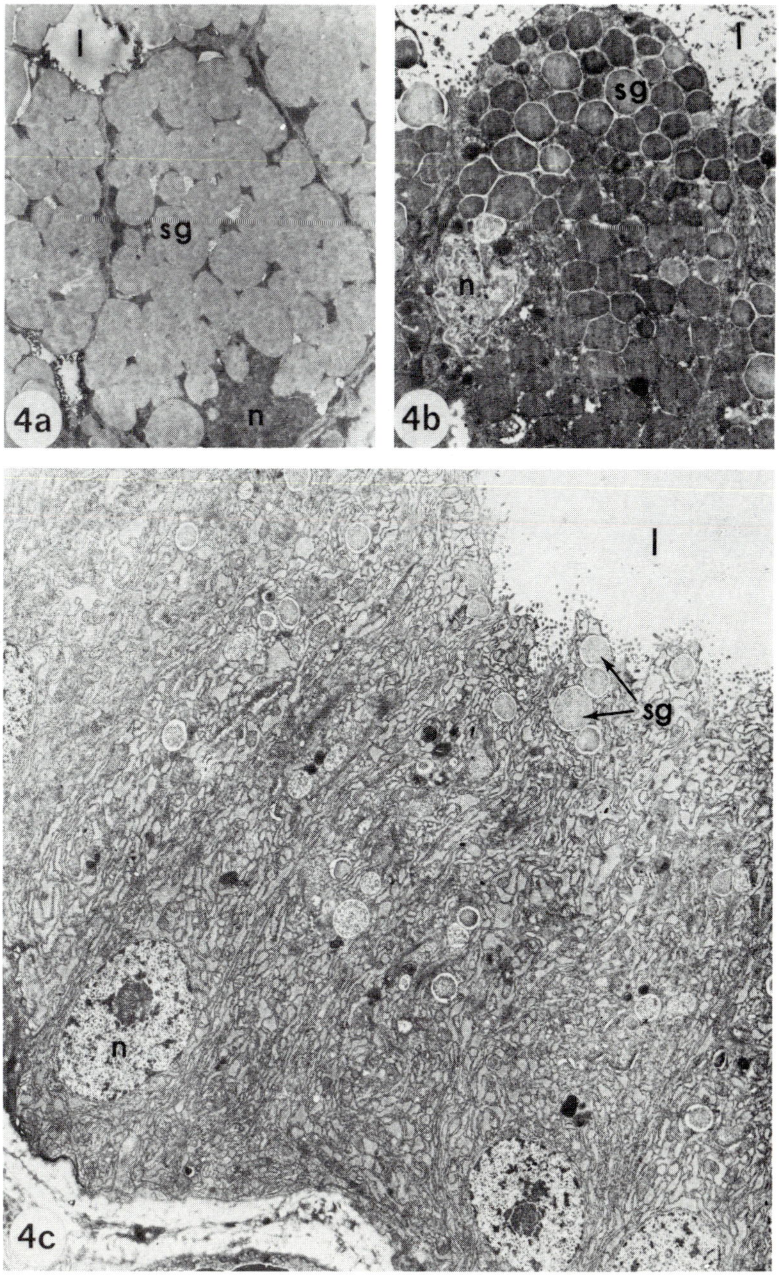

Fig. 4. Electron micrographs of oral glands. a) Duvernoy's gland of *Dispholidus typus*; approx. 4000x. b) Venom gland of *Naja melanoleuca*; approx. 5000x. c) Venom gland of *Vipera palaestinae*; approx. 3000x. 1 - lumen; n - nucleus. sg - secretory granules.

The major differences between the pancreas and the viperid venom gland, thus, lie in the storage of secretion in the glands. While in the pancreas and salivary glands the secretion is stored intracellularly in the so-called zymogen granules, in the viperid venom gland secretion is mainly accumulated in the extended lumina of the gland. After manual extraction of the venom (milking) there is an increased rate of secretion which is a result of a high rate of venom synthesis and of intracellular transport. As the gland lumina become filled with venom, both processes slow down considerably (Oron and Bdolah 1978b). The secretion cycle in the Elapidae venom gland is virtually unknown.

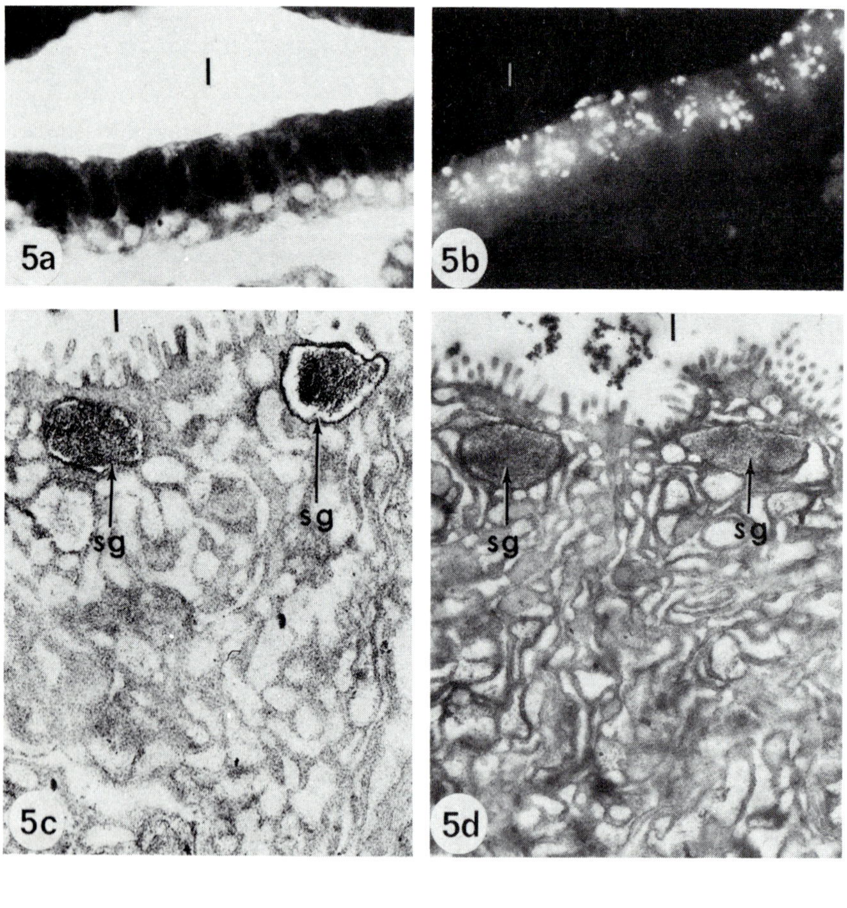

Fig. 5. Localization of venom components in *Vipera palaestinae*. a) Histochemical staining for L-amino acid oxidase; approx. 900x. b) Immuno-fluorescence staining for the two-component toxin; approx. 800x. c) Immuno-peroxidase staining for phosphodiesterase; approx. 14000x. d) Immuno-peroxidase staining for L-amino acid oxidase; approx. 8000x. l - lumen; sg - secretory granule.

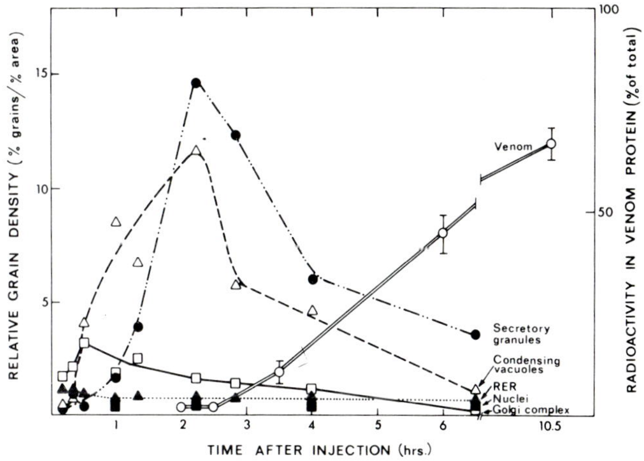

Fig. 6. Labelling kinetics of cell organelles and of secreted venom in the active venom gland of *Vipera palaestinae*. The snakes were labelled by a chronic cannulation of the left systemic arch (Oron and Bdolah 1978a) and sacrificed at the indicated intervals. Relative grain densities were calculated from radioautographs of the glands and the radioactivity in the secreted venom was monitored at various intervals after milking (Oron and Bdolah 1978b).

EVOLUTION

From what has been said so far, it appears that the compound oral glands of snakes have preserved some basic characteristics of other exocrine glands, such as the pancreas, glands that have appeared early in vertebrate evolution. These characteristics are more evident in the non-venomous, colubrid snakes, but are also found in the Elapidae. In the latter group, the venom apparatus in general is in a less advanced stage of development as compared to the Viperidae, which show a high specialization of both the venom glands and skull components related to the venom injecting mechanism (Kochva, 1978b). It is therefore interesting to note that some of the elapid venom components - cardiotoxins, short and long neurotoxins - are considered to be the last step in toxin evolution, while the phospholipase-containing toxins appear to be their predecessors (Strydom, 1977).

In the two-component toxin system of *Vipera palaestinae*, both components, the basic, non-enzymic protein and the acidic phospholipase A are required for lethality. The first point we would like to stress is that the phospholipase can be replaced effectively by heterologous enzymes taken from venoms of elapid and viperid snakes, but not by the enzyme from pig pancreas (Table 1; Simon, Bdolah and Kochva, 1980). The second point deals with the anti-toxic factor found in the blood serum of *Vipera* and of other snakes, a factor that inhibits phospholipase activity and, at the same time, abolishes the toxicity of the venom (Table 2). The anti-toxic factor(s) that is found in the blood serum of venomous and non-venomous snakes and in some mammals neutralizes a variety of venoms except elapid venoms (Table 3, Ovadia and Kochva, 1977).

These data in the context of the current ideas on the evolution of venom (Eaker, 1975; Heinrikson, Krueger, and Keim, 1977; Strydom, 1977) suggest the following hypothesis: The ancestors of snakes had a pancreas that secreted a phospholipase and had also a phospholipase-inhibitor in their blood. When compound glands appeared in the lower jaw of some lizards and in the upper jaw of snakes, they carried with them, among other things, a phospholipase. This enzyme has been found so far in the lizard *Heloderma* (Shier and co-workers, 1979) and in the colubrid snakes *Malpolon* (unpublished) and *Leptodeira* (Mebs, 1968), but not in *Thelothornis* (Kornalik, Taborska and Mebs, 1978). The presence of the phospholipase inhibitor made it possible for the enzyme to become toxic by preventing damage to the snake in case the toxin should find its way into the blood stream. We thus present here a scheme of molecular co-evolution of two proteins, enzyme and inhibitor, toxin and anti-toxin, that had obvious functions in the ancestors, without having to involve "preadaptation" or "neutral" mutations as a way of explanation.

TABLE 1 Substitution of Phospholipase (PLA) of the *Vipera palaestinae* Two-Component Toxin by Heterologous Enzymes (Simon, Bdolah and Kochva, 1980)

Source of PLA		Mixture injected: PLA (μg)	Mixture injected: A (μg)	Toxicity (surviving mice)
V. palaestinae	pI 4.5	10	10	10/18
Pseudocerastes fieldi	pI 7.2	20	10	3/18
	pI 5.5	20	10	2/18
Walterinnesia aegyptia	pI 7.8	50	20	1/6
	pI 4.5	25	20	1/6
Sus scrofa, pancreas		100	10	6/6

A - basic, non-enzymic component of *Vipera*

TABLE 2 Inhibition of Phospholipase A (PLA) Activity by *Vipera palaestinae* Antitoxic Factor (Simon, Bdolah and Kochva, 1980)

Incubation mixture	Lecithin splitting (%)	Lethality (surviving mice)
Exp. I		
Toxin	92	0/10
Toxin + antitoxic factor 1:100	39	10/10
Toxin + bovine albumin 1:100	96	0/10
Toxin + rabbit serum 1:100	88	0/10
Exp. II		
Isolated PLA	90	-
Isolated PLA + antitoxic factor	20	-
Isolated PLA + antihemorrhagic factor	60	-

TABLE 3 Neutralization of *Viperidae* and *Elapidae* venoms by Sera of Different Animals (Ovadia and Kochva, 1977)

Origin of sera	Origin of venom: Viperidae				Elapidae	
	Vipera palaestinae	*Echis colorata*	*Pseudocerastes fieldi*	*Aspis cerastes*	*Walterinnesia aegyptia*	*Naja nigricollis*
	No. surviving mice / No. injected mice					
Snakes						
Viperidae						
Vipera palaestinae	9/10	8/10	7/10	10/10	0/10	0/10
Pseudocerastes fieldi	10/10	9/10	10/10	10/10	0/10	1/10
Vipera ammodytes	10/10	8/10	10/10	10/10	0/10	0/10
Elapidae						
Walterinnesia aegyptia	10/10	9/10	7/10	10/10	0/10	10/10
Naja nigricollis	10/10	0/10	10/10	5/10	0/10	10/10
Colubridae						
Malpolon monspessulanus	9/10	8/10	2/10	10/10	0/10	0/10
Natrix tessellata	9/10	3/10	8/10	4/10	0/10	0/10
Mammals						
Herpestes ichneumon	0/10	7/10	1/10	10/10	0/10	0/10
Mesocricetus auratus	8/10	4/10	1/10	1/10	0/10	0/10

ACKNOWLEDGEMENTS

We thank Dr. H. Gainer for comments and Mrs. M. Wollberg, Mr. A. Shoob and Mrs. C. Meyer for help in the preparation of the manuscript.

REFERENCES

Adelson, J.W. (1971). Enterosecretory proteins. Nature, 229, 321-325.
Brasileiro, I.L.G. (1976). Investigacões morphológicas sobre granulos nas cisternas do reticulo endoplasmático rugoso das células secretoras de veneno da cascavel sulamericana (*Crotalus durissus terrificus*), ao longo de um ano durante o ciclo secretor. Dissertation presented to the Faculty of Medicine, University of São Paulo at Riberão Preto. Brasil.
Dayhoff, M.O., P.J. McLaughlin, W.C. Barker, and L.T. Hunt (1975). Evolution of sequences within protein superfamilies. Naturwissenschaften, 62, 154-161.
Eaker, D. (1975). Structural nature of presynaptic neurotoxins from Australian elapid venom. Toxicon, 13, 90-91.
Heinrikson, R.L., E.T. Krueger, and P.S.Keim (1977). Amino acid sequence of phos-

pholipase A_2-α from the venom of *Crotalus adamanteus*. J. Biol. Chem., 252, 4913-4921.
Isenman, L.D., and S.S. Rothman (1979). Diffusion-like processes can account for protein secretion by the pancreas. Science, 204, 1212-1215.
Ivanov, Ch.P., and O. Ivanov (1979). The evolution and ancestors of toxic proteins. Toxicon, 17, 205-220.
Kochva, E. (1978a). Evolution and secretion of venom and its antidotes in snakes. Period. biol., 80 (Suppl. 1), 11-23.
Kochva, E. (1978b). Oral Glands of the Reptilia. In C. Gans (Ed.), Biology of the Reptilia, Vol. 8, Academic Press, London and New York. pp. 43-161.
Kornalik, F., E. Taborska, and D. Mebs (1978). Pharmacological and biochemical properties of a venom gland extract from the snake *Thelotornis kirtlandi*. Toxicon, 16, 535-542.
Marchi, F., A. Haddad, and F.L. de Lucca (1978). Radioautographic and biochemical studies of secretion of venom protein in the south American rattlesnake *Crotalus durissus terrificus*. J. Exp. Zool., 203, 429-442.
Mebs, D. (1968). Analysis of *Leptodeira annulata* venom. Herpetologica, 24, 338-339.
Palade, G.E. (1975). Intracellular aspects of the process of protein synthesis. Science. 189, 347-358.
Oron, U., and A. Bdolah (1978a). Chronic cannulation of left systemic arch of the snake, Lab. Anim. Sci., 28, 219-220.
Oron, U., and A. Bdolah. (1978b). Intracellular transport of proteins in active and resting secretory cells of the venom gland of *Vipera palaestinae*. J. Cell Biol., 78, 488-502.
Ovadia, M., and E. Kochva (1977). Neutralization of Viperidae and Elapidae snake venoms by sera of different animals. Toxicon, 15, 541-547.
Simon, T., A. Bdolah, and E. Kochva (1980). The two component toxin of *Vipera palaestinae*: Contribution of phospholipase A to its activity. Toxicon,(in press).
Shier, W.T., J.P. Durkin, J.T. Trotter, and G.V. Pickwell (1979). Phospholipase A_2 electrophoretic variants in reptile venoms. Toxicon, 17, 167.
Strydom, D.J. (1977). Snake venom evolution. South African J. Sci. 73, 70-71.
Takeda, M., H. Yoshida, and N. Tamiya (1974). Biosynthesis of erabutoxins in the sea snake, *Laticauda semifasciata*. Toxicon, 12, 633-641.

PHARMACOLOGY OF VENOMS

F. E. Russell

Lab. Neurol. Res., Univ. Southern California, Los Angeles County-Univ. Southern California Medical Center, Los Angeles, California, USA

ABSTRACT

The action of a venom on an organism is dependent upon a number of variables: the route of administration, absorption, distribution, passage across a succession of membranes, accumulation at receptor site(s), metabolism, and excretion. In addition, in determining the action of a venom, such factors as autopharmacological changes, the action of venom metabolites, and the importance of different animal and tissue kinds must be considered. These various influences on the pharmacological activities of animal venoms are discussed.

KEYWORDS

Route of administration; absorption; distribution; passage across membranes; accumulation at receptor site(s); metabolism, excretion; autopharmacology; lethality; immunity.

INTRODUCTION

It would be nice to think that Kipling had the International Society on Toxinology in mind when he wrote:

"It is unjust that when we have done
All that a serpent should,
You gather our poisons, one by one,
And break them down to your good."

Man's interest in breaking down venoms is several fold. Firstly, he is interested in what these diversified and intriguing substances are composed of. Secondly, he is interested in how these substances exert their deleterious effects, as well as their beneficial ones. Thirdly, he is interested in why these poisons have evolved as they did. Finally, he is interested in the potential of venoms as drugs for the treatment of disease states, and as tools in biology for the study of cellular and subcellular function, as well as for general physiopharmacologic processes.

The pharmacologist, in formulating his investigations, should exercise the consciousness of a fundamental biologist by seeking to understand how and why venoms came into being, and how the evolution of their function and chemistry relates to the evolution of the anatomical development of the venom apparatus. In his investigative work he must be concerned with the biological activities of the isolated and characterized fractions of the venom. He must know the techniques for screening the individual venom components for their specific pharmacologic properties and, hopefully, he should be wise enough to screen for the wide spectrum of activities that has been endowed in the venoms.

He must be aware of the potential for any autopharmacologic responses precipitated by the release of normal tissue components, and he must also be cognate of the possibility that venom fraction metabolites might be formed within the envenomated organism and might, in themselves, produce deleterious reactions. Most importantly, he must be conscious of the fact that synergistic and, possibly, antagonistic reactions might occur as a result of interaction between individual venom components. It seems wise to keep in mind that there is no piece of experimental evidence which demonstrates that the total pharmacologic effect of a whole venom is equal to the sum of the properties of the individual fractions or functions nor, from a philosophical posture, does such a conclusion seem plausible.

It is one of the unfortunate facts in the study of the chemistry and pharmacology of venoms that the structure and design are most easily investigated by taking the venom apart. This has two shortcomings; it means that a destructive process must be substituted for a constructive, progressive and integrative one; and, secondly, the essential quality of the whole venom may be destroyed before one has made a suitable acquaintance with it. Often times the process of examination becomes so exacting that the end is lost sight of in our preoccupation with the means, so much so that in some cases the means becomes substituted for the end.

A few of us may still recall the decided attempt in 1954 to press for a classification of snake venoms based solely on their enzyme content. Today, the pendulum appears to have swung to the opposite pole. The basis for classifying snake venoms should be founded on data derived from all biological considerations, including those presented by systemics, taxonomy, biology, anatomy, physiology, pharmacology, biochemistry, immunology and clinical medicine with, perhaps, a dash of philosophical adventure thrown in. We should be exceedingly conscious of the possibility that our experiments, however well performed, may not be a true reflection of the manner in which nature herself went about constructing the properties of venoms.

MECHANISMS

In general, it can be said that the disposition of a venom, that is, what is done with it (not what it does) is associated with the chemical nature of its component parts. The action of the function of a venom, on the other hand, is dependent upon the pharmacologic properties of the individual and collective components, as well as their metabolites, and on any autopharmacologic changes the combined properties produce. Although much emphasis has been placed on receptor sites, it must be remembered that some components, such as enzymes, may attack any macromolecule in any tissue within their enzymatic specificity: combination with a receptor site is not necessary.

The fate of a venom or venom component in an organism is dependent upon a number of variables, including its route of administration, absorption, distribution, passage across a succession of membranes, accumulation at receptor site(s), metabolism, and excretion. All of these factors play some role in determining the effect of a venom or venom component within the organism. During the past two decades it has become increasingly clear that there are very significant variations in the roles of these factors in different species of animals. Differences which, in some cases, are more important than the differences usually attributed solely to the weight of the experimental animal.

The toxinologist, as the pharmacologist, is confronted with the question of whether or not a particular difference between animals of various kinds is due to variations in the effectiveness of the toxin at a receptor site or to its passage across membranes, absorption, distribution, accumulation, metabolism, or to its excretion. Of equal importance is the consideration of the possible conversion of toxins to less or, perhaps, more pharmacologically active metabolites.

With respect to the route of administration of a venom and its bioavailability, this not only affects the latent period and duration of an effect but also the toxicity. The physico-chemical property of the sample, its pH, the vehicle, the particle size, and the concentration are important considerations in the distribution and absorption within the organism. The route of administration has different values in different animals. As seen in Table 1, the LD_{50} of a venom is usually less when the toxin is injected intravenously than when given subcutaneously, intramuscularly, or intraperitoneally. However, with some venoms there may be exceptions to this in mice, while in cats and dogs the intravenous route almost always appears to be the far more life-threatening.

TABLE 1 Variations in LD_{50} by Different Routes of Injection

VENOM	INTRAVENOUS	INTRAPERITONEAL	SUBCUTANEOUS
Crotalus viridis helleri	1.29	1.60	3.65
Crotalus adamanteus	1.68	1.90	13.73
Crotalus atrox	4.18	3.71	17.75
Crotalus scutulatus	0.21	0.23	0.31
Agkistrodon piscivorus	4.17	5.10	25.10
Agkistrodon contortrix	10.92	10.50	26.10
Sistrurus miliarius	2.91	6.89	25.10

All determinations in 20 g female mice of the same group, done within a one-hour period and observed for 48 hours.

As seen in Table 1, closely related venoms may display marked differences related to the route of administration. For instance, the subcutaneous LD_{50} for *Crotalus viridis helleri* venom is approximately three times the intravenous LD_{50}, while with *Sistrurus* venom the difference is almost nine fold. Surprisingly, the intraperitoneal LD_{50} for *Agkistrodon contortrix* venom is less than the intravenous LD_{50}. The route of administration and bioavailability is thus an important factor in determining its pharmacologic activity.

Before a venom can be absorbed it must be in a form suitable for passage through several membranes prior to reaching the circulation or some specific site. The membranes through which it may pass act as semipermeable barriers to its penetration. They may selectively permit the passage of certain venom fractions, while blocking the permeation of others.

When a venom is injected into a vein its primary target will be the blood-vascular system, although, obviously, every tissue may be affected in one way or another. When the same venom is injected into subcutaneous tissues, absorption through lymph channels, as well as through the capillary bed and other membranes may affect the toxin's activity, as well as its target tissue or tissues. When the toxin is injected into the peritoneum, again, different membranes become involved.

Some venoms and venom fractions have been injected intraventricularly or directly into the cerebrum. Such studies have elicited considerable academic interest, as well they might. Some reports attempt to show properties of the blood-brain barrier as it relates to the diffusion of venoms. However, the delicacy of this barrier and the factors which can influence it by the very nature of an experimental technique may invalidate the experimenter's results. Such factors as mechanical force, volume of injectable, concentration, pH, and vehicle can greatly affect results, and are too frequently minimized. In addition, the amounts of venom or venom fraction that have been applied to the central nervous system in some experiments are far in excess of physiological parameters or the amount of toxin that could reach the center following parenteral injection or injection by a snake.

Another difficulty relating to bioavailability and absorption is sometimes reflected in disagreements relating to whether or not a venom fraction exerts its effect on a neuromuscular junction, a heart fiber, a vascular strip or some other site. It is not unusual to hear this point debated. The difficulty lies in the fact that it is not possible, in studying the effect of a specific dose of snake venom or venom fraction on various *in vitro* preparations, to come to unequivocal conclusions on an *in vivo* effect. In the *in vivo* preparation the concentration of the toxin reaching the various sites will be different; the amount of toxin needed to elicit specific responses will be different; the ability of the site receptor to absorb, metabolize and excrete the toxin will be different; and the ability of the whole organism, by its own physiopharmacology, to adjust to the action of the poison can be very different. If one compares the doses of venom used in some nerve-muscle or coagulation preparations with those that are administered in *in vivo* studies, or compares the data with changes seen in humans following envenomation, it is obvious that the factors which may affect the biological activity of a venom may be altered considerably by the physiopharmacology of the intact animal.

Nowhere is this more evident than in studies on venoms and neuromuscular transmission. The investigator who uses a dose of "neurotoxin" isolated from three adult cobras to elicit a particular in vitro neuromuscular phenomenon (and one not seen in the in vivo animal preparation or in humans), and who seeks to project his data to conclusions on humans (which frequently occurs), does little but confuse our understanding of the development of venom poisoning. Although the experimenter's interest may not directly relate to this concern, he has the moral responsibility to oversee the use of his data and its application. Finally, it is a matter of grave concern that few toxinologists attempt to pursue the several possible sites of mechanisms of action of a single venom fraction.It hardly seems valid to accept the dogma that venom fractions are organ specific ("neurotoxins, cardiotoxins or hemotoxins"), based on single studies of isolated tissue preparations, but the hypothesis is so deeply rooted in traditional toxinology that it persists, in spite of strong evidence to the contrary.

In considering the passage of toxins across membranes, this can be accomplished by one or several mechanisms: passive diffusion, facilitated diffusion, active transport, or pinocytosis. Studies to date would seem to indicate that passive diffusion and perhaps facilitated diffusion are the principal mechanisms by which venom components reach their target sites. In passive diffusion the drug is transported across the membrane by the concentration gradient of the solute. The rate of diffusion is proportional to the gradient and is dependent upon lipid solubility, degree of ionization, molecular size, and the area of the absorptive surface. The rate of entry into the vascular bed is usually determined for lipid soluble venom fractions by their water-oil partition coefficients, and for lipid-insoluble fractions by their molecular size.

The various membranes of the body are remarkably similar in their chemical structure and spatial arrangement, regardless of their location. This is sometimes overlooked, when such terms as "cytotoxin," "myotoxin," " nephotoxin," "necrotoxin," and the like are used. Primarily, membranes are composed of proteins, phospholipids, and cholesterol. It is thought that the membrane protein is primarily involved in the transport process of venom fractions, although recent work appears to indicate that the phospholipids may play a role. The lipids confer both hydrophilic and hydrophobic properties thereby giving stability to the membrane and providing the characteristics of permeability.

In cases of facilitated diffusion it has been suggested that a "carrier component" combines reversibly with the venom molecule at the membrane's outer surface and that the carrier-substrate complex diffuses more rapidly across the membrane, releasing the molecule (or toxin) at the membrane's inner surface. For certain drugs it is known that this process of facilitated diffusion is highly selective, accepting only those substances which have a relatively specific molecular configuration. There is some evidence to believe that some fractions of venoms are transported by facilitated diffusion.

A third way in which a drug may be transported across a membrane involves active transport, that is, the cell expends energy, and substrates may be accumulated intracellularly against a concentration gradient. The fourth manner of transport, pinocytosis, is a process by which a cell engulfs particles or fluids by invaginating, forming a vesicle that later buds off within the interior of the cell. There is some evidence that several venom components can be transported by pinocytosis.

The site of action and metabolism of a toxin depends on its being distributed to, and partitioned in, various tissues once it has entered the circulation. In the case of most venoms and venom fractions so far studied, distribution is rather unequal, being affected by protein binding, variations in pH, and membrane permeability, among other factors. Once the toxin reaches a particular site its entry is dependent upon the rate of blood flow into that tissue, the mass of the tissue, and the partition characteristics between the toxin and that particular tissue. Some venom components have a high affinity for certain tissues and exert their most deleterious effects on these sites. The point at which they act is the receptor. The various receptor sites have a highly variable degree of sensitivity. It has been shown that the differences in the rate of metabolism of a drug at a receptor site varies considerably in mammals. The differences observed in effective dosages of drugs between man and laboratory animals does not usually reflect any increased sensitivity on the part of man's target organs but is more directly related to the differences in specific rates of metabolism for the drug. The same is probably true for most venoms.

A venom produces its pharmacological effect when the quantity of the toxin attains a critical minimum level at a receptor site. In the case of such complex mixtures as snake venoms there may be several, if not many receptor sites. There may also be considerable variability in the sensitivity of these sites to the different components.

A venom may be metabolized in several or many different tissues. In some cases, it may be more important in experimental work to evaluate to what extent each tissue contributes to the venom's metabolism, as demonstrated by the level of the toxin or its metabolites in the plasma or urine, than to rely solely on the dose given. The amount of a toxin which the tissues of various species of animals can metabolize without endangering the organism varies considerably. To demonstrate a specific tissue's ability to metabolize a venom, tissue slices or hemogenates and subcellular fractions of different tissues should be studied. However, in evaluating such data it must be remembered that organs usually consist of several different kinds of tissues, each of which may contain enzymes which catalyze different reactions. Enzymes which oxidize venoms by oxygenase mechanisms are, for the most part, localized in the parenchymal cells of the liver, while other enzymes may be found somewhat unevenly distributed in many tissues. Thus, a difference in species of animals may play an important role in determining the metabolism of a toxin, on the simple basis that the relative population of a particular cell type in an organ or tissue varies from animal to animal.

The major organ for excretion of snake venoms is the kidney. The intestines play a minor role and the contribution of the lungs and biliary system has not yet been demonstrated. The excretion rate of some snake venoms is complicated by several factors affecting the kidneys, one of the most important of which is the direct effect of the venom on blood cells, and the resulting obstruction of the tubules. In addition, some venom may have a direct effect on the kidneys.

THE EXPERIMENTAL ANIMAL

The choice of experimental animal is very important and I know of few other areas of the pharmacology of venoms that have elicited more controversy and, perhaps, misunderstanding. It cannot be expected that the effective or lethal dose of a venom in any one kind of animal be qualitatively or even quantitatively equal to that found in another kind of animal. Reasonable similarities among some animal kinds may be expected and, indeed, do occur. However, when the data need to be applied to another animal and, in particular, to man, extreme caution must be exercised.

With most drugs man appears to differ more from the other animal kinds than they do among themselves. However, it is too early in our knowledge on venom poisoning to generalize on the relationships between, for example, the rat and the human, but those who deal with both creatures are aware of some similarities and some very important differences in venom dosages. Investigators and physicians who work at this interface will never grow bored for lack of problems but they will need to be prudent in their exercise of comparative data for man and the different animal kinds.

Many investigators have assumed that by merely multiplying the mouse LD_{50} by x, one can arrive at the LD_{50} for the hippopotamus or the fruit fly. Unfortunately, there is an overabundance of such extrapolations in the literature on toxins, some of which attempt to prove that certain animals are 100 times more "immune" than the mouse to a certain snake venom; or that the opossum, mongoose or some other creature is "immune" to a particular venom or venoms. Based on the mouse LD_{50}, and only the size of the animal, plus a dash of rueful conclusion-jumping, one might place the jack rabbit of eastern Arizona and the tarantula high among the "immune" animals to *Crotalus scutulatus* venom, while the kangaroo rat and the wasp are worse off than the laboratory mouse. However, I trust we will not be encouraged by these examples to look for the immune elixir in tarantula hemolymph, which might somehow protect the human against rattlesnake venom, or that we encourage the biologist to cross the tarantula with the rabbit for the production of such an antidote.

Aside from the shortcomings in the design of such questionably thoughout experiments that purport to show immunity in various animals, most of the data are more easily explained by the differences in venom bioavailability, membrane transport, absorption, metabolism, and excretion. Unfortunately, the possibility of finding an immune elixir in the blood or tissues of some snimal is sufficiently tantalizing to encourage a good many studies in search of some universal remedy, even today.

In a series of recent experiments it was suggested that "the combined action of horse antivenin, rattlesnake and wood rat sera could be more effective in snakebite treatment than antivenin alone." The tests on which this conclusion is based are adequately controlled and the results of individual experiments are valid but the conclusions, in my opinion, again seem somewhat short of concern for the differences in the absorption, distribution, metabolism and excretion of a venom with the different experimental agents, and under the conditions of the experiment. Further, there is no reason to believe that the human would react along the line of the theory proposed. Indeed, it would be a very unusual human if it did.

The differences in effective and lethal doses for most drugs in several kinds of animals are well known. Doses are well established for almost all substances which come in contact with animals and, in particular, with humans. Table 2 shows some lethal dose data in different kinds of animals for a representative drug, alpha napthol thio urea, a pesticide and rodenticide.

TABLE 2 Lethality of ANTU

Animal	LD_{50} (mg/kg)
Rat, strain I	2.5
Rat, strain II	6.25
Dog	16.0
Mouse	56.0
Guinea Pig	350.0
Monkey	175.0
Rabbit	400.0
Chicken	2550.0

(Modified from Dicks and Richter, 1946)

The LD_{50} for one strain of rat is 2.5 mg/kg, while that for a different strain is 3 times greater. That for the mouse is 25 times greater, and that for the chicken is 1000 times greater. The toxic dose for humans is between 0.5 g and 5 g/kg. These data again indicate the care that must be exercised in applying information on one kind of animal to another kind of animal.

While the choice of the experimental animal is of primary concern, its weight is also of importance for any specific determination of the lethal or effective dose of a venom. As Trevan has pointed out, the LD_{50} is the most reliable dose level for experimental work. The minimal lethal dose has "in practice...no value, because of the wide variations in the sensitivity of individual animals" (Trevan, 1927).

It is, of course, necessary to compensate for variations in body weight by adjusting individual doses. However, when the body weights of a given group of mice vary more than eight grams, we have found that a straight-line plot is not always reliable for venom testing. Sixteen-gram mice are more sensitive than 25 gram mice, at least for most of the animal venoms.

In determining the LD_{50} of a venom, the sex of the animal must be taken into account. We have found that female mice are more susceptible to snake venoms than male mice. Increasing the environmental temperature of the mice from 15° to 27° decreases the number of deaths. In all LD_{50} determinations, mice of the same sex should be used, and the environmental temperature should be held constant for one hour before the experiment and until well after its completion.

SUMMARY

In this short review I have tried to touch upon a few of the principles and some of the problems that beset the pharmacologist working with venoms. He must be mindful of the pharmacologic principles relating to the route of administration of a toxin, its bioavailability, passage across membranes, absorption, distribution, metabolism, and excretion. He must be aware of the possibility of the formation of metabolites in the envenomated organism. He must keep in mind the probability of autopharmacologic responses secondary to the release of natural-occurring tissue substances, through the direct action of the venom. He must be mindful of synergisms between the venom components and, possibly, antagonisms. He must be cognate of the considerable difference in the manner in which different animals, including man, react to a venom or a venom fraction. He must give attention to the importance of the test animal's body weight and sex. Finally, he should always keep in mind the role the poison plays in the animal's armament.

ACKNOWLEDGEMENT

Work on the pharmacology of venoms is supported by grants NS11476-05 and GM24141-01, of the USPHS, and a gift from the Gould Family Foundation.

REFERENCES

Dieke, S. H. and C. P. Richter (1946). Age and species variation in the acute toxicity of alpha-naphthyl thiourea. Proc. Soc. Exter. Biol. Med., 62, 22-

Trevan, J. W. (1927). The error of determination of toxicity. Proc. R. Soc. (London), B101, 483-

Pathophysiology of Envenomation

STUDIES ON SNAKEBITES IN THE ASIAN AREAS

Y. Sawai

The Japan Snake Institute, Gunma, Japan

ABSTRACT

In the Asian areas snakebites are an occupational hazard in both agriculture and fishing. More than ten thousand deaths are reported annually. The mortality rate in snakebite depends on the species and the density of venomous snakes in each area. Thus, the mortality rate is higher in the Philippines, Thailand, Burma, Sri Lanka and India, where bites by species of Naja naja and Vipera ruselli are predominant in number, whereas lower rates are recorded from bites in Japan, Korea, Hong Kong, Taiwan, Malaysia and Indonesia where bites by pit vipers of Agkistrodon and Trimeresurus species predominate. Sea snakes (Hydrophis ssp) are also a problem among fishermen in Malaysia and Thailand. This report concerns epidemiologic and clinical aspects of snakebites in those areas.

KEYWORDS

Snakebite, Asian areas, epidemiology, clinical symptoms, Naja naja, Agkistrodon, Trimeresurus, Vipera, Bungarus, Hydrophis.

EPIDEMIOLOGICAL ASPECTS OF SNAKEBITES

Venomous snakes responsible for bites in India and Southeast Asia are species of Agkistrodon, Trimeresurus, Naja, Ophiophagus, Bungarus and Hydrophis. However, the distribution of these snakes varies among the different countries, as shown in Table 1. Thus, the mortality rates of bites, which depend on the kind and population of venomous snakes, are higher in the Philippines, Thailand, Burma, Sri Lanka and India, where bites by Naja naja and Vipera russelli species are predominant in number. Lower rates are recorded from Japan, Korea, Hong Kong, Taiwan, Malaysia and Indonesia, where bites by pit vipers such as Agkistrodon and Trimeresurus species predominate, as shown in Table 2. Sea snake bites are also a problem among fishermen in Malaysia and Thailand (Reid and others, 1963; Lim and Abu Bakar, 1970; Sawai and others, 1972, 1976, 1978; Kawamura and others, 1975; de Silva, 1976).

Seasonal patterns in snakebites depend upon the atmospheric temperature and the agricultural activity in each area. Thus, the period of high incidence of bites in Korea or the Japanese mainland, which are located in the northern part of the region, is shorter than the snakebite period in the warmer countries to the south.

In the Philippines, Thailand and Burma bites by species of Naja naja or Vipera russelli increase during rice-planting and harvest time, although the variation in atmospheric temperature throughout a year is not so marked in those areas.

Table 1. Distribution of Venomous Snakes Responsible for Bites

	Agkistrodon	Trimeresaurus	Vipera	Naja	Ophiophagus	Bungarus	Hydrophis
Japan	++*	++*	(-)	(-)	(-)	(-)	(-)
Korea	++	(-)	(-)	(-)	(-)	(-)	(-)
Hong Kong	(-)	++	(-)	+	+	+	+
PROC***	++*	++	+	+*	+	+	+
Taiwan	+*	++*	+	+*	(-)	+*	(-)
Philippines	(-)	+	(-)	++*	+	(-)	+
Thailand	++*	++*	+*	++*	+*	+*	+
Malaysia	++**	+	(-)	+**	+	+	++**
Burma	(-)	+	++*	+*	+	+	+
Indonesia	+*	++	+	+*	+	+*	+
Sri Lanka	+	(-)	++**	++**	(-)	+**	+
India	+	+	++*	++*	+	+*	+

* Antivenin is produced. ** Antivenin is imported. ++ Very common. + Common. (-) Not found. *** People's Republic of China.

Table 2. Mortality per 100,000 Population due to Snakebites

	Bites*	Deaths	Fatality rates (%)	Mortality
Japan[6)]	610 ***	5.6	0.9	0.57
Hong Kong[2)]	203	1.3	0.65	0.09
Thailand[1)]	3,985	302	6.6	0.86
Burma[3)]	8,508	759	8.9	2.7
Malaysia[1)]	2,480	16	0.6	0.18
Taiwan[1)]		36		0.27
Sri Lanka[4)]		318 **		3.9
Philippines[1)]		294		0.77
India[5)]		1,093 ***		2.1

[1)] Sawai and others, 1972. [2)] Sawai and others, 1978. [3)] Report from the Government of Burma, 1978. [4)] de Silva, 1976. [5)] Sawai and Honma, 1976. [6)] Sawai and others, 1976. * Average number per year. ** Maharashtra State of India. *** Habu bites.

Bites show a characteristic frequency distribution with regard to the age of the victim and the geographic location of the incident (Sawai and others, 1972). The bites extend over a wide range of ages from the teens to the fifties, and most occur in cultivated fields, near residences and on roads, where there is frequent close contact between humans and snakes. Although most of the snakes are nocturnal, two-thirds of the bites occurred during daylight, when the snakes lie hidden under cover.

The extremities are the most frequent sites of bites, although the ratio of bites between the upper and lower extremeties varies with the habits and species of the snakes. Thus bites on the lower extremities occurred two to four times more often than bites on upper extremities in the case of rhodostoma and Naja naja species. In contrast, bites on the upper extremities were more frequent with the mamushi (A blomhoffi), whereas bites by Trimeresaurus species (green pit viper and the habu, T flavoviridis) occurred about equally at both extremities.

CLINICAL ASPECTS OF SNAKEBITE

Toxicity of Venom and Envenomation

Fatality due to snakebite depends on the toxicity and the amount of venom injected into victims. The amount of venom ejected by a snake depends on the amount of venom in the venom gland and on the aggressiveness of the snake, and also on the part of the body of the victim penetrated by the fangs. Thus, the equal fatality rates observed in bites by A acutus and B multicinctus of very different toxicity can be explained as follows: the venom of multicinctus is highly lethal, as shown in Table 3, but the amount of venom ejected is small and the snake is less aggressive than A acutus, which injects much larger amounts of less lethal venom through larger fangs by aggressive attack. The difference between fatality rates in bites by T mucrosquamatus and T stejnegeri is due to the larger amount of venom and more aggressive habit of the former, although the toxicity of mucrosquamatus is rather low as compared to that of stejnegeri.

Table 3. Toxicity of Venomous Snakes of Taiwan

Snakes	Mice (sc) * LD_{50} (μg/g)	Fatality rate ** (percent)
B. multicinctus	0.16	23.0
A. acutus	9.2	24.2
T. stejnegeri	4.0	0.9
T. mucrosquamatus	8.6	8.4
N. n. atra	0.67	14.7
V. russelli	1.4	2.2

* Lee and others, 1962. ** To, 1941.

Local lesions: Swelling, Hemorrhages and Necrosis

Swelling at the locus of the bite is one of the most characteristic symptoms of bites by snakes of Agkistrodon, Trimeresurus, Vipera, Ophiophagus and Naja species. Extensive swelling is often accompanied by vesicles. Hemorrhage is another characteristic symptom of bites by Agkistrodon, Trimeresurus and Vipera species. In severe envenomation, both swelling and hemorrhage extend not infrequently far from the locus of the bite. Although necrosis of tissue does not always occur in these bites, it often results in motor disturbances after the wound has healed, as seen in bites by T flavoviridis or N n atra (Figs. 1 and 2).

Systemic Symtoms: Paralysis, Systemic Hemorrhage and Prolonged Coagulation of Blood and Acute Chronic State of Shock

Drowsiness, ptosis of eyelids, blurred vision, drooling of saliva, difficulty of speaking, dyspnea and unconsciousness appear in bites by Naja, Bungarus and Hydrophis species. Blurred vision or drowsiness were also observed in some bites by V

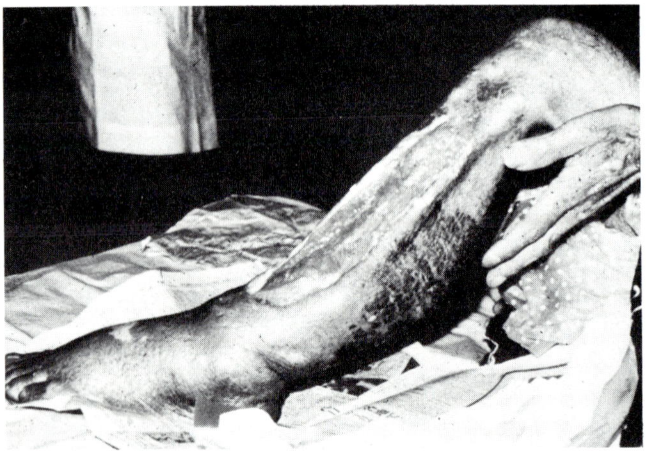

Fig. 1. Bite by T flavoviridis (Sawai and others, 1976).

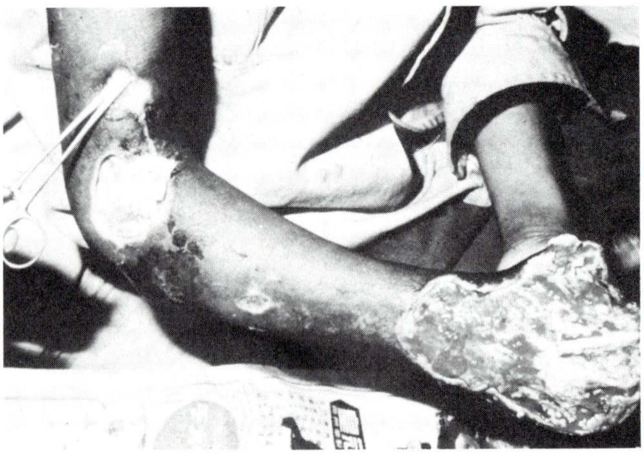

Fig. 2. Bite by N n atra (Kuo and Wu, 1972).

russelli, A blomhoffi, A b brevicaudus, etc. (Sawai and Lah, 1978; Sitprija and others, 1976). Systemic hemorrhage such as ecchymosis, hemoptysis, hematemesis, bleeding from gums, hematuria and prolonged coagulation of blood occur also in severe envenomation by species of Agkistrodon (rhodostoma and acutus) and Vipera (V russelli and Echis carinatus). More serious effects of venoms are hemorrhagic and necrotic lesions in internal organs such as kidney, lung and heart in fatal bites of V russelli or A blomhoffi (Sitprija and others, 1976; Tateno and others, 1963). In such cases patients expire after three to ten days of subacute disease. In fatal bites by the habu (T flavoviridis) most deaths occur within 24 hours. Vomitting, hypotension, cyanosis and rapid and formicant pulse are the characteristic symptoms.

Bites by Naja naja species

About 300 deaths were reported annually from the Philippines, mainly due to bites by N n philippinensis. Most of the deaths may be attributable to inadequate supplies of venoms at hospitals and inadequate treatment by medicine men. Thus, the fatality rate among treated patients was 12.5 percent, as compared to 63.6 percent among victims who died outside hospitals without receiving any medical treatment. By contrast, the fatality rate was only 7.7 percent among victims of N n kauothia bites treated in hospitals in Thailand, where the supply of antivenins seems fairly good. About 60 percent of the snakebites reported annually in Thailand are due to cobras. About 34 percent of 318 deaths by snakebite in Sri Lanka were due to N n naja (de Silva, 1976). Swelling at the loci of bites and the frequent ensuing necrosis of tissue are difficult to prevent by antivenin, and patients needed long periods of hospitalization to receive tissue homografts.

Bites by Bungarus and Ophiophagus Species

B multicinctus occurs in Taiwan, Hong Kong and mainland China and accounts for 20 percent of the total bites in Taiwan, where the fatality rate is a rather high 23 percent (Kuo and Wu, 1972). Fatal cases have also been reported from Hong Kong (Sawai and others, 1978). The antivenin is produced only in Taiwan, but tiger snake (Notechis scutatus) antivenin has been reported to neutralize the venom of B multicinctus (Minton, 1967).

B caeruleus is also a cause of fatal bites in India and Sri Lanka. The symptoms of the bites are similar to those of B multicinctus. Antivenin is available from India. Bites by B fasciatus occur widely in Thailand, Malaysia, Indonesia and other countries. However, the frequency is relatively low owing to the placid disposition of the snake, and the fatality is also low (1.5 %) compared to that in bites by multicinctus and caeruleus, owing to the considerably lower toxicity of the venom (Ganthavorn, 1969). No bites by B candidus or B flaviceps have been reported. The antivenins are produced in Thailand and Indonesia.

The king cobra, Ophiophagus hannah, is widely distributed throughout Southeast Asia. However, reports of bites are infrequent owing to the jungle habitat of the snake. The antivenin is produced in Thailand. A large amount (1150 ml) of the antivenin was used in the treatment of a patient who had been bitten accidentally by a king cobra while working in a snake farm (Ganthavorn, 1971). Artificial respiration contributed decisively to the rescue of the patient.

Vipera Species

Bites by V russelli make an important if not predominant contribution to the high fatality rate among snakebite victims in Burma, India, Sri Lanka and Thailand. It has been reported that more than 90 percent of 800 deaths by snakebite reported annually from Burma are caused by russelli. V russelli accounts for about 40 percent of the 318 deaths by snakebite occurring annually in Sri Lanka. The fatality rate is 2.7 percent in Thailand (Sawai and others, 1978), whereas a high rate of 10 percent was reported from Burma and 11.3 percent from India (Ahuja, 1954). In fatal cases systemic hemorrhage and drowsiness are observed in addition to local swelling and cellulitis, and most of the deaths occur within 24 hours of the bite. On the other hand, anuria or oligouria caused by renal failure often resulted in chronic death within a few days after the bite.

Echis carinatus viper bites are reported in India. The fatality rate is not higher than that in V russelli bites owing to the smaller size of the snake. A characteristic symptom is systematic hemorrhage, such as gum bleeding, although local signs are not marked. India is the only source of antivenin (Sawai and Honma, 1976).

Agkistrodon Species

More than 70 percent of the total bites in West Malaysia occurred in the northwest area of the Malay Peninsula, where 75 percent of the bites were by A rhodostoma. The same species accounted for 49.3 percent of the total bites in Thailand. Swelling is very common, with subcutaneous bleeding and vesicle formation. Local necrosis of tissues occurred in 11 percent of cases. Systemic symptoms, such as prolonged coagulation of the blood, occurred in 27 percent and hemorrhagic diathesis in 12 percent of cases. The fatality rate is less than one percent (Reid and others, 1963). Although monovalent antivenins are imported from Thailand, the application is limited only to severe cases in Malaysia.

A acutus bites are reported from southern areas of Taiwan (Sawai and others, 1972; Kuo and Wu, 1972). In severe bites both local and systemic hemorrhage and prolonged coagulation of the blood are characteristic sequellae. The fatality rate is high (14-16 %) compared to that (4 %) for all bites. Monovalent antivenin is produced, but most patients are treated by herb medicine.

Bites by A blomhoffi (mamushi) are common in Japan apart from the Amani and Okinawa Islands. Bites by A b brevicaudus, A caliginosus and A saxatilis are reported from Korea. Bites by A b brevicaudus also occur in PROC (Tateno and others, 1963; Sawai and Lah, 1978). Regional lymphadenopathy and swelling of the bitten area are the major signs of envenomation, but blurred vision and drowsiness were observed in some cases. A prolonged state of shock and acute renal failure were the main causes of death.

Trimeresurus Species

Bites by T flavoviridis (habu) are very common on the Amani and Okinawa Islands of Japan. Bites by T okinavensis are one-tenth as frequent. Bites by T elegans are limited to the Yaeyama Islands in Okinawa. Bites by T tokarensis occur on the Tokara and Kodakara Islands in Kagoshima. The number of habu bites averaged 610 annually during the nine years from 1962-1970. The highest morbidity rate per 1000 population was 4.5 in the Tokunoshima Islands. Necrosis at the loci of bites occurred in 6.8 percent of cases, and the incidence of motor disturbances after the wound had healed was 4.5 percent. The fatality rate was 0.9 percent. All of the patients received 20-40 ml of purified antivenin. A fatal outcome is very rare in the case of bites by elegans, tokarensis and okinavensis.

More than 60 percent of the total bites in Taiwan are by T mucrosquamatus and T stejnegeri (Sawai and Tseng, 1973). Most of the patients are treated by herb medicine, although divalent antivenin against both venoms are produced.

T albolabris, T popeorum and T erythrurus are called green pit vipers and are very difficult to distinguish clinically. About 30 percent of the total bites in Thailand are due to green pit vipers. Fatal cases are very rare, although the bites are widely distributed over Southeast Asia. Antivenin is not used for the treatment of these bites except in Thailand, where antivenin against albolabris is produced. Bites by T purpureomaculatus, T wagleri and T sumatranus are not common, although some are reported from Malaysia (Reid and others, 1963; Sawai and others, 1978).

Hydrophis Species

During eight years from 1957 to 1964, eight (7.9 %) of 101 patients died from sea snake bites in Malaysia (Reid, 1975). During five years from 1966-1969, five (3.2 %) of 158 victims died; and two (1.9 %) of 105 patients died during the period 1970-1975 in Malaysia (Sawai and others, 1972, 1978). Although both the incidence and the fatality rate have decreased yearly, the number of bites by land snakes has not decreased.

Small fang marks are observed at the loci of bites without pain or swelling. Motor disturbances, convulsions, difficulty of speaking, trismus, ptosis of eyelids and dyspnea are systemic symptoms which appear within 30 minutes after the bite. Myalgia and myoglobinuria are also characteristic in bites by Enhydrina schistosa.

Antivenin against the venom of E schistosa prepared in Australia became available in 1961. Intravenous administration of 3000-10000 units of the antivenin has been recommended for serious bites (Reid, 1975). Although E schistosa is mainly responsible for the bites in Malaysia, bites by Lapemis hardwickei and Hydrophis cyanocinctus occur in Thailand, Hong Kong, Indonesia and other countries (Sawai and others, 1978; Tu, 1974; Okonogi, 1973). Antivenin against the venom of Notechis scutatus is reported to effectively neutralize the venoms of schistosa, hardwickei, cyanocinctus and others (Baxter and others, 1974). Antivenin against the venom of schistosa also neutralized the venom of cyanocinctus (Tu and Ganthavorn, 1969).

CONCLUDING REMARKS

More detailed epidemiological and clinical analyses of snakebites in the Asian areas should be promoted to decrease the severity and fatality rate of bites. The effectiveness and method of distribution of antivenins should be re-investigated to improve the medical treatment of bites. In parallel with the improvement of treatment of bites, development of prophylactiv toxoid against cobra and Russell's viper bites should be encouraged to decrease the fatality rate.

REFERENCES

Ahuja, M. L. (1954). Snake bite in India. Ind. J. Med. Res., 42, 661-686.

Baxter, E. H., and H. A. Gallicho (1974). Cross-neutralization by tiger snake (Notechis scutatus) antivenene and sea snake (Enhydrina schistosa) antivenene against several sea snake venoms. Toxicon, 12, 273-278.

De Silva, A. (1976). The patterns of snake bite in Sri Lanka. Snake, 8, 43-51.

Ganthavorn, S. (1969). Toxicity of Thailand snake venoms and neutralization capacity of antivenin. Toxicon, 7, 239-241.

Ganthavorn, S. (1971). A case of king cobra bite. Toxicon, 9, 293-294.

Kawamura, Y., H. Chinzei, and Y. Sawai (1975). Snakebites in Indonesia. Snake, 7, 73-78.

Kuo, T-P., and C-S. Wu (1972). Clinicopathological studies on snakebites in Taiwan. Snake, 4, 1-22.

Lee, C. Y., C. C. Chang, and Y. W. Chen (1962). The toxicity and thermostability of Formosan snake venom. J. Formosan Med. Assoc., 61, 239-244.

Lim, B. L., and Abu Bakar bin Ibrahim (1970). Bites and stings by venomous animals with special reference to snake bites in West Malaysia. Med. J. Malaysia, 25, 128-141.

Minton, S. A. (1967). Paraspecific protection by elapid and sea snake antivenins. Toxicon, 5, 47-55.

Okonogi, T. (1963). Venomous sea snake bite. Snake, 5, 156-161.

Reid, H. A. (1975). Epidemiology of sea-snake bites. J. Trop. Med. and Hyg., 78, 106-113.

Reid, H. A., P. C. Thean, and W. T. Martin (1963). Epidemiology of snake bite in north Malaya. Brit. Med. J., 1, 992-997.

Report on snakebite situation and research in Burma. Report to Director-General, Department of Medical Research, Burma, 1978.

Sawai, Y., and M. Honma (1976). Snakebites in India. Animal, Plant and Microbial Toxins, Vol. 2, pp. 451-460. Plenum, New York.

Sawai, Y., K. Koba, T. Okonogi, S. Mishima, Y. Kawamura, H. Chinzei, Abu Bakar bin Ibrahim, T. Devaraj, S. Phong-Aksara, C. Puranananda, E. S. Salafranca, J. S. Sumpaico, C. S. Tseng, J. F. Taylor, C. S. Wu, and T. P. Kuo (1972). An epidemiological study of snakebites in the Southeast Asia. Japan. J. Exp. Med., 42, 283-307.

Sawai, Y., M. Makino, Y. Kawamura, T. Fukuyama, H. Chinzei, T. Okonogi, Z. Hokama, and M. Yamakawa (1976). Epidemiological study of habu bites on the Amami and Okinawa Islands of Japan. Animal, Plant and Microbial Toxins, Vol. 2, pp. 439-450. Plenum, New York.

Sawai, Y., and K-Y. Lah (1978). Snakebites in the South Korea. Snake, 9, 39-47.

Sawai, Y., S. Mishima, C. S. Tseng, M. Toriba, B-L. Lim, C. P. Ramachandran, T. Devaraj, S. Phong-Aksara, and J. D. Romer (1978). Study on seasnakes and the bites in Malaysia, Thailand and Hong Kong. Snake, 9, 48-62.

Sawai, Y., and C. S. Tseng (1973) Snakebites in Taiwan. Toxins of Animal and Plant Origin, Vol. 3, pp. 985-991. Gordon and Breach, New York.

Sitprija, V., C. Benyajati, and V. Boonpucknavig (1976). Renal involvment in snakebite. Animal, Plant and Microbial Toxins, Vol. 2, pp. 483-495. Plenum, New York.

Tateno, I., Y. Sawai, and M. Makino (1963). Current status of mamushi snake (Agkistrodon halys) bites in Japan with special reference to severe and fatal cases. Japan. J. Exp. Med., 33, 331-346.

To, S. (1941). Statistical studies on victims poisonous snakebites in Formosa. J. Med. Assn. of Formosa, 40, 1477-1502; 1795-1824.

Tu, A. T. (1974). Sea snake investigation in the Gulf of Thailand. J. Herpetologica, 8, 201-210.

Tu, A. T., and S. Ganthavorn (1969). Immunological properties and neutralization of sea-snake venoms from Southeast Asia. Am. J. Trop. Med. and Hyg., 18, 151-154.

CROTALID VENOM SHOCK: MECHANISM AND TREATMENT

F. E. Russell

Lab. Neurol. Res., Univ. Southern California, Los Angeles County-Univ. Southern California Medical Center, Los Angeles, California, USA

ABSTRACT

The various mechanisms that may be involved in the production of crotalid venom-induced hypotension and shock are reviewed. Specific therapeutic measures for combating shock are outlined and their efficacy is discussed.

KEYWORDS

Crotalid venoms; shock; cardiovascular dynamics; blood cell changes; autopharmacology; circulating blood volume; capillary permeability; intravenous fluids; isoproterenol hydrochloride; ventilation; steroids.

INTRODUCTION

The problem of hypotension and shock in snake venom poisoning is often a difficult one to delineate and treat, since the etiology can be, and often is, multiple and complex. In crotalid venom shock the etiology may certainly be multiple but in most cases the parameters can now be defined, and the advances in the therapeutics of shock during the past decade have been such that the deleterious consequence of a hypotensive crisis can now be minimized.

Experimental and clinical studies in animals have shown that several modes of action may be implicated in crotalid venom shock. These are listed in Table 1.

TABLE 1 Suggested Etiology for Crotalid Venom Shock

Cardiac failure	Electrolyte imbalance
Decreased venous return	Autopharmacology
Blood cell changes	CNS depression
Pooling of blood	Neurogenic reflexes
Thromboemboli	Decreased or increased peripheral resistance
Loss in circulating blood volume	

Cardiac failure was once thought to be the principal cause of the hypotensive crisis. However, more recent work has shown that while direct cardiac changes may sometimes be involved, the amounts of venom necessary to affect these changes, or produce sufficient cardiac damage to induce shock, are considerably greater than those that evoke other vascular changes which, in turn appear to be more directly responsible for the hypotension. Clinically, serious tissue changes and blood loss may occur and lead to shock without evidence of cardiac dysfunction, except for those changes reflecting alterations in dynamics secondary to a decrease in circulating blood volume.

A deficit in venous return to the heart has also been implicated as the primary cause of shock following crotalid venom poisoning. Certainly, a deficiency in venous return occurs in this type of shock but that appears to be an effect rather than the primary cause of the hypotension.

Changes in the configuration of the blood cells certainly occur following some crotalid bites. These alterations can lead to a shock state by affecting blood viscosity, among other things, thus requiring an increased stroke force which may not always be possible. Altered blood cells may also occlude the tubules, or the capillary bed of the lungs or other organs, and thus sufficiently embarrass cardiovascular dynamics to the point where shock results. Like cardiac failure, however, this plugging effect is usually a later finding in the hypotensive state, or is seen when lethal or near lethal injections of venom have been given to experimental animals.

The pooling of blood in the major organs of the body, particularly in the lungs and larger vessels of the chest, as occurs in both man and the cat, and in the abdominal organs in the dog, has been cited as a cause of shock following rattlesnake venom poisoning. The pooling has been attributed to altered resistance within these organs or to increased resistance in the immediate vascular structures. In cats, when a bolus injection of *Crotalus* venom is given, there is an immediate pooling of blood, as evidenced by an increase in lung weight and pulmonary artery pressure, and a decrease in blood flow. Visual observation of the lungs during this period shows vascular engorgement (Russell, Buess, and Strassberg, 1962).

The mechanism involved in these changes is probably related to alterations on the post-capillary side of the lungs, probably in the smaller venules, where either constriction or a decreased viscosity of the blood, or possibly both, occur and lead to pooling proximally. Such a mechanism may not be very common following bites on humans, unless the venom is injected directly into a blood vessel, or a very large amount is injected. Nevertheless, it is interesting to observe that post-mortem examinations in humans usually note lung changes that are remarkably similar to those seen in cats given a lethal dose of rattlesnake venom. One can assume that if the poisoning is severe enough, these changes will occur and that they can be an important contributing factor to hypotension, shock, and death.

The formation of thromboemboli in the pulmonary vascular bed has been suggested as a possible mechanism for the shock state (Halmagyi, Starzecki, and Horner, 1965). Multiple pulmonary emboli may be found in animals receiving a fatal dose of rattlesnake venom. However, the production of thromboembolism within a minute after receiving a bolus injection, or even after a 30-minute infusion of rattlesnake venom, might be a difficult explanation for the rapid onset of pulmonary hypertension and the precipitous fall in systemic arterial pressure seen in animals given the venom by injection, or via the bite of a rattlesnake. Clumping of blood cells in the lungs, thrombosis, or even multiple pulmonary emboli might conceivably cause pulmonary hypertension within this short period, but it seems unlikely that thromboembolism could be responsible for the immediate circulatory failure. Another finding that must add question to this proposed mechanism is that in post-mortem reports on patients who survived less than three hours following the bite of a rattlesnake, there has been no evidence of pulmonary thromboembolism.

Although electrolyte imbalance has been implicated as a cause of shock, the imbalance seen following crotalid envenomation is an effect rather than a cause, and it is not usually observed until the period of hypotension or shock is well advanced.

The release of autopharmacologic substances - histamine, serotonin, bradykinin, and others, is sometimes noted as being responsible for shock following snake venom poisoning (Roche e Silva, Berald, and Rosenfeld, 1949). For the most part, the supposition is based upon data from *in vitro* studies and its interpolation to the intact animal and man is dependent upon questionable assumptions. The several *in vivo* studies in which autopharmacological substances have been studied in venom-poisoned animals or envenomated humans do not indicate that the mechanism of autopharmacology plays an important role in venom poisoning. Of the 700 cases of snake venom poisoning treated by our staff, we have not seen a case of shock that could be attributed to the release of normal tissue vasoactive substances in a non-sensitized patient.

Depression of the central nervous system has been suggested as a possible mechanism for shock in both animals and man. In studies which purport to implicate the central nervous system, the doses of venom injected are usually so great that almost all organs of the body are affected. Thus, the validity of data relating to the central nervous system in such studies must be held in question. The changes observed in central nervous activity in these experiments is more easily explained on the basis of a decreased blood supply to the brain, resulting in cerebral anoxemia, secondary to the ischemic anemia. In cats receiving doses of *Crotalus* venom sufficient to cause shock, recordings from chronically implanted electrodes fail to show significant central nervous system involvement. One of the most remarkable and consistent findings in patients severely envenomated by rattlesnakes is their extremely clear sensorium, even in those cases in which they eventually lapse into coma and die. This might seem inconsistent with any postulate that implicates the central nervous system as the prime organ.

Neurogenic reflex mechanisms have been presented as modes by which shock might be induced but there is no experimental evidence to support such a proposal.

Decreased or increased peripheral resistance have also been noted as the cause for hypotension following *Crotalus* bites. However, the mechanisms responsible for the resistance changes have not been made clear, and much of the data are too highly dependent upon *in vitro* studies to be easily interpreted in either *in vivo* or clinical terms. Furthermore, there is no agreement as to whether the principal effect is increased or decreased peripheral resistance. The changes depicted appear to reflect both dosage and tissue-segment specificity. None the less, resistance changes probably exert some influence.

Recent work by our group, particularly by Carlson and Schaeffer, has shown that when *Crotalus* venom is given intravenously and slowly over a 30-minute period, there is marked hypovolemia characterized by hemoconcentration, lactacidemia, and hypoproteinemia. This occurs in both rats and cats; it is also seen in clinical cases. The decrease in circulating blood volume leading to shock is reflected in both experimental studies and clinical findings. When the poisoning is particularly severe, blood cell changes and even hemolysis may also occur early in the course of the poisoning. It appears that while pooling, blood cell changes, and even changes in vascular resistances and cardiac dynamics may play a role in the hypotensive crisis, the basic and most important change is an alteration in capillary permeability leading to the loss of circulating blood fluid, protein and, when the envenomation has been severe, a loss of erythrocytes.

The loss in circulating blood volume and protein is dose related and can be demonstrated as a loss in protein in the blood and as an increase in tissue protein outside the blood vascular system. The lactacidemia reflects oxygen lack and the inability to metabolize lactic acid.

In both animals and patients there is early hemoconcentration, due to the decrease in circulating fluid volume without the concomitant loss of blood cells. Subsequently, if, and when, blood cells are lost, there is a fall in hematocrit, causing further embarrassment of the circulation. If the period is prolonged, as in controlled experimental studies, the depth of the hypotension becomes more severe, the animal becomes oliguric, rales develop, and the animal dies.

The evidence for the loss of blood from capillary beds was first demonstrated by S. Wier Mitchell (1886). He showed clumping of capillary hemorrhages in the gut, as frequently seen in experimental studies. Ohsaka (1974) has shown that erythrocytes, changed in form, may spurt through a partially disrupted junction in the vascular endothelium exposed to a crotalid venom (Fig. 1.).

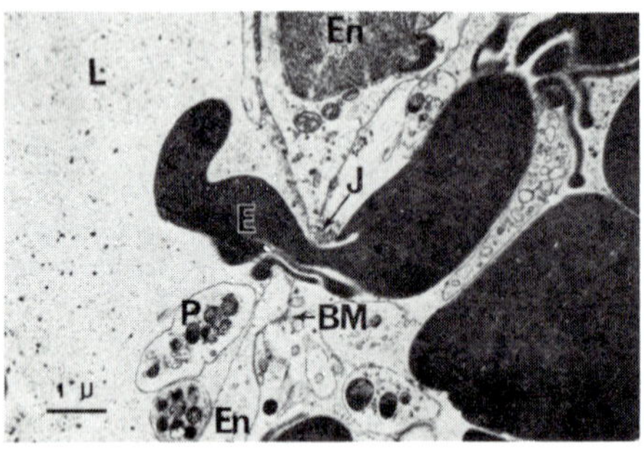

Fig. 1. Electron micrograph showing spurting of an erythrocyte through a junction of the vascular endothelium exposed to *Trimeresurus flavovirdis* venom. Erythrocyte (E), basement membrane (BM), junction (J), lumen (L), endothelial cell (En), platelet (P). (From Ohsaka, 1974.)

Recent studies in our laboratory indicate that the increase in capillary permeability and the loss of protein, is due, for the most part, to the peptide content of the venom. This peptide, as isolated and characterized by Pattabhiraman, Buffkin, and Russell, (1974), and by Maeda and colleagues (1978), has a molecular weight of 4990, has 43 amino acid residues, 6 half-cystine residues, and other than 5 amino acid substitutions and one residue addition at the C-terminus, it is similar to the "neurotoxin" crotamine. This peptide appears to alter the permeability of the capillary wall (and I might entertain the possibility that it also alters physiochemical relationships in other membranes). Apparently, when the amounts of venom are great enough, membrane permeability properties are altered and allow the passage of red blood cells. However, the hemolytic property appears more closely related to certain other proteins of the venom than to the peptide. Venom in which the peptide has been removed produces far less blood protein loss; whole venom also produces a much lesser protein loss (Schaeffer and colleagues, 1978a; Schaeffer and colleagues, 1979). The suggested sequence of events in the shock produced by a crotalid venom is shown in Table 2.

TABLE 2 Suggested Sequence Following Injection of *Crotalus viridis helleri* Venom

Pharmacology	Chemistry	Clinical	Laboratory
Increased capillary permeability	*C.v.h.* Peptide I	Hypotension	Hypoproteinemia, lactacidemia, and hemoconcentration
Loss of blood fluid and protein		Shock	
Loss of further fluid, protein, and erythrocytes	Plus Protein	Hemorrhagic manifestations, rales, oliguria, and other findings	Decreased hematocrit, lysis, abnormal clotting screen, electrolyte imbalance, thrombocytopenia

TREATMENT

What do we do about the patient in shock following a rattlesnake bite? Fortunately, the incidence of shock following crotalid venom poisoning has been greatly reduced through the early use of antivenin. Shock usually develops only in those cases when antivenin is not used or its use is delayed, when the envenomation is unusually severe, or when venom has been injected directly into a blood vessel. The loss of circulating blood fluid throughout the capillary bed in the general area of the bite, in the lungs, and in other tissues initiate the hypotension. We have seen patients in whom there was a reduction of approximately 25%-45% in total circulating blood volume within eight hours of envenomation. These patients were hypotensive, had cool and moist skin, a rapid and feeble pulse, rales, and oliguria.

The patient who has been bitten by a snake and arrives at the hospital prostrate, with cold and moist skin, pallor, collapsed superficial vessels, and hypotension presents a serious medical problem. The immediate treatment must be directed at treating the shock, and then treating the mechanism responsible for the shock. In all such cases, the VIP treatment: ventilation, infusion and pumping should be instituted. In shock, a secondary cause of death is a failure in respiratory gas exchange, with cardiac arrest often developing as a consequence of acute anoxemia. In the case of snake venom poisoning the primary deficit is perfusion failure, caused by a reduction in cardiac output, usually due to a decrease in circulating blood volume. However, shock which follows within 30 minutes of an envenomation may not be entirely due to the loss in fluid volume; it may be caused by a defect in blood distribution, presumably caused by intravascular pooling, or by the other factors that have been noted.

While hemoglobin and hematocrit determinations should be obtained on admission of all patients with snake venom poisoning, they are imperative when the patient is in shock. However, it must be borne in mind that these measurements can be misleading when there has been insufficient time for transcapillary refilling. In such cases, and whenever available, the use of multiple measurements of blood volume by radioisotopes or dye dilution methods are indicated.

In our experience, of particular value in evaluating the patient's circulatory state has been determinations of the central venous pressure (CVP) or, preferably, pulmonary artery and pulmonary wedge pressures (PAWP). The use of these procedures as a guide for the competence of the heart to bear fluid challenge is advised in all cases of severe envenomation or in shock states. The PAWP and CVP are not direct indicators of vascular tone or blood volume but, rather, they reflect cardiac competence, i.e., the heart's ability to serve as a pump for the movement of blood. In essence, such measurements are indicative of left ventricular function. It is always advisable to measure colloidal osmotic pressure (COP) during CVP or PAWP procedures.

In both moderate and severe envenomations, an electrocardiogram or electrocardiographic monitoring should be done during the first several hours following the bite. Whatever the cause of shock, oxygen is of primary and immediate importance. In all cases of shock the airway should be checked and freed of any obstruction before mechanical ventilation assistance is initiated. Measurements of blood pH, arterial carbon dioxide pressure (PCO_2) and oxygen saturation (PO_2) in arterial blood, are of value in providing quantitative information for the regulation of inhalation therapy. When the pH is less than 7.35 and PCO_2 is in excess of 46 torr, the patient is in respiratory acidosis. When the PO_2 of arterial blood is less than 70 torr there is a deficiency in oxygen exchange.

Following initiation of ventilation, fluid infusion should be started. We have found 5% albumin solution to be superior to isotonic saline or dextrose solutions for the replacement of fluid volume both in the immediate and delayed shock states (Schaeffer and colleagues, 1978b). If the pulmonary artery wedge pressure (PAWP) is less than 11 torr, the fluid is infused at 20 ml/minute, and if over 18 torr, 0.5 ml/minute. If the PAWP increases by more than 7 torr above the initial pressure and remains there for more than one minute, the infusion is discontinued. If the pressure increases more than 3 torr but less than 7 torr, it is discontinued at the end of 10 minutes.

The CVP may be used in place of the PAWP if the latter is not available. Baseline measurements should be obtained over a period of 10 minutes. If the CVP is less than 9 torr, fluid is infused at 20 ml/minute for 10 minutes. If the CVP increases by more than 4 torr, fluid challenge is discontinued. If it does not exceed the initial pressure by more than 2 torr the challenge is continued. If the CVP increases by more than 2 but no more than 4 torr the infusion is discontinued for 10 minutes. Fluid challenge is restarted after the 10 minute delay if CVP declines to within 2 cm of the initial measurement.

The pharmacologic treatment of snake venom poisoning shock, regardless of the species of snake involved, is open to a considerable difference of opinion. In spite of their wide use, both adrenergic vasoconstrictor drugs and adrenergic blocking agents are more likely to be detrimental than beneficial in some shock states. When responses to fluid perfusion are unsuccessful, use of isoproterenol hydrochloride, or low doses of epinephrine or dopamine can be tried.

There are indications that synthetic corticosteroids may improve myocardial contractility but without adequate controlled studies the controversy over their benefits and hazards in shock remains unresolved. Their once lauded value as potentiators of vasopressor amines has been reputed. In shock following both viper and pit viper bites, they should be avoided. In the presence of an already potentially dangerous poisoning typified by coagulation defects the use of these drugs seems unwise. On reviewing reports following deaths attributed to crotalid venom poisoning I have found that most of the patients had been maintained on steroids during the greater period of their early illness. In these cases it was obvious that the steroids were masking the unfolding of the deleterious changes occurring in the lungs, heart and kidneys, which were associated, in part, with hypovolemia. The steroids have no significant vasopressor effect and decrease peripheral resistance, although they may increase cardiac output, at least in some shock states. Perhaps, in supporting blood pressure the physcian was led to believe that the patient was "doing well." However, the steroids do not alleviate the hypovolemia nor do they block or reverse the effects produced in the blood vessels, lungs, or kidneys; nor do they alter the deleterious action on the blood cells. All of these factors contribute to death in the patients I have noted. In each case, dependency on the corticosteroids seemed misguided.

It must be remembered that in most cases of rattlesnake venom poisoning the principal cause of shock is the loss of plasma and blood cells into the tissues in the area of the injury, as well as into the lungs, peritoneum and other parts of the body. This can occur within a very short period of time. However, it is most often seen between the 6th and 26th hour following envenomation. Hypovolemic shock may be further complicated by hemolysis, with a decrease in red cell mass, and with renal and pulmonary failure. This may occur early, or as late as three or four days after the envenomation. It should be kept in mind that blood fluid loss can be rapid and extensive: an increase of just over 2 cm in the circumference of a thigh may represent the extravasation of half the total blood volume.

In shock, antivenin should always be given, and Antivenin (Crotalidae) Polyvalent should always be given intravenously. Although antivenin may not reverse a severe or prolonged shock state in itself, it will prevent shock from worsening, as well as limit those changes that contribute to the shock. The combination of antivenin, fluids, ventilation and, possibly, isoproterenol hydrochloride appear, at the present time, to be the most satisfactory method of combating the shock of rattlesnake venom poisoning.

ACKNOWLEDGEMENT

The author wishes to thank H. Gonzalez, T.R. Pattabhiraman, and W. Wingert for their advice in the preparation of this manuscript. Work on venom shock is supported by grants NS11476-05, USPHS, GM24141-01 TOX, USPHS, and a gift from the Gould Foundation.

REFERENCES

Halmagyi, D.F.J., Starzecki, B., and Horner, G.J. (1965). Mechanism and pharmacology of shock due to rattlesnake venom in sheep. J. Appl. Physiol., 20, 709-718.

Maeda, N., Tamiya, N., Pattabhiraman, T.R., and Russell, F.E. (1978). Some chemical properties of the venom of the rattlesnake, Crotalus viridis helleri. Toxicon, 16, 431-441.

Mitchell, S.W., and Reichert, E.T. (1886). Researches Upon the Venoms of Poisonous Serpents. Smithsonian Contributions to Knowledge. No. 26.

Ohsaka, A. (1974). An approach to the physiological mechanisms involved in hemorrhagic principles as a useful analytical tool. In A. Ohsaka, K. Hayashi, and Y. Sawai (Eds.) Animal, Plant, and Microbial Toxins, Vol. 1, Plenum Press, New York. pp. 123-136.

Pattabhiraman, T.R., Buffkin, D.C., and Russell, F.E. (1974). Some chemical and pharmacological properties of the toxic fractions from the venom of the Southern Pacific rattlesnake Crotalus viridis helleri, II. Proc. West. Pharmacol. Soc., 17, 227-232.

Roche e Silva, M., Berald, W.T., and Rosenfeld, G. (1949). Bradykinin: a hypotensive and smooth muscle stimulating factor released from plasma globulin by snake venoms and by trypsin. Am. J. Physiol., 156, 261-273.

Russell, F.E., Buess, F.W., and Strassberg, J. (1962). Cardiovascular response to Crotalus venom. Toxicon, 1, 5-18.

Schaeffer, R.C., Jr., Carlson, R.W., Whigham, H., Weil, M.H., and

Russell, F.E. (1978a). Acute hemodynamic effect of rattlesnake, *Crotalus viridis helleri*, venom. In P. Rosenberg (Ed.), *Toxins Animal, Plant and Microbial*. Pergamon Press, Oxford. pp. 383-391.

Schaeffer, R.C., Jr., Carlson, R.W., Puri, U.K., Callahan, G., Russell, F.E., and Weil, M.H. (1978b). The effects of colloidal and crystalloidal fluids on rattlesnake venom shock in the rat. *J. Pharmacol. Exptl. Therap.*, *206*, 687-695.

Schaeffer, R.C., Jr., Pattabhiraman, T.R., Carlson, R.W., Russell, F.E., and Weil, M.H. (1979). Cardiovascular failure produced by a peptide from the venom of the Southern Pacific rattlesnake, *Crotalus viridis helleri*. *Toxicon*, *17*, 447-453.

RENAL DISEASES IN SNAKEBITE

V. Sitprija

Department of Medicine, Chulalongkorn Hospital Medical School, Bangkok, Thailand

ABSTRACT

The spectrum of renal diseases was studied in 42 patients bitten by tropical poisonous snakes. Mild mesangial proliferative glomerulonephritis was noted in the majority of patients. Severe glomerulonephritis with crescent and fibrin deposition was observed in only one patient bitten by a Russell's viper. Arteritis of interlobular arteries was noted in Russell's viper cases. Thrombophlebitis of arcuate veins and their tributaries was demonstrated in both Russell's viper and green pit viper cases. Tubular necrosis was a constant finding in Russell's viper-bite and sea snake-bite, being responsible for acute renal failure. There was mild interstitial change. However, acute interstitial nephritis was observed in one patient bitten by a Russell's viper. Clinically, acute renal failure was noted only in patients bitten by sea snake and Russell's viper. Myoglobinuria was observed in sea snake poisoning. Hematuria was common in viper cases. Occasionally there was mild hemoglobinuria. Proteinuria was benign and transient.

KEYWORDS

Russell's viper; sea snake; cobra; green pit viper; renal failure; proteinuria; hematuria; hemoglobinuria; myoglobinuria; glomerulonephritis; arteritis; thrombophlebitis; interstitial nephritis; tubular necrosis.

INTRODUCTION

There is a broad spectrum of renal involvement in snakebite. Commonly described is renal failure following sea snake-bite and viper-bite (Sitprija et al, 1971, 1973, 1976; Marsden and Reid, 1961; Chugh et al, 1975). The other renal manifestations include hematuria, myoglobinuria, hemoglobinuria and proteinuria. Nephrotic syndrome has been reported (Steinbeck, 1960). Renal pathological changes ever described consist of glomerulonephritis (Sitprija and Boonpucknavig, 1977), arteritis (Sitprija et al, 1974), interstitial nephritis (Sant and Purandare, 1972), tubular necrosis (Sitprija et al, 1971, 1973, 1976, 1977) and cortical necrosis (Chugh et al, 1975; Varagunam and Panabokke, 1970). In experimental models renal infarct and even severe forms of glomerulonephritis have been shown (Raab and Kaiser, 1966; Pearce, 1909). In Chulalongkorn Hospital Medical School, over a period of 12 years from 1965 to 1977, a total of 400 cases of snakebite were admitted in the hospital. The types of snakes included cobra, green pit viper, Russell's viper, Agkistrodon rhodostoma, sea snake and unidentified snakes (Table 1).

Table 1 Snakebites in Chulalongkorn Hospital (1965-1977)

Snake	Cases	Percent
Cobra	154	38.50
Green pit viper	147	36.75
Russell's viper	25	6.25
Agkistrodon rhodostoma	3	0.75
Sea snake	2	0.50
Unidentified snakes	69	17.25
Total	400	100.00

In this review, an account of recently published data (Sitprija and Boonpucknavig, 1977) and additional data will be presented.

RENAL MANIFESTATIONS

The spectrum of renal manifestations included renal failure, proteinuria and gross hematuria (Table 2). Myoglobinuria was observed only in sea snake-bite, and hemoglobinuria was occasionally seen in Russell's viper-bite.

Table 2 Renal Manifestations

Renal failure	5.5%
Proteinuria	4.0%
Gross hematuria	35.0%

Renal Failure

Of 400 patients, renal failure was noted in 22 cases or 5.5%. Two of these patients were bitten by sea snake, and 20 were bitten by Russell's viper. It should be pointed out that among 25 patients bitten by Russell's viper, renal failure was observed in 20 patients. The other 5 patients had only gross hematuria without impaired renal function. They were rapidly treated from the health centers with specific antivenom within less than 30 minutes after the bite.

The course of renal failure in snakebite did not differ from that of renal failure due to other causes. Dialysis was required in severe cases. Oliguria was prolonged when renal failure was associated with acute interstitial nephritis or extracapillary glomerulonephritis. These 2 pathological entities were noted in 2 patients bitten by Russell's viper. In sea snake-bite hyperkalemia secondary to myonecrosis can be alarming and requires prompt treatment. Hemodialysis has been shown to improve muscular symptoms, perhaps due to potassium removal (Sitprija et al, 1971). Hyperuricemia may be observed if myonecrosis is severe. Severe intravascular hemolysis may occasionally occur in Russell's viper-bite, and exchange blood transfusion has been reported to be fruitful in the patient management (Peiris et al, 1969). In our experience, massive intravascular hemolysis has not been found. Furthermore, cortical necrosis reported in India in Russell's viper-bite (Chugh et al, 1975) has not been observed. This could reflect early treatment in our patients. The use of heparin in severe disseminated intravascular coagulation and adequate hydration could have prevented the development of cortical necrosis.

Proteinuria

Mild proteinuria of less than 500 mg/24 h was observed in 4% of cases. This was noted mostly in cobra-bite. The urinary sediment was not remarkable, but there was hematuria in green pit viper and Russell's viper cases. Proteinuria was detectable only for a few days. The pathological counterpart was mild mesangial proliferative glomerulonephritis. Severe proteinuria has not been observed, and this has raised a serious doubt about a report of nephrotic syndrome developing after the bite of a brown coloured snake, presumed to be Demansia textilis (Steinbeck, 1960). Since the cause-effect relationship was not shown, nephrotic syndrome could merely be an associated phenomenon.

Hematuria

Gross hematuria was noted in 35% of cases. They were green pit viper and Russell's viper cases. Gross hematuria disappeared within a few days, but microscopic hematuria persisted for several days. Coagulation defect, thrombocytopenia and vascular changes are responsible for bleeding. Although renal infarction, as shown in experimental animals, could be a cause of gross hematuria, clinical manifestation of renal infarction was not revealed in the patients with gross hematuria. Another cause of hematuria; namely renal vein thrombosis, although a possibility, seems remote. Hematuria was in no case severe enough to be troublesome.

RENAL FUNCTION

Renal function was studied in the patients without renal failure using creatinine and para-aminohippurate clearances. The results are shown in Table 3.

Table 3 Renal Function

	Creatinine clearance (ml/min)		PAH clearance (ml/min)	
	Range	Mean	Range	Mean
Cobra-bite (n=5)	116-132	123.4	596-624	611.2
Green pit viper-bite (n=5)	110-131	118.2	386-422	401.6

In cobra cases both creatinine and para-aminohippurate (PAH) clearances were within the normal limits averaging 123.4 ml/min and 611.2 ml/min, respectively. In green pit viper cases creatinine clearance was also normal having a mean of 118.2 ml/min, but PAH clearance was decreased with a mean of 401.6 ml/min. The decrease in PAH clearance was attributable to mild tubular degeneration. There was thus good structural and functional relationship.

In cases with renal failure renal blood flow was measured by ^{133}Xe using the technique previously described (Sitprija et al, 1977). There was a decrease in renal cortical blood flow. The pattern was not different from that observed in acute renal failure due to other causes. In these patients creatinine and PAH clearances were also determined during the recovery phase, and were found to be normal 2 to 4 months after hospital discharge.

RENAL PATHOLOGY

Glomerular Lesion

Glomerular changes in all cases were mild. The findings were consistent with mesangial proliferative glomerulonephritis, characterized by proliferation of mesangial cells and occasionally endothelial cells. Segmental thickening of the basement membrane was observed in cobra cases. Epithelial proliferation was present in one case, indicating disruption of the basement membrane with fibrin deposition. This patient was bitten by a Russell's viper and had severe renal failure with a prolonged period of oliguria. Similar findings have been observed in a patient bitten by *Bitis arietans* (Seedat, Reddy and Edington, 1974).

By electron microscopy, narrowing of glomerular capillary lumen was noted. This was due to the increase in amount of basement membrane-like matrix and the swelling of the attenuate portion of the endothelial cytoplasm. Electron-dense deposition was demonstrated in the basement membrane-like matrix. There was irregular thickening of the basement membrane in cobra cases. On occasions, there was striated membranous structure in the basement membrane. Focal absence of epithelial foot processes was observed in the area where the basement membrane changes were prominent. Fibrin deposition in the paramesangial area was demonstrable in green pit viper and Russell's viper cases.

By immunofluorescence, granular deposition of C_3 and IgM was noted in the glomerular mesangium and along the capillary wall. This was observed irrespective of antivenom therapy. The deposition of IgM appeared to be denser in Russell's viper cases than it did in green pit viper and cobra cases. On the other hand, cobra cases were found to have more C_3 deposition than the others. This is interesting in view of the recent suggestion that cobra venom protein and C_3 have cross immunologic reactivity (Alper, 1979). Of pathogenetic significance is the absence of C_3 and IgM deposition in the Russell's viper case with extracapillary glomerulonephritis.

The mechanism responsible for the development of glomerular changes is not clear. Several hypotheses have been proposed (Sitprija and Boonpucknavig, 1979). Granular deposition of C_3 and IgM in the glomeruli and the decrease in serum C_3 as shown in our previous report (Sitprija and Boonpucknavig, 1977) suggest an immunologic process. Whether this is immune complex glomerulonephritis or glomerulonephritis which results from a reaction between the venom antigen already fixed in the glomeruli and the antibody remains to be clarified. It is also possible that the venom causes direct glomerular injury along with complement activation, and that both C_3 and IgM are trapped by the injured glomeruli. In one Russell's viper case an attempt was made to detect C_4 in the glomeruli, but C_4 was not demonstrable. Although more data are required, this would suggest complement activation by the alternative pathway. Extracapillary glomerulonephritis in one Russell's viper case is interpreted to indicate rupture of the basement membrane with fibrin deposition and secondary epithelial proliferation. The absence of C_3 and IgM deposition in the glomeruli in this interesting case serves as supporting evidence in favour of glomerulotoxicity of Russell's viper's venom. In the clinical setting, it seems that both immunologic mechanism and direct glomerulotoxicity are at work and that intravascular coagulation plays a contributing role in the pathogenesis of glomerular lesion in severe cases.

Vascular Lesion

Vascular changes were noted in Russell's viper-bite and green pit viper-bite. Necrotizing arteritis was observed in the interlobular arteries in Russell's viper cases. The finding could be easily missed if the renal biopsy is not deep enough. Thrombophlebitis of arcuate veins and their tributaries was demonstrated in both Russell's viper and green pit viper cases.

Immunofluorescent study showed deposition of C_3 in the arterial lesion. Of interest is the presence of C_3 in the wall of afferent and efferent arterioles without any change in histological structure by light microscopy. It is believed that the venoms of Russell's viper and green pit viper are vasculotoxic.

Interstitial Lesion

Interstitial changes are usually secondary to tubular degeneration, and mild interstitial changes are often observed in the patient with tubular necrosis. However, acute interstitial nephritis has been observed in one patient bitten by a Russell's viper. There was mononuclear cellular infiltration in the interstitium especially in the perivascular area. Since interstitial nephritis is uncommon in snakebite, the question is therefore raised of the possibility of drug hypersensitivity. However, the patient was not on any drug known to cause interstitial nephritis. Furthermore, eosinophilia and eosinophiluria which are characteristic of interstitial nephritis due to hypersensitivity were not observed. The patient had prolonged course of renal failure, but finally recovered. Immunofluorescent study did not show any deposition of immunoglobulins. Interstitial nephritis is probably a direct effect of the venom, a rare and severer form of nephrotoxicity.

Tubular Lesion

Tubular necrosis was noted in sea snake and Russell's viper cases. Tubular degeneration appeared more striking in the distal tubules. There were edema and mild cellular infiltration in the interstitium. Hemoglobin casts were occasionally seen in Russell's viper cases (Sitprija and Boonpucknavig, 1979). In sea snakebite myoglobin casts were demonstrable (Sitprija et al, 1973). Tubulorhexis was noted in some areas in severe cases of renal failure. There was mild tubular degeneration in green pit viper cases. Immunofluorescent study was unrevealing.

In sea snake-bite myoglobinemia and myoglobinuria secondary to myonecrosis are responsible for tubular lesion and renal failure (Sitprija et al, 1973). Hyperuricemia, which may occur when myonecrosis is severe, may be a contributing factor. In Russell's viper-bite tubular necrosis with acute renal failure is likely due to direct tubulotoxicity of the venom for 2 reasons. First, the onset of oliguria is abrupt after the bite without any change in vital signs. Second, under the same clinical setting of intravascular coagulation and bleeding tendency in green pit viper-bite, Agkistrodon rhodostoma-bite and Russell's viper-bite, renal failure with tubular necrosis was observed only in Russell's viper poisoning.

Besides the above mechanisms, nonspecific factors must always be taken into consideration in the pathogenesis of renal failure in snakebite. Among these factors are cardiotoxicity of the venom, vasodilatation, hemorrhage and hypovolemia which could lead to hypotension and decrease renal blood flow. Hemorrhage attributed to coagulation defect, thrombocytopenia and vascular damage is common in viper-bite. Apart from bleeding, hypovolemia could be due to the effects of chemical mediators released during the process of inflammation (Graeme and Majno, 1977). These substances include histamine, serotonin, kinins, anaphylatoxins, fibrinopeptides, fibrin degradation products and prostaglandins. These chemical mediators, by their effects on increasing vascular permeability, allow the leakage of fluid and protein out of the intravascular compartment resulting in hypovolemia. Hypovolemia and catecholamine release secondary to hypotension and kinin stimulation could compromise renal blood flow in sufficient degree to cause tubular necrosis and renal failure.

In conclusion, all renal structures can be involved in snakebite depending upon the type of snakes. The mechanisms are multiple including immunologic reactions, direct nephrotoxicity and nonspecific effects of the venom.

REFERENCES

Alper, C. A. (1979). Snakes and the complement system. In C. Y. Lee (Ed.), Snake Venoms, Springer-Verlag, Berlin Heidelberg New York. Chap. 22, pp.863-880.

Chugh, K. S., Aikat, B. K., Sharma, B. K., Dash, K. C., Mathew, M. T., and Das, K. C. (1975). Acute renal failure following snakebite. Amer.J.Trop.Med.Hyg., 24, 692-697.

Graeme, R. B., and Majno, G. (1977). Acute inflammation. A review. Amer.J.Path., 86, 185-276.

Marsden, A. T. H., and Reid, H. A. (1961). Pathology of sea-snake poisoning. Brit.Med.J., 1, 1290-1293.

Pearce, R. M. (1909). An experimental glomerular lesion caused by venom (Crotalus adamanteus). J.Exp.Med., 11, 532-540.

Peiris, O. A., Wimalaratne, K. D. P., and Nimalasuriya, A. (1969). Exchange transfusion in the treatment of Russell's viper bite. Postgrad.Med.J., 45, 627-629.

Raab, W., and Kaiser, E. (1966). Nephrotoxic action of snake venom. Mem.Inst. Butantan, 33, 1017-1020.

Sant, S. M., and Purandare, N. M. (1972). Autopsy study of cases of snake bite with special reference to renal lesions. J.Postgrad.Med., 18, 181-188.

Seedat, Y. K., Reddy, J., and Edington, D. A. (1974). Acute renal failure due to proliferative nephritis from snake bite poisoning. Nephron, 13, 455-463.

Sitprija, V., Sribhibhadh, R., and Benyajati, C. (1971). Haemodialysis in poisoning by sea-snake venom. Brit.Med.J., 3, 218-219.

Sitprija, V., Sribhibhadh, R., Benyajati, C., and Tangchai, P. (1973). Acute renal failure in snakebite. In A. de Vries and E. Kochva (Eds.), Toxins of Animal and Plant Origins, Vol. III. Gordon and Breach, London. pp. 1013-1028.

Sitprija, V., Benyajati, C., and Boonpucknavig, V. (1974). Further observations of renal insufficiency in snakebite. Nephron, 13, 396-403.

Sitprija, V., Benyajati, C., and Boonpucknavig, V. (1976). Renal involvement in snakebite. In A. Ohsaka, K. Hayashi and Y. Sawai (Eds.), Animal, Plant, and Microbial Toxins, Vol. II. Plenum, New York. pp. 483-495.

Sitprija, V., and Boonpucknavig, V. (1977). The kidney in tropical snakebite. Clin.Nephrology, 8, 377-383.

Sitprija, V., Vongsthongsri, M., Poshyachinda, V., and Arthachinta, S. (1977). Renal failure in malaria: a pathophysiologic study. Nephron, 18, 277-287.

Sitprija, V., and Boonpucknavig, V. (1979). Snake venoms and nephrotoxicity. In C. Y. Lee (Ed.), Snake Venoms, Springer-Verlag, Berlin Heidelberg New York. Chap. 28, pp. 997-1018.

Steinbeck, A. W. (1960). Nephrotic syndrome developing after snakebite. Med.J. Aust., 1, 543-545.

Varagunam, T., and Panabokke, R. G. (1970). Bilateral cortical necrosis of the kidneys following snakebite. Postgrad.Med.J., 46, 449-451.

ULTRASTRUCTURAL CHANGES IN THE LUNGS, KIDNEYS AND ERYTHROCYTES AFTER *NAJA NIGRICOLLIS* BASIC PHOSPHOLIPASE ADMINISTRATION

C. Svalander*, G. Eggertsen, C. Hellerström***, D. Eaker**** and J. Fohlman*******

**Dept. Clin. Pathol., Sahlgren's Hospital, S-413 45 Göteborg, Sweden*
***Dept. Med. Physiol. Chem., Box 575, S-751 23 Uppsala, Sweden*
****Dept. Histol., Box 571, S-751 23 Uppsala, Sweden*
*****Inst. Biochem., Box 576, S-751 23 Uppsala, Sweden*
******Dept. Cell Res., box 562, S-751 22 Uppsala, Sweden*

ABSTRACT

The in vivo effect of a basic phcspholipase from the venom of Naja nigricollis was investigated. Purified phospholipase was administered intravenously into mice, and the lungs, kidneys and blood cells were examined by electronmicroscopy. Distinct pathological changes appeared in mice receiving 400 µg/kg or more. The erythrocytes underwent transformation to spherocytes, fragmentation and hemolysis. The endothelial cells in the pulmonary capillaries showed focal swelling with development of small processes from the cell membranes and pinching off of small membrane fragments. There was a general congestion of the blood vessels. In the kidneys the endothelial cells of the peritubular vessels underwent changes similar to those observed in the lung. Characteristic lesions appeared in the proximal and distal tubular cells with dissolution of the vasal labyrinthic membrane structure. Animals receiving porcine phospholipase showed slight ruptures in the endothelium of the peritubular vessels, but no other pathological changes were observed. The significance of these findings is discussed.

KEYWORDS

Phospholipase; snake venom; kidney; lung; erythrocytes; hemolysis;

INTRODUCTION

The fangs of the West African black-necked spitting cobra Naja n. nigricollis are formed with a frontward opening which permits venom to be expelled out several meters, usually aimed at the eyes of the victim (Bogert, 1943; Freyvogel and Honegger, 1965). This behavioural specialization is a defense against territorial intruders and has nothing to do with feeding. Human encounters with this species can thus result in eye damage (Warrell and Ormerod, 1976) or serious local reactions following a "regular" bite (Warrell and co-workers, 1976).

Although N. nigricollis venom contains postsynaptic neurotoxins (e.g., toxin α) (Karlsson, Eaker and Porath, 1966) the most serious sequellae are local necrosis and rarely (if ever) are signs of neurotoxicity present (Warrell and co-workers, 1976). This indicates that other venom components should be implicated in the pathogenesis. Recently a basic phospholipase was isolated from this venom by gel filtration and ion exchange chromatography on Bio Rex 70 (Eaker, 1975). It is a single chain protein of 118 amino acid residues crosslinked by 7 disulfide bridges and has an intravenous LD_{50} of 300 µg/kg in mice. The peculiar effects of this phospholipase in vivo were strikingly different from those of the neurotoxic phospholipases (Eaker and co-workers, 1976) which we have previously studied. Therefore, we decided to use electron microscopy to examine the pathophysiology and to correlate the morphological data with the different modes of action exhibited by different phospholipases A2.

MATERIALS AND METHODS

The study was performed using white mice weighing between 18-30 grams. Freeze-dried purified phospholipase from Naja nigricollis was dissolved in physiological buffered saline. The material was administered in a single injection into the tail vein, and the amount given varied from 200 to 6000 µg/kg. Purified porcine phospholipase was obtained from Bert Verheij, Utrecht, and was administered in the same manner. Mice which received physiological saline without any phospholipase were used as controls. The animals were then killed by cervical dislocation after different periods of time, from 13 minutes to 5 hours following injection. Specimens from the kidneys, lungs and centrifuged blood were processed for electron microscopy by immersion first in a combined paraformaldehyde-glutaraldehyde fixative and then in osmium tetroxide. The material was subsequently embedded in Epon, sectioned on a LKB Ultrotome III and contrasted with uranyl and lead. Intravascular hemolysis was estimated by spectrophotometric recording of free hemoglobin in serum at 412 nm. A homologous fraction of normal mouse red blood cells was obtained by centrifugation of whole heparinized blood in a selfgenerating gradient of Percoll (Pharmacia Fine Chemicals, Uppsala, Sweden) (density 1.085 g/cm^3). The erythrocytes were suspended in phosphate buffered saline to a concentration of 3×10^6 cells/ml and were incubated with Naja nigricollis phospholipase for 60 minutes at +37°C. The incubation was stopped by addition of fixative, after which the specimens were processed for electron microscopy.

RESULTS

Reproducible and distinct structural changes were obtained in mice receiving doses of 400 µg/kg and larger. Injection of 1500 µg/kg of phospholipase was rapidly lethal. The individual response was reflected in the different survival times, ranging from 20 to 60 minutes for the latter dose. Control animals receiving physiological saline were unaffected during two hours' observation.

The general effects appearing after injection of the phospholipase were lethargy, immobilization, paresis of hindlimbs, superficial respiration, edema of paws and nasal bleeding. The internal organs showed moderate congestion. The kidneys were swollen and hyperemic. Patchy lungbleeding and cardiac dilatation with ventricular fibrillation were seen. There was no general hemorrhagic diathesis, and no gross alterations in the liver, spleen, intestines, endocardium and serosal cavities or brain (1500 µg/kg) were observed. There was an early hemolysis with a dose-dependent increase of free hemoglobin spectrophotometrically demonstrable in serum (Fig. 1).

In the kidneys a dose of 400 µg/kg gave reproducible morphological changes in the tubuli and peritubular vessels. The basal labyrintic structure of both the proximal and distal tubular cells showed signs of damage with dissolution of the membrane structure (Figs. 2-4,6). The mitochondria looked contracted, probably indicating a state of low energy potential. In the tubular lumina there was accumulation of electron dense material, probably hemoglobin (a spectrophotometric scan on

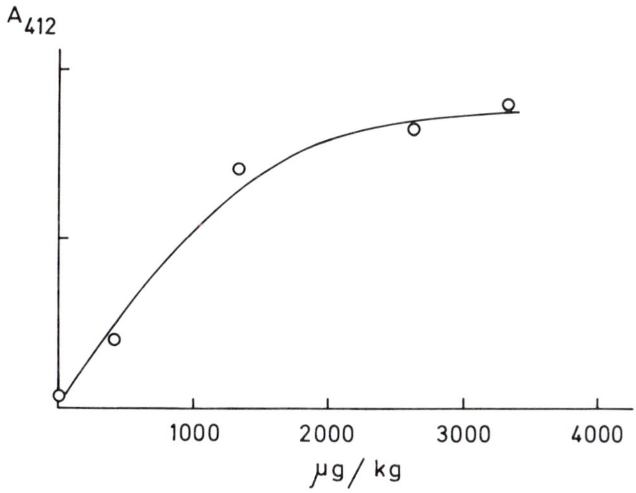

Fig. 1. The amount of free hemoglobin in serum (estimated as the absorption at 412 nm) of mice injected with Naja nigricollis phospholipase plotted against the dose of enzyme given.

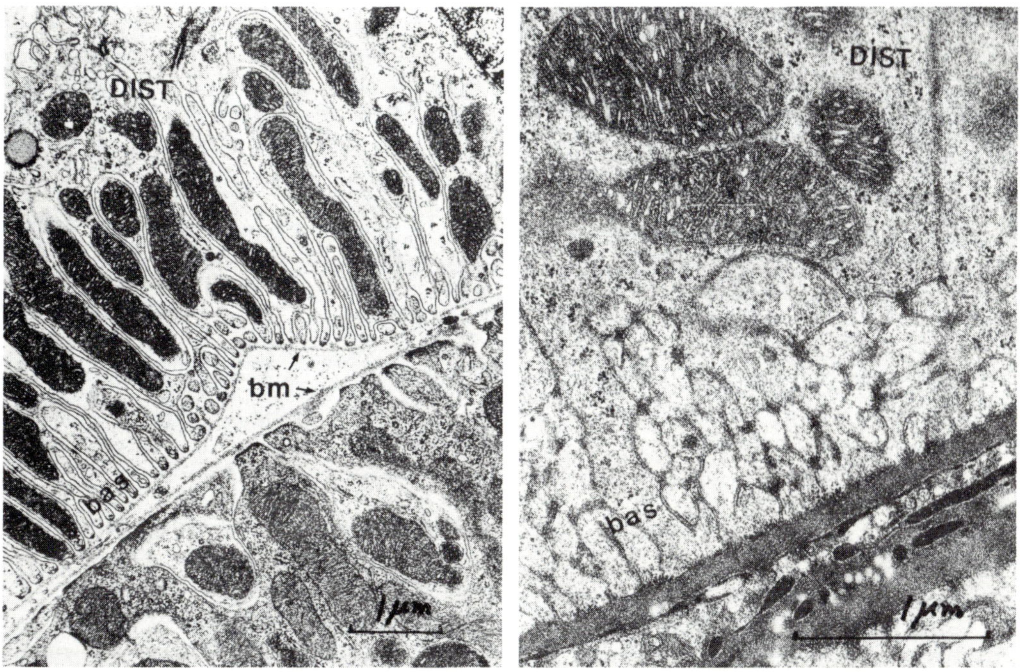

Figs. 2 and 3. Distal tubule epithelial cells (DIST) with basal portions (bas) close to the basement membrane (bm) demonstrating the normal labyrinth structure in a control mouse (Fig. 2) and labyrinth alteration in a mouse 50 minutes after a single injection of basic phospholipase, 400 μg/kg (Fig. 3).

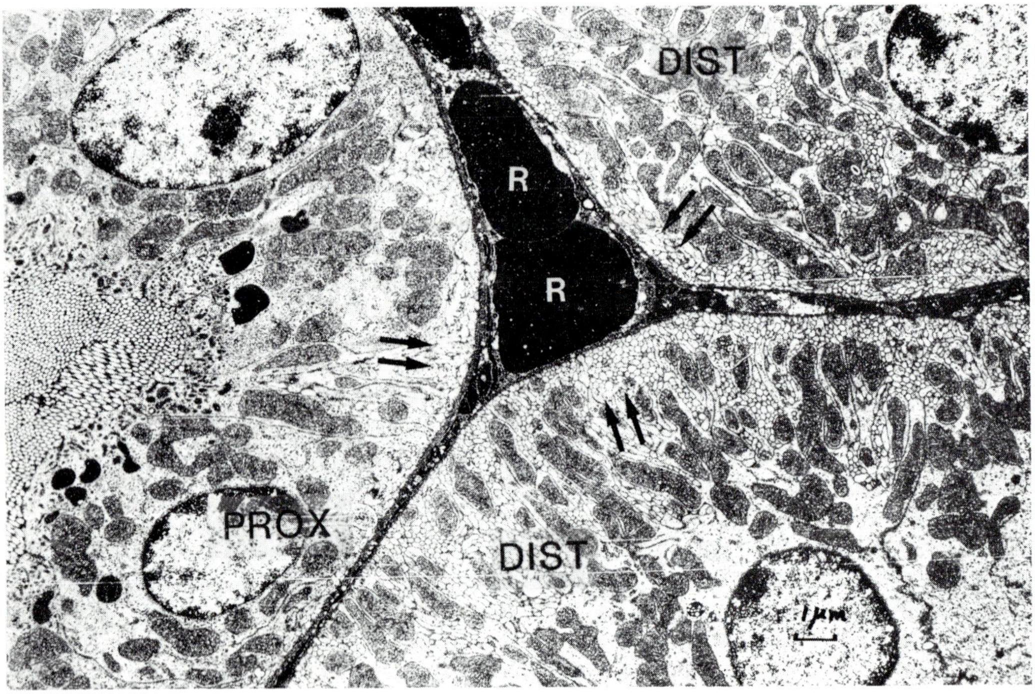

Fig. 4. Survey of three adjacent tubules with obvious dissolution of basal labyrinth structure (arrows). Similar changes occur in proximal (PROX) and distal (DIST) parts of the nephron. Peritubular vessel occupied by erythrocytes (R). Basic phospholipase, 400 μg/kg; 50 min. specimen.

a urine specimen showed an absorption peak at 412 nm). Focal epithelial cell necrosis could also be seen within one hour following injection of the enzyme. In the peritubular vessels interstitial edema was present and the endothelial cells displayed focal disruptions and slender cytoplasmic projections into the lumina with pinching off of membrane material. The mice injected with porcine phospholipase (Fig. 6) or saline did not show any significant pathological changes in their kidneys.

In the glomeruli only minor endothelial changes were seen. The capillary lumina contained abnormal erythrocytes (see below), but fibrin or platelet thrombi were not observed.

In the lung vessels a slight intracellular edema was present in the endothelial cells after injection of saline (Fig. 8). After administration of the higher doses of phospholipase there was a pronounced endothelial swelling with appearence of pathological membrane structures (Fig. 9). In the lumina of the vessels an obvious accumulation of abnormally shaped erythrocytes and ghosts was present, suggesting intravascular hemolysis, which was, in fact, observed (see Fig. 1). In the surrounding plasma numerous small dense particles could be seen. Intravenous injection of porcine phospholipase caused no change in the shape of the red blood cells and no endothelial lesions.

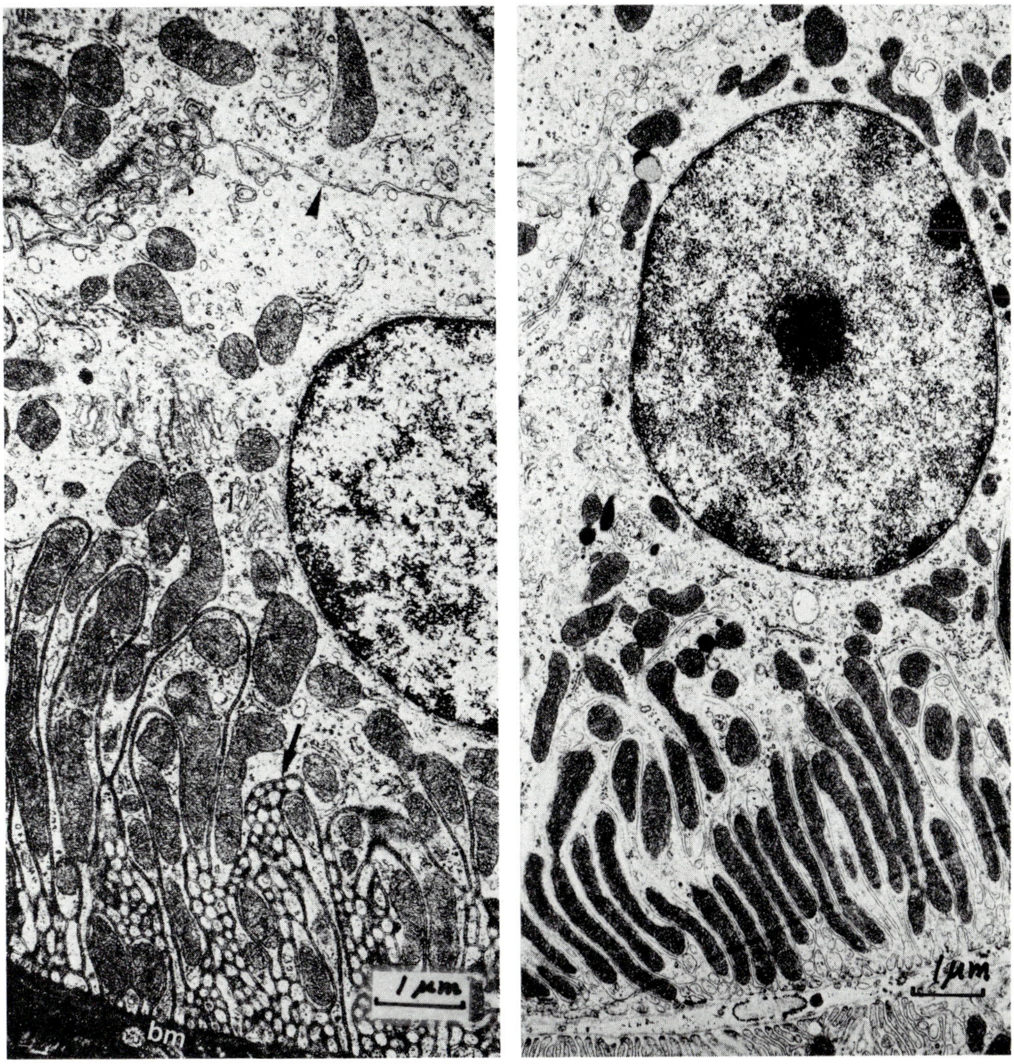

Figs. 5 and 6. Distal tubule epithelium 13 minutes after single injection of basic phospholipase, 6000 μg/kg (Fig. 5). Note that the basal labyrinth is broken into spherical profiles with electron dense material in extracellular compartments (arrow) and in basement membrane (bm). Apical plasma membrane (arrowhead) and internal membrane systems are intact. Compare to Fig. 6, which shows no such changes after porcine phospholipase, 1900 μg/kg; 40 min. specimen.

The erythrocytes in all of the tissue sections from animals treated with the higher doses of the Naja nigricollis phospholipase appeared seriously deformed, the majority having the shape of spherocytes (Figs. 10-12). Many showed crenations and projections from the cell surface, suggesting budding of small membrane fragments (Fig. 13). The dense particles observed in the plasma could then represent shedded pieces of erythrocyte membranes. The erythrocytes in blood specimens drawn at different times showed the same morphological changes with spherocytic transformation

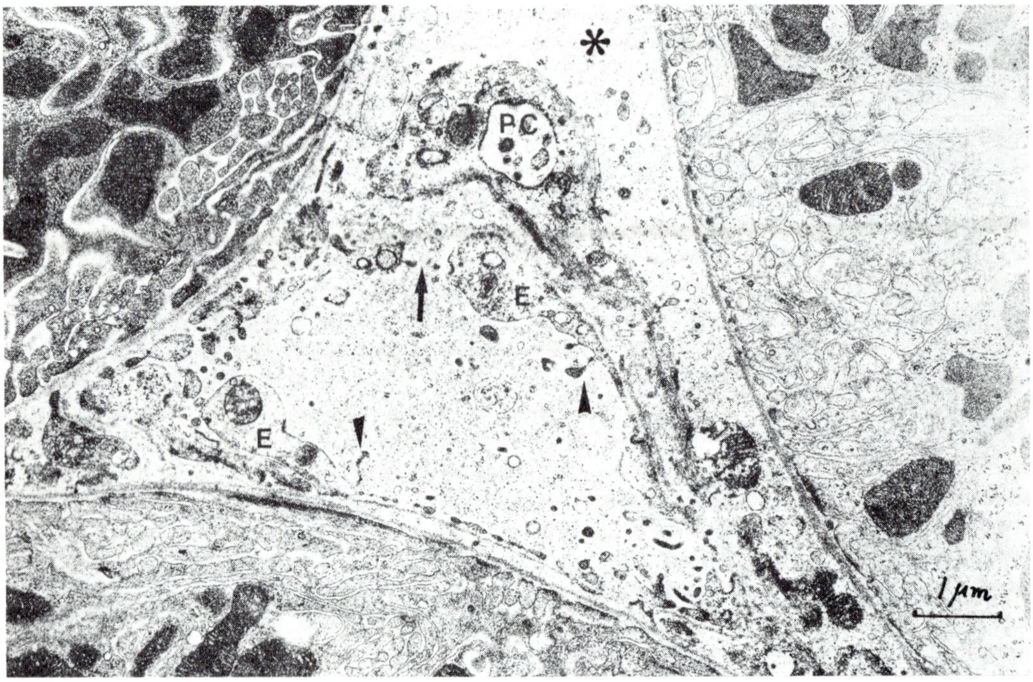

Fig. 7. Mouse kidney peritubular vessel demonstrating the endothelium (E) with focal disruption (arrow) and slender cytoplasmic processes (arrowheads) projecting into vessel lumen. Note interstitial edema (*) and autophagic vacuole (PC) in perivascular cell and slight labyrinth change in basal portions of neighbouring tubule epithelium. Basic phospholipase, 400 μg/kg: 55 min. specimen.

and crenation and projection phenomena (Figs. 14,15). Lower doses of the phospholipase induced only minor changes (Fig. 14). Similar changes were also seen after *in vitro* incubation of fractionated normal mouse erythrocytes with *Naja nigricollis* phospholipase in phosphate buffered saline (Fig. 16).

DISCUSSION

Our study in mice shows that within minutes after i.v. injection of phospholipase in doses of 400 μg/kg and larger, there is extensive membrane damage in the red blood cells, endothelial cells in the lungs and peritubular vessels and tubular epithelium of the kidneys. This effect is morphologically localized to certain cytomembranes, most clearly demonstrated in the tubular epithelium of the kidney, where only the basal cytoplasma membranes are affected. Similarly the vascular endothelium seems to be variably affected, with only minor lesions in the glomeruli, while the peritubular endothelium is focally disrupted. The hemolytic effect on red blood cells is also a very constant phenomenon, whereas leukocytes and platelets seem to be unaffected. It also seems to be a direct (non-mediated) effect of the enzyme, since the same morphological changes could be produced in a serum-free system. The amount of free hemoglobin released was slight, but increased markedly after addition of small quantities of serum (Eggertsen, unpublished observations), most probably due to production of lysolecithin.

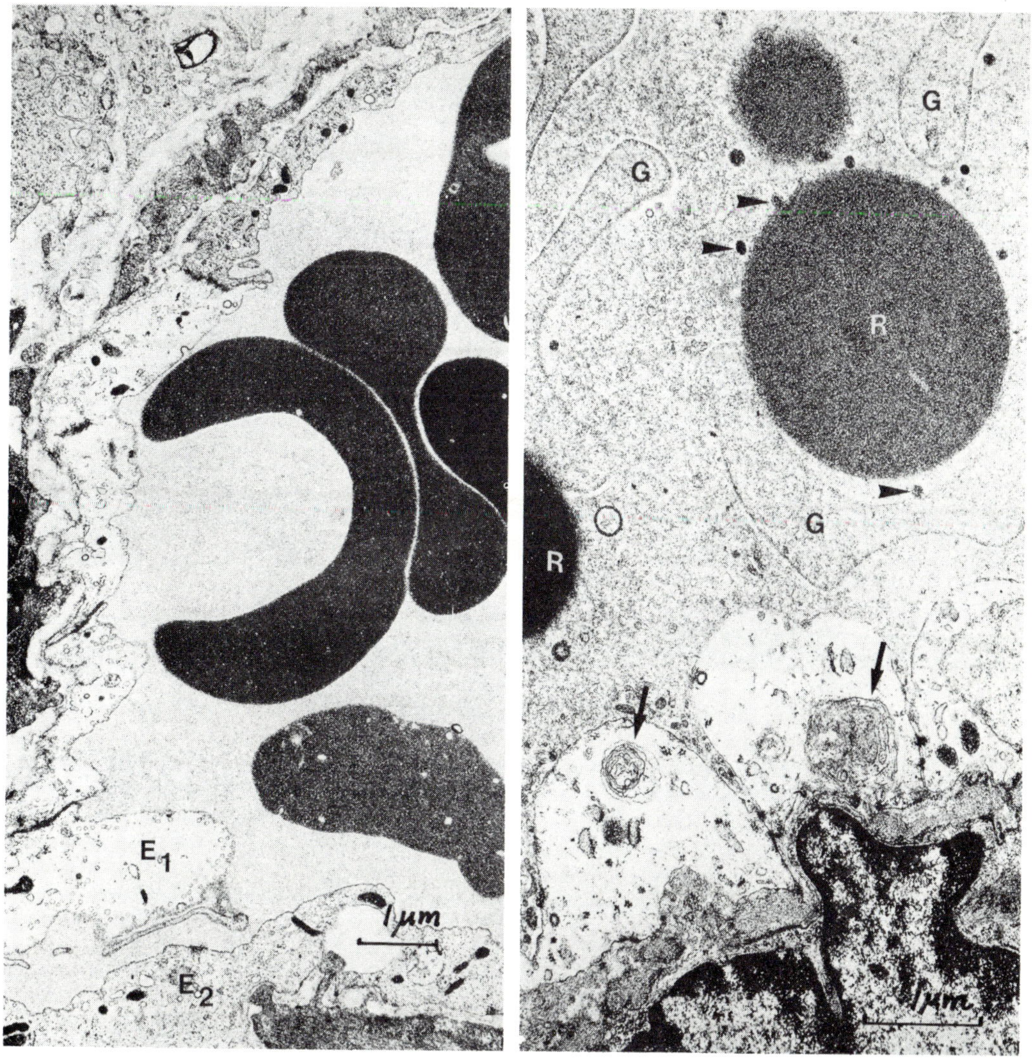

Figs. 8 and 9. Structure of lung artery endothelium. After saline injection, 50 μl, 120 min., (Fig. 8) endothelial cells (E_1 and E_2) demonstrate variable cytoplasm density compatible with slight focal intracellular edema. Note normal configuration of erythrocytes in vessel lumen. After single injection of basic phospholipase, 6000 μg/kg: 13 min. (Fig. 9) there is severe endothelial cytoplasm swelling with abnormal membrane profiles (arrows). Note erythrocytes (R) with variable density, ghosts (G) and dense particles (arrowheads) accumulated in lumen.

At doses of 1500 μg/kg and larger, the animals succumb within 20-60 minutes. The lethal effect is most probably associated with hemolysis and insufficiency of the vascular system, especially of the lungs. However, pathophysiologically this is a very complicated situation and the specific biochemical pathogenesis involved remains to be investigated.

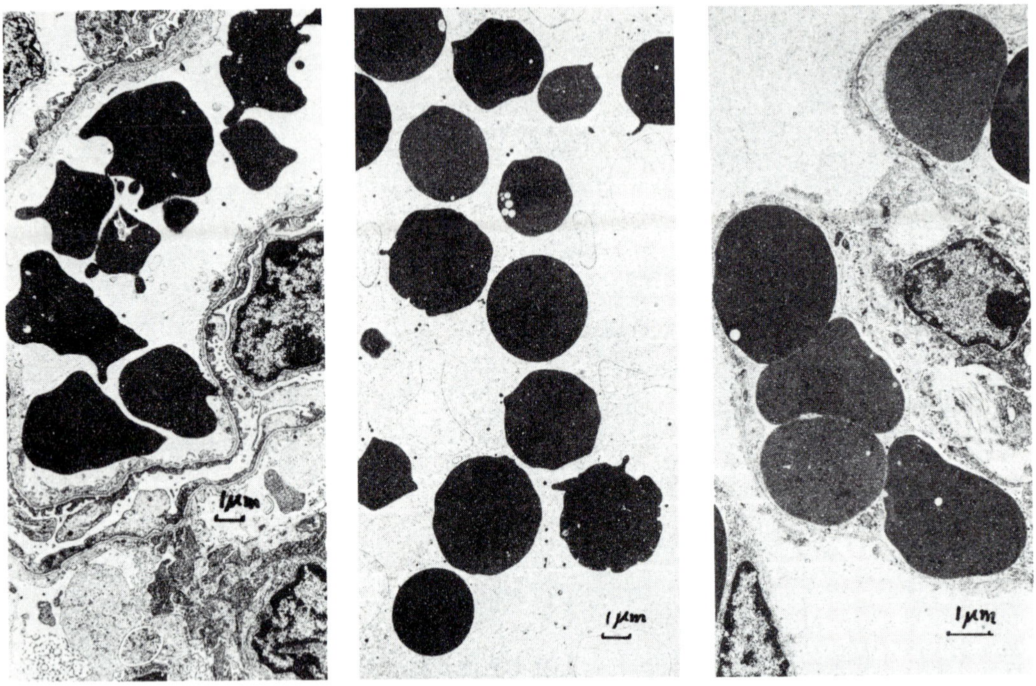

Figs. 10, 11 and 12. Erythrocyte deformation intravascularly. Crenated cells in glomerular capillary (Fig. 10) from mouse given phospholipase 400 μg/kg, 120 min. Spherocytes with single spicula, ghosts and small dense particles in lung artery (Fig. 11) and lung capillaries (Fig. 12) after phospholipase, 3000 μg/kg: 13 min. specimen.

The dual function of the venom. i.e., immobilization of prey and damage to the eyes of offenders might be reflected in a bimodial action of venom components. The postsynaptic neurotoxin and cardiotoxins thus can kill prey rapidly and the main function of the basic phospholipase might be to cause ocular lesions. Our results show, however, that many organ systems are sensitive to the venom phospholipase. Particularly the red blood cells are seriously affected, which probably both will lead to impaired organ perfusion due to rheological phenomena and to decreased oxygen supply to the tissues. These effects will probably help in both the immobilization and the killing of a prey, since the doses needed for an adequate effect (40-100 μg/mouse) could well be delivered in a single bite. The effects of the phospholipase might be further exaggerated by synergistic action with neurotoxins and cardiotoxins. In larger animals (or humans) local necrosis with severe loss of skin, nerves and blood vessels of an extremity and a hemorrhagic tendency might be the consequence of a subcutanous or intramuscular injection of phospholipase. Local necrosis can be caused by such enzymes, an effect which is enhanced by cardiotoxin (Fohlman, unpublished observations). Prominent local necrosis is also associated with bites of Naja naja (Reid, 1964), and both venoms contain the same principal components. Necrosis of muscular tissue is caused by phospholipases from the venoms of Enhydrina schistosa and Notechis s. scutatus (Fohlman and Eaker, 1977; Harris and co-workers, 1975). Neuromuscular paralysis in humans is not observed until 100-250 mg is injected, an amount which hardly can be injected in a single bite from even a large specimen of Naja nigricollis.

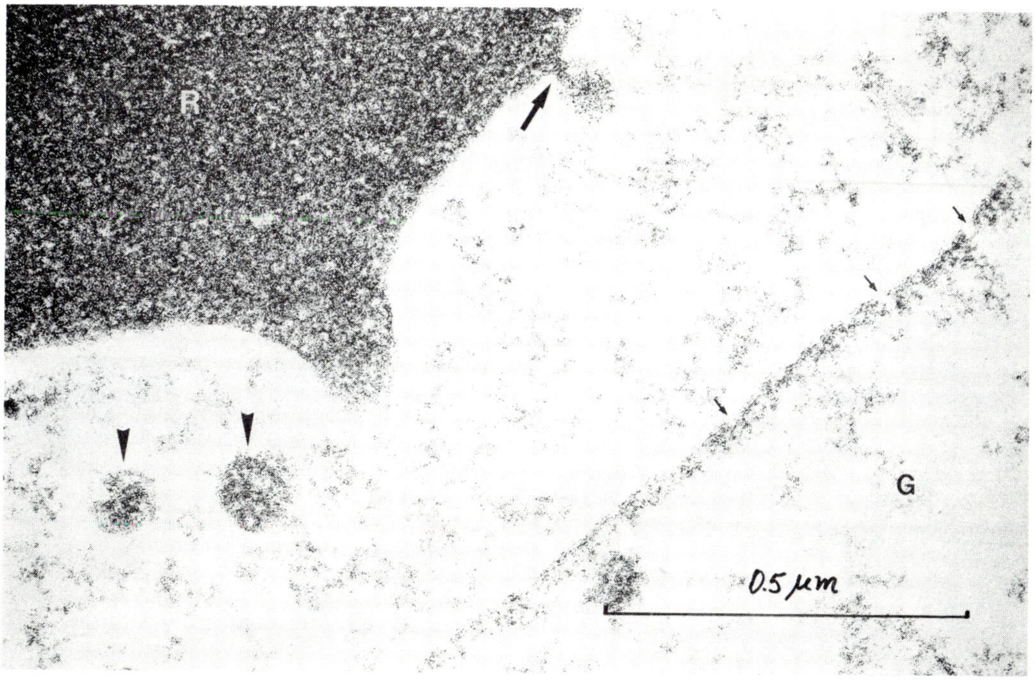

Fig. 13. Erythrocytes in lung vessel 13 minutes after basic phospholipase, 3000 μg/kg intravenously. Note projections from erythrocyte (R) suggesting budding from cell surface (arrow). Dense particles in surrounding plasma (arrowheads). Ghost cell (G) with defects (small arrows) in plasma membrane.

Possibly venom gland phospholipases had originally a digestive function to supplement alimentary tract enzyme juices. In the case of snake venoms, phospholipases have clearly evolved new functions. The high evolutionary "turnover" of phospholipases is reflected in the number of mutations per time unit (Dayhoff, 1978), and probably also in the fact that many snake venoms clearly contain large numbers of iso-phospholipases. An evolutionary tree has been constructed (Barker, Young and Dayhoff, 1978), and the astonishing result is that elapid snakes have evolved more sophisticated phospholipases than mammals. This probably should be interpreted to indicate that the main evolution of poisonous snakes occurred in the venom gland, requiring more changes in the part of chromosome coding for these enzymes. As a consequence phospholipases have many more functions than would be expected for a digestive enzyme. Among these are presynaptic neurotoxicity, myotoxicity, anticoagulation activity, necrotizing activity and perhaps a primary "oculotoxicity".

All elapid and hydrophid venoms investigated so far contain postsynaptic "curaremimetic" neurotoxins which show lethal doses in the vicinity of 100 μg/kg upon intravenous injection into mice. Some elapid venoms, notably those of *Bungarus multicinctus* (β-bungarotoxin), *Notechis scutatus scutatus* (notexin and notechis II-5) and *Oxyuranus scutellatus scutellatus* (taipoxin), and probably several other Australian elapids contain, in addition, pre-synaptic neurotoxins with intravenous mouse lethal doses in the vicinity of 20-2 μg/kg. These are by far the most lethal substances present in the venoms in which they occur. In the absence of the considerably more potent pre-synaptic neurotoxins, the postsynaptic curaremimetic

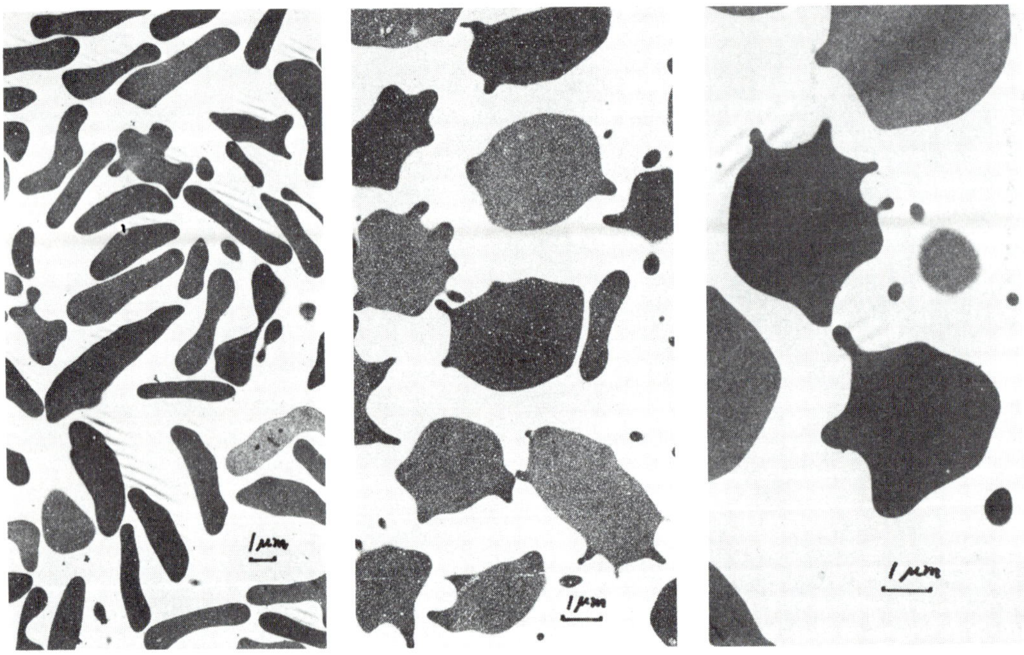

Figs. 14, 15 and 16. Erythrocyte structure in centrifuged blood. From mouse 120 minutes after intravenous injection of phospholipase 11 µg/kg with minor changes (Fig. 14). Compare to severe crenation and spherocyte transformation 120 minutes after 400 µg/kg (Fig. 15). Similar change after in vitro incubation for 60 minutes at +37°C with phospholipase 40 µg/ml (Fig. 16).

neurotoxins are otherwise the most lethal substances present in the venoms, and owing to their very selective binding properties they have emerged during the last decade as extremely valuable tools for the isolation and study of the nicotinic acetyl choline receptor. During the last 5 years the more recently characterized pre-synaptic neurotoxins have received increasing attention in connection with studies of the mechanism of neurotransmitter release.

Unfortunately, our vastly improved knowledge of the chemical natures and modes of action of these two types of neurotoxins has given little joy to clinicians confronted with the problem of treating patients who have been envenomated by these snakes. In the case of the Australian "killer" snakes, a penetrating bite seems always to be accompanied by injection of a lethal quantity of pre-synaptic neurotoxin, and since these cause structural damage to the nerve terminal, the prognosis is very bad unless antiserum is given before the toxin reaches a lethal concentration in the circulation.

In the case of venoms containing only post-synaptic neurotoxins the situation is quite different. Although all cobra venoms, for example, contain substantial amounts of these toxins, human victims of accidental cobra bite rarely exhibit a serious degree of the peripheral paralysis that results upon blockade of peripheral nicotinic receptors, apparently because the amount of venom injected, usually rather superficially, is too little to allow the build-up of a paralytic concentration in the circulation. Instead, the clinician is often confronted with delayed local necroses and other unpleasant chronic sequellae similar to those caused by the purified basic N. nigricollis phospholipase.

Probably many snake venoms contain phospholipases with similar properties. Although the LD_{50} of the purified nigricollis enzyme is rather high (ca 400 μg/kg) compared to those of neurotoxins, one can expect that most of its effects on susceptible membranes - especially hemolysis - would be greatly enhanced in the presence of the cardiotoxins and/or direct lytic factors that invariably occur in cobra venoms. By the same token, phospholipases which exhibit no significant lethality on their own might make very important contributions to the pathology of snakebite in combination with the latter and other constituents of the venoms. Biochemists engaged in the fractionation of snake venoms should thus remember that the most lethal fractions are not necessarily the most interesting ones from the clinical point of view.

ACKNOWLEDGEMENT

The authors wish to express their appreciation to Mrs. Anita Olofsson for skilful technical assistance.

REFERENCES

Barker, W. C., C. L. Young, and M. O. Dayhoff (1978). In Atlas of Protein Sequence and Structure, Vol. 5, Suppl. 3. National Biomedical Research Foundation, Washington D.C., USA, pp. 95-130.

Bogert, C. M. (1943). Bull. Am. Mus. Nat. Hist., 81, 285-360.

Dayhoff, M. O. (1978). In Atlas of Protein Sequence and Structure, Vol. 5, Suppl. 3. National Biomedical Research Foundation, Washington D.C., USA, pp. 1-8.

Eaker, D., J. Halpert, J. Fohlman, and E. Karlsson (1976). In Animal, Plant and Microbial Toxins, Vol. 2. Plenum Press, New York, USA, pp. 27-45.

Fohlman, J., and D. Eaker (1977). Toxicon, 15, 385-393.

Freyvogel, T. A., and C. G. Honegger (1965). Acta Trop., 22, 289-302.

Harris, J. B., M. A. Johnson, and E. Karlsson (1975). Clin. Exp. Pharmacol. Physiol., 2, 383-404.

Karlsson, E., D. L. Eaker, and J. Porath (1966). Biochim. Biophys. Acta, 127, 505-520.

Reid, H. A. (1964). Brit. Med. J., 2, 540-545.

Warrell, D. A., B. M. Greenwood, N. McD. Davidson, L. M. Ormerod, and C. R. M. Prentice (1976). Q. J. Med. (N. S.), XLV, 1-22.

Warrell, D. A., and L. D. Ormerod (1976). Am. J. Trop. Med. Hyg., 25, 525-529.

SIGNS, SYMPTOMS AND TREATMENT OF SEVERE SCORPION POISONING IN CHILDREN

J. A. Campos*, O.S. Silva, M. Lopez** and L. Freire-Maia*****

**Dept. Pediatrics, Faculty of Medicine, UFMG, and Center of Intoxication Control, Hospital Joao XXIII, Belo Horizonte, Brazil*
***Intensive Care Unit, Faculty of Medicine, UFMG, Belo Horizonte, Brazil*
****Dept. Physiology, ICB, UFMG, Belo Horizonte, Brazil*

ABSTRACT

The authors describe the signs and symptoms observed in 40 children severely poisoned by brownish-yellow scorpion Tityus serrulatus. The treatment in a Intensive Care Unit consisted of symptomatic measures, support of vital functions and neutralizing of circulating venom. From the total of 1.173 adults and children stung by scorpions, in a 7 years period, only 3 patients died, with a mortality rate of 0.26%.

KEYWORDS

Tityus serrulatus; scorpion venom; scorpion sting; treatment of scorpion poisoning.

INTRODUCTION

The Brazilian scorpion Tityus serrulatus induces severe clinical manifestations, mainly in children, leading to death in 3.5% of cases (Magalhães, 1938).

Investigations reported by our group since 1970 have shown that the effects induced by scorpion toxin in the rat, such as cardiac arrhythmias, arterial hypertension, pulmonary edema, respiratory arrhythmias, gastric secretion, excessive salivation, and contraction of gut smooth muscle, are due to stimulation of peripheral nervous system (Catanzaro and co-workers, 1978; Cunha-Melo and co-workers, 1973; Freire-Maia and Diniz, 1970; Freire-Maia and co-workers, 1978; Freire-Maia, Azevedo and Lima, 1976; Freire-Maia, Pinto and Franco, 1974; Gonzaga and co-workers, 1979). Based on these experimental data we decided to improve the clinical treatment of children, severely poisoned by scorpions, in the Intensive Care Unit of the "Hospital das Clínicas UFMG", Belo Horizonte, Brazil.

Preliminary results were published elsewhere (Campos and co-workers, 1975 and 1979).

METHODS

One thousand one hundred and seventy three patients stung by scorpions were admitted at the "Hospital João XXIII", in Belo Horizonte, between January 1972 and December 1978 (an average of 168 cases per year).

The majority of stings occured in Summer time. For instance, in the 7 years period, the total number of stings in the months of December-January-February (Summer) was 326, whereas the number in June-July-August (Winter) was 240.

From the total number of patients, 323 were children below 12 years old. As the clinical symptoms in adults were always benign, only the cases of children were included in this paper. The majority of cases was treated in children infirmary, whereas 40 severe cases (25 male and 15 female) were treated at Intensive Care Unit.

The children were examined soon after their admission to hospital and in majority of cases blood samples were taken out for biochemical and hematologic tests. Electrocardiograms consisting of 3 standard, 3 unipolar limb and 6 precordial leads were taken in the supine position. At Intensive Care Unit the children were monitored by a bipolar chest lead. The chest roentgenography was taken in some cases in order to observe the size of heart and detect pulmonary edema.

Based on informations of the patients or their relatives, the scorpions were identified as belonging to the species Tityus serrulatus, of the Family Buthidae and Subfamily Titynae. The venom of this scorpion is of a protein nature and does not present hemolytic effects (Diniz and Gonçalves, 1960). A purified toxin with a molecular weight of about 7000 daltons (tityustoxin), obtained from the crude scorpion venom (Gomez and Diniz, 1966), induces the same effects of the venom in laboratory animals (Freire-Maia and Diniz, 1970; Freire-Maia and co-workers, 1978).

RESULTS

Clinical Findings

The most prominent clinical findings in severe scorpion envenomation in children treated at Intensive Care Unit, are shown in Table 1.

TABLE 1 The Most Prominent Clinical Findings of Severe Scorpion Poisoning in Children (40 cases)

CLINICAL FINDINGS	PERCENTAGE
Pain at site of sting	100.0
Tachycardia	95.0
Vomiting	92.5
Hyperthermia	62.5
Tachypnea	35.0
Profuse sweating	32.5
Dyspnea	25.0
Congestive heart failure	25.0
Arterial hypertension	17.5
Pulmonary Edema	15.0
Dehydration	15.0
Shivering	15.0
Prostation	15.0
Excessive salivation	15.0

The following findings were also observed: restlessness (12.5%), convulsion (12.5%), shock (7,5%), cardiac arrest (7.5%), bradycardia (5.0%), bradypnea (5.0%), diarrhea (5.0%), abdominal pain (2.5%), coma (2.5%), opisthotonos (2.5%) and muscle spasm (2.5%).

The most serious clinical findings in these children were congestive heart failure, arterial hypertension, pulmonary edema, dehydration, convulsion, cardiac arrest, shock and coma.

Electrocardiographic Findings

Table 2 shows the electrocardiographic findings in this group of children, and Fig. 1 and 2 show examples of some ECG abnormalities.

TABLE 2 Electrocardiographic Findings of Severe Scorpion Poisoning in Children (40 cases)

ELECTROCARDIOGRAPHIC FINDINGS	PERCENTAGE
Sinus Tachycardia	80.0
Prominent U wave	40.0
T wave inversion and ST deviations	25.0
LABBB*	2.5
Ventricular ectopic beats	2.5
Complete A-V heart block	2.5
Sinus arrest	2.5
Sinus bradycardia	2.5
Wandering pacemaker	2.5

*Left Anterior Bundle Branch Block

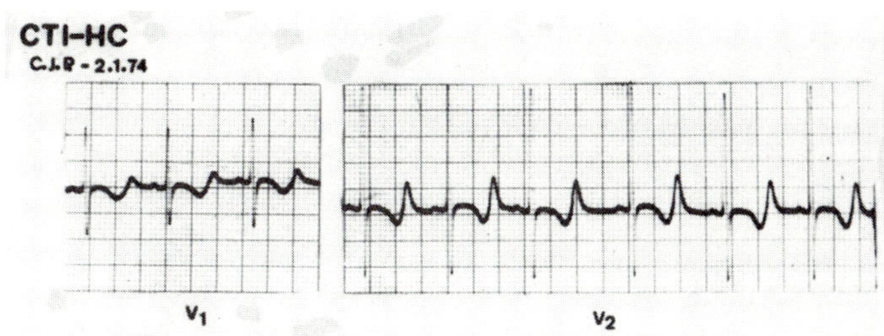

Fig. 1. Electrocardiogram of a 2 years old child, stung by a scorpion Tityus serrulatus, at January 2, 1974. Leads V_1 and V_2. Sinus rhythm. Negative T wave followed by prominent U wave.

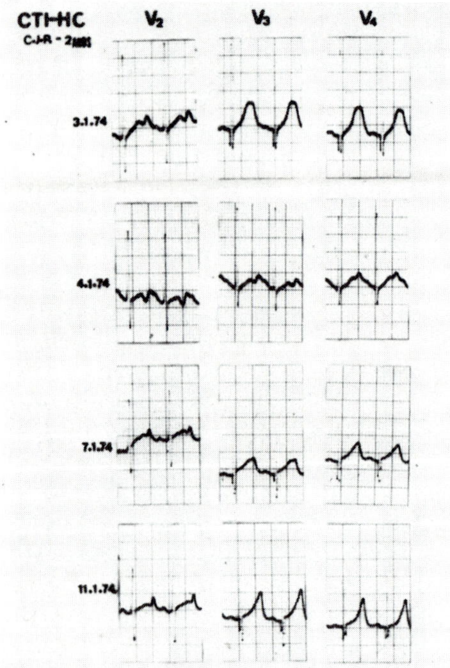

Fig. 2. Electrocardiographic evolution of patient C.J.P. (Fig. 1), from January 3 to January 11, 1974. Leads V_2-V_4. T wave became positive at V_2. Sometimes there is fusion of T and U waves, resulting in a combination wave which resembles a tall and wide T wave.

Laboratory Findings in Severe Scorpion Poisoning

Hematologic findings. Table 3 shows that the mean values of hemoglobin, hematias and hematocrit are within the normal limits, when they are compared with Brazilian populations of same age (0-12 years old). A striking neutrophil leukocytosis is found in all cases.

In some cases it was possible to follow the course of leukocytosis in the children. For instance, patient J.A.S., 5 years old, presented a marked leukocytosis (44.400 cells per mm^3) at the day of the scorpion sting (March 19, 1977). Hyperglycemia (202 mg%) and tachycardia (140 bpm) were also observed. Fourty-eight hours later, the leukocyte count had fallen to 10.100 cells per mm^3, returning to normal values (7.400 cells per mm^3) at the third day after the sting, when the heart rate and glycemia were also normal.

TABLE 3 Hematologic Findings in Severe Scorpion Poisoning

HEMATOLOGIC EXAMINATIONS	N	Mean ± S.E.	Range
Hemoglobin (g%)	10	11.9 ± 0.5	9.2 - 14.2
Hematias (mm^3)	10	3.959.000 ± 187.000	3.1×10^6 - 4.7×10^6
Hematocrit (%)	07	34 ± 2	27 - 42
Leukocytes (mm^3)	10	20.080 ± 3.602	10.400 - 44.400
Differential count	10		
Neutrophils (young) %		4 ± 1	1 - 8
Neutrophils (adult) %		81 ± 2	66 - 92
Lymphocytes %		10 ± 2	2 - 24
Monocytes %		3 ± 1	0 - 5
Eosinophils %		2 ± 1	0 - 11*
Basophils %		0	0

*In only one case it was observed 11% of eosinophils. In the other cases, the figures were 3% or below.

Biochemical findings. Table 4 shows that glycemia varied from 65 to 400mg%, with a mean of 153 ± 19. In 12 out of 20 cases the glycemia was higher than 120 mg%. The serum amylase levels were higher than normal, oscillating from 60 to 360 units per cent, with a mean of 211 ± 38 units per cent. The mean values of urea, creatinine, serum sodium and serum chlorides were within the normal limits. The serum potassium levels varied from 4.0 to 4.6 mEq/L in 5 cases; from 3.0 to 3.9 mEq/L in 7 cases and from 2.1 to 2.9 mEq/L in 3 cases. The mean value was 3.6 ± 0.2 mEq/L.

TABLE 4 Biochemical Findings in Severe Scorpion Poisoning

BIOCHEMICAL EXAMINATIONS	N	Mean ± S.E.	Range
Blood glucose (mg%)	20	153 ± 19	65 - 400
Serum amylase (units %)	08	211 ± 38	60 - 360
Blood urea (mg%)	12	32 ± 4	18 - 63
Serum creatinine (mg%)	11	1.1 ± 0.1	0.6 - 1.9
Serum sodium (mEq/L)	09	138 ± 2	128 - 146
Serum chlorides (mEq/L)	10	110 ± 2	100 - 120
Serum potassium (mEq/L)	15	3.6 ± 0.2	2.1 - 4.6

Calcium determinations in blood of 4 patients showed the following results: 8.0-9.0-10.5-12.0 mg%.

Treatment of Severe Scorpion Poisoning

The patients with high risk or main physiological system instability were admitted at Intensive Care Unit and underwent constant clinical evaluation and continuous electrocardiographic monitoring. The treatment was symptomatic, supportive of vital functions and neutralizing of circulating venom.

Pain is usually insupportable and could lead to a state of shock. It is treated by injection of dipirone or propoxifeno, in doses of 40-80 mg/kg/day. When possible, pain is abolished by anesthesia of sting site with lidocaine. Vomiting, present in more than 90% of cases, could induce electrolyte and acid-base imbalances, or even dehydration, and is treated by intravenous injection of metoclopramide (0.5mg/kg), followed by oral administration of the same drug, 2-3 times per day. Hyperthermia is controlled with dipirone (40-80 mg/kg/day).

For the support of vital functions, the following should be charted: pulse rate, arterial blood pressure, respiration rate and urine flow. All patients underwent continuous electrocardiographic monitoring to permit the early diagnosis and treatment of cardiac arrhythmias, and ventilatory support through oxygentherapy or positive pressure respiration. In cases of cardiac failure, digitalis and a diuretic agent (furosemide) should be used besides oxygentherapy. If the patient presents pulmonary edema the treatment consists of oxygen, digitalis, furosemide and limb tourniquet to decrease the venous return.

Neutralizing of circulating venom: intravenous injection of 20-40ml of antivenom, specific for scorpions of genus Tityus (Butantan Institute, São Paulo, Brazil), is made in all patients.

The mild cases of intoxication were treated with symptomatic measures and/or antivenom, in adults or children infirmaries at Emergency Hospital.

DISCUSSION

Human beings stung by scorpions presented electrocardiographic signs of myocardites (Poon-King, 1963) or "infarct of myocardium" (Gueron, Stern and Cohen, 1967; Gueron and Yaron, 1970). On the other hand, our data showed that the most prominent electrocardiographic findings in 40 severely intoxicated children, stung by Brazilian scorpion Tityus serrulatus, were sinus tachycardia (80%), prominent U wave (40%) and T wave inversion and ST deviations (25%). It seems likely that tachycardia is due to actions of catecholamines, released by scorpion venom, on SA node, as it was shown in laboratory animals (Freire-Maia, Pinto and Franco, 1974). As far as the T wave, ST segment and U wave changes, Lepeschkin and co-workers (1960) have shown that infusion of epinephrine in human beings may induce inversion of T wave, deviations of ST segment and elevation of U wave, which showed partial or complete fusion with T wave. These changes were explained by effects of epinephrine on ventricular action potential. Therefore, the same changes, observed in children stung by scorpions, could be explained by effects of epinephrine, released by venom, on the heart. Part of these effects could also be due to a local myocardial hypoxia, induced by intensification of oxygen consumption, evoked by epinephrine (Raab, 1960). It seems likely that the prominent U wave, observed in 40% of our cases, is not due to hypopotassemia, since in the majority of cases the potassium levels were within the normal limits. However, in 3 patients the serum potassium varied from 2.1 to 2.9 mEq/L and this, of course, could contribute to the U wave changes (Lepeschkin, 1955).

In all patients severely poisoned by scorpions a remarkable leukocytosis (10.400-44.400 cells per mm^3) was observed. Leukocytosis has also been reported during hypertensive crises in patients suffering of pheochromocytoma (French and Campagna, 1961; Radtke and co-workers, 1975). Therefore, it seems likely that the increase in white cells count in cases of scorpion venom intoxication could also be due to an effect of catecholamines, released by venom.

Many patients severely intoxicated by scorpion venom die with pulmonary edema (Barros, 1938; Gueron, Stern and Cohen, 1967; Gueron and Yaron, 1970; Magalhães, 1946; Reddy and co-workers, 1972; Stahnke, 1950; Waterman, 1938). In the present study we confirm that pulmonary edema is one of the most serious complications of scorpion poisoning, since the three children who died after the stings presented pulmonary edema. Experimental data have shown that the edema in laboratory animals is related, at least in part, to heart failure, induced by catecholamines released by venom (Freire-Maia and co-workers, 1978). It seems worthwhile to keep this in mind during the treatment of severe scorpion intoxications.

Mortality rate. Waterman (1938) reported in Trinidad 698 cases of patients stung by scorpion Tityus trinitatis, in a 4 years period, with a mortality rate of 4.7%. But in children under 5 years old, the rate was about 25%. Later, Poon-King (1963) reported 45 cases in the same country, without deaths. At least two reasons could explain the lack of deaths in the latter report, that is, the use of antivenom therapy and the age of the patients (over 9 years old). Many other scorpion species cause also death in children (see reviews in Efrati, 1978; Stahnke, 1978). For instance, Gueron and Yaron (1970) in Israel reported 82 cases of patients stung by scorpion Buthus quinquestriatus, in a 9 years period, with a mortality rate of 10.9%. But, all cases of death occurred in children below 9 years of age. In Brazil, Magalhães (1938) reported 6.668 cases of scorpion sting with a mortality rate of 3.5%. But, after the use of antivenom therapy the rate decreased to 1.8%. Silva (1950) reported 985 cases of scorpion sting in Ribeirão Preto region, with a mortality rate of 0.71%. Usually, the severe cases of intoxication in Brazil are caused by Tityus serrulatus. Around the city of São Paulo, G. Rosenfeld reported 701 cases of patients stung by Tityus bahiensis, from 1954 to 1965, with only two deaths (Rosenfeld, personal communication to W. Bücherl, 1978).

According with Bücherl (1971) the Brazilian scorpion Tityus serrulatus may cause the death of 0.8-1.4% of the adults and 3-20% of children, depending on the age. The method used by our group of treating mild cases with symptomatic measures and/or antivenom therapy in Emergency Hospital Infirmaries and severe cases with symptomatic measures, suport of vital functions and antivenom in an Intensive Care Unit decreased these rates to 0.26%.

ACKNOWLEDGEMENT

One of the Authors (L.Freire-Maia) express his gratitude to the Brazilian Agency CNPq for a fellowship.

REFERENCES

Barros, E.F. (1938). Aspectos clínicos da intoxicação escorpiônica. Mems Inst.Biol. Ezequiel Dias, 2, 101-287.

Bücherl, W. (1971). Classification and biology of scorpions. In W. Bücherl, and E.D.Buckley (Ed.), Venomous animals and their venoms. Vol. 3, Venomous invertebrates, Academic Press, New York. pp 339-342.

Bücherl, W. (1978). Venoms of Tityinae. A. Systematic, Distribution, Biology, Venomous Apparatus, etc. of Titynae; Venom Collection, Toxicity, Human Accidents and Treatment of Stings. In S. Bettini (Ed.). Arthropod Venoms, Springer-Verlag, Berlin. pp 371-379.

Campos, J.A., O.A.Silva, P.V. Guimarães, M. Lopez, and L. Freire-Maia (1975). Tratamento de intoxicação escorpiônica em seres humanos. Abstracts XII Congress Assoc.Med. Minas Gerais, Belo Horizonte, 131-132.

Campos, J.A., O.A.Silva, M. Lopez, and L. Freire-Maia (1979). Signs, symptoms and treatment of severe scorpion sting in children. Toxicon, 17 (suppl. 1), 19.

Catanzaro, O.L., R.A.S. Santos, O.M. Parra, R.M. Santos, L. Freire-Maia, and W.T. Beraldo (1978). Effect of scorpion toxin (tityustoxin, TsTX) on the salivary gland of the rat, in vivo and in vitro. Agents Actions, 8, 119-124.

Cunha-Melo, J.R., L. Freire-Maia, W.L. Tafuri, and T.A. Maria (1973). Mechanism of action of purified scorpion toxin on the isolated rat intestine. Toxicon, 11, 81-84.

Diniz, C.R. and J.M. Gonçalves (1960). Separation of biologically active components from scorpion venoms by zone electrophoresis. Biochem.Biophys.Acta., 41, 470-477.

Efrati, P. (1978). Venoms of Buthinae. B. Epidemiology, symptomatology and treatment of Buthinae stings. In S. Bettini (Ed.), Arthropod Venoms, Springer-Verlag, Berlin. pp 312-317.

Freire-Maia, L., H.O. Almeida, J.R. Cunha-Melo, A.D. Azevedo, and J. Barroso (1978). Mechanism of the pulmonary edema induced by intravenous injection of scorpion toxin in the rat. Agents Actions, 8, 113-118.

Freire-Maia, L., A.D.Azevedo, and E.G.Lima (1976). Pharmacological blockade of the cardiovascular and respiratory effects produced by tityustoxin in the rat. In A. Ohsaka, K. Hayashi, and Y. Sawai (Ed.), Animal, Plant, and Microbial Toxins, Vol. 2, Plenum, New York. pp. 287-298.

Freire-Maia, L., and C.R. Diniz (1970). Pharmacological action of a purified scorpion toxin in the rat. Toxicon, 8, 132.

Freire-Maia, L., G.I. Pinto, and I. Franco (1974). Mechanism of the cardiovascular effects produced by purified scorpion toxin in the rat. J. Pharmac. exp. Ther., 188, 207-213.

French, C. and F.A. Campagna (1961). Pheochromocytoma with shock, marked leukocytosis, and unusual electrocardiograms: case report and review of the literature. Ann.Intern.Med., 55, 127-134.

Gomez, M.V., and C.R. Diniz (1966). Separation of toxic components from the Brazilian scorpion - Tityus serrulatus - venom. Mems Inst. Butantan, 33, 899-902.

Gonzaga, H.M.S., F. Alzamora, J.R. Cunha-Melo, and L. Freire-Maia (1979). Gastric secretion induced by scorpion toxin. Toxicon, 17, 316-318.

Gueron, M., J. Stern, and W. Cohen (1967). Severe myocardial damage and heart failure in scorpion sting. Am.J.Cardiol., 19, 719-726.

Gueron, M., and R.Yaron (1970). Cardiovascular manifestations of severe scorpion sting.Chest, 57, 156-162.

Lepeschkin, E. (1955). The U wave of the electrocardiogram. Arch. Intern. Med., 96, 600-617.

Lepeschkin, E., H. Marchet, G. Schroeder, R. Wagner, P. Paula e Silva, and W.Raab (1960). Effect of epinephrine and norepinephrine on the electrocardiogram of 100 normal subjects. Am.J.Cardiol., 5, 594-603.

Magalhães, O.C. (1938). Scorpionism. J.Trop.Med.Hyg., 41, 393-399.

Magalhães, O.C. (1946). Escorpionismo. Monography. Monog.Inst.Oswaldo Cruz, 3,1-220.

Poon-King, T. (1963). Myocarditis from scorpion stings. Brit. Med. J., 1, 374-377.

Raab, W. (1960). Key position of catecholamines in functional and degenerative cardiovascular pathology. Am.J.Cardiol. 5, 571-578.

Radtke, W.E., F.J. Kazmier, B.D. Rutherford, and S.G. Sheps (1975). Cardiovascular complications of pheochromocytoma crisis. Am.J.Cardiol., 35, 701-705.

Reddy, C.R.R.M., G. Syvarnakumari, C.S. Devi, and C.N. Reddy (1972). Pathology of scorpion venom poisoning. J.Trop.Med.Hyg. 75, 98-100.

Silva, T.L. (1950). Escorpionismo em Ribeirão Preto. Notas sobre epidemiologia e profilaxia. Arch. Hig.Saude Pública (São Paulo), 15, 79-90.

Stahnke, H.L. (1950). The Arizona scorpion problem. Ariz.Med., 7, 23-29.

Stahnke, H.L. (1978). The genus Centruroides (Buthidae) and its venom. In S.Bettini (Ed.), Arthropod Venoms, Springer-Verlag, Berlin. pp 277-307.

Waterman, J.A. (1938). Some notes on scorpion poisoning in Trinidad. Trans.R.Soc. Trop.Med.Hyg., 31, 607-624.

HISTOPATHOLOGY AND PHYSIOLOGICAL ACTION OF VENOM FROM THE BROWN RECLUSE SPIDER, *LOXOSCELES RECLUSA*

B. R. Norment and L. D. Foil

Department of Entomology, Mississippi State University, Mississippi Agricultural and Forestry Experiment Station, Mississippi State, Mississippi, USA

ABSTRACT

Experiments with Loxosceles reclusa venom upon invertebrate hosts have revealed both localized and systemic manifestations. Bioassays have yielded LD_{50} values of 0.42 μg/g (Acheta domesticus); 0.33 μg/g (Galleria mellonella) and 0.26 μg/g (Musca domestica). Evidence for a lytic effect on fat and muscle tissue of Heliothis virescens larvae, hemolymph proteins (H. virescens) and hemocytes (H. virescens, A. domesticus) has been demonstrated. Observations histochemically showed stronger reactions of protease, lipase, esterase and alkaline phosphatase activity in envenomized H. virescens and M. domestica. L. reclusa venom was separated by gel filtration into three 280 nm absorbing peaks two of which contained components lethal to insects. Peak 1 (high molecular weight) and peak 2 (low molecular weight) produced above control mortality in M. domestica; whereas, only whole venom and peak 2 aliquots induced increases in the endogenous activity of the ventral nerve cord in Periplaneta americana. When maximally lethal samples of peaks 1 and 2 were combined, observed mortalities were 88% greater than predicted, suggesting either synergism or dependent joint action.

KEYWORDS

Loxosceles reclusa; spider venom; histochemical; cytotoxicity; enzymes; synergism; neurotoxicity.

INTRODUCTION

The brown recluse spider, Loxosceles reclusa, is considered to be one of the most dangerous venomous spider species in the United States. There are several other Loxosceles species present in the U.S. but are considered to be of lesser importance to public health. In the Continental United States, infestations of L. reclusa are currently known to occur in 17 midwestern and south central states. This species is found in both outdoor and indoor environments, however its importance to public health is amplified by the large populations which frequently occur indoors in undisturbed areas (Foil and Norment, 1979).

Adult female L. reclusa will vary from 7-12 mm in total length and average 9 mm; whereas, the males average 8 mm. A dark brown violin-shaped band on the cephalothorax of both males and females is a distinguishing feature; the body coloration varies from light tan to dark brown.

The first authentic case of loxoscelism in North America was reported in 1929 (Schmaus, 1929). The significance of this report was long overlooked and it was not until 1957 that circumstantial evidence first associated L. reclusa with the "necrotic spider bite" syndrome (Atkins and coworkers, 1957). Then in 1958, there was conclusive evidence that L. reclusa was the specific spider producing the bite syndrome (Atkins and coworkers, 1958).

SYMPTOMOLOGY

An individual bitten by L. reclusa will normally experience cytotoxic reactions accompanied by localized cutaneous responses (Atkins and coworkers, 1958; Dillaha and coworkers, 1963; Anderson, 1971). One may experience a mild stinging at the time of the bite or be unaware that a bite has occurred; initially, pain is minimal until 2-8 hours following the bite. At the wound site a small bleb or blister quickly follows a transient erythema and an irregular area of ischemia surrounds the bleb. Shortly, a hemorrhagic zone may develop, the individual may become restless, feverish, and have difficulty in sleeping. A physician would generally be consulted at this point. The central ischemic area becomes stellate and turns dark over the next several days. Generally, between 1-2 weeks, the central area becomes depressed, the edges become demarcated with the locally affected tissue gradually sloughing, forming an open ulcer. Healing is a very slow process often requiring several weeks to months, and in some instances graft surgery is necessitated.

More infrequently are systemic responses which may include fever, headache, malaise, nausea, vomiting, joint pain and a generalized rash within 24-48 hours following envenomation (Dillaha and coworkers, 1964; Micks, 1963). These effects are generally worse in children. A definite hematological involvement in fatal cases has included hemolytic anemia and thrombocytopenia with further circulatory involvement including hemoglobinuria and renal failure (Madrigal and coworkers, 1972).

PHYSICAL PROPERTIES

L. reclusa venom is a clear, viscous fluid; the wet weight of the venom is approximately 1 mg/μl; the protein content ranges from 200 to 215 μg/μl (whole venom average of adult female - 0.36 μl; male - 0.25 μl).

The venom has been separated into high and low molecular weight components by gel filtration (Geren and coworkers, 1973). The low molecular weight components reportedly contain at least two polypeptides and multiple nucleotides (Geren and coworkers, 1975; Jong and coworkers, 1979a). The high molecular weight components which have been examined for enzymatic activities are not reflective of the normal enzyme patterns in vertebrate toxins. L. reclusa venom is devoid of phospholipase A, C and D, acetylcholinesterase, ribonuclease, deoxyribonuclease, phosphodiesterase, dipeptidase, collagenase, catalase, amylase or acid phosphatase activity (Hall, 1970; Wright, 1973; Nazhat, 1968; Wright and coworkers, 1973; Elgert and coworkers, 1974; Norment and coworkers, 1979). Thus far, detectable enzymes include hyaluronidase, protease, lipase, alkaline phosphatase, aliesterase, arylesterase, 5'-nucleotidase and sphingomyelinase D (Wright, 1973; Wright and coworkers, 1973; Jong and coworkers, 1979b; Norment and coworkers, 1979; Heitz and Norment, 1974; Geren and coworkers, 1976; Forrester and coworkers, 1978; Hall, 1970).

In establishing the effects of *L. reclusa* venom, it is important to determine not only its activity on man and other higher animals but also upon invertebrate species. *Loxosceles* spp. normally feed upon small insects such as firebrats, flies, cockroaches, and others that may frequent its irregularly spun web.

HISTOPATHOLOGY

Initially, evidence of a toxic effect of *L. reclusa* venom against hemocytes of adult *Acheta domesticus* was demonstrated (Norment and Smith, 1968). Results indicated a mean total hemocyte count of 53,345 for normal specimens; whereas 2.4-fold and 2.9-fold reductions, respectively were observed in 24 hr and 48 hr venom treated groups. Subsequently, protease activity of *L. reclusa* venom was indicated by electrophoretic assay of hemolymph from *Heliothis virescens* larvae (Norment and Vinson, 1969). There were 7 protein bands resolved from normal *H. virescens* larvae, whereas 6 of 7 bands that appeared were variously affected at 2, 6 and 8 hours post-injection.

Further evidence for tissue level protease activity of the venom and additionally for monoamine oxidase and polysaccharides has been demonstrated histochemically in *Heliothis virescens* larvae (Eskafi and Norment, 1976). Monoamine oxidase activity was observed in the epidermal layers of envenomized *H. virescens* (Table 1). This enzyme has been suggested to activate protease in snake venom, however, it is normally found in the mitochondrial system of various animal tissues. It has been postulated that the enzyme functions only inside mitochondria-like particles in animals and man, but several factors, including histamine can disturb its location and hence its function in affected cells. Millon's test detected tyrosine, a useful marker for most proteins, in muscles of control and envenomized specimens. Muscle tissues of control *H. virescens*, however, stained darker than those of envenomized larvae. Conversely, an increased protein concentration was observed in the hemolymph. This reversal of color intensity strongly suggested that lysed proteins or their simpler breakdown products, in envenomized larvae, diffused into the hemolymph. Extensive granular patches were stained with PAS in fat cells of control *H. virescens*, but little staining of these granular patches was observed in envenomized specimens. It has been reported that materials positive with PAS, but negative after acetylation, contain carbohydrates, most likely polysaccharides.

TABLE 1 Histochemical Reactions Observed in *Heliothis virescens* Larvae Envenomized by *Loxosceles reclusa*

Substrate	Stain method	Control	Envenomized	Activity
Epidermis	Tryptamine oxidation	- a/	+ b/	Monoamine oxidase
Fat Body	PAS	++ c/	+	Polysaccharide
Longitudinal and transverse muscle	Millon's test	++	+	Protease
Hemolymph	Millon's test	+	++	Protease

a/ - Negative.
b/ - Positive.
c/ - Strong positive.

PHYSIOLOGICAL ACTIVITY

Bioassays of selected insect species injected with 1 µl or less *L. reclusa* venom, using an Isco model M microapplicator, have yielded LD_{50} values of 0.42 µg/g for *Acheta domesticus* (house cricket) and 0.33 µg/g for *Galleria mellonella* (wax moth) larvae (Foil, 1978). The LD_{50} of *L. reclusa* venom in house flies was calculated at 0.26 µg/g, i.e. 18-fold more toxic to house flies than to mice. Upon electrical stimulation, adult female spiders normally yield about 70 µg of venom protein. Thus, the venom from a single spider is enough to kill 50% of 13,460 injected house flies. The house fly, therefore, is a very sensitive assay for the study of toxinological manifestations of *L. reclusa* venom. House flies injected with sub LD_{50} doses of whole venom first develop uncoordinated leg movements and loss of wing movements within an hour. Within 4 hours total paralysis ensues which is frequently accompanied by excessive salivation. House flies injected with *L. reclusa* venom doses above the LD_{50} are often knocked down within 5 minutes, indicating possible neurotoxicity.

Conventional electrophysiological techniques (Roeder and Roeder, 1939) were used to record the activity of *L. reclusa* upon the ventral nerve cord of the American cockroach, *Periplaneta americana*. The nerve cords were extricated and placed in a plexiglass recording chamber containing a 200 µl saline bath. The endogenous electrical activity of the ventral nerve cords was monitored by a suction electrode (Flory and Kriebel, 1966) and subsequently amplified and recorded on magnetic tape for further analysis. Application of *L. reclusa* venom (2.5-10 µg) induced dramatic increases in both the amplitude and frequency of the endogenous activity of the cockroach ventral nerve cord (Foil and coworkers, 1979b).

Analysis of spikes recorded greater than 33 µV revealed increases up to 680-fold above the control level, usually reaching maximum activity between 1 and 2 minutes after application and producing a complete block of endogenous activity within 3 minutes. This block was reversed within 45 minutes by saline infusion with rhythmic bursting activity observed during the saline wash. The increase in frequency and amplitude observed in the ventral nerve cords indicates the presence of invertebrate neurotoxins, however, it does not correspond to the symptomology of a flaccid paralysis produced in injected insects.

To further characterize the effects of *L. reclusa* venom upon invertebrate nervous systems, the venom was applied to the cercal nerve-giant fiber synapse in the sixth abdominal ganglion of *P. americana*. *L. reclusa* venom blocks this synaptic transmission which has previously been reported to be cholinergic (Shankland and coworkers, 1969).

Additionally, we have recorded the effects of *L. reclusa* venom upon the cockroach metathoracic leg kick response. The crural nerve was severed between the metathoracic ganglion and the leg and stimulated using suction electrodes. The kick response of the leg was monitored by transduction and venom was applied to the coxal stump. The kick response was blocked within 3 minutes by 25 µg of venom and higher concentrations blocked the response in less than 3 minutes.

We have recently begun studies of the effects of *L. reclusa* venom upon the intact cockroach heart and have found that the venom blocks the normal heartbeat in an innervated heart prep. Large abdominal wall muscle contractions and cessation of heartbeat normally followed venom application within 30 seconds. Further studies comparing innervated vs. denervated insect heart should contribute further to the knowledge of the mode of action of *L. reclusa* venom upon invertebrate nervous systems.

To date, we have observed an increase in amplitude and frequency of the VNC endogenous activity, a block of the sixth abdominal ganglion giant fiber-cercal nerve synaptic transmission, a block of intact heartbeat; and a block of crural nerve stimulated metathoracic leg kick. All of these effects have been observed using whole venom.

Before proceeding to more refined neurophysiological studies in the description of the mode of action of the invertebrate neurotoxins, the multicomponent venom was separated to eliminate possible error derived by the presence of more than one neurotoxin in the venom. The venom was separated by Sephadex G-50 gel filtration into three 280 nm absorbing peaks. Peak 1 contains an insect lethal factor which is in the heavy molecular weight void volume of the G-50 column. Peak 2 contains another insect lethal factor of less than 10,000 mw; peak 3 contains nucleotides which appear to have no biological activity in insects. Peak 1 and peak 2 are both polypeptides as their lethal activity is eliminated by trypsin digestion. Additionally, treatment of the peak 1 fraction at 70°C for 30 minutes eliminated activity; whereas, heating at 90°C for 1 hr did not inactivate peak 2 activity. Peak 2 produces rapid knockdown followed within a few hours by death. Peak 1 produces knockdown between 20 and 24 hours post-injection and is rapidly followed by death.

When the fractions separated by gel filtration were analyzed against the endogenous activity of the cockroach ventral nerve cord, the only aliquots which produced greater than control responses were in peak 2. When these aliquots were heat treated at 90°C, they did not lose their neuroactivity; trypsin digestion, however, did inactivate these components.

The lethal components found in the gel filtration elution scheme are in peak 1 [high molecular weight (HMW)] and peak 2 [low molecular weight (LMW)] and before proceeding to further characterization of the mode of action of these two components, we investigated the possibility of interactions between them. Since *L. reclusa* venom is multicomponent, the testing of possible combinations between all venom components was not feasible, therefore, combinations of whole venom and the gel filtration fractions were tested for greater-than-additive mortality in injected house flies. No fractions were found to produce mortality above saline diluted whole venom control other than those previously reported producing lethal activity in peaks 1 and 2.

Assuming independent action of the LMW and HMW lethal components on the basis of differences in time of action and symptomology, the observed mortality, produced by mixtures of the maximally lethal fraction from peak 1 and peak 2, were compared to predictive values. If the venom components acted independently and were not synergistic in action, the observed mortality of the fraction mixtures should have been approximately the same as the sum of the fractions tested separately (Rosenberg and Coon, 1958). However, the observed mortality was 88% greater than that predicted (Table 2) indicating that these two components either work via synergism or in a dependent mode of action (Foil and coworkers, 1979a).

The possibility of dependent mode of action was investigated by expressing the observed mortality produced by one component as a function of expected concentration of the other component (Dubois, 1961). By summing the observed and calculated doses the expected mortality via dependent action can be determined. For instance, mortality via HMW action can be predicted by transposing the LMW observed mortality to HMW equivalents using the HMW dosage vs. mortality regression line. The HMW equivalent and the HMW alone dosage are then summed and the expected percent mortality of the summed dosages calculated from the HMW regression line. Subsequently, the expected percent mortality can be compared to the observed percent mortality of the combined fractions.

TABLE 2 Predicted vs. Observed Mortality of Combined *L. reclusa* Venom Sephadex G-50 Fractions Compared as Dissimilar Acting Compounds

	N	% Mortality
0.5 LMW (peak 2)	300	21.5
0.5 LMW (peak 1)	300	18.3
LMW + HMW Predicted[a/]		36.5
LMW + HMW Observed	300	68.5
Observed less predicted		32.0[b/]

a/ (0.5 HMW/100) (100 - 0.5 LMW) + 0.5 LMW.
b/ Student's t-test; t = 11.0, d.f. = 5; $p < 0.01$).

When predicted via HMW activity, the observed mortality was 67% greater than the predicted mortality (Table 3). Conversely, when the observed mortality of the HMW component was converted to LMW lethal activity, the observed mortality was only 3% greater than the predicted. Therefore, the HMW and LMW lethal components either work independently as synergists or dependently via the LMW activity.

TABLE 3 Observed vs. Predicted Mortalities of Mixtures of LMW and HMW Sephadex G-50 Fractions of *L. reclusa* Venom Compared via Dependent Action

	N	% Mortality
LMW + HMW observed	250	67.2
Predicted via HMW[a/]		40.2
Observed less predicted		27.0[b/]
Predicted via LMW[c/]		65.0
Observed less predicted		2.2[d/]

a/ Predicted by converting LMW-alone mortality to HMW equivalents, summation of dosages, and calculation of expected mortality from the summed dosages using the HMW dosage vs. mortality regression line.
b/ Mean difference highly significant ($p < 0.01$) according to t-test.
c/ Predicted as in a/ except reversing LMW and HMW.
d/ Not significantly different ($p > 0.4$).

HMW components from brown recluse venom that produce systemic death without producing lesions have been reported (Elgert and coworkers, 1974). Additionally, there have been reported changes in the heartbeats of patients exhibiting hemolytic anemia (Nance, 1961). Therefore, the possibility of a HMW neurotoxin in *L. reclusa* venom cannot be eliminated. Further biochemical separation and component mode of action studies will be required to describe the interaction between *L. reclusa* venom components. The fractions contained in peak 1 and peak 2 cannot be considered pure components by this means of separation; however, either venom component synergism or dependent joint action as LMW activity in invertebrates must be considered in future studies involving biochemical separation of *L. reclusa* venom components.

SUMMARY

L. reclusa venom is a multicomponent biological product which causes complex interactions between animals and venom at the organism, tissue and cellular level. The local and systemic complications in vertebrates induced by L. reclusa envenomation are manifestations of both venom mass action and immunopathological contributions. In venom-injected insects, lysis of hemocytes, fat and muscle tissue and an effect on hemolymph proteins have been demonstrated.

Additionally, our research has provided information concerning previously undescribed brown recluse venom component interactions and neurotoxicities in insects. Comparative vertebrate studies, however, will be required to determine the implications of these basic facts. Regardless of whether these venom activities are homologous, analogous or non-existent in vertebrate systems, the basic knowledge of L. reclusa venom has been expanded by these studies incorporating insect assay systems.

REFERENCES

Anderson, P. C. (1971). Treatment of severe loxocelism. Mo Med., 68, 609-618.

Atkins, J. A., C. W. Wingo, and W. A Sodeman (1957). Probable cause of necrotic spider bite in the Midwest. Science, 126, 73.

Atkins, J. A., C. W. Wingo, W. A. Sodeman, and J. E. Flynn (1958). Necrotic arachnidism. Am. J. Trop. Med. Hyg., 7, 165-184.

Dillaha, C. J., G. T. Jansen, and W. M. Honeycutt (1963). The gangrenous bite of the brown recluse spider in Arkansas. J. Arkansas Med. Soc., 60, 91-94.

Dilleha, C. J., G. T. Jansen, W. M. Honeycutt, and C. R. Hayden (1964). North American loxocelism. J. Am. Med. Assoc., 188, 33-36.

Dubois, K. P. (1961). Potentiation of the toxicity of organophosphorus compounds. Adv. Pest Control Res., 4, 117-151.

Elgert, K. D., M. A. Ross, B. J. Campbell, and J. T. Barrett (1974). Immunological studies of brown recluse spider venom. Infect. Immun., 19, 1412-1419.

Eskafi, F. M., and B. R. Norment (1976). Physiological action of Loxoceles reclusa (G & M) venom on insect larvae. Toxicon, 14, 7-13.

Flory, E. and M. E. Kriebel (1966). A new suction electrode system. Comp. Biochem. Physiol., 18, 175-178.

Foil, L. D. (1978). Venom gland ultrastructure, venom neurotoxicities and venom component interactions of the brown recluse spider, Loxoceles reclusa (Gertsch and Mulaik). Dissertation, Mississippi State University, 104 p.

Foil, L. D., H. W. Chambers, and B. R. Norment (1979a). Loxoceles reclusa venom component toxicity and interaction in Musca domestica. Toxicon, in press.

Foil, L. D., J. L. Frazier, and B. R. Norment (1979b). Partial characterization of lethal and neuroactive components of the brown recluse spider (Loxoceles reclusa) venom. Toxicon, 17, 347-354.

Foil, L. D., and B. R. Norment (1979). Envenomation by Loxoceles reclusa. J. Med. Entomol., 16, 18-25.

Forrester, L. J., J. T. Barrett, and B. J. Campbell (1978). Red blood cell lysis induced by the venom of the brown recluse spider: The role of sphingomyelinase D. Arch. Biochem. Biophys., 187, 355-365.

Geren, C. R., T. K. Chan, B. C. Ward, D. E. Howell, K. Pinkston, and G. V. Odell (1973). Composition and properties of extract of fiddleback (Loxoceles reclusa) spider venom apparatus. Toxicon, 11, 471-479.

Geren, C. R., T. K. Chan, D. E. Howell, and G. V. Odell (1975). Partial characterization of the low molecular weight fractions of the extract of the venom apparatus of the brown recluse spider and its hemolymph. Toxicon, 13, 233-238.

Geren, C. R., T. K. Chan, D.E. Howell, and G. V. Odell (1976). Isolation and characterization of toxins from brown recluse spider venom (Loxoceles reclusa). Arch. Biochem. Biophys., 174, 90-99.

Hall, J. E. (1970). A Study of Protein and Peptide Components of Venom of Loxosceles reclusa (G&M) and Dugesiella hentzi (Girard). M.S. Thesis, Oklahoma State University, 49 p.

Heitz, J. R. and B. R. Norment (1974). Characteristics of an alkaline phosphatase activity in brown recluse venom. Toxicon, 12, 181-187.

Jong, Y. S., B. R. Norment, and J. R. Heitz (1979a). Separation and characterization of venom components in Loxosceles reclusa. I. Preparative-disc electrophoresis. Toxicon, 17, 307-312.

Jong, Y. S., B. R. Norment, and J. R. Heitz (1979b). Separation and characterization of venom components in Loxosceles reclusa. II. Protease enzyme activity. Toxicon, In Press.

Madrigal, G. C., R. L. Ercolani, and J. E. Wenzl (1972). Toxicity from a bite of the brown spider (Loxosceles reclusa). Clin. Pediatr., 11, 641-644.

Micks, D. W. (1963). The current status of necrotic arachnidism in Texas. p. 153-157. In: Keegan, H. L. and W. V. Macfarlane, eds., Venomous and Poisonous Animals and Noxious Plants of the Pacific Region, Pergamon Press, Oxford.

Nazhat, N. (1968). Venom of Loxosceles reclusa Protein Components. M.S. Thesis, Oklahoma State University, 32 p.

Nance, W. E. (1961). Hemolytic anemia of necrotic arachnidism. Am. J. Med., 31, 801-807.

Norment, B. R., Y. S. Jong, and J. R. Heitz (1979). Separation and characterization of venom components in Loxosceles reclusa. III. Hydrolytic enzyme activity. Toxicon, 17, 539-548.

Norment, B. R. and O. E. Smith (1968). Effect of Loxosceles reclusa Gertsch and Mulaik venom against hemocytes of Acheta domesticus (Linnaeus). Toxicon, 6, 141-144.

Norment, B. R. and S. B. Vinson (1969). Effect of Loxosceles reclusa Gertsch and Mulaik venom on Heliothis virescens (F.) larvae. Toxicon, 7, 99-101.

Roeder, K. D. and S. Roeder (1939). Electrical activity in the isolated ventral nerve cord of the cockroach. J. Cell Comp. Physiol., 14, 1-9.

Rosenberg, P. and J. M. Coon (1958). Potentiation between cholinesterase inhibitors. Proc. Soc. Exp. Biol. Med., 97, 836-839.

Schmaus, L. F. (1929). Case of arachnidism (spider bite). J. Am. Med. Assoc., 92, 1265-1266.

Shankland, D. L., J. A. Rose, and C. Donninger (1969). The cholinergic nature of the cercal nerve-giant fiber synapse in the sixth abdominal ganglion of the American cockroach, Periplaneta americana (L.). J. Neurobiol., 2, 247-262.

Wright, R. P. (1973). Enzymic characterization of brown recluse spider venom. Bull. Mo. Acad. Sci., Suppl., 2, 94 p.

Wright, R. P., K. D. Elgert, B. J. Campbell, and J. T. Barrett (1973). Hyaluronidase and esterase activities of the venom of the poisonous brown recluse spider. Arch. Biochem. Biophys., 159, 415-426.

EPIDEMIC OF STINGS BY THE JELLYFISH *PELAGIA NOCTILUCA* IN THE ADRIATIC

Z. Maretić, F. E. Russell, and J. Ladavać

Medical Center, Pula, Yugoslavia and Lab. Neurol. Res., Univ. Southern California, Los Angeles, California, USA

ABSTRACT

During the summers of 1977, 1978 and 1979, large swarms of the coelenterate Pelagia noctiluca appeared in the northern Adriatic Sea. An estimated 250,000 persons were stung along northern Yugoslavian coasts during the summer months of 1978. These scyphomedusa also caused occupational difficulties by fouling the driving parts of boat motors and fishing gear.

KEYWORDS

Jellyfishes; Pelagia noctiluca; stings; nematocysts; lesions; treatment; etiology; Anemonia sulcata.

INTRODUCTION

Jellyfish stings in the waters of the northern Adriatic Sea appear to have been relatively uncommon and seldom reported to public health officials along the Istrian coast during the past 50 years. In the period 1947 - 1975, one of us (Z.M.) observed less than 10 cases of jellyfish stings on bathers in the Pula area of Yugoslavia (Maretić, 1975). However, during the summers of 1977 and 1978, swarms of the coelenterate Pelagia noctiluca appeared in such large numbers inshore that the sea around Pula sometimes appeared appeared yellowish-brown or violet from their presence.

During the three-month period of 1978, inquiries in the vicinity of Pula indicated that more than 50% of the bathers had been stung one or more times by this scyphomedusa. Although the total number of stingings cannot be known, since many of the bathers were not residents of the area, and in most cases the injuries were probably of such minor medical significance that they did not warrant medical care, a conservative estimate of 250,000 cases for the northern Adriatic coast of Yugoslavia seems reasonable.

CLINICAL FINDINGS

Most of the stings were inflicted on the extremities, particularly the forearms. The pattern of the lesions indicated that the majority of injuries were caused by the nematocysts of the oral arms or tentacles (Fig. 1A.), but in some cases the sting pattern showed that the umbrella nematocysts were involved (Fig. 1B.). The victims complained of immediate and sometimes sharp pain, followed by intense pruritis, which, in some cases, persisted for more than a week.

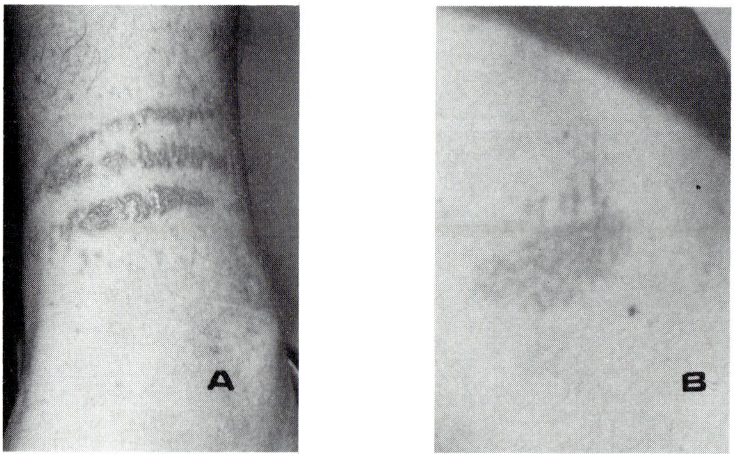

Fig. 1. Appearance of typical linear lesions on ankle at 36 hours following *Pelagia noctiluca* sting (A), and unusual sting pattern produced by animal's umbrella (B).

The injured sites appeared as blanched papules surrounded by erythema. The lesion sometimes appeared in discontinuous lines and in some cases proceeded to vesiculation and pustulation, with desquamation occurring in a few cases. The wounds tend to heal slowly; some secondary infections occurred. Hyperpigmentation of the healed lesions was observed in some patients. The clinical appearance of the wounds was similar to that described for other jellyfishes by Russell (1965), Halstead(1965), and Russell (1978). Systemic manifestations occurred in a few patients. These included syncopy, nausea, and vomiting. Primary shock was reported in some patients.

TREATMENT

Treatment by the victims was usually ineffective. In view of the fact that these stingings were not known to the people of the areas, nor was information on first aid available, a number of home remedies were tried. These seem to have been equally ineffective, although bathing of the injured areas with alcohol appeared to give some relief. Rubbing the area with sand or oil was tried but these procedures only worsen the injury (Russell, 1965). Fortunately, the lesions were of such minor significance, as compared with certain Cubomedusae and other Semaeostomae stings, as well as those by the Medusae, that the clinical course was unaltered by first aid.

Many years of experiences with thousands of jellyfish stings along the southern California coast (Russell, 1965), as well as off the northern coast of Australia (Barnes, personal communication, 1965) has provided a therapeutic protocol for both the first aid and medical treatment of coelenterate stings. When the offending animal is known to produce relatively minor lesions or, as in most cases, the injury is slight, washing the area with the cold salt water at hand and then applying alcohol, weak ammonia or meat tenderizer over the area offers some relief. Fresh water should be avoided. An analgesic-antihistamine cream can then be applied. In most cases, these simple measures will suffice, particularly in *Pelagia* stings.

In the more serious coelenterate stingings, ocean water should be poured over the injured parts to remove any tentacle pieces. Alcohol should then be applied to the area, care being taken not to rub or otherwise traumatize the injured part. Flour, baking powder or shaving soap should then be put over the lesions and the surrounding area. Use dry sand only if none of these are available. The powder or soap should then be scraped free, using a sharp knife or instrument. The area should then be washed with salt water and a corticosteroid-analgesic-antihistamine balm applied, preferably by aerosol. Systemic manifestations should be treated empirically, and should be directed at maintenance of ventilation, circulating blood volume, and cardiac performance. Ulcerating lesions should be cleansed three times a day and painted with an aqueous dye, consisting of brilliant green 1:400, gentian violet 1:400, and n-acriflavine 1:1000. Secondary infections are relatively rare; the use of antibiotics should be limited to those patients in whom a large cutaneous area is injured. A combination of aspirin and codeine is the drug of choice for more than trivial pain (Russell and Carlson, 1976).

DISCUSSION

Pelagia noctiluca is a Scyphomedusae with a somewhat saucer-shaped unbrella lacking coronal groove and pedalia, and having eight marginal tentacles and four simple oral arms with frilled lips (Fig.2) It was first described by Forskål as *Medusa noctiluca* in 1775. It ranges in diameter from several cm in the juvenile form, in which they are usually yellowish-brown, to 10 cm in the adult form, where they are rose to pink tinged, particularly on the tentacles, gonads and nematocyst warts (Russell, 1970).

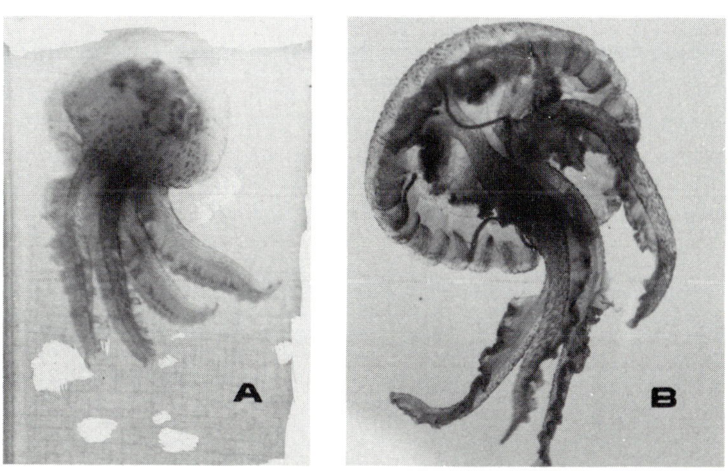

Fig. 2. Adult *Pelagia noctiluca* swimming in tank (A), and preserved specimen showing underside of umbrella with 4 oral arms and tentacles (B). Approximate diameter of umbrella, 6 cm.

The species is widely distributed in warm waters of the Atlantic, Pacific and Indian Oceans, and the Carribean and Mediterranean Seas. In some years it is found around the British Isles, in the Bay of Biscay, and the North Sea. This jellyfish breeds in summer and fall, and probably into the winter in some instances. Full development takes about one year. Swarms of *Pelagia* may be seen in the open sea and, in some cases, appear to occur at boundaries between oceanic currents, where they can be seen in long rows. Swarms may also occur in shoals and estuaries. Although the factors which may influence their appearance are not well defined, changes in weather conditions that bring about upwellings or other disturbances in water masses, changes in nutrient salt concentrations, water temperature or sunlight, and those factors which affect water turbulence and illumination probably play some role in reproduction and swarming. The importance of water pollution as a factor in their reproduction and swarming is not known but in some instances it would seem to play a role.

As previously noted, these jellyfish appear to have been relatively uncommon along the northern Adriatic coast of Yugoslavia prior to 1977, and stings by them were rarely reported. In the spring and summer of that year, however, they appeared in great numbers along the Istrian coast, and they continued through the winter months. In the spring of 1978, swarms of juvenile forms were observed, and by summer the number of adults exceeded that seen in 1977. Their ability to fluoresce made it possible to see 4 or 5 specimens per square meter of water on most nights during the summer months. Their appearance was not limited to Istria. According to Piccinetti (personal communication, 1979) they were also found in increased numbers at all Italian marine stations from Gargano in the south to the northern Adriatic seaboard. They were also seen off the coast of Sicily. Reports for 1979 indicate their continued presence in large numbers. Riedl (1963) notes that swarms of these scyphaozoa are sometimes seen during some years in the southern Adriatic Sea.

Histological examination of the oral arms and tentacles showed the typical cnidoblasts of cnidarians, containing the capsuled nematocyst with a long coiled hollow thread. The nematocysts measured approximately 5 microns and appeared more numerous in the oral arms than in the tentacles (Fig. 3.) They were also found in the umbrella.

As repeated stingings in a single individual by *Pelagia* were common (one of us, Z.M., was stung on seven different occasions), the question of developing a sensitivity or an immunity to the venom may thus arise. In southern California, with the advent of board surfing and increased body surfing during the past decade and a half, an increasing number of persons have become sensitive to the stings of jellyfishes. Repeated stingings have precipitated increasing reactions to the point of anaphylactic shock. Surfers so sensitized have been advised to avoid swimming when the jellyfishes are prevalent, or to wear wet suits while in the ocean. Lifeguards who have been exposed to jellyfishes over many years do not seem to have become sensitive to the animal's venom, although they are occasionally stung in the course of their duties. Some lifeguards report they have little or no reaction to such stings. However, they avoid excessive swimming or exposure, when swarms of jellyfish are close inshore. The exposure in the series reported herein has been too short to evaluate the possibility of sensitivity or immune reactions. One fisherman, who had been stung many times by the anemone Anemonia sulcata, and was not affected by their stings, had a severe reaction when stung by P. noctiluca. There is also the danger of stings to the eyes or mouth, which can be more serious, and have been reported in Pula during the past two years.

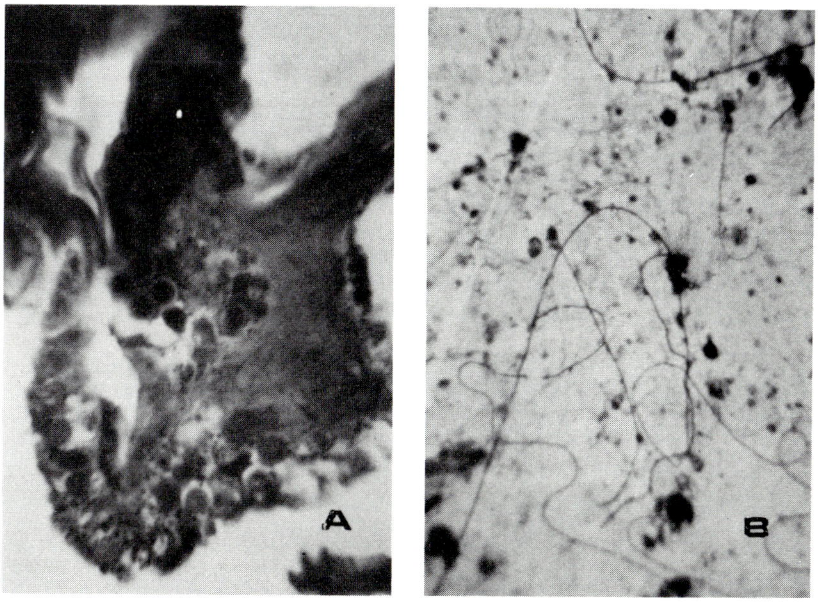

Fig. 3. Section through oral arm of Pelagia noctiluca (400x), showing cnidoblasts with encapsulated nematocysts, some of which have already discharged (A). Discharged and undischarged nematocysts (800x); note long hollow threads (B).

In addition to injuries by the scyphozoa Pelagia, stings by anthozoa, particularly the anemone Anemonia sulcata, are sometimes reported(Fig. 4.). Other coelenterates, such as Cotylorhiza tuberculata may produce minor reactions and although Aurelia aurita has been observed, particularly around Kotor and Vis during some years, few stings have been reported by this Palagiidae (Maretić, 1975). Rhizostoma pulmo, Chrysaora hysoscella, and Nausithoe punctata are also seen in the Adriatic Sea (Riedl, 1963) but apparently they are of little medical importance. The Portuguese man-o-war is rarely seen in northern Adriatic waters. Its sting can be unusually severe (Russell, 1966).

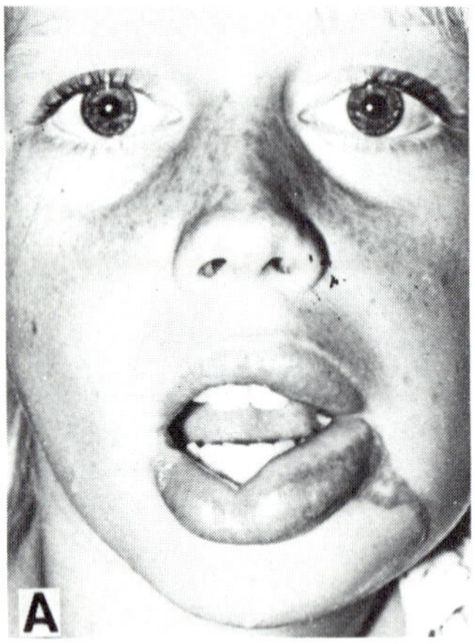

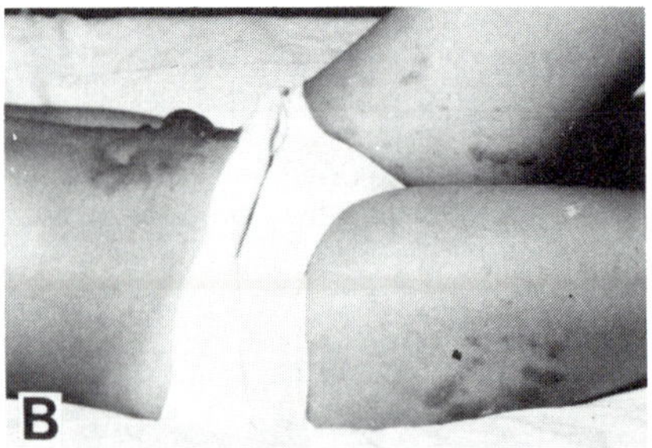

Fig. 4 Stings by Anemonia sulcata on lips and face(A), over body and legs 24 hours after sting (B), and on hip at 48 hours (C).

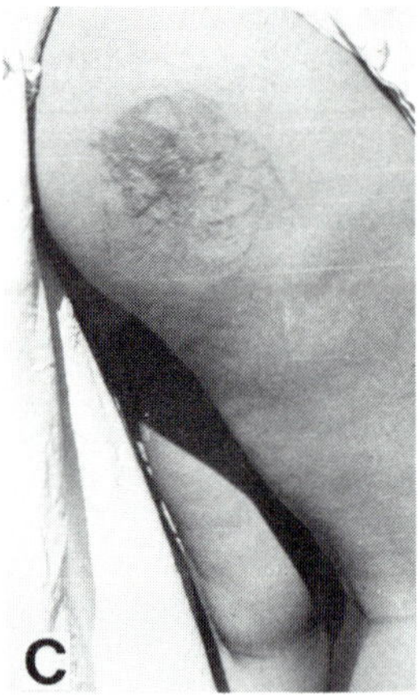

Aside from their medical importance, the over abundance of *P. noctiluca* off Pula caused economic and occupational difficulties. Small trawlers and fishing boats had to frequently disengage masses of jellyfish from the screws or submerged driving parts of their engines. Trawlers also found their nets full of these animals, not only causing damage to their gear, and a decrease in number of hauls, but a marked increase in the number of stingings among fishermen. In some instances, more than 1000 kilograms of the jellyfish, mostly juveniles, would be taken in a single haul.

ACKNOWLEDGEMENT

Supported by GM24141-01 TOX, USPHS, and a contract from the Office of Naval Research. The authors appreciate the advice of Sir F.S. Russell, and the technical assistance of S. Premate.

REFERENCES

Halstead, B. W. (1965). Poisonous and Venomous Marine Animals of the World, Vol. 1, U. S. Government Printing Office, Washington, D.C.

Maretić, Z. (1975). Živitinje otrovnice i otrovne živitinje Jadranskog mora. J. A. Z. U., Zagreb, pp. 11-22.

Riedl, R. (1963). Fauna und Flora der Adria., P. Pareu. Hamburg.

Russell, F. E. (1965). Marine toxins and venomous and poisonous marine animals. In: F. S. Russell (Ed.), Advances In Marine Biology, Vol. 3, Academic Press, London, pp. 256-284

Russell, F. E. (1966). Physalia stings: a report of two cases. Toxicon, 4, 65-67.

Russell, F. E. (1978). Hazardous marine life. Part 1; Venomous marine animals. Hyperbaric and Undersea Medicine, 1, 1-18.

Russell, F. E., and R. W. Carlsson (1976). Jellyfish stings. In: W. Conn (Ed.), Current Therapy, W. B. Saunders, Philadepphia, pp.835-836.

Russell, F. S. (1970). The Medusae of the British Isles. University Press. Cambridge.

Venom Toxins and the Immune System

STUDY ON IMMUNOLOGICAL RELATIONSHIPS AMONG VENOMS OF THE ASIATIC AGKISTRODON

Y. Sawai and Y. Kawamura

The Japan Snake Institute, Gunma, Japan

ABSTRACT

This report concerns toxicity and immunological relationships among venoms of the following Agkistrodon species: A blomhoffi from Japan, A caliginosus, A b brevicaudus and A saxatilis from Korea and A Halys caucasicus from Iran. As controls, the venoms of A rhodostoma from Malaysia and A acutus from Taiwan were also investigated.

KEYWORDS

Immunological relationships, Agkistrodon venoms, A blomhoffi, A caliginosus, A b brevicaudus, A saxatilis, neutralization, immunodiffusion test, fatal toxicity, hemorrhagic toxicity.

MATERIALS AND METHODS

Venoms and Antivenins

Venoms of A blomhoffi, A caliginosus, A b brevicaudus and A saxatilis were supplied by the Japan Snake Institute. Venom of A caucasicus was supplied by the Razi Institute, Iran, and A acutus venom was obtained from NAMRU No 2, Taipei, Taiwan and the Snake and Venom Institute, Penang, Malaysia. As shown in Table 1, the antivenins used were prepared at the Institute of Medical Science, University of Tokyo (A blomhoffi, horse origin); Japan Snake Institute (A caliginosus, A b brevicaudus and A saxatilis, rabbit origin); Razi Institute (A h caucasicus, horse origin); Taiwan Serum and Vaccine Laboratory (A acutus, horse origin); and the Queen Saovabha Memorial Institute, Bangkok (A rhodostoma, horse origin).

Measurement of Venom Toxicity

LD_{50}-values were calculated according to Litchfield and Wilcoxon (1949) after intravenous injection into mice of 0.1 ml of venom diluted in M/60 phosphate buffered saline. Minimum lethal dose (mld)was calculated by intramuscular injection of 0.1 ml of venom solution into mice. Minimum hemorrhagic dose (mhd) was determined by intramuscular injection into mice (Sawai and others, 1967, 1972) or by intradermal injection with rabbits (Kondo and others, 1960).

Table 1. List of Antivenins Used

Producers	Name of Product	Name of Venom
Razi State Serum and Vaccine Inst., Iran	Monovalent Antivenin A halys	A h caucasicus
Queen Saovabha Memorial Inst., Bangkok, Thailand	Antivenin Serum Pit viper	A rhodostoma (Malayan pit viper)
Taiwan Serum & Vaccine Laboratory, Taipei, Taiwan, ROC	Agkistrodon Monovalent	A acutus (100-pacer)
Institute of Medical Science, Univ of Tokyo, Tokyo, Japan	Mamushi Antivenin	A blomhoffi
Japan Snake Institute, Gunma, Japan	Monovalent* Agkistrodon ssp	A caliginosus A b brevicaudus A saxatilis

*rabbit origin

Neutralization Test of Antivenins and Immunodiffusion Test

Undiluted antivenin (0.1 ml) was mixed with an equal volume of venom dilution, and after incubation for one hour at 37° C the mixture was injected intramuscularly into the legs of 4 mice. Twenty-four hours after the injection, the amount of venom neutralized was calculated on the basis of survival or death of the mice injected. The degree of local hemorrhage was examined in surviving mice and the amount of venom neutralized with respect to hemorrhagic activity was calculated. Ouchterlony's double diffusion method was used for immunodiffusion tests (Ouchterlony, 1948).

RESULTS

Fatal and Hemorrhagic Toxicity of the Venoms

The $LD_{50}s$ of the venoms used are shown in Table 2. The most lethal venom was that of A h caucasicus, and the venom of A rhodostoma was the least toxic. The minimum hemorrhagic doses of the venoms in mice and rabbits are shown in Table 3. The hemorrhagic toxicities of the venoms of blomhoffi, caliginosus, brevicaudus and saxatilis were higher than those of caucasicus, rhodostoma and acutus.

Neutralizing effect of anti-Agkistrodon antivenins against homologous and heterologous venoms

Anti-blomhoffi antivenin: As shown in Table 4, 0.1 ml of the antivenin neutralized the lethal effect of 600 µg (2 mlds) and the hemorrhagic effect of 300 µg (512 mhds) of the homologous venom. The same amount of the antivenin also neutralized the lethal activity of all heterologous venoms excepts caucasicus and rather effectively neutralized the hemorrhagic effects of all except acutus and rhodostoma.

Table 2. Lethal Toxicity of Venom on Mice

Venoms	LD_{50} (μg/mouse)
Agkistrodon h. caucasicus	15.2 (14.3-16.2)
A. caliginosus	20.5 (21.6-30.1)
A. saxatilis	30.2 (26.8-34.2)
A. blomhoffi	30.6 (25.9-36.2)
A. b. brevicaudus	36.8 (34.6-38.9)
A. acutus	71.7 (62.5-82.2)
A. rhodostoma	91.2 (78.2-105.5)

Mice: dd-strain, 18 g. LD_{50}: Litchfield-Wilcoxon method. Number in parenthesis denote confidence limits. Route of injection: iv.

Table 3. Minimum Hemorrhagic Dose of Venoms on Mice and Rabbits

Venoms	Mice (im)	Rabbits (ic)
A. blomhoffi	0.5	0.5
A. b. brevicaudus	0.5	0.5
A. caliginosus	0.5	0.5
A. saxatilis	1.0	0.5
A. h. caucasicus	2.0	1.0
A. acutus	2.0	4.0
A. rhodostoma	2.0	2.0

im: intramuscular injection. ic: intracutaneous injection. Doses in μg.

Anti-brevicaudus, caliginosus and saxatilis antivenin: The same amount of each of these antivenins neutralized 300 μg (1 mld) of all three venoms plus that of blomhoffi with regard to lethality and 18.7-75 μg (32-128 mhds) of the same four venoms with regard to hemorrhagic activity. On the other hand, none of these antivenins neutralized the lethal effects of caucasicus, acutus and rhodostoma, although some degree of antihemorrhagic activity against these latter three venoms was observed.

Anti-caucasicus antivenin: The antivenin (0.1 ml) neutralized the lethal effects corresponding to 600 μg (1-2 mlds) of the homologous and all heterologous venoms and neutralized the hemorrhagic effects of 37.5-300 μg (16-128 mhds) of all venoms except acutus.

Anti-acutus antivenin: The same dose of antivenin neutralized the lethal effects corresponding to 300-600 μg (1 mld) of the homologous and all heterologous venoms except caucasicus. However, the anti-hemorrhagic activity of the antivenin against heterologous venoms was poor.

Anti-rhodostoma antivenin: The antivenin (0.1 ml) neutralized 600 μg (2 mlds) and 75 μg (16 mhds) of the homologous venom with regard to lethal and hemorrhagic effects, respectively. On the other hand, the same dose of the antivenin did not neutralize the lethal toxicity of any heterologous venom except blomhoffi, and its neutralizing effect against the hemorrhagic activity of heterologous venoms was

Table 4. Neutralizing Ability of Antivenins against Venom of Agkistrodon

Venoms	Antivenins:	blomhoffi	brevicaudus	caliginosus	saxatilis	caucasicus	acutus	rhodostoma
A.blomhoffi	MLD	2 (600)	1 (300)	1 (300)	1 (300)	2 (600)	1 (300)	1 (300)
	MHD	512 (300)	64 (37.5)	64 (37.5)	32 (18.7)	128 (75)	32 (18.7)	4 (2.3)
A.b.brevicaudus	MLD	2 (600)	1 (300)	1 (300)	1 (300)	2 (600)	1 (300)	0
	MHD	156 (150)	128 (75)	64 (37.5)	32 (18.7)	64 (37.5)	64 (18.7)	2 (1.1)
A.caliginosus	MLD	1 (300)	1 (300)	1 (300)	1 (300)	2 (600)	1 (300)	0
	MHD	128 (75)	64 (37.5)	128 (75)	32 (18.7)	64 (37.5)	32 (18.7)	2 (1.1)
A.saxatilis	MLD	1 (300)	1 (300)	1 (300)	1 (300)	1 (300)	1 (300)	0
	MHD	16 (18.7)	16 (18.7)	16 (18.7)	32 (37.5)	32 (37.5)	16 (18.7)	4 (4.6)
A.h.caucasicus	MLD	0	0	0	0	1 (300)	0	0
	MHD	128 (300)	16 (37.5)	16 (37.5)	8 (18.7)	128 (300)	16 (37.5)	0
A.acutus	MLD	1 (300)	0	0	0	1 (300)	1 (300)	0
	MHD	8 (18.7)	16 (37.5)	8 (18.7)	16 (37.5)	1 (2.3)	64 (150)	8 (18.7)
A.rhodostoma	MLD	1 (600)	0	0	0	1 (600)	1 (600)	1 (600)
	MHD	4 (18.7)	16 (75)	16 (75)	16 (18.7)	16 (75)	1 (4.6)	16 (75)

MLD, MHD: The first figure in each column is the number of minimum lethal doses (MLD) or minimum hemorrhagic doses (MHD) neutralized by 0.1 ml of the antivenin. The second figure in parentheses is the quantity of venoms neutralized in μg.

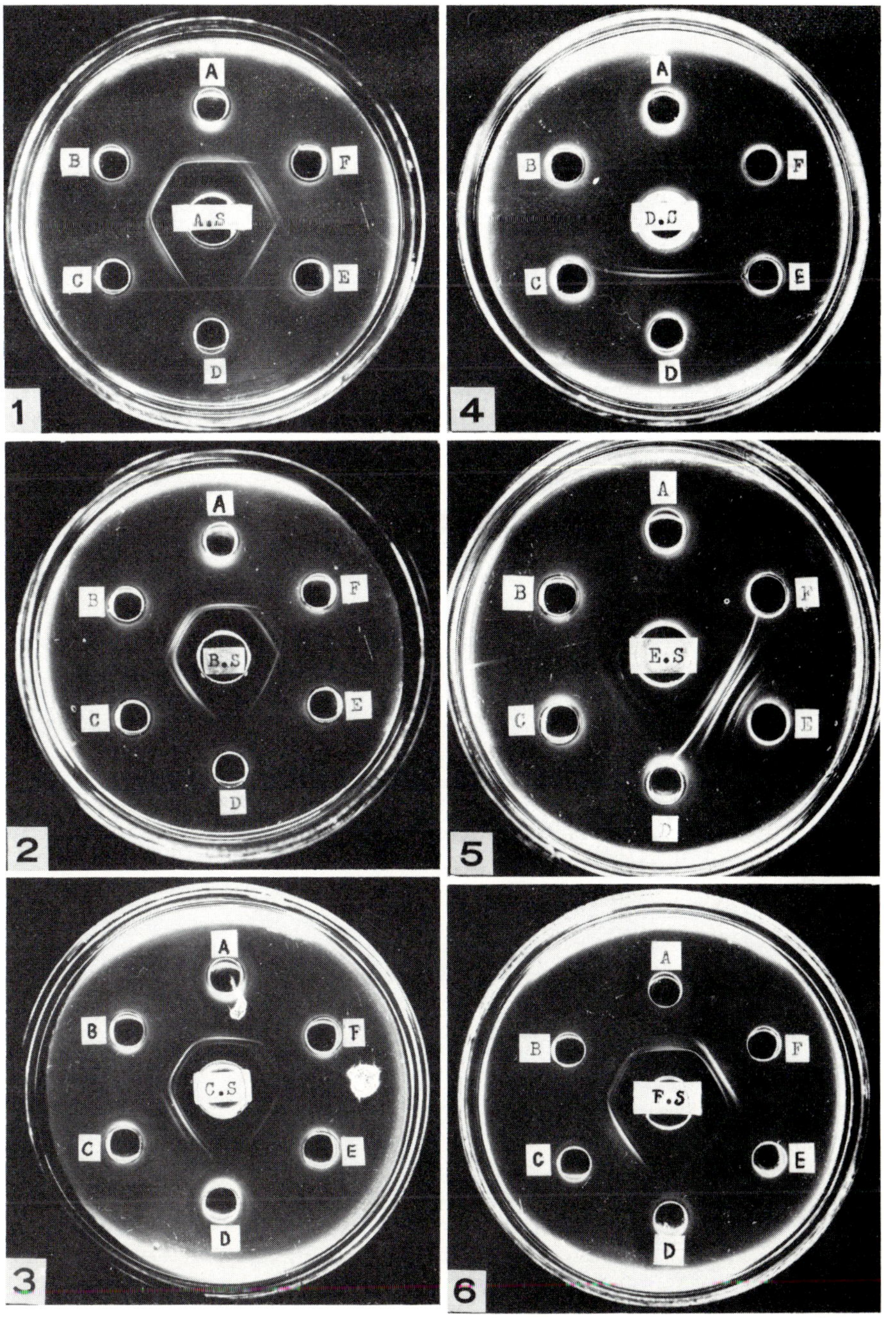

Fig. 1. Ouchterlony Reaction. Venom in peripheral wells are (A) blomhoffi, (B) caliginosus, (C) brevicaudus, (D) rhodostoma, (E) acutus, (F) caucasicus. Antivenin in center wells are (1) blomhoffi, (2) caliginosus, (3) brevicaudus, (4) rhodostoma, (5) acutus, (6) caucasicus.

poor.

Immunological Relationships Among the Venoms by Ouchterlony Reaction

As shown in Fig. 1, the precipitin lines between the antivenins of blomhoffi (A), caliginosus (B), brevicaudus (C), caucasicus (F) and all four venoms fused together. The same results were obtained with saxatilis. On the other hand, the antivenins of rhodostoma (D) and acutus (E) gave precipitin lines only against their homologous venom. The results suggest that all of these venoms except rhodostoma and acutus are antigenically similar.

DISCUSSION

These results demonstrate the presence of certain common antigens in the venoms of five of the seven Asiatic Agkistrodon species studied, and should thus contribute both to the taxonomy of snakes and to medical treatment of the bites by antivenins. Anti-mamushi (blomhoffi) antivenin produced in Japan is thus effective for the medical treatment of snakebites in Korea, where no effective antivenin has been used until now. It is interesting that the Iranian Agkistrodon proved to have the highest paraspecific activity of the seven Agkistrodon antivenins tested.

SUMMARY

Studies of the immunological relationships among the venoms of A blomhoffi, A caliginosus, A b brevicaudus, A saxatilis, A caucasicus, A acutus and A rhodostoma indicated that the venoms of A blomhoffi from Japan and caliginosus, brevicaudus and saxatilis from Korea were closely related immunologically with regard to the cross-neutralizing activities of the four antivenins against the lethal and hemorrhagic effects of all four venoms. Common antigens were also detected in venoms of the Asiatic Agkistrodon blomhoffi, caliginosus, brevicaudus, saxatilis and caucasicus by the Ouchterlony technique.

REFERENCES

Kondo, H., A. Kondo, H. Ikezawa, R. Murata, and A. Ohsaka (1960). Studies on the quantitative method for determination of hemorrhagic activity of habu snake venom. Japan J. Med Sci. Biol., 13, 43-51.

Litchfield, J. T., Jr., and F. Wilcoxon (1949). Simplified method of evaluating dose effect experiments. J. Pharmacol., 96, 99-113.

Ouchterlony, O. (1948). In vitro method for testing the toxin-producing capacity of diphtheria bacteria. Acuta Path. Microbiol. Scand., 25, 186-191.

Sawai, Y., H Chinzei, Y. Kawamura, T. Fukuyama, and T Okonogi (1972). Studies on the improvement of habu (Trimeresurus flavoviridis) bites. 9. Studies on the immunogenicity of the purified habu venom toxoid by alcohol precipitation. Japan J. Exp. Med., 42, 155-164.

Sawai, Y., Y. Kawamura, T. Fukuyama, and H. L. Keegan (1967). Studies on the inactivation of snake venoms by dihydrothiotic acid. Japan J. Exp. Med., 37, 121-128.

ANTIGENICITY-DETERMINING AMINO ACID RESIDUES OF ERABUTOXIN b

N. Tamiya and T. Abe

Department of Chemistry, Tohoku University, Aobayama, Sendai, Japan

ABSTRACT

Anti-erabutoxin b sera were prepared by injecting native erabutoxin b into rabbits. The antibodies were fractionated into 'specific antibody' and 'common antibody' by use of erabutoxin b-Sepharose and toxin astrotia stokesii a-Sepharose columns. Inhibitory activities of erabutoxin b derivatives and of other snake neurotoxins on the binding of erabutoxin b, [^{3}H]-acetylated at the N-terminal, were measured by radioimmunoassay. The acetylation of the amino groups at N-terminal, 15-Lys, 27-Lys and 47-Lys did not affect the binding. [26-Asn]-erabutoxin b (erabutoxin a) also showed the same binding activity. The acetylation of 51-Lys or its replacement with Asn (erabutoxin c), however, resulted in decreased binding activity. An erabutoxin b derivative without a hexapeptide portion (33-Arg - 38-Glu) and seven toxins from other snakes, except cobrotoxin, cross-reacted with the antibodies to varying extents, but reduced and S-carboxymethylated erabutoxin b and the hexapeptide (33-Arg - 38-Glu) gave no cross-reactions. From a comparison of the amino acid sequences of the toxins and the toxin derivatives, 9 residues out of 62 residues of erabutoxin b were pointed out as candidate residues to be involved in the specificity determination. Residues 1-Arg, 12-Gln, 28-Gln, 57-Ser and 58-Glu may participate in the binding with 'specific antibody', whereas residues 11-Pro, 23-Ser, 51-Lys and 52-Leu may participate in the binding with 'common antibody'. It is of interest that none of these residues are located on the receptor binding side of the small flat erabutoxin molecule and six of them (1-Arg, 12-Gln, 28-Gln, 51-Lys, 57-Ser and 58-Glu) are found on the surface of the other side of the molecule.

KEYWORDS

Erabutoxin b; neurotoxin; antigenicity of erabutoxin b; immunology of neurotoxins

INTRODUCTION

Sea snake and cobra venom neurotoxins are low molecular weight proteins (60-74 amino acid residues) with immunogenicity. As there are more than 60 examples of established amino acid sequences, the neurotoxins are good sample proteins for the study of immunological specificity. The present paper describes an attempt to locate the specificity determining amino acid residues of erabutoxin b, a sea snake neurotoxin. The results are discussed in relation to the stereo structure of the molecule.

MATERIALS AND METHODS

Sea snake neurotoxins, namely, erabutoxins a, b (Tamiya and Arai, 1966; Sato and Tamiya, 1971) and c (Tamiya and Abe, 1972), laticotoxin a (Sato et al, 1969, further separated into components a and a', A. Sato and N. Tamiya, unpublished), aipysurus laevis a (Maeda and Tamiya, 1976) and astrotia stokesii a (Maeda and Tamiya, 1978) were prepared as described previously. Toxin hydrophis ornatus '75 a was prepared from the venom of sea snake *Hydrophis ornatus* captured in Philippines in the year 1975 and sequenced (N. Maeda and N. Tamiya, unpublished). Toxin B from *Naja naja naja* and cobrotoxin from *Naja naja atra*, and toxin α from *Naja nigricollis* were kind gifts from Dr. K. Hayashi and Dr. P. Boquet, respectively.

Anti-erabutoxin b antisera were prepared by injecting subcutaneously into male rabbits an equivolume mixture of erabutoxin b solution (1 mg/ml) in saline and Freund's complete adjuvant. The first dose was 0.05-0.06 mg/kg and the successive increasing doses were given at intervals of 1-3 weeks for 10-11 times during 3-4 months. One week after the final dose (0.5 mg/kg), the sera were collected. The antisera (No. 701, CT-2 and TA-1) were added with sodium azide (0.02%, w/v) and kept at 4°C. Antisera NO. 701, CT-2 and TA-1 neutralized about 190, 160 and 130 μg erabutoxin b/ml, respectively, when tested on mice.

Immunoadsorbent was prepared by coupling erabutoxin b or astrotia stokesii a to cyanogen bromide-treated Sepharose 4B (Cuatrecasas and Anfinsen, 1971). Erabutoxin b-Sepharose and astrotia stokesii a-Sepharose contained 2.4 mg/ml and 2.3 mg/ml gel, respectively.

Monoacetyl erabutoxin b derivatives, acetylated at one of the five amino groups of the toxin molecule, were prepared and separated from one another as described by Hori and Tamiya, 1976. Mono-[^{3}H]-acetyl erabutoxin b ([1-*N*$^\alpha$-acetylarginine]-erabutoxin b), used for the radioimmunoassay, was prepared with radioactive acetic anhydride. The specific radioactivity of the preparation was 2 Ci/mmole.

Partial peptic digestion products of erabutoxin b were prepared and isolated as described elsewhere (Abe and Tamiya, 1979).

Radioimmunoassay was carried out essentially according to the method of Herbert et al (1965). Antiserum or purified antibody (see RESULTS) was dissolved in 0.05M phosphate buffer, pH 7.4, containing 1%(w/v) bovine serum albumin and 0.02%(w/v) sodium azide. The solution (0.1 ml) was mixed with a sample solution (0.1 ml) in the same buffer and the mixture incubated at 37°C for 1 hr. *N*-Terminal mono-[^{3}H]-acetyl erabutoxin b solution (20 μl, 5 pmole, 20000 dpm) in the same buffer was added to the mixture. After standing at 4°C for 15-20 hr, a bovine immunoglobulin G solution (2.5%, w/v, 0.5 ml) in the same buffer and 'charcoal solution' (see below, 0.2 ml) were further added successively to the mixture. The final mixture was kept at room temperature for 40 min and centrifuged (3000 rev/min for 10 min) at 4°C. The supernatant was mixed with Bray's scintillator solution (13 ml, Bray, 1960) and counted for the radioactivity with a scintillation counter (Unilux II-A, Nuclear Chicago, Des Plains, Ill.). 'Charcoal solution' was prepared as follows: Dextran T-70 (0.1 g) solution in 0.05M phosphate buffer, pH 7.4 (20 ml) was mixed with an activated charcoal (1.0 g) suspension in the same buffer (20 ml) and stirred for 30 min at room temperature. 'Charcoal solution' was prepared daily and used while stirring.

RESULTS

Fractionation of Anti-Erabutoxin b Antibody

Anti-erabutoxin b serum (No.701, 18.5 ml) was fractionated into its components by ammonium sulfate precipitation (Heide and Schwick, 1973) and the immunoglobulin G precipitate was dissolved in 0.02M borate buffer, pH 8.0 (4 ml), containing 0.15M sodium chloride and 0.02%(w/v) sodium azide. The solution was dialyzed against the buffer (3x3 l) for 3 days. The solution thus obtained (8.5 ml) contained 36.5 mg immunoglobulin G/ml and gave a single precipitin line with erabutoxin b on double diffusion test (Ouchterlony and Nilsson, 1973). The immunoglobulin G solution was diluted with 0.02M borate buffer, pH 8.0, containing 0.15M sodium chloride to give a concentration of 7 mg protein/ml, and the diluted solution (10 ml) applied on an erabutoxin b-Sepharose column (1.5 x 5 cm) in the borate buffer. The column was washed with the borate buffer (43 ml) and with 0.02M borate buffer, pH 8.0, containing 1M sodium chloride (50 ml), which eluted 60% and 1% of the charged protein, respectively. The column was then treated with 5.3M formic acid, pH 1.3, containing 1M sodium chloride. The eluate (40 ml) was collected in an ice-chilled flask, neutralized immediately to pH 4 with 25% (w/w) ammonia and placed in a Diaflo apparatus with UM-10 filter (Amicon Corp., Lexington, Mass.). The eluate was concentrated and the solvent medium was converted into 0.02M borate buffer, pH 8.0, containing 0.15M sodium chloride (7 ml) in the apparatus. The anti-erabutoxin b immunoglobulin solution thus obtained contained 0.87 mg protein/ml, which bound 1.9 nmole erabutoxin b/mg as measured by radioimmunoassay.

TABLE 1 Inhibitory Activities of Erabutoxin b Derivatives on the Binding of N-Terminal Acetylated Erabutoxin b

Erabutoxin b Derivative	Serum No. 701 I_{max} (%)	Serum No. 701 Relative Conc. at 50% Inhibition	Serum CT-2 I_{max} (%)	Serum CT-2 Relative Conc. at 50% Inhibition
Erabutoxin b	100	1.0	100	1.0
α-Ac-Eb	100	1.1	90	1.2
15-Ac-Eb	100	1.0	102	1.0
27-Ac-Eb	99	1.0	101	1.0
47-Ac-Eb	97	1.0	91	1.0
51-Ac-Eb	98	1.5	101	1.4
[26-Asn]-Eb	96	1.0	N.D.	
[51-Asn]-Eb	98	1.4	N.D.	
Component C-2	95	1.0	N.D.	
Hexapeptide	0	-	N.D.	
RCM-Eb	0	-	N.D.	
Lysozyme	0	-	N.D.	

Abbreviations: I_{max}, maximum inhibition (see text); α-Ac-Eb, [1-N^{α}-acetylarginine]-erabutoxin b; 15-Ac-Eb, [15-N^{6}-acetyllysine]-erabutoxin b and so on; [26-Asn]-Eb, erabutoxin a; [51-Asn]-Eb, erabutoxin c; Component C-2, erabutoxin b whose peptide bond between 32-Phe and 33-Arg is cleaved; Hexapeptide, hexapeptide which corresponds to 33rd to 38th residues of erabutoxin b (Arg-Gly-Thr-Ile-Ile-Glu); RCM-Eb, reduced and S-carboxymethylated erabutoxin b; N.D. not determined.

The solution (7 ml, 6 mg protein) was then passed through an astrotia stokesii a-Sepharose column (1.3 x 4 cm) in 0.02M borate buffer, pH 8.0, containing 0.15M sodium chloride, and the column was eluted with the same buffer (22 ml). The eluate, which contained 60% of the charged protein, was concentrated to 6 ml in a

Diaflo apparatus. A solution of anti-erabutoxin b immunoglobulin G, without common antibody toward astrotia stokesii ('specific antibody') was thus obtained. The 'specific antibody' solution contained 0.18 mg protein/ml, which bound 1 nmole erabutoxin b/mg.

Another portion of the immunoglobulin G solution (36.5 mg/ml) was diluted with 0.02 M borate buffer, pH 8.0 containing 0.15M sodium chloride to give a 10 mg protein/ml solution and the diluted solution (10 ml) was applied to an astrotia stokesii a-Sepharose column (1.3 x 4 cm) in the same buffer. The column was washed with the buffer (126 ml) and then eluted with 5.3M formic acid, pH 1.3, containing 1M sodium chloride (30 ml). The eluate was treated similarly to the above described erabutoxin b-Sepharose column eluate. The fraction of anti-erabutoxin b immunoglobulin G, that can also bind astrotia stokesii a ('common antibody') was thus obtained in solution. The solution (8 ml) contained 0.26 mg protein/ml, which bound 1.5 nmole erabutoxin b/mg.

Antibody Binding Activities of Erabutoxin b Derivatives

The results of radioimmunoassay of the inhibitory effect of erabutoxin b derivatives on the binding of N-terminal mono-[^{3}H]-acetyl erabutoxin b to the antibodies are shown in Fig. 1. Duplicate control experiments without the addition of erabutoxin

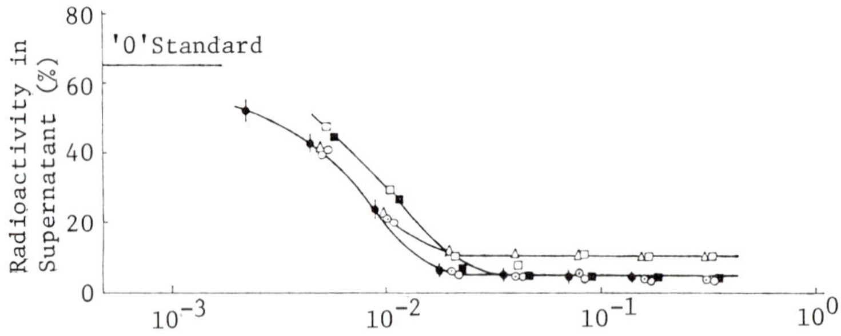

Fig. 1. Radioimmunoassay of antibody binding activities of monoacetylated erabutoxin b derivatives.

Serum CT-2 was used at the final dilution of 660 times. Radioimmunoassay was carried out as described in MATERIALS AND METHODS. Each point gives the average of five assays with erabutoxin b (●) and the average of two assays with α-Ac-Eb (□), 15-Ac-Eb (o), 27-Ac-Eb (⊙), 47-Ac-Eb (△) and 51-Ac-Eb (■). ' 'Standard value is an average of eight assays.

b derivatives were also performed. Relative maximal inhibition (I_{max}) values were calculated for each derivative as follows (Hunter, 1973) with erabutoxin b as a standard,

$$I_{max} = 100 \times ('0'St - S_{min})/('0'St - E_{min})$$

where '0'St stands for the % radioactivity remaining in the supernatant in control experiments, and S_{min} or E_{min} stand for the % radioactivity in the supernatant when it reached its minimal value by the addition of a sample protein or nonlabeled erabutoxin b, respectively. When it was difficult to obtain S_{min} value for a derivative or a toxin, the % radioactivity value in the supernatant in the presence of 2.3 nmole sample/ml was used and I' value calculated in the same way. The results are summarized in TABLE 1. Concentration of an erabutoxin b derivative at its 1/2 I_{max} value relative to that of erabutoxin b was also calculated (TABLE 1).

The erabutoxin b derivatives, except reduced and S-carboxymethylated erabutoxin b and fragment hexapeptide, reacted with anti-erabutoxin b sera, giving I_{max} values higher than 90%. 51-Substituted derivatives required, however, a higher concentration to give the same extent of immunological reaction as native erabutoxin b.

Antibody Binding Activities of Toxins from Other Snakes

The results of radioimmunoassay experiments are summarized in TABLE 2.

TABLE 2 Inhibitory Activities of Toxins on the Binding of N-Terminal Acetylated Erabutoxin b to Antibodies

Toxin	Whole serum I'(%)	'Common antibody' I'(%)	'Specific antibody I'(%)	Double diffusion ppt.
Erabutoxin b	100	100	100	+*
Erabutoxin c	98¶	90†	N.D.	+*
Laticotoxin a	43	65	12	+*
Toxin α	41	60	4	±*
H. ornatus '75 a	37	42	0	-
A. stokesii a	38	35	0	-*
A. laevis a	22	18	0	-*
Cobrotoxin	1	2	1	-*
Toxin B	14	8	0	-*
A. stokesii b	9	8	0	N.D.
Component E	46	31	99	-

Abbreviations: I', inhibition at the final concentration of 2.3 nmole toxin/ml; Component E, erabutoxin b from which a hexapeptide fragment (33-Arg - 38-Glu) is removed; N.D., not determined.
*Results with TA-1 serum.
¶Maximum inhibition (I_{max}).
†Inhibition at the final concentration of 0.46 nmole toxin/ml.

Cobrotoxin did not cross-react with erabutoxin b antibody, whereas other toxins tested, including two long-chain neurotoxins (Toxin B and A. stokesii b), cross-reacted to varying extents. The cross-reactivities of toxins with whole serum and with 'common antibody' are very similar. 'Specific antibody' reacted only with component E and to smaller extents with laticotoxin a and toxin α. The circular dichroism spectrum of component E was very different from that of erabutoxin b, although the component reacted well with antibodies, especially with 'specific antibody'.

DISCUSSION

Sea snake and cobra neurotoxins are basic proteins consisting of 60-74 amino acid residues. There are two main groups of them, namely short-chain neurotoxins (60-62 amino acid residues with four disulfide bridges) and long-chain neurotoxins (70-74 residues with five disulfide bridges). The only exception so far known is toxin laticauda semifasciata III (Maeda and Tamiya, 1974), which consists of 66 amino acid residues with five disulfide bridges and is one tenth as active as most of the other toxins. The three dimensional structures of erabutoxins a and b, short-chain neurotoxins, have been elucidated (Low et al, 1976; Tsernoglou and Petsko, 1976, 1977) The sequence similarity and structure prediction by Chou and Fasman (1974) method suggest similar stereo structures for all the neurotoxins (Dufton and Hider, 1977; Menez et al, 1978).

Although all the neurotoxins have essentially the same physiological activity and similar structure sharing 12 so-far invariant residues, they do not always cross-react immunologically (Boquet, 1973, 1977). The present paper describes an attemt to locate amino acid residues, which are involved in the immunological specificity determination.

The results on single amino acid replacement derivatives of erabutoxin b (TABLE 1) suggest that residue 51-Lys is involved in the binding to the antibody, because its modification or replacement reduced the affinity to the antibody.

The amino acid sequences of the toxins used in the present experiments are given in TABLE 3. 'Common antibody' reacted more or less with all the short-chain neurotoxins, except cobrotoxin. 'Common antibody' is a fraction of anti-erabutoxin b antibodies, that can also react with toxin astrotia stokesii a. There are eight

TABLE 3 Amino Acid Sequences of the Neurotoxins Used in the Present Study

		5 10 15 20 25 30
1.	Erabutoxin b	RICFNQHSSQPQTTKTCPSGESSCYHKQWS
2.	[51-Asn]-erabutoxin b	==============================
3.	Component E	==============================
4.	Laticotoxin a	=R===HP======N=S==P==N===N===R
5.	Toxin α	LE=H==Q====P====== ==TN==K=V=R
6.	H. ornatus '75 a	MT=C==Q====K==TN= A =====K=T=R
7.	A. stokesii a	MT=C==Q====K==TN= A= N===K=T==
8.	A. laevis a	LT=C==Q====K==TD= A DN===K=T=Q
9.	Cobrotoxin	LE=H==Q===TP==TG=SG==TN==K=R=R
10.	Toxin B	IR== ITP DI=S=D==N= HV==T=T=C
11.	A. stokesii b	LS=Y LGY KSH Q===P==NV=FV=T=C

	35 40 45 50 55 60 65 70	
1.	D FRGTIIERGC GCPTVKPGIKLSCCESEVCNN	(Sato and Tamiya, 1971)
2.	= ========== =========N===========	(Tamiya and Abe, 1972)
3.	= = === =====================	(Abe and Tamiya, 1979)
4.	= H========= ===========T==Q==D===	
5.	= H========= ===========N==TTDK===	(Eaker et al, 1967)
6.	= ====R===== ===Q=======E==HTNE===	
7.	= H========= ===Q==S====E==HTNE===	(Maeda and Tamiya,1978)
8.	= H===R===== ===Q=======E==KTNE===	(Maeda and Tamiya,1976)
9.	= H==YRT==== ===S==N==EIN==TTDR===	(Yang et al, 1969)
10.	=GFCSS==KRVDL==AAT====RT=VDIQ==STDD=DPFPTRKRP	(Nakai et al, 1971)
11.	=GFCNT==ER=IM==AAT===A=S=VNIA==STDN=HIYAKWGS*NH2*	(Maeda and Tamiya,1978)

= The same residue as in erabutoxin b.
Abbreviations: [51-Asn]-erabutoxin b, erabutoxin c; Component E, erabutoxin b less 33-38 residues. One letter symbols for amino acids: A,Ala; R,Arg; N,Asn; D,Asp; C,Cys; Q,Gln; E,Glu; G,Gly; H,His; I,Ile; L,Leu; K,Lys; M,Met; F,Phe; P,Pro; S,Ser; T,Thr; W,Trp; Y,Tyr; V,Val.

residues, which are present commonly in erabutoxin b and astrotia stokesii a but not in cobrotoxin. Out of the eight residues, four are not always found in other neurotoxins tested and in component E. Therefore, the remaining four residues, namely 11-Pro, 23-Ser, 51-Lys and 52-Leu, are the most probable candidate residues to be involved in the specificity determination in the reaction with 'common antibody'.

'Specific antibody', which was prepared from an anti-erabutoxin b serum by removing 'common antibody' with an astrotia stokesii a column, reacted with erabutoxin b and its derivative without a hexapeptide portion (component E) and to a smaller extent with laticotoxin a (Toxin α showed also a very small reaction.). The residues which are common to erabutoxin b and laticotoxin a and not present in other non-reacting toxins are 1-Arg, 12-Gln, 28-Gln, 57-Ser and 58-Glu. They are considered to be candidate residues to be involved in the reaction with 'specific antibody'.

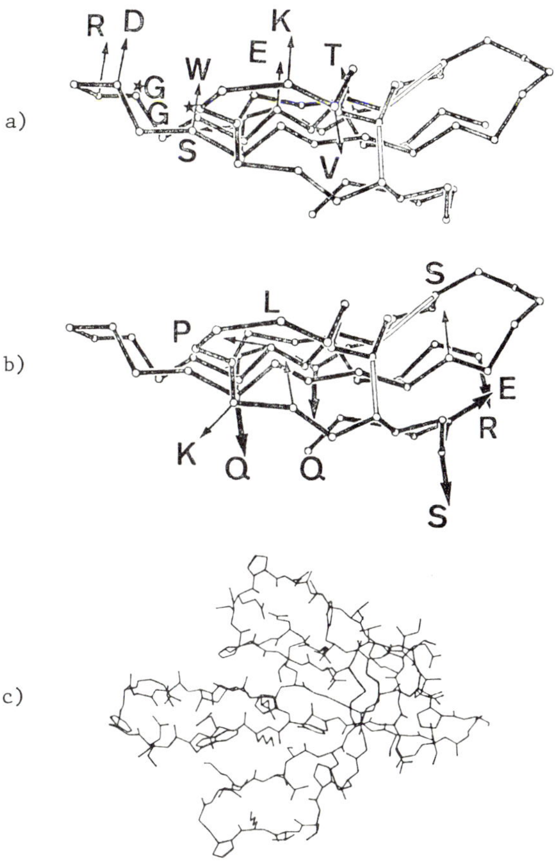

Fig. 2. Skeleton of erabutoxin b molecule.

a) Side view of the molecule. Arrows indicate the candidate residues to be involved in the binding with acetylcholine receptor (Ishikawa et al, 1977).
b) Side view of the molecule. Arrows indicate the candidate residues to be involved in the binding with 'specific antibody'(➡) and 'common antibody'(→).
c) Front view of the molecule.

Erabutoxin b is a flat, three-toed duck-foot like molecule with β-structure in and among the toes. Many of the residues are, therefore, directed either upwards or downwards of the flat molecule. Based on the data presented by Ishikawa et al (1977), Tamiya and Maeda (1978)assumed that erabutoxin b bound to acetylcholine receptor by one side of the flat surface (Fig.2.a)). In the present paper, nine residues were pointed out as candidate residues to be involved in the antibody binding. It is of interest that six out of the nine residues are found on the surface of other side of the molecule than the acetylcholine binding side. Out of three remaining candidate residues, two are buried in the molecule and one (11-Pro) is on the rim of the flat molecule. The neurotoxin molecule seems have head and tail, by which it attaches to the acetylcholine receptor and to antibodies, respectively (Fig. 2. b)). The residues to be involved in the attachment of the antibodies are 1-Arg, 12-Gln, 28-Gln, 51-Lys, 57-Ser and 58-Glu.

REFERENCES

Abe, T., and N. Tamiya (1979). Toxicon, 17, 571-582.

Boquet, P., G. Poilleux, C. Dumarey, Y. Izard and A.-M. Ronsseray (1973) Toxicon,11 333-339.

Boquet, P., C. Dumarey, and D. Joseph (1977). C. r. hebd Séanc. Acad. Sci. Paris, 284, Serie D, 2439- 2445.

Chou, P. Y., and G. D. Fasman (1974) Biochemistry, 13, 222-245.

Cuatrecasas, P., and C. B. Anfinsen (1971) Affinity Chromatography. In: Method in Enzymology Vol. 22 p.345-378, (Jakoby, W. B., Ed.). New York, Academic Press.

Dufton, M. J., and R. C. Hider (1977).J. Mol. Biol. 115, 177-193.

Eaker, D. L., and J. Porath (1967). Japanese J. Microbiol. 11, 353-355.

Heide, K., and H. G. Schwick (1973). Salt Fractionation of Immunoglobulins. In: Handbook of Experimental Immunology, 2nd edn. Ch. 6 (D.M. Weir, Ed.) Oxford: Blackwell Scientific Publications.

Herbert, V., K.S. Lau, C.W. Gottlieb, and S.J. Bleicher (1965). Coated Charcoal Immunoassay of Insulin, J. Clin. Endocrin. Metab. 25 1375

Hori, H., and N. Tamiya (1976). Biochem. J., 153, 217-222.

Hunter, W. M. (1973). Radioimmunoassay. In: Handbook of Experimental Immunology 2nd edn. Ch. 17 (D. M. Weir, Ed.) Oxford: Blackwell Scientific Publications.

Ishikawa, Y., A. Menez, H. Hori, H. Yoshida, and N. Tamiya (1977). Toxicon 15, 477-488.

Low, B. W., H. S. Preston, A. Sato, L. S. Rosen, J. E. Seal, A. D. Rudko, and J. S. Richardson (1976). Proc. Natl. Acad. Sci. U.S.A. 73, 2991-2994.

Maeda, N., and N. Tamiya (1974). Biochem. J. 141, 389-400.

Maeda, N., and N. Tamiya (1976). Biochem. J. 153, 79-87.

Maeda, N., and N. Tamiya (1978). Biochem. J. 175, 507-517.

Menez, A., G. Langlet, N. Tamiya, and P. Fromageot (1978). Biochimie 60, 505-517.

Nakai, K., T. Sasaki, K. Hayashi (1971). Biochem. Biophys. Res. Comm. 44, 893-897.

Ouchterlony, O., and L. A. Nilsson (1973). Immunodiffusion and Immunoelectrophoresis In: Handbook of Experimental Immunology 2nd edn. Ch. 19 (D. M. Weir, Ed.) Oxford: Blackwell Scientific Publications.

Sato, S., and N. Tamiya (1971). Biochem. J. 122, 453-461.

Sato, S., H. Yoshida, and N. Tamiya (1969). Biochem. J. 115, 85-90.

Tamiya, N., and H. Abe (1972). Biochem. J. 130, 547-555.

Tamiya, N., and H. Arai (1966). Biochem. J. 99, 624-630.

Tamiya, N., and N. Maeda (1978). Chemical Taxonomy of Snake Neurotoxins. In: Evolution of Protein Molecules p.297-310.

Tsernoglou, D., and G. A. Petsko (1976). FEBS Lett. 68, 1-4.

Tsernoglou, D., and G. A. Petsko (1977). Proc. Natl. Acad. Sci., U. S. A. 74, 971-974.

Yang, C. C., H. J. Yang, and J. S. Huang (1969). Biochim. Biophys. Acta 188, 65-77.

ANTISERA AGAINST WEEVER AND SCORPION FISH VENOMS A PRELIMINARY REPORT

D. Matić-Piantanida*, V. Vidaković-Bival*, V. Radman* and Z. Maretić**

**Institute of Immunology, Zagreb, Yugoslavia*
***Medical Center, Pula, Yugoslavia*

ABSTRACT

Specific antisera against extracts of the venom glands of Trachinus draco, Scorpaena scrofa, Scorpaena porcus and Scorpaena ustulata were obtained by immunization of rabbits. Gel-chromatography of the venom on Sephadex G-100 yielded two major peaks: one with main toxic components having molecular weight about 150,000 or more, and a low molecular dialysable fraction. The toxin could be separated in four fractions in cellulose acetate electrophoresis. The toxicity of venoms was tested in vivo and expressed as LD_{50}. Antigenic identity of S. scrofa, S. porcus and S. ustulata venoms was proved by means of immunoelectrophoresis and gel-diffusion. On the contrary the toxins from weever and scorpionfish were antigenically different. A minimal degree of cross-reactivity between heterologous systems of venoms and antisera was due to the presence of non-specific tissue antigens in venom extracts. In neutralization tests in mice a good protection was achieved with homologous toxins, while antisera mixed with heterologous toxins failed to give any protection. On post-mortem examination of mice inoculated with toxin, alterations in lung and heart were found. The final purpose of this work however was the investigation of possible successfull application of the respective antisera in humans. During the past 15 years, 24 cases, more or less severe, were treated with rabbit antisera against weever or scorpionfish venom with good results. On the basis of clinical experience it appears that the antivenom antisera are very effective in the treatment of severe or special cases of specific poisoning.

KEYWORDS

Trachinus draco, Scorpaena scrofa, Scorpaena porcus, Scorpaena ustulata, weever, scorpionfish, venom, antisera, antigens.

INTRODUCTION

Weever and scorpionfish belong to the most venomous fishes of the Adriatic Sea.

Among the people who have been stung by them, there is always a certain number of severe cases. It is very probable that at least a part of complications caused by envenomation could be eliminated by application of the respective antisera. That was the reason why Maretić (1970, 1975) started as early as 1963 a series of experiments aimed at producing and applying antisera against Adriatic Scorpaenidae and Trachinidae. At the beginning he immunized rabbits by direct sting from the venom apparatus of weever, scorpionfish and star-gazer. The polyvalent antisera protected guinea-pigs from direct sting of weever and scorpionfish. In the same way a monovalent antitrachinic antiserum was produced in 1965. It was for the first time that the antisera against weever and scorpionfish toxin were used for therapeutic purposes in humans. In fact both antisera were successfully applied in 8 patients

The protective value of antisera against envenomation with weever toxin was first reported by Briot (1902), who found that the sera of immunized rabbits would protect other rabbits against venom of the weever. Later, an antivenin against stonefish venom with a high degree of potency was produced and described by Wiener (1959). Another way of protection against weever toxin was proposed by Skeie (1962), who described the possibility of active immunization. All these data confirm the antigenicity of piscine venoms, and - accordingly - the possibility of production of antisera with protective action against these venoms.

The greatest problem in the production of such antisera is the lack of knowledge concerning the composition and the mode of action of the venom components. Fish venoms, in fact, are complex mixtures (Russell, 1971; Saunders, 1960), which vary considerably in their chemical composition in spite of the similarity of some clinical symptoms, amongst which the most pronounced are the toxic effect, the pain-producing property and the necrotic effect. Also, it is not known whether all the principal components of a venom are at the same time antigens at all. In addition, the most pronounced characteristic of fish venoms is their great instability, especially temperature dependent.

Taking all these facts into consideration we have tried to make a preliminary evaluation of our antisera by testing them in 3 ways: 1. immunochemically, against weever and scorpionfish venom antigens, 2. in animals, measuring their protective value against the lethal effect of the toxin, and 3. investigating their positive effect as therapeutical agents. The subject work presents a study of antisera against the following venomous fishes of the Adriatic: T. draco, S. scrofa, S. porcus and S. ustulata.

MATERIALS AND METHODS

Venoms. Venom apparatus were taken from fresh fish, immediatelly frozen and kept at -20° C. Venom gland extracts were prepared by maceration of venom apparatus of T. draco, S. scrofa, S. porcus and S. ustulata with cold distilled water. After centrifugation at 18,000 r.p.m. for 30 min at 5°C the clear supernatant was used either immediately for immunization and experiments or frozen after addition of 15% glycerol. Non-specific tissue extract was prepared from muscles and skin of scorpionfish on the same way as the venom gland extract.

Antisera. Groups of 3 - 7 chinchilla rabbits, weighing more than 3 kg were immunized with venom or tissue extracts in Freund's complete adjuvant, and boostered after 4 weeks with the same extract in Freund's incomplete adjuvant. Each rabbit received approximately 1 - 5 LD_{50} in mice of the respective venom. The dosis was 2 ml and was injected into foot pads and into hind limbs intramuscularly. One week afterwards the blood was collected and the antiserum either frozen or purified. The antisera were purified by precipitation with 39% ammonium sulphate. The precipitate was washed twice with the corresponding solution of ammonium sulphate, dialysed and sterile filtered. The antisera for human use were tested for sterility, inocuity and pyrogenicity.

Laboratory methods. The immunoelectrophoresis (Scheidegger, 1955) and the Ouchterlony double diffusion technique (Ouchterlony, 1953) were used to detect precipitating antibodies. Electrophoresis on cellulose acetate was performed according to Thompson (1977). Gel-chromatography on Sephadex G-100 was used for fractionation of crude venom or tissue extracts. Samples of 2 - 5 ml were chromatographed on a 2.5 x 100-cm column in phosphate-buffered saline, pH 7.1, at a flow rate of 20.4 ml per hour. Eluate absorbance was measured at 280 nm.

Tests on animals. The toxicities of the toxins were assayed by intravenous application of the respective toxins into white mice of 14 - 16 g weight, Bethesda B/S NIH strain. The mice were injected intravenously with 0.5 ml of two-fold dilutions of the respective venom extracts in saline. Four mice were injected with each dilution. The toxicity determination was repeated twice and on the basis of the lethal effect the LD_{50} dose was calculated. The neutralization capacities of the respective antisera were also tested in mice. A constant amount of the antiserum was mixed with various amounts of the respective toxin. The mixture in a total volume of 0.5 ml was injected intravenously into mice and the dose-response was followed over a period of 48 hours.

RESULTS

Physico-Chemical and Immunochemical Analyses

The complexity of the venom gland extract was confirmed by separation of the components according to their electrophoretic mobility on the cellulose acetate strips, as shown in Table 1.

TABLE 1 CAE Analysis of T. draco Venom Extract

Fractions	%
alpha-1	2.1
alpha-2	25.0
beta	56.3
gamma	16.7

The same sample of the T. draco venom gland extract was fractionated on Sephadex G-100 to examine the molecular weight distribution of its components (Fig. 1).

The non-specific tissue surrounding the venom gland was obviously included in the venom extracts and could contribute to the antibody formation in rabbits. In Fig. 1

the gel-chromatographic separation of the tissue extract compared with the venom gland extract is presented. Both had common maxima in the first peak (exclusion in void volume) containing components of molecular weight of about 150,000 or more, and in the last peak with the low molecular components having obviously high absorption in the UV region. Fractions No. 28 and No. 70 - 72 of both samples A. and B. were concentrated. In immunoelectrophoresis against appropriate antisera only fraction No. 28 of the T. draco venom gave precipitation lines in alpha and beta regions, while no precipitation lines were formed with the other 3 samples.

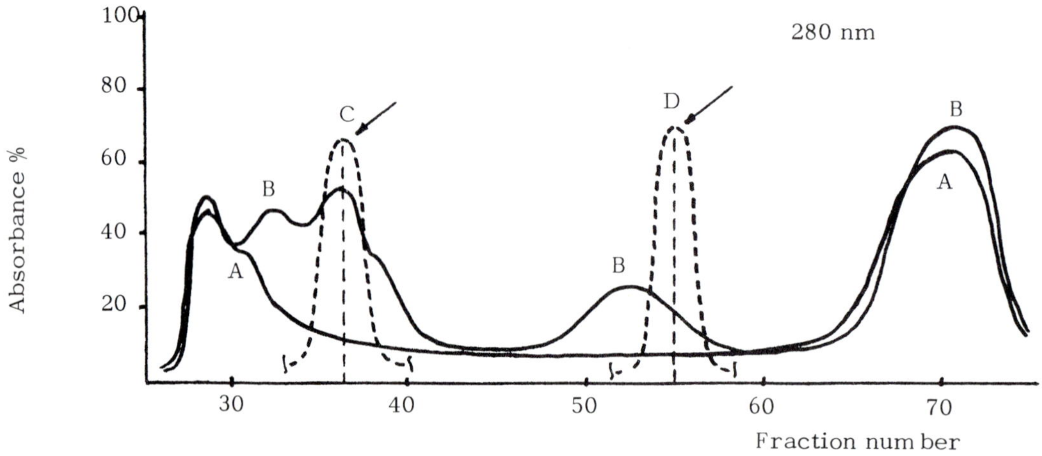

Fig. 1. Gel-chromatography on Sephadex G-100 of the following samples: A = T. draco venom gland extract, B = non-specific tissue extract, C = human serum albumin monomer, D = human myoglobin. Column size: 2.5 x 100 cm, PBS buffer, pH 7.1, flow rate: 20.4 ml/hour, fraction volume: 6.8 ml. Arrows indicate the molecular weight of the respective fraction: mol w_C = 66,300, mol w_D = 17,800.

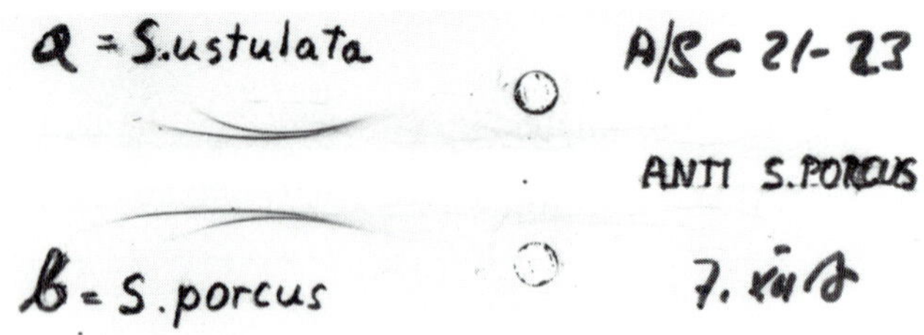

Fig. 2. Immunoelectrophoretic pattern of a = S. ustulata venom and b = S. porcus venom. In the troughs antiserum against S. porcus venom.

The specificities of the antisera against S. scrofa, S. porcus, S. ustulata and T. draco were tested both immunoelectrophoretically and by gel-diffusion. These analyses served to prove the antigenic identity among various apecies of Scorpaenidae and the antigenic differences between Scorpaenidae and Trachinidae.

The results are presented in Fig. 2 and 3.

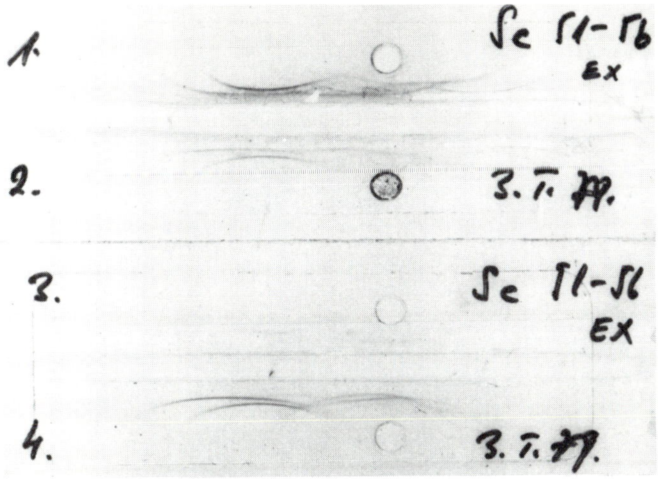

Fig. 3. Immunoelectrophoretic analysis of scorpionfish and weever venom. Samples were placed in wells: 1 = S. scrofa, 2 = S. porcus, 3 = T. draco, 4 = S. ustulata. Antiserum against S.scrofa was placed in both troughs.

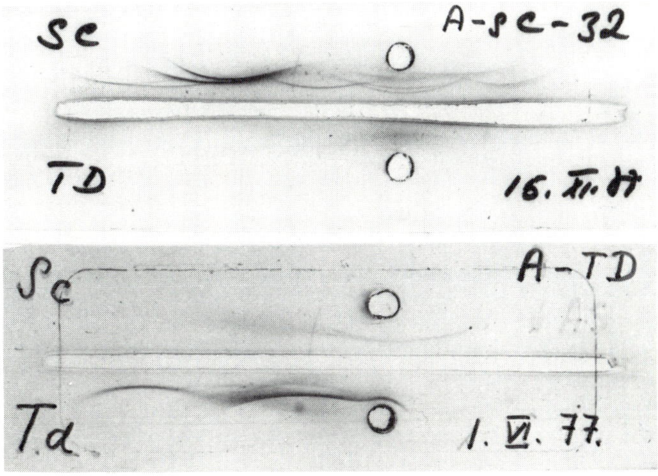

Fig. 4. Immunoelectrophoretic pattern showing the antigenic difference between the scorpionfish (SC) and weever (TD) toxins. Venom gland extracts were placed the respective wells. In the upper troughs antiserum against scropionfish venom, in the lower troughs antiserum against weever venom.

Antigenic heterogeneity between scorpionfish and weever venoms is clearly demonstrated in the Fig. 4. The same results obtained in gel-diffusion are presented in Fig. 5.

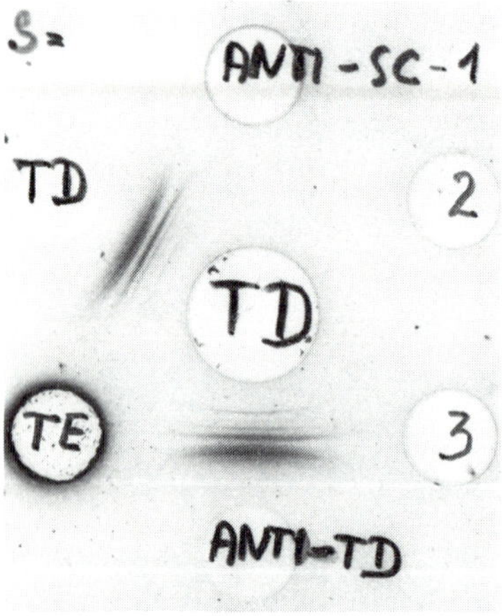

Fig. 5. Double diffusion in gel. T. draco venom in the central well. In the peripheral wells antisera against: S. scrofa (Anti Sc-1), S. porcus (2), S. ustulata (3), tissue extract (TE) and T. draco (Anti-TD).

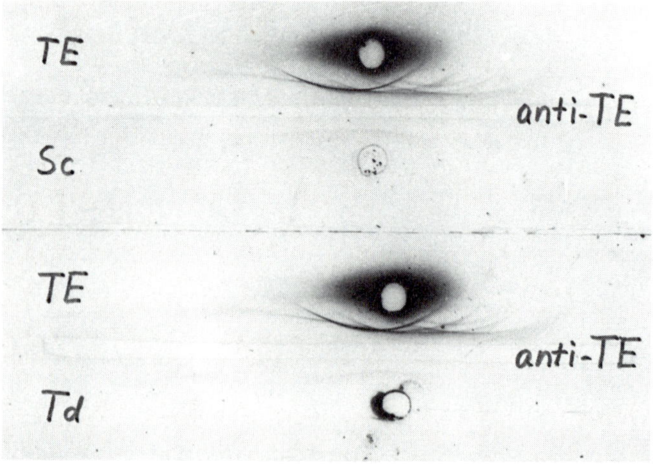

Fig. 6. Immunoelectrophoretic pattern of non-specific tissue, respectively venom extracts, against tissue extract antiserum. TE = tissue extract, Sc = scorpionfish venom extract, Td = weever venom extract. In both troughs antiserum against tissue extract (anti TE).

The presence of non-specific tissue antigens in venom extracts was tested by specially prepared antiserum against the non-specific tissue extract, as shown in Fig. 5 and 6.

In Vivo Tests

Toxicity. The original toxin samples contained approximately the venom from 1 spine extracted in 1 ml saline. Different doses were injected in mice. Toxins diluted 1 : 2 killed mice in 60 minutes. The next dilution 1 : 4 was lethal for 50% mice, and in lower concentrations there was no lethal effect at all. Thus the LD_{50} dose for weever and scorpionfish venom extracts was 0.125 ml of the venom extract.

The neutralization capacity. The efficiency of the specific antisera to protect mice against the toxic effect of respective toxins is presented in Tables 2 and 3. All mice survived except the control group which also received 2 LD_{50} of the respective toxin, but without the antiserum.

TABLE 2. Neutralization Test "In Vivo"

Anti-TD serum		Toxin TD	Results	S/N
0.25 ml	+	2 LD_{50}	- - - -	4/4
0.25 ml	+	1 LD_{50}	- - - -	4/4
0.25 ml	+	0.5 LD_{50}	- - - -	4/4
-		2 LD_{50}	+ + + +	0/4

TD = *T. draco* toxin
S = survival, N = total number of mice

TABLE 3. Neutralization Test "In Vivo"

Anti-SC serum		Toxin SC	Results	S/N
0.25 ml	+	2 LD_{50}	- - - -	4/4
0.25 ml	+	1 LD_{50}	- - - -	4/4
0.25 ml	+	0.5 LD_{50}	- - - -	4/4
-		2 LD_{50}	+ + + +	0/4

SC = Scorpionfish (S. scrofa + S. porcus + S. Ustulata)
S = survival, N = total number of mice

Using the heterologous antisera the results were different: when mixed with 2 or 1 LD_{50} dose of toxins they failed to give any protection, as is shown in Table 4.

TABLE 4. Neutralization Test "In Vivo"

Anti-TD serum		Toxin SC	Results	S/N
0.25 ml	+	2 LD_{50}	+ + + +	0/4
0.25 ml	+	1 LD_{50}	- + + +	1/4
Anti - SC serum		**Toxin TD**		
0.25 ml	+	2 LD_{50}	+ + + +	0/4
0.25 ml	+	1 LD_{50}	- - + +	2/4

TD = weever toxin, SC = scorpionfish toxin
S = survival, N = total number of mice

Histological Findings

On postmortem examination of mice inocculated with T. draco toxin alterations in the lung and heart were found. The lungs and pulmonary vessels were congested. The lungs parenchyma showed perivascular hemorrhages and oedema (Fig. 7). The right and left heart ventricles were distended and vessels were congested. There was increased capillary permeability.

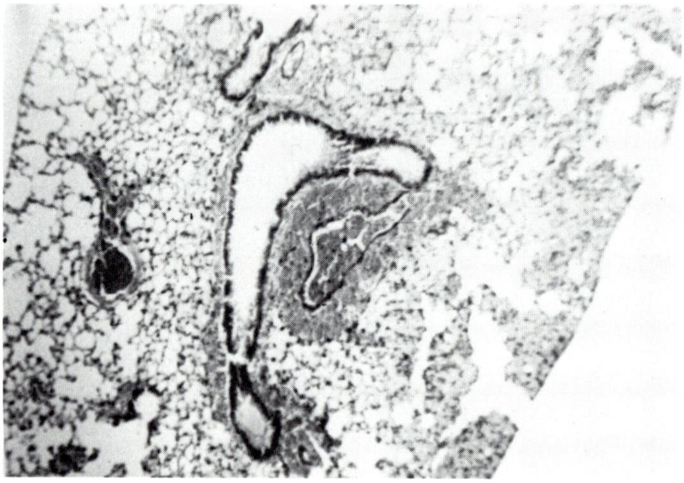

Fig. 7. The lung of mouse. Perivascular haemorrhages and oedema. H-E stain. Magnification 76x.

Human Application

As already stated, the main purpose of the present work has been the investigation of possible successful application of the specific antisera in humans. A total of 24 patients (20 stung by weever and 4 by scorpionfish) were treated with the specific antisera. All of them suffered severe pain and developed large oedema. The usual hot water treatment did not help. The patients received 2 - 5 ml of the immunoglobulin fraction of the respective antisera intramuscularly. The pain ceased within 20 minutes - 2 hours. The oedema still persisted in a light form for a few hours after. There were some cases, where the painful oedema persisted for some 4 - 6 days in spite of the intensive treatment with hot water, calcium and antihistaminics, but after the application of the antiserum, the pain as well as oedema practically disapeared in about 10 hours.

DISCUSSION

It is not known, as yet, which components of the fish toxins have a deleterious effect in envenomation. In our work the venom extracts were prepared by maceration of the whole venom gland apparatus. In this way all components which could possibly enter the human organism by action of a sting were present in extracts used for immunization of rabbits.

The venom extract gave 4 fractions when submitted to electrophoresis on cellulose acetate (Table 1), but in immunoelectrophoresis 8 or 9 precipitation lines were detected (Fig. 3 and 4). Russell and Emery (1960) and Saunders (1960) established the existence of high molecular toxic components with deleterious effects, and low molecular dialysable fractions containing pain-producing components (Carlisle, 1962). These results confirm our findings presented in Fig. 1, where gel-chromatographic separation of T. draco toxin into two main fractions is shown.

Although no basic structure for the toxin of any venomous fish has been established, it is already known (Russell, 1971) that toxins of different families differ markedly, and that the toxin within the same family and species can vary considerably. In our study, we have compared specific antisera against 3 species of Scorpaenidae. The results shown in Fig. 2 and 3 suggest that the particular venom extracts of scorpaena species are of the same antigenic composition. The slight differences in the intensity of precipitation lines were obviously caused by the variability of the toxin sample. In Fig. 4 and 5 a distinct antigenic difference between scorpionfish and weever venom extracts was proved.

In the previous experiments specific antigen-antibody systems for weever and scorpionfish could be demonstrated, but the question that still remains open is, how and to what extent could the presence of non-specific tissue antigens in venom extracts influence the antibody formation in rabbits, and thus possibly lead to false conclusions. Therefore, a non-specific tissue extract and a corresponding antiserum were prepared. In immunoelectrophoretic and gel-diffusion patterns (Fig. 5 and 6) the appearance of only two weak precipitation lines could be proved, which means that all the other antibodies were raised against the respective toxic components. The non-specific tissue extract was also fractionated on Sephadex G-100 (Fig. 1) yielding 5 peaks. The first peak contained components of molecular weight of 150,000 or more, but they were not identical with the first peak of the T. draco venom extract (Fig. 1) as confirmed by immunoelectrophoresis with specific antisera.

In vivo tests in mice indicated that venom and respective antisera are highly specific for a given genus. However, in view of the great instability of the toxins, and the lack of adequate standard toxin preparations, a continuation of testing is suggested, with repeated tests of toxicity and of neutralization capacity. The use of the same toxin sample in the neutralization tests in vivo is indispensable.

The specific antisera, when applied to humans after envenomation, exhibited a satisfactory protection effect. Still, one could ask which is the practical value of the antiserum application, when usually the treatment with hot water is sufficient. Of course, the antisera should not be applied routinely, but are to be reserved only for cases of severe intoxication, where oedema is persistent, and when general symptoms are prolonged. Their use is also recommendable when treating patients suffering from other serious chronic diseases, as their condition could change for the worse as a result of a sting by a venomous fish.

ACKNOWLEDGEMENT

We wish to thank Professor Findlay E. Russell for his valuable suggestions concerning our work.

REFERENCES

Briot, A. (1902). Sur l'action du venin de la vivre (Trachinus draco). C. R. Soc. Biol., 54, 1169-1171.
Carlisle, D. B. (1962). On the venom of the lesser weeverfish, Trachinus vipera. J. Mar. Biol. Ass. U. K., 42, 155-162.
Maretić, Z., and B. Marzan (1970). O otrovanjima izazvanim ribama Jadrana. Medicina, 7, 167-170.
Maretić, Z. (1975). Zivotinje otrovnice i otrovne zivotinje Jadranskog mora. JAZU, Zagreb, p. 80.
Ouchterlony, Ö. (1953). Antigen-antibody reactions in gels. IV. Types of reactions in coordinated systems of diffusion. Acta Pathol. Microbiol. Scand., 32, 231-240.
Russell. F. E., and J. A. Emery (1960). Venom of the weevers Trachinus draco and Trachinus vipera. Ann. N. Y. Acad. Sci., 90, 805-819.
Russell, F. E. (1971). Marine Toxins and Venomous and Poisonous Marine Animals, T. H. F. Publications, Inc., 109-151.
Saunders, P. R. (1960). Pharmacological and chemical studies of the venom of the stonefish (genus Synanceja) and other scorpionfishes. Ann. N. Y. Acad. Sci., 90, 798-804.
Scheidegger, J. J. (1955). Une micro-méthode de l'immunoélectrophorese. Int. Arch. Allergy Appl. Immunol., 7, 103-
Skeie, E. (1962). Weeverfish toxin. Acta Pathol. Microbiol. Scand., 56, 229-236.
Thompson, R. A. (1977). Techniques in Clinical Immunology, Blackwell Scientific Publications, Oxford, p. 26.
Wiener, S. (1959). The production and assay of stonfish antivenene. Med. J. Australia, 2, 715-719.

Substances Affecting Blood Coagulation and Fibrinolysis

SNAKE VENOM PROTEASES AFFECTING BLOOD COAGULATION AND FIBRINOLYSIS

K. Stocker

Pentapharm Ltd., CH-4002 Basle, Switzerland

ABSTRACT

Numerous snake venoms, due to the action of their proteases, may affect blood coagulation by either activating or damaging platelets, factors V, X, XIII, prothrombin or fibrinogen; some venoms may cause fibrinolysis by activating plasminogen or by direct digestion of fibrin. Several venom proteases have found practical application in coagulation research and control and some fibrinogen clotting enzymes, isolated from Crotalinae venoms, are used as potential agents for therapeutic defibrinogenation. A species-dependent interaction with fibrinogen and serum protease inhibitors of different mammals was recognized for ancrod and batroxobin, two well characterized thrombic proteases being used for defibrinogenation in man.

KEYWORDS

Blood coagulation; fibrinolysis; ancrod; batroxobin; ecarin; thrombocytin; fibrinopeptide release; therapeutic defibrinogenation.

INTRODUCTION

Blood coagulation is an important contribution to haemostasis, the mechanism which prevents the escape of blood from injured vessels, whereas fibrinolysis is the enzymatic way to dissolve a thrombus and to render occluded vessels patent. However, pathologic activation of these mechanisms causes danger to life by intravascular coagulation or bleeding. Many snake venoms owe part of their toxicity to proteases which affect blood coagulation and fibrinolysis, causing either thromboembolism or haemorrhage.

Both coagulation and fibrinolysis result from the harmonic interaction of plasma- and tissue proteins in presence of lipids and low molecular plasma components in a balanced electrolyte medium. Blood, circulating in an intact vessel-system, contains, protected by protease inhibitors, the precursors of coagulation and fibrinolysis factors. Initiated by surface contact at the site of a vessel injury or initiated by pathological events, these precursors become activated. The major part of these precursors are zymogens of proteases, and their activation is effected by a limited proteolysis which splits off one or several activation peptides, thereby exposing the active centers. Thus, in the course of coagulation and of fibrinolysis, a protease activates a zymogen yielding a further protease which in turn activates another zymogen. At the end of this activation cascade, the protease thrombin causes the transformation of fibrinogen to a fibrin clot or, in case of fibrinolysis, the protease plasmin catalyzes the degradation of fibrin to soluble fragments and thereby the dissolution of the clot. It is evident that such a balanced system of zymogens and substrates may easily be disturbed by extraneous proteases like those contained in snake venoms.

In the beginning of this century, when Morawitz (1905) defined the essential mechanism of blood coagulation, Lamb (1901), Noc (1904) and others concluded that the ability of snake venoms to coagulate blood, to render it unclottable or to dissolve coagulated blood, and the ability of these venoms to digest meat, egg-white, casein and other proteinous material, are due to the presence of proteolytic enzymes. At that time it was not possible to isolate and purify a single protease out of the complex protein mixture that represents a snake venom. Trials to characterize venom proteases and their modes of action were based on experiments with crude venom fractions, using unspecific test systems. The presence of more than one protease in the same venom, synergistic or antagonistic reactions among several enzymes, and the ability of single enzymes to act on different substrates led during a long period to contradictory statements concerning the procoagulant, anticoagulant and fibrinolytic effects of snake venoms.

Our knowledge of venom proteases acting on coagulation and fibrinolysis has improved thanks to the application of efficient protein separation techniques which allow to isolate and purify individual enzymes from crude venom, and to the availability of plasma fractions and purified plasma proteins which allow to investigate pure enzymes, venom fractions or even crude venoms in highly specific test systems.

MODE OF VENOM PROTEASE ACTIONS

Platelets

Snake venom enzymes like thrombocytin from *Bothrops atrox* (Niewiarowski and coworkers, 1977) may act like thrombin on platelets, causing aggregation and release reactions as well as activation of their contractile system. This kind of enzyme may contribute to the venoms toxicity by triggering intravascular coagulation. However, it is difficult to understand why the same *Bothrops atrox* venom contains another protease, the fibrinogen clotting enzyme batroxobin, which exerts just the opposite effect, impairing platelet functions (Markwardt and Nowak, 1979). Ecarin too, the coagulant prothrombin activating enzyme from *Echis carinatus* exerts, according to Kornalik (pers. comm., 1978) a damaging effect on platelets by reducing their aggregability. (Fig. 1)

Coagulation

Transformation of blood from the fluid state to a gel is due to the conversion of fibrinogen to fibrin which is initiated by the limited proteolytic action of thrombin on fibrinogen. (Fig. 2)

Thrombin generation. Thrombin is a serine protease which is generated from the inactive precursor prothrombin by the proteolytic action of factor Xa in presence of calcium ions. The action of factor Xa is strongly accelerated by factor Va, a protein which, in turn needs first to be activated by a protease from its inactive precursor

The conversion of factor X to factor Xa occurs via two different pathways: The intrinsic pathway, requiring factors VIII, IX and platelet factor 3, and the extrinsic pathway, requiring a tissue lipoprotein and factor VII. Snake venom proteases, like the coagulant protease of Russell's viper venom (Furie and Furie, 1976) may cause thrombin generation by activating factor X in presence of Ca^{++}. Other venom enzymes, like ecarin (Kornalik and Blombäck, 1975) are capable of activating prothrombin directly. Several venoms, like Notechis scutatus venom, contain proteases which activate factor V (Andersson, 1971). The venom of Naja naja has been found to contain a protease which inhibits thrombin generation, probably by degradation of one or more of the involved proteins.

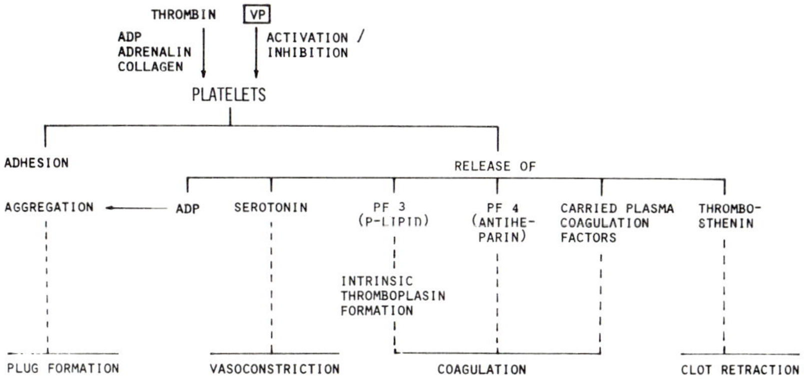

Fig. 1. Venom proteases (VP) and platelets.

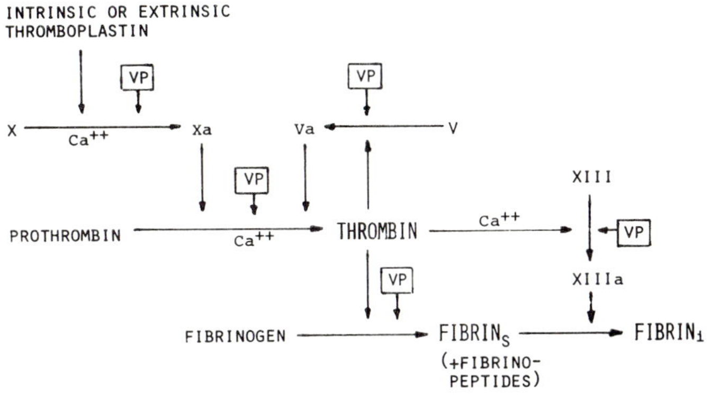

Fig. 2. Venom proteases (VP) and blood coagulation.

Fibrin formation. (Fig. 3) Fibrinogen is a dimer of a protein unit consisting of three chains, Aα, Bβ and γ, interlinked at the N-terminus by disulfide bonds. Thrombin, by cleaving Arg-Gly bonds, splits off two small peptides, fibrinopeptide A and B, from the Aα- and Bβ-chains, exposing reactive groups. The resulting product is fibrin in a monomeric form which rapidly aggregates to a polymer. This process of aggregation is reversible and the formed $fibrin_s$ is still soluble in 1% monochloracetic acid. Many venom proteases are capable of splitting fibrinopeptides from fibrinogen. A protease of Bitis gabonica venom (Gaffney and coworkers, 1973), like thrombin, splits off fibrinopeptides A and B and causes the formation of monomers which aggregate "end-to-end" and "side-to-side" forming a firm fibrin clot. In contrast to thrombin, a large number of proteases from Crotalinae venoms, like ancrod and batroxobin, split off exclusively fibrinopeptide A from fibrinogen. The resulting monomers only aggregate "end-to-end", forming a soft fibrin gel which is particularly susceptible to fibrinolysis. A protease from Agkistrodon contortrix venom (Herzig and coworkers, 1970) catalyzes predominantly the release of fibrinopeptide B from fibrinogen and the resulting new molecule is unable to form a true clot unless fibrinopeptide A is removed, too. Several venom proteases (e.g. Ecarin) may degrade fibrinogen to nonpolymerizable fragments.

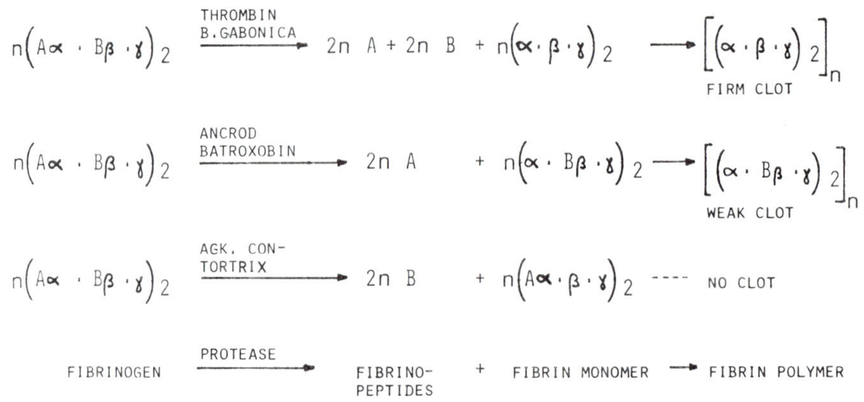

Fig. 3. Conversion of fibrinogen into fibrin, induced by thrombin and different snake venom enzymes.

Fibrin stabilization. Factor XIIIa, (Curtis and Lorand, 1976) generated by the action of thrombin or of a venom protease like thrombocytin from the inactive precursor factor XIII, is a transamidase which causes the formation of a covalent bond between a lysyl residue in one fibrin molecule and a glutamyl residue in a neighbour molecule. Fibrin cross-linked by the action of factor XIIIa, $fibrin_i$ (Fig. 2), is insoluble in monochloracetic acid 1%.

Fibrinolysis (Fig. 4)

Fibrinolysis, as the counter-part of coagulation, effects the transformation of clotted blood back to a liquid state again. This is achieved by a chain of proteolytic reactions which lead to the formation of plasmin, the protease which degrades fibrin (and fibrinogen) to soluble fragments. Fibrin(ogen) degradation products (FDP) exert an anticoagulant effect by inhibiting fibrin polymerization. Under normal conditions no fibrinolytic activity is present in circulating blood; plasmin has first to be generated from its inactive precursor plasminogen. The activation of plasminogen is a proteolytic process mediated by urokinase or by numerous other activators occuring in tissues and body fluids. Snake venom proteases may also act as plasminogen activators or may directly degrade fibrin and / or fibrinogen.

Table 1 provides a survey on snake venoms and their protease actions on blood coagulation and fibrinolysis, as summarized from our own laboratory findings and bibliographic data (Davey and Lüscher, 1965; De Vries and Cohen, 1969; Denson and coworkers, 1972; Gaffney, 1977; Kaiser and Michl, 1958; Stocker, 1978; Seegers and Ouyang, 1979; Rosenfeld and coworkers, 1968; Andersson, 1971).

TABLE 1 Coagulant, anticoagulant and fibrinolytic actions of snake venoms

Species	Activation / Coagulation of						Inhibition of		Lysis of		
	Platelet functions	Fibri-nogen	Pro-thrombin	F.V	F.X	F.XIII	Platelet functions	Prothrombin activation	Fibri-nogen	Fibrin non heated	Fibrin heated
Colubrinae											
Dispholidus typus		0	+		+	+					
Thelotornis kirtlandi		0	+		0						
Elapinae											
Acantophis antarcticus			+	+							
Demansia textilis			+								
Naja Naja		0						+	+	0	0
N. nigricollis		0	+						+		
Notechis scutatus		0	+	+							
Oxyuranus scutellatus		0	+								
Viperinae											
Bitis gabonica		+								0	+
B. lachesis	0								+	+	+
Causus rhombeatus				+							
Cerastes cerastes		0			+				+	0	0
Echis carinatus	+	0	+	+	+		+		+	0	0
E. coloratus		0	+		+		+		+		+
Vipera ammodytes		+		+					+		
V. aspis		0		+						0	0
V. berus				+							
V. lebetina										0	0
V. xanthina							+	+			
V. russellii		0		+	+					0	0
Crotalinae											
Agkistrodon acutus		+							+	+	+
A. bilineatus		+	0		0					+	
A. contortrix	0	+	0							+	
A. halys		+	0		0					+	+
A. piscivorus		+							+	+	
A. rhodostoma	0	+				+			0	+	

TABLE 1 (Continued)

Species	Activation / Coagulation of: Platelet functions	Fibri- nogen	Pro- thrombin	F.V	F.X	F.XIII	Inhibition of: Platelet functions	Prothrombin activation	Lysis of: Fibri- nogen	Fibrin: non heated	Fibrin: heated
Crotalinae (cont.)											
Bothrops alternatus		+							+	+	+
B. andianus		+								+	+
B. asper		+			+	+				+	+
B. atrox	+	+			+	+				+	+
B. bilineatus		+								+	+
B. castelnaudi		+								0	+
B. cotiara		+									
B. erythromelas		+									
B. hyoprorus		+								0	+
B. jararaca	+	+			+					+	+
B. jararacussu		+								+	+
B. lanceolatus	0	+								+	+
B. microphthalmus		+								+	
B. moojeni	+	+			+	+	+			+	+
B. neuwiedi	+	+							+	+	+
B. nummifer		+									
B. pradoi		+								+	+
Crotalus adamanteus	0	+	0		0					+	+
C. atrox		+	0		0					+	
C. durissus durissus		+	0		0					+	
C. durissus terrificus	+	+									
C. horridus	0	+									
C. scutulatus		0	0		0					+	
C. viridis	0	+	0		+					0	
Lachesis muta		+									
Sistrurus miliarius	+	+	0		0					+	
Trimeresurus erythrurus	+	+								+	
T. flavoviridis	0	+	0		0					0	0
T. gramineus		+						+	0		
T. mucosquamatus								+	+	+	+
T. okinavensis		+									
T. popeorum	+	+								+	
T. purpureo-maculatus	+	+			0						

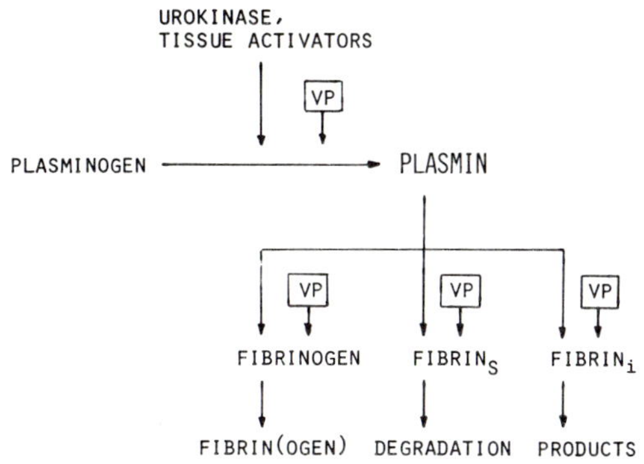

Fig. 4. Venom proteases and fibrinolysis

PRACTICAL USE OF VENOM PROTEASES

The best characterized venom proteases are those which have been isolated from relatively easy available venoms for current practical application as a drug or as a research or test reagent (table 2).

TABLE 2 Practical application of purified snake venom proteases

Protease	Origin	Use	Reference
RVV coagulant protease (Stypven®)	V. russellii	F.X determination	Furie and Furie (1976)
Ecarin	E. carinatus	Prothrombin determination	Kornalik and Blombäck (1975)
Ancrod (Arvin®, Arwin®)	A. rhodostoma	Therapeutic defibrinogenation	Bell (1974)
Batroxobin (Defibrase®)	B. moojeni	Therapeutic defibrinogenation	Egberg (1973)
Batroxobin (Reptilase®-R)	B. atrox	Testing fibrin formation	Funk and coworkers (1971)
A. contortrix thrombic protease	A. contortrix	Testing fibrin formation	Herzig and coworkers (1970)
Thrombocytin	B. atrox	Testing platelet functions	Niewiarowski and coworkers (1977)

The coagulant protease from Russell's viper venom, according to Kisiel and colleagues (1976) is a double-chain glycoprotein with a molecular weight of 78'000. This enzyme cleaves an Arg-Ile bond in the heavy chain of factor X which yields an activation peptide and factor Xa (Furie and Furie, 1976). The highly purified venom enzyme in addition to factor X, activates also factor IX.

Ecarin, the direct prothrombin activator of *Echis carinatus* venom is used for the determination of prothrombin in plasma and plasma fractions (Franza and Aronson, 1976). The prothrombin activating enzymes of *Dispholidus typus* (Atkinson and coworkers, 1978) and of Oxyuranus scutellatus (Denson, 1969) have been tried for the same purpose.

Thrombocytin a platelet activating enzyme has recently been discovered by Niewiarowski and coworkers, (1977) as a contaminant in semipurified batroxobin preparations. It was then isolated from crude Bothrops atrox venom by means of affinity chromatography on insolubilized heparin. It was characterized as a single-chain serine protease with a molecular weight of 36'000 and a carbohydrate content of 5,6%. A comparison of activities of thrombocytin, thrombin and batroxobin is given in Table 3.

TABLE 3 Thrombocytin: Comparison of activities

	Thrombin	Thrombocytin	Batroxobin
Platelet aggregation and release	+	+	-
Clot retraction	+	+	-
Clotting of fibrinogen	+	weak	+
Activation of: Factor XIII	+	+	-
Factor VIII	+	weak	-
Factor X	-	weak	-
Factor V	+	+	-
Degradation of fibrinogen α-chain	-	+	-
Cleavage of prothrombin to Intermediate I	+	+	-
Inhibition by: DFP	+	+	+
antithrombin III-heparin	+	+	-
hirudin	+	-	-
α_1-antitrypsin	-	-	-

(Niewiarowski and co-workers, 1979)

Thrombocytin is used in platelet research as a thrombin like agent which does not clot the test mixture in presence of fibrinogen.

Fibrinogen coagulant proteases like ancrod and batroxobin are used for therapeutic defibrinogenation in humans (Stocker, 1978). Injection of these enzymes causes the transformation of fibrinogen to an unstable fibrin derivative which is rapidly degraded by fibrinolysis and eliminated in form of fragments by the urine. Blood deprived from fibrinogen becomes unclottable, its viscosity decreases and its antiplasmin level is reduced; clotting factors other than fibrinogen as well as platelet count, remain unaffected. Ancrod and batroxobin are applied in the treatment of peripheric arterial occlusions, retinal vein thrombosis, deep vein thrombosis, prevention of postoperative thrombosis and other related conditions. (Egberg, 1973; Bell, 1974).

Both, ancrod and batroxobin are antigens and patients develop resistance upon prolonged treatment. However, the two enzymes are immunologically not cross reactive; a subject resistant to the one may successfully be treated further with the alternate preparation. (Barlow and coworkers, 1973).

Highly or semipurified thrombin-like enzymes of Agkistrodon acutus (Ouyang and coworkers, 1971), Bothrops jararaca (Kelen and coworkers, 1978), Lachesis muta (Chamone and coworkers, 1979), Crotalus adamanteus (Markland and Damus, 1971), Crotalus horridus (Bonilla, 1975), Trimeresurus gramineus (Ouyang and Yang, 1974) and of Trimeresurus okinavensis (Andersson, 1972) were found to be capable of inducing a benign defibrination in laboratory animals.

SPECIES DEPENDENCE OF VENOM PROTEASES, THEIR SUBSTRATES AND INHIBITORS

A survey on Bothrops venoms for presence of fibrinogen coagulant proteases as shown in table 4, revealed important quantitative differences as well as different electrophoretic mobilities of the coagulant enzymes even within the closely related species B. atrox, B. asper, B. moojeni and B. pradoi.

TABLE 4 Fibrinogen coagulant and amidolytic activities in some Bothrops venoms

Species	Origin	Fibrinogen coagulant activity		Amidolytic activity (mU/mg)	
		NIH (thrombin) u/mg	relative electrophoretic mobility	Cbo-Gly-Pro-Arg·pNA	Bz-Pro-Phe-Arg·pNA
B. alternatus	Brazil	1,5	0,30	162	21
B. andianus	Peru	< 0,1	0,11	105	333
B. asper	Costa Rica	3,1	0,09	90,5	21
B. atrox	Columbia	24,0	0,11	242	193
B. atrox	Venezuela	22,5	0,13	228	160
B. atrox	Maranhao, Brazil	14,8	0,17	141	45
B. atrox	Peru I	13,4	0,19	209	40,5
B. atrox	Peru II	23,5	0,13	140	69
B. moojeni	Brazil	5,6	0,06	266	69
B. bilineatus	Peru	< 0,1	0,49	112	106
B. castelnaudi	Peru	< 0,1	0,12	227	0
B. hyoprorus	Peru	< 0,1	0,12	229	29
B. jararaca	Brazil	8,3	0,27	214,5	327
B. jararacussu	Brazil	1,4	0,20	262,0	132
B. lanceolatus	Martinique	< 0,1	0,12	421	60
B. microphthalmus	Peru	7,0	0,34	273	207
B. neuwiedi	Brazil	5,5	0,10	182	54
B. pradoi	Brazil	10,5	0,03	355	122

A further indication for species related characteristics may be recognized in the immunochemical behaviour of fibrinogen coagulant proteases. Thus, a specific antibody preparation against batroxobin (B. atrox Maranhao, Brazil) forms precipitating antigen-antibody complexes with a large number of Bothrops venoms. As shown in table 5, this antibatroxobin preparation displays a very different neutralizing capacity towards the fibrinogen coagulating activity of the investigated venom species. It is of special interest that the activity of B. asper (Hoge) (= B. atrox asper Morfin) is completely neutralized, whereas the activity of the B. atrox-related B. pradoi (Hoge) (= B. atrox Amaral) and B. moojeni (Hoge) (commonly B. atrox in South-Central Brazil) is only partially neutralized.

TABLE 5 Inhibition of fibrinogen coagulant activity of crude Bothrops venoms by a specific anti-batroxobin preparation

Species	mg crude venom per ml test solution (ct 15 - 30 seconds)	% inhibition (from reciprocal clotting times)
B. atrox (Columbia)	0,07	> 92 %
B. atrox (Maranhao, Brazil)	0,1	> 92 %
B. atrox (Venezuela)	0,3	> 92 %
B. asper	0,2	> 92 %
B. moojeni	0,5	71,4%
B. pradoi	0,33	40,7%
B. lanceolatus	5,0	3,1%
B. alternatus	10,0	0
B. andianus	5,0	> 92 %
B. bilineatus	10,0	9,5%
B. hyoprorus	3,3	0
B. jararaca	0,33	> 92 %
B. jararacussu	1,25	0
B. microphthalmus	0,4	7,6%
B. neuwiedi	0,5	> 92 %

Clotting test: 2,2 ml venom solution, 0,05 ml antibody or saline/10 min. 37°C/0,2 ml bovine fibrinogen 0,4%/clotting time 37°C.

The fibrinogen coagulant enzymes isolated from the venoms of B. atrox, B. moojeni and B. asper, as listed in table 6, showed distinct physical and chemical properties and defibrinogenating preparations thereof caused a reduction of plasma fibrinogen in man which differed in degree and duration.

TABLE 6 Properties of purified thrombic proteases from Bothrops venoms

	B. atrox Maranhao	B. asper	B. moojeni
Molecular weight (SDS PAGE, reduced and alkylated)	41 600	32 000	35 800
Specific activity (BU/mg protein, bovine fibrinogen)	1 900	2 000	500
Carbohydrate content	~ 10 %	---	~ 5 %
Electrophoretic mobility pH 2,5, B. moojeni = 1,0	0,77	1,2	1,0
pH 8,6 Bromphenol blue = 1,0	0,2	0,15	0,1
Inactivation by human serum (24 hrs. 37°C)	83,3 %	---	56,7 %
Inactivation by elastase (24 hrs. 37°C)	0 %	---	100 %
Elution from insolubilized heparin (NaCl-concentration)	0,1 M	---	0,25 M
In vivo defibrinogenating effect	weak, short	---	strong, long-lasting

Laboratory animals undergoing batroxobin treatment showed species dependent dose response. Whereas the dog is defibrinogenated by an amount of batroxobin which approximately corresponds to the human dose, rabbit, rat and pig require several hundred times a human dose. Comparable observations on ancrod have been reported. The reason for these differences in dose response must be the fact that protein structure is species-specific. This is true for the thrombin-like venom enzymes as well as for fibrinogen, for the serum protease inhibitors and for the enzymes responsible for the metabolic degradation of the injected venom enzyme. A complex affinity- and reactivity relationship will finally determine the dose response.

Species differences in enzyme-fibrinogen interaction are shown in table 7 (Enzyme solutions adjusted to equal potency on bovine fibrinogen were assayed on fibrinogens of four other species). Variations of inhibitory capacity of serum of three species towards the venom enzymes of three snake species are given in table 8. As demonstrated by Egberg, (1973) α2-macroglobulin is the major serum inhibitor for batroxobin.

TABLE 7 Species dependent interaction of coagulant proteases and fibrinogen

4 NIHu (bovine fibrinogen / US-standard thrombin)	NIH units determined on fibrinogen of:			
	Man	Pig	Rabbit	Rat
Human thrombin	5,5	4,9	19,0	3,7
Bovine thrombin	4,2	4,7	18,6	4,0
Ancrod	6,2	5,3	15,1	5,8
Batroxobin (B. moojeni)	1,9	6,3	4,5	4,9
Batroxobin (B. atrox Maranhao)	6,4	4,0	2,2	1,75

TABLE 8 Species dependent inhibition of fibrinogen coagulant venom enzymes by serum

Enzyme	Inhibition of fibrinogen clotting activity (NIH thrombin units) by 24 hrs. incubation (37°C) with serum of		
	Man	Rabbit	Rat
Ancrod	78,2 %	94,3 %	90,7 %
Batroxobin (B. moojeni)	56,7 %	41,7 %	97,5 %
Batroxobin (B. atrox Maranhao)	83,3 %	30,0 %	95,8 %

This species dependent interaction of thrombic venom proteases, serum inhibitors and fibrinogen may stand as an example for similar interrelations between other venom enzymes and other substrate- and inhibitor proteins in the body of a prey- or victim species. The investigation of species characteristics of venom enzymes may provide important contributions for phylogenetic considerations, for the toxonomical classification of poisonous snakes and for the production of antivenoms.

REFERENCES

Andersson, L. (1971). A study of the coagulant action of some snake venoms. Coagulation, 4, 309.

Andersson, L. (1972). Isolation of thrombin-like activity from the venom of Trimeresurus okinavensis. Haemostasis, 1, 31-43.

Atkinson, P.M., B.A. Bradlow, E.D. Gomperts, and M. Feesey (1978). The coagulant action of boomslang venom Dispholidus typus. (Abstract) XVII Cong. Int. Soc. Haematol. Paris.

Barlow, G.H., L.J. Lewis, R. Finley, D. Martin, and K. Stocker (1973). Immunochemical identification of Ancrod and Reptilase (Defibrase). Thromb. Res., 2, 17-22.

Bell, W.R. (1974). Defibrinogenation with arvin in thrombic disorders. In S. Sherry, A. Scriabine (Eds.), Platelets and Thrombosis, Munich, Berlin, Vienna, Urban-Schwarzenberg. pp. 274-298.

Bonilla, C. (1975). Defibrinating enzyme from timber rattle snake (Crotalus horridus horridus) venom: A potential agent for therapeutic defibrination. I. Purificatic and properties. Thromb. Res., 6, 151-169.

Chamone, D.A.F., A. Magalhaes, C.R. Diniz, L.T.V. Milo, and M. Jamra (1979). The effect of Lachesis muta venom (Clotase) on blood coagulation factors. (Abstract) Thromb. and Haemostasis, 42, 400.

Curtis, C.G., and L. Lorand (1976). Fibrin stabilizing factor (Factor XIII). In L. Lorand (Ed.), Proteolytic Enzymes, Academic Press, New York, San Francisco, London. pp. 177-191.

Davey, M.G., and E.F. Lüscher (1965). Action of some coagulant snake venoms on blooc platelets. Nature, 207, 730-732.

Denson, K.W.E. (1969). Coagulant and anticoagulant action of snake venoms. Toxicon, 7, 5.

Denson, K.W.E., F.E. Russell, D. Almagro, and R.C. Bishop (1972). Characterization of the coagulant activity of some snake venoms. Toxicon, 10, 557-562.

De Vries, A., and I. Cohen (1969). Haemorrhagic and blood coagulation disturbing action of snake venoms. In L. Poller (Ed.), Recent Advances in Blood Coagulatio J. and A. Churchill, London. pp. 277-297.

Egberg, N. (1973). Experimental and clinical studies on the thrombin-like enzyme fr the venom of Bothrops atrox. On the primary structure of fragment E. Acta physi Scand. Suppl. 400.

Franza, B.R., and D.L. Aronson (1976). Detection and measurement of low levels of prothrombin. Use of a procoagulant from Echis carinatus venom. Thromb. Res., 8, 329-336.

Funk, C., J. Gmür, R. Herold, and P.N. Straub (1971). Reptilase-R - A new reagent i blood coagulation. Brit. J. Haematol., 21, 43.

Furie, B.C., and B. Furie (1976). Coagulant protein of Russell's viper venom. In L. Lorand (Ed.), Proteolytic enzymes, Academic Press, New York, San Francisco, Lon don. pp. 191-205.

Gaffney, P.J. (1977). Report of the task force on standards for thrombin and thromb like enzymes. Thromb. and Haemostasis, 38, 562-566.

Gaffney, P.J., N.A. Marsh, and B.C. Whaler (1973). A coagulant enzyme from gaboon v per venom: some aspects of its mode of action. Biochem. Soc. Transactions, 1, 1

Herzig, R.H., O.D. Ratnoff, and J.R. Shainoff (1970). Studies on a procoagulant fra tion of southern copperhead snake venom: the preferential release of fibrinopep tide B. J. Lab. and Clin. Med., 76, 451.

Kaiser, E., and H. Michl (1958). Die Biochemie der tierischen Gifte. Deuticke, Wien

Kelen, E.M.A., G. Rosenfeld, M. Vainzof, and Z.C. Machado (1978). Experimental defi brination with bothropase. Haemostasis, 7, 35-45.

Kisiel, W., M.A. Hermondson, and E.W. Davie (1976). Factor X activating enzyme from Russell' viper venom. Biochem., 15, 4901.

Kornalik, F., and B. Blombäck (1975). Prothrombin activation induced by ecarin - a prothrombin converting enzyme from Echis carinatus venom. Thromb. Res., 6, 53-63.
Lamb, G. (1901). On the action of snake venoms on the coagulability of the blood. Ind. Med. Gaz., 36, 443-455.
Markland, F.S., and P.S. Damus (1971). Purification and properties of a thrombin-like enzyme from the venom of Crotalus adamanteus. J. biol. Chem., 246, 6460-6473.
Markwardt, F., and G. Nowak (1979). The influence of drugs on disseminated intravascular coagulation (DIC). IV. Effects of the thrombin-like enzyme batroxobin on thrombin-induced DIC in rats. Thromb. Res., in press.
Morawitz, P. (1905). Die Chemie der Blutgerinnung. Ergeb. Physiol., 4, 307.
Noc, F. (1904). Sur quelques propriétés physiologiques des différents venins de serpents. Ann. Inst. Pasteur, 18, 387-406.
Niewiarowski, S., E. Kirby, and K. Stocker (1977). Thrombocytin - a novel platelet activating enzyme from Bothrops atrox venom. Thromb. Res., 10, 863-869.
Niewiarowski, S., E.P. Kirby, T.M. Brudzynski, and K. Stocker (1979). Thrombocytin: A serine protease from Bothrops atrox venom. II Interaction with platelets and plasma clotting factors. Biochemistry, in press.
Ouyang, C., I.S. Hong, and Ch. Teng (1971). Purification and properties of the thrombin-like principle of Agkistrodon acutus and its comparison to bovine thrombin. Thromb. Diath. Haem., 26, 224-234.
Ouyang, C., and F.Y. Yang (1974). Purification and properties of the thrombin-like enzymes from Trimeresurus gramineus venom. Biochim. Biophys. Acta (Amsterdam), 351, 354-464.
Rosenfeld, G., L. Nahas, and M.A. Kelen (1968). Coagulant, proteolytic and hemolytic properties of some snake venoms. In W. Bücherl, E. Buckley, and V. Deulofeu (Ed.), Venomous Animals and their venoms, Vol. I, Academic Press, New York, London. pp. 229-273.
Seegers, W.H., and Ouyang, C. (1979). Snake venoms and blood coagulation. In C.Y. Lee (Ed.), Snake venom, Springer-Verlag, Berlin, Heidelberg, New York.
Stocker, K. (1978). Defibrinogenation with thrombin-like snake venom enzymes. In F. Markwardt (Ed.), Fibrinolytics and Antifibrinolytics, Springer-Verlag, Berlin, Heidelberg, New York. pp. 451-484.

BACTERIAL ACTIVATORS OF PROTHROMBIN

J. Jeljaszewicz*, L. M. Switalski*, Z. Wegrzynowicz and G. Pulverer*****

**National Institute of Hygiene, Warsaw, Poland*
***Institute of Nuclear Research, Warsaw, Poland*
****Institute of Hygiene, University of Cologne, Cologne, Federal Republic of Germany*

ABSTRACT

Extracellular substances produced by anaerobic and aerobic bacteria interact with blood-clotting factors by prothrombin activation. Two of them act by formation of stable complexes with prothrombin (staphylothrombin and peptothrombin) which are able to polymerize fibrinogen and produce fibrin and blood clotting without involvement of other blood-clotting factors necessary for physiological clotting. These substances are: staphylocoagulase produced by some strains of *Staphylococcus aureus* and peptocoagulase excreted by some strains of *Peptococcus indolicus*. However, it has been demonstrated that non-specific activation of prothrombin may occur due to proteolytic enzymes produced by some staphylocci, *Bacteroides melaninogenicus* and *Pseudomonas aeruginosa*. It seems that these enzymes act by activation of prothrombin through limited proteolysis and generation of thrombin. Proteolytic enzymes exerting such effects are produced by strains of *Bacteroides* and *Pseudomonas* species and have been extensively studied and mechanisms of action have been proposed. Staphylococcal proteases can simulate the action of staphylocoagulase. A test has been elaborated which enables a clear-cut demonstration as to whether clot formation by staphylococcal extracellular proteases is due to staphylocoagulase or staphylococcal proteases.

KEYWORDS

Blood clotting; staphylocoagulase; peptocoagulase; prothrombin activation; clotting activities of bacteria.

INTRODUCTION

Bacteria and their extracellular products can interact with the blood-clotting system in several different ways. They can activate prothrombin, initiating the fibrinogen-fibrin conversion; activate other blood-clotting factors (directly or through mediation by other factors such as complement); or precipitate fibrinogen in a non-enzymatic way (paracoagulation). Many bacteria possess also an ability to activate plasminogen, which leads to active plasmin formation and fibrinolysis.

Several bacterial species have been reported to be able to clot citrated plasmas obtained from different animal species. At present, it is clear that different mechanisms of action of the clotting pathway may be involved, but data presented by different authors are quite contradictory. This is partly due to the use of different classification systems for bacteria and different methods of testing for clotting and fibrinolytic activity. In some cases, the application of inadequate or even primitive methods to the study of these phenomena has led to the accumulation of false information.

Despite these problems, one can try to summarize the data concerning the clotting activities of bacteria (Table 1). This information was collected from the literature and has not been subjected to critical evaluation.

TABLE 1 Production of Prothrombin Activators by Different Bacterial Species

UNKNOWN MECHANISM OF ACTIVATION[1)]	
Bordetella pertussis	Billaudelle, 1955
Pasteurella pestis	Jawetz & Meyer, 1944; Eisler, 1961
Escherichia coli	Krech, 1952
Serratia marescens, *Bacillus subtilis*, *Actinomyces*, *Streptococcus faecalis*, *Streptococcus durans*[2)]	Wood, 1959
ACTIVATION OF PROTHROMBIN PRESENT IN CITRATED PLASMA BY CITRATE UTILIZATION[3)] (liberation of Ca^{2+} and unblocking of physiological clotting)	
Enterobacter, *Citrobacter* *Salmonella*	Mushin & Kerr, 1954
FORMATION OF A COMPLEX CONSISTING OF BACTERIAL PRODUCT AND PROTHROMBIN	
Staphylococcus aureus	Zajdel and others, 1976
Peptococcus indolicus	Switalski and others, 1978
PROTEOLYTIC ACTIVATION OF PROTHROMBIN BY BACTERIAL ENZYMES	
Bacteroides melaninogenicus	Pulverer and others, 1977 Wegrzynowicz and others, 1978
Pseudomonas aeruginosa	Pulverer and others, 1980
Staphylococcus aureus	Wegrzynowicz and others, 1979

1) Old data which require complete re-investigation. Some clotting may be due to citrate utilization, as is most probably the case with the reported effects of *Streptococcus faecalis* and *Streptococcus durans*. *Bordetella pertussis* effect may be similar to that produced by staphylococcal clumping factor (nonenzymatic paracoagulation by fibrinogen precipitation). Other bacteria may produce proteolytic enzymes causing effects established for products listed in section four of the table.

2) Effects resulting from interference of streptococci with fibrinogen require further studies because of demonstrated interactions of proteins M and T of *Streptococcus pyogenes* with this substrate.

3) In some instances, citrate utilization seems a clear cause. However, re-investigation is required to demonstrate the absence of extracellular substances which may quickly interact with prothrombin in a non-specific way.

The aim of our studies during the last few years has been to re-investigate some extracellular products of anaerobic and aerobic bacteria which are able to interact with prothrombin and to convert it into an active complex with the capacity to initiate conversion of fibrinogen into fibrin. These products are: staphylocoagulase and proteolytic enzymes produced by *Staphylococcus aureus*, peptocoagulase of *Peptococcus indolicus*, and proteolytic enzymes of *Bacteroides melaninogenicus* and *Pseudomonas aeruginosa*.

PEPTOCOAGULASE

Sørensen (1973, 1974) was the first to describe the production of a plasma-clotting factor by strains of *Peptococcus indolicus*, anaerobic cocci isolated most frequently from animals. This phenomenon has been studied by us in detail (Switalski and others, 1978). Our studies indicate that most strains of this microorganism are able to produce an extracellular substance capable of clot production in vitro. This substance, named by us peptocoagulase, is produced during the stationary growth phase and can occur also in cell-bound form. Peptocoagulase has been purified by ammonium sulphate precipitation followed by DEAE-Sephadex chromatography and ultrafiltration. It does not possess any proteolytic (amidolytic) activity when tested on natural protein substrates or synthetic chromogenic substrates. The activity of purified peptocoagulase is limited to prothrombin activation. The mechanism of its action is similar to that previously described for staphylocoagulase, although both substances are completely different chemically, physically and immunologically.

STAPHYLOCOAGULASE AND PROTEASES OF *Staphylococcus aureus*

Strains of *S. aureus* produce an extracellular substance which clots plasmas of different animal species. A full account of the properties and mode of action of this substance has been presented elsewhere (Zajdel and others, 1976). It has been demonstrated that staphylocoagulase reacts stoichiometrically with prothrombin. This results in active complex formation and the emergence of the ability to convert fibrinogen into fibrin. However, the situation became more complex after discovery of the role of proteolytic enzymes produced by some staphylococci. It is quite evident that these can interact with prothrombin and perhaps other blood-clotting factors.

Staphylococci are known to produce at least three proteolytic enzymes. Some of them have been extensively purified and characterized (Arvidson and others, 1973; Björklind and Jörnvall, 1974; Drapeau, 1976). Interaction of these enzymes with the blood-clotting system has been studies by us on 245 strains of *S. aureus* (Wegrzynowicz and others, 1979). It appeared that all but eight strains clotted rabbit plasma within 18 hours. When Trasylol (protease inhibitor) and/or heparin was added to plasma the percentage of clotting-positive strains decreased markedly, whereas the number of strains exhibiting weak clotting activity increased. These observations indicate that, in some cases, clotting of plasma by staphylococcal extracellular products may be due to the action of factors other than staphylocoagulase. We have also observed an extension of clotting time in the presence of these inhibitors. This may be considered as additional evidence for the view that other factors besides staphylocoagulase are involved in the clotting effect produced by staphylococci. These observations point up the need for a new test for the detection of "true" staphylocoagulase.

Pseudomonas aeruginosa ENZYME

Strains of these bacteria produce several extracellular enzymes possessing proteolytic activity (Morihara, 1974). One protease and elastase of *P. aeruginosa* has been purified and characterized. It was postulated many years ago that some extracellular substances of this microorganism can induce clotting of plasma (Pulverer and Korth, 1962).

In our studies (Pulverer and others, 1980) 101 out of 136 strains of *P. aeruginosa* isolated from clinical sources produced such an effect. The enzyme responsible for this phenomenon has been isolated and purified by ammonium sulphate precipitation. Active fractions were subjected to ion exchange chromatography and preparative flat bed isoelectric focussing. The activity of this purified enzyme was determined by the use of chromogenic substrates. It has been demonstrated that the investigated strain of *P. aeruginosa* produces as least five proteases, one of which activates prothrombin. This process occurs within 3 minutes, and the clotting effect is well demonstrable for the next 30 minutes. The clotting activity of *P. aeruginosa* is inhibited by EDTA. Other inhibitors, such as diisopropylfluorophosphate, N-ethylmaleimide, ε-aminocaproic acid and soybean trypsin inhibitor have no effect.

Bacteroides melaninogenicus ENZYME

Another bacterial species has been recognized as being able to interact with the blood-clotting system. Early observations concerning this property exhibited by *Bacteroides melaninogenicus* (Pulverer, 1958; Pulverer and Heinrich, 1960) have been recently confirmed (Pulverer and others, 1977; Wegrzynowicz and others, 1978).

Our observations indicate that most strains of the *B. melaninogenicus* species produce extracellular substances exhibiting clotting activity. This property is more common among strains belonging to subspecies *asaccharolyticus* (76 out of 87 strains tested were positive) than among subspecies *intermedius* (7 out of 19 strains tested were positive). The kinetics of *B. melaninogenicus* clotting factor parallel the bacterial growth curve. When incubated with prothrombin the enzyme can activate the substrate within a few minutes, but after reaching the peak of clotting activity the activity decreases. This is quite different from the action of substances of the staphylocoagulase type, where the activity of the staphylocoagulase-prothrombin complex (staphylothrombin) remains stable. We postulate that the disappearance of clotting activity of the *Bacteroides* enzyme-prothrombin mixture is related to a completely different mechanism of action. Probably in the first step of prothrombin activation limited proteolysis occurs which is similar, but not identical with that observed during physiological clotting. However, an active form of prothrombin (activated by the *Bacteroides* enzyme) is digested later by proteases produces by the same strain, which, in turn, results in prothrombin/thrombin inactivation.

REFERENCES

Arvidson, S. T. Holme, and B. Lindholm (1973). Studies on extracellular proteolytic enzymes from *Staphylococcus aureus*. I. Purification and characterization of one neutral and one alkaline protease. Biochim. Biophys. Acta, 302, 135-148.

Billaudelle, H. (1955). Studien am *Haemophilus pertussis* (Bordet-Gengou). II. Die Koagulase bei *Haemophilus pertussis*. Acta Pathol. Microbiol. Acand., 37, 5-13.

Björklind, A., and H. Jörnvall (1974). Substrate specificity of three different extracellular proteolytic enzymes from *Staphylococcus aureus*. Biochim. Biophys. Acta, 370, 524-529.

Eisler, D. M. (1961). Coagulation of human plasma by *Pasteurella pestis*. J. Bacteriol., 81, 241-245.

Jawetz, E., and K. F. Meyer (1944). Studies on plague immunity in experimental animals. II. Some factors of the immunity mechanism in bubonic plague. J. Immunol., 49, 15-30.

Krech, U. (1952). Untersuchungen über di Koagulation von menschlichen und tierischen Plasma durch Bacterium coli. Ztschr. Immunitätsforsch., 109, 206-209.

Morihara, K. (1974). Comparative specificity of microbial proteinases. In: A. Meister (ed.), Advances in Enzymology, Academic Press, New York, pp 179-243.

Mushin, R, and V. J. Kerr (1954). Clotting of citrated plasma and citrate utilization by intestinal Gram-negative bacilli. J. Gen. Microbiol., 10, 445-451.

Pulverer, G. (1958). Zur Morphologie, Biochemie und Serologie des *Bacteroides melaninogenicus*. Ztschr. Hyg. Infekt., 145, 293-303.

Pulverer, G., and S. Heinrich (1960). Infektionsversuche an Laboratoriumstieren und in vitro Untersuchungen zur Fermentausstattung des *Bacteroides melaninogenicus*. Ztschr. Hyg. Infekt., 146, 341-349.

Pulverer, G., H. L. Ko, Z. Wegrzynowicz, and J. Jeljaszewicz (1977). Clotting and fibrinolytic activities of *Bacteroides melaninogenicus*. Zbl. Bakt. Hyg., I. Abt. Orig. A, 239, 510-513.

Pulverer, B., and H. Korth (1962). Zur Biochemie und Fermentstruktur von *Pseudomonas aeruginosa*. Zbl. Bakt. Hyg., I. Abt. Orig. A, 186, 36-54.

Pulverer, G., Z. Wegrzynowicz, H. Hl Ko, and J. Jeljaszewicz (1980). Prothrombin and plasminogen activators produced by *Pseudomonas aeruginosa*. Zbl. Bakt. Hyg., I. Abt. Orig. A, in press.

Sørensen. G. H. (1973). *Micrococcus indolicus*. Some biochemical properties and the demonstration of six antigenically different types. Acta Vet. Scand., 14, 301-326.

Sørensen, G. H. (1974). Studies on the aetiology and transmission of summer mastitis. Nord. Veterinärmed., 26, 122-132.

Switakski, L. M., O. Schwan, C. J. Smyth, and T. Wadström (1978). Peptocoagulase: clotting factor produced by bovine strains of *Peptococcus indolicus*. J. Clin. Microbiol., 7, 361-367.

Wegrzynowicz, Z., P. B. Heczko, J. Jeljaszewicz, M. Neugebauer, and G. Pulverer (1979). Pseudocoagulase activity of staphylococci. J. Clin. Microbiol., 9, 15-19.

Wegrzynowicz, Z., H. L. Ko, G. Pulverer, and J. Jeljaszewicz (1978). The nature of clotting and fibrinolytic activities of *Bacteroides melaninogenicus*. Zbl. Bakt. Hyg., I. Abt., Orig. A, 240, 106-111.

Wood, M. (1959). The clotting of plasma by group D streptococci. J. Gen Microbiol. 21, 385-388.

Zajdel, M., Z. Wegrzynowicz, J. Sawecka, J. Jeljaszewicz, and G. Pulverer (1976). Mechanism of action of staphylocogulase. In: J. Jeljaszewicz (ed.), Staphylococci and Staphyloccal Diseases. Gustav Fischer Verlag, Stuttgart, pp. 549-575.

CLASSIFICATION OF PHOSPHOLIPASES A_2 BASED UPON THEIR ANTICOAGULANT ACTIVITY AND PENETRATION ABILITY INTO PHOSPHOLIPID MONOLAYERS

M. C. Boffa*, C. Rothen, H. M. Verheij***, R. Verger** and G. H. De Haas*****

**Laboratoire d'Hémostase, C.N.T.S., 6 rue Alexandre Cabanel, 75739 Paris Cedex 15, France*
***CNRS, Centre de Biochimie et Biologie Moléculaire, 13274 Marseille Cedex 2, France*
****Laboratory of Biochemistry, State University, University Center of Uithof, Utrecht, The Netherlands*

ABSTRACT

The anticoagulant effect and the penetration ability into phospholipid monolayers of purified phospholipases A_2 were analysed. This study enabled the distinction of two groups of enzymes : one group of strongly anticoagulant phospholipases exhibiting high penetration ability into tightly packed phosphatidyl-choline monolayers and another group of phospholipases without anticoagulant activity and with weak penetrating ability.
The anticoagulant enzymes were all basic proteins. However this cannot by itself explain the anticoagulant effect : some non anticoagulant phospholipases possess likewise a basic character.
Among the basic enzymes, two groups were strikingly separated : one group of basic anticoagulant phospholipases known as moderately toxic, and able to bind to erythrocytes, and another group of non anticoagulant phospholipases with low penetrating ability and highly neurotoxic activity.
The proposed classification of the phospholipases according to their anticoagulant effect may help towards a better understanding of the different biological effects of these lipolytic enzymes.

KEY WORDS

Phospholipase A_2, anticoagulant; phospholipid monolayer; neurotoxin.

INTRODUCTION

An anticoagulant factor displaying phospholipase A_2 activity has previously been purified from the venom of *Vipera berus orientale* (Boffa G.A., Boffa M.C. and Winchenne, 1976). Both phospholipase and anticoagulant properties seemed to be related : it was not possible to separate them by temperature and pH changes or by photo-oxydation as well as by immunological inhibition (Boffa M.C. and Boffa G.A., 1976). In contrast, phospholipases A_2 purified from the venom of *Vipera aspis* (Boffa and co-workers, 1971) did not show any anticoagulant effect.

It was therefore interesting to examine the anticoagulant properties of a relatively large number of purified phospholipases A_2 and to study the relation between the anticoagulant and the enzymatic activities.

As demonstrated previously, kinetics of lipolytic enzymes, at the air-water interface, can be successfully analysed by a monolayer technic at constant lipid surface pressure (Verger, Mieras and de Haas, 1973). The ability of an enzyme to penetrate into the lipid monolayer can be evaluated by measuring at different pressures, the induction time of lipolysis and under steady state conditions, the hydrolysis velocity (Verger and de Haas, 1976).

In this work we report the effect on clotting of 26 highly purified phospholipases A_2 and the relationship between their anticoagulant activities and their ability to penetrate into phospholipid monolayers.

MATERIAL AND METHODS

Phospholipases A_2 : Pig pancreas phospholipase was purified in Utrecht (Nieuwenhuizen, Kunze and de Haas, 1974) and *Vipera berus* and *aspis* phospholipases in Paris, as described above. Twenty-three other purified enzymes were kindly provided by different laboratories, as listed in table I. Crotapotin, devoid of phospholipase activity was included in the study because it is part of the crotoxin complex, formed with a basic phospholipase A_2 and the acidic crotapotin as reviewed by Habermann and Breithaupt (1978).

Clotting Assays : Recalcification times were measured at 37°C on human platelet poor plasma, obtained from human citrated (1 : 9, v/v) blood (Boffa, Delori and Soulier, 1972). Veronal buffer : 0.026 M sodium barbital /0.026 M sodium acetate/ 0.1 M NaCl, pH 7.3, was used for control and for diluting phospholipases.

Kinetics Studies on Phospholipid Monolayers : Didodecanoyl phosphatidyl-choline was prepared by reacylation of glyceryl phosphocholine according to Cubero-Robles and van Den Berg (1969). A zero order trough with 2 compartments and a fully automatized barostat was used as previously described (Verger and de Haas, 1973).

After spreading the phospholipid film at the desired pressure, the enzyme was injected into the stirred subphase and hydrolysis recorded. After an induction time during which the rate of hydrolysis progressively increased, the hydrolysis became linear. The induction time was then measured and plotted for each different surface pressure (Verger, Mieras and de Haas, 1973).

RESULTS

Anticoagulant Properties of Phospholipases A_2 (fig. 1 and table I)

As seen in fig. 1, phospholipases could be separated into 3 groups, according to their anticoagulant properties. *Group I* : 5 anticoagulant phospholipases which delayed indefinitely the plasma recalcification time, at the concentration of 2,5 µg of enzyme/ml of plasma. *Groups III* : 15 non anticoagulant phospholipases. At the same concentration, they did not modify the plasma clotting time while the 6 phospholipases listed in *group II*, delayed it moderately (5 to 15 min.) and constituted an intermediary group. There was no clear cut separation between the 3 groups. The enzymes are listed from the most active (the basic phospholipase from *Naja nigricollis*) to the least active (the acidic component of crotoxin, crotapotin).

Fig. 1 : Recalcification times obtained with the phospholipases A_2 at different concentrations.

Clotting assay

0.2 ml of plasma

+ 0.1 ml of phospholipase.

Incubation 37°C - 60 sec.

+ 0.2 ml of $CaCL_2$ 0.025 M

Control time (buffer instead of phospholipase) = 3'45 ± 10 sec.

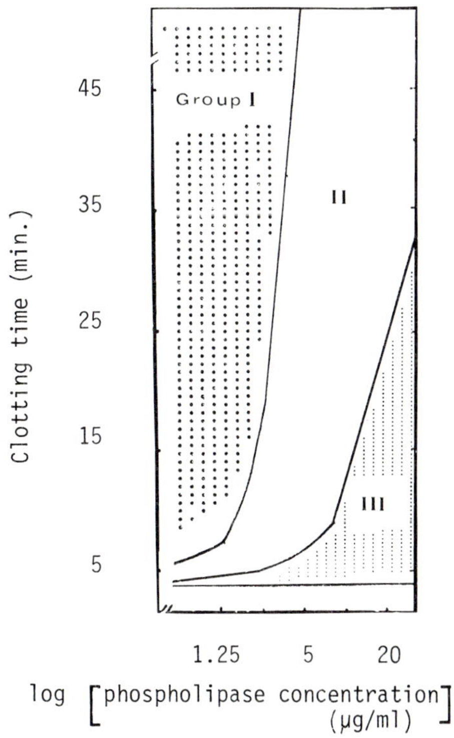

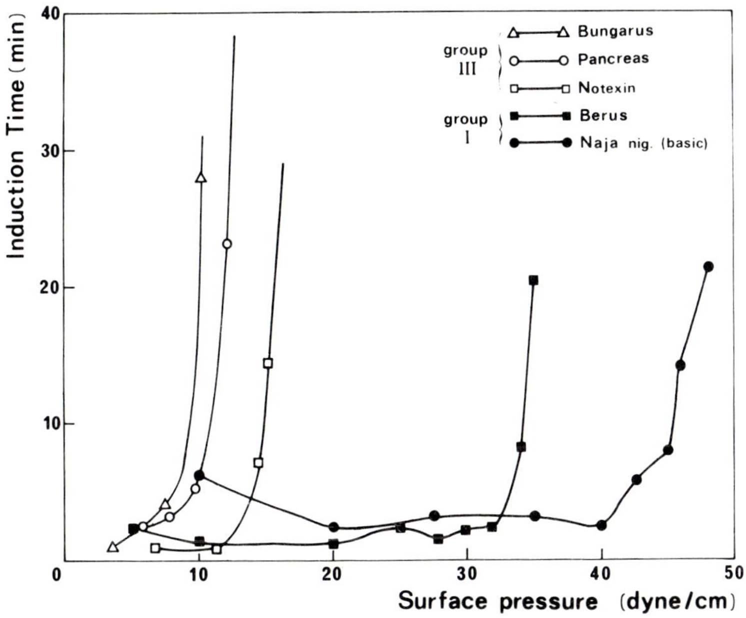

Fig. 2: Variation of induction time with surface pressure:didodecanoyl phosphatidyl choline monolayer hydrolysis by phospholipases A_2 from different origins : per ml; β-bungarotoxin,100 µg. Pancreas,8 µg. Notexin,2.5 µg. *Vipera berus*, 0.6 µg. *Naja nig* (basic, 0.1 µg. Experimental details in Verger and de Haas (1973).

TABLE I. Classification of phospholipases A_2 according to their anticoagulant properties.

	Animal origin of the venom	Phospholipase (Venom fraction)	Purified fraction kindly provided by	Isoelectric point
GROUP I	NAJA *nigricollis*	Basic	Eaker, Uppsala Boquet, Paris	> 9.5
	NAJA *mossambica moss.*	(CM III)	Joubert, Pretoria Rochat, Marseille	> 9.5
	AGKISTRODON *halys blom.*	Basic	Hanahan, San Antonio	> 9.5
	VIPERA *berus orient.*		Boffa, Paris	> 9.5
	CROTALUS *durissus terr.*		Habermann, Giessen	> 9.5
GROUP II	APIS *mellifera* (bee)		Shipolini, London	> 9.5
	NAJA *mossambica moss.*	(CM II)	Joubert, Pretoria	8.8
	NAJA *nigricollis*	Acid	Boquet, Paris	
	AGKISTRODON *halys blom.*	Neutral	Hanahan, San Antonio	6.7
	ENHYDRINA *schistosa*	Myotoxin (VI:5)	Lind-Eaker, Uppsala	> 9
	OXYURANUS *scutellatus*	Taipoxin	Lind-Eaker, Uppsala	10 - 7 - 2.5 *
GROUP III	HAEMATACHUS *haematachus*	(DE I)	Joubert, Pretoria	
	NAJA *moss. moss.*	(CM I)	Rochat, Marseille	
	NAJA *naja naja*		Dennis, La Jolla	5
	BITIS *gabonica*		Viljoen, Pretoria	
	NAJA *melanoleuca*	(DE III)	Joubert, Pretoria	
	NAJA *melanoleuca*	(DE II)	Joubert, Pretoria	
	CROTALUS *adamanteus*		Wells, Tucson	4.6
	CROTALUS *durissus terr.*	Crotoxin	Habermann, Giessen	5
	NOTECHIS *scutatus scut.*	(II-5)	Eaker, Uppsala	> 9
	PIG PANCREAS		De Haas, Utrecht	6.45
	AGKISTRODON *halys blom.*	Acid	Hanahan, San Antonio	4
	CROTALUS *atrox*		Kleps-Kezdy, Chicago	4.5
	VIPERA *aspis B*		Boffa, Paris	7.2
	NOTECHIS *scutatus scut.*	Notexin	Lind-Eaker, Uppsala	> 9
	BUNGARUS *multicinctus*	β-bungarotoxin	Abe, Niigata City Strong, London	> 9
	CROTALUS *durissus terr.*	Crotapotin	Habermann, Giessen	3.6

* Taipoxin consists of 3 chains.

It can be noticed that group I contains exclusively basic enzymes. However all basic phospholipases are not anticoagulant. This is particularly noticeable for neurotoxins such as notexin or β-bungarotoxin. These basic enzymes had no effect on clotting, even at the concentration of 10 µg/ml of Plasma.

Ability of Phospholipases A_2 to Penetrate Phospholipid Monolayers Films (fig. 2).

Figure 2 illustrates kinetic studies obtained on monolayer film of didodecanoyl phosphatidylcholine with 5 enzymes : 2 anticoagulant from group I and 3 non-anticoagulant : the neutral porcine pancreas phospholipase and 2 basic enzymes from group III. Two distinct patterns are clearly distinguishable : one corresponding to anticoagulant enzymes and the other to non anticoagulant ones. When the surface pressure of the film reaches a critical pressure (higher than 15 dynes/cm) the non anticoagulant enzymes can no longer penetrate into the phospholipid layer and no hydrolysis can take place. The maximum velocity for these enzymes was observed for surface pressures lower than 15 dynes/cm. At the opposite for anticoagulant enzymes, the maximum velocity corresponded to high pressures around 30 dynes/cm. At 40 dynes/cm, the anticoagulant phospholipase from *Naja nigricollis* still displayed a marked enzymatic activity.

New data, obtained with other phospholipases, again showed a penetration ability and an anticoagulant activity well correlated with the proposed classification : in group I *Crotalus durissus terr.* phospholipase (component B of the crotoxin complex) behaved the same as *Vipera berus* phospholipase, in group III, both the *Notechis* phospholipase (II-5) and the Crotoxin complex exhibited a weak penetrating capacity, slightly higher than that of βbungarotoxin.

DISCUSSION - CONCLUSION

The anticoagulant effect of snake venoms, known for a long time (Tu, 1977) may result essentially from two distinct mechanisms, either defibrination by a thrombin-like or a fibrino/fibrinogenolytic agent or inhibition of the pro-coagulant activity of phospholipid. The role of the phospholipases in the anti-coagulant effect was already suspected in the fifties, by Kruse and Dam (1950) for *Naja naja* venom and by Habermann (1954) for bee venom. More recently, the main anti-coagulant factor in the venom of *Vipera berus* was shown (Boffa M.C. and Boffa G.A., 1976) to be a phospholipase A_2, such is the case for the anticoagulant factor isolated from *Trimeresurus mucrosquamatus* (Ouyang and co-workers, 1978). In spite of extensive kinetic and structural studies on phospholipases A_2, their role in the anticoagulant effect as well as in the neuro toxicity remains unclear.

From this work, it appears that five enzymes (Group I) out of the 26 studied enzymes possess marked anticoagulant activity. They belong to 3 different families of venomous snakes : elapidae, crotalidae and viperidae. They are all basic proteins. They are able to penetrate rapidly into monolayers of phospholipid, packed at such high pressure as 30 dynes/cm. By this last property, they can be distinguished from the non anticoagulant enzymes (Group III), unable to do so and thereby incapable of hydrolysing rapidly such packed phospholipid. Thirty to thirty-five dynes/cm correspond roughly to the lipid packing of phospholipid in membranes of red cells (Demel and co-workers, 1975) and platelets (Chap, Zwaal and Van Deenen, 1977). Phospholipids active in clotting come from platelet. Released from the membrane, as lipoprotein complexes, they probably keep their original packing structure. In this hypothesis, only group I phospholipases would be able to hydrolyse these procoagulant phospholipids.

The importance of the velocity of the enzyme penetration in the lipid layer has to be emphazised. Indeed the formation of the clot is the result of a rapid sequential activation of clotting enzymes. In this process, phospholipids are well known to play a major speed-amplifying role. The anticoagulant phospholipases, at the concentration of 2,5 μg/ml of plasma, complete their hydrolytic action during the 3-4 minutes which are necessary to clot formation, after calcium addition to citrated plasma. For this reason only phospholipases from group I can be designated as "anticoagulant"; phospholipases from group III such as pig pancreas phospholipase at similar concentration, were also able to prevent clot formation, but only if they were incubated overnight with the plasma (unpublished results). Because of such a long delay,this cannot be considered as an efficient anticoagulant effect.

The anticoagulant activity and highly penetrating capacity of the group I phospholipases cannot be directly related to the basic character of these proteins : the basic phospholipases,βbungarotoxin and notexin,are non anticoagulant and have weak penetrating ability (see fig. 2), even when using negatively charged phospholipid monolayers (didodecanoyl phosphatidyl serine or glycerol) at different surface pressures (data not shown). The basic character of a phospholipase and/or a toxin is not "per se" required for a strong penetration capacity, even into negatively charged phospholipids. However the anticoagulant property and the penetration ability are two non dissociable characters of all the phospholipases we have studied so far.

From the biological standpoint, this classification of phospholipases shows two groupsof basic enzymes strikingly separated. On one hand, the basic anticoagulant phospholipases which could display moderately toxic, cardiotoxin-like, hemolytic activity (Dumarey and co-workers, 1975; Lee, Ho and Eaker, 1977) on the other hand, the non anticoagulant, presynaptic neurotoxins such as β-bungarotoxin (Strong and co-workers, 1976), notexin (Halpert, Eaker and Karlsson, 1976) and crotoxin (Hendon and Fraenkel-Conrat, 1971; Habermann and Breithaupt, 1978) with weak penetrating capacity. It seems that the most powerful neurotoxin : taipoxin (Fohlman and co-workers, 1976) and the myotoxin from *Enhydrina schistosa* (Fohlman and Eaker, 1977), outstanding for its lethal and myonecrotic effect, both present in group II, have to be distinguished from the other group III neurotoxins.

The case of crotoxin is worth particular attention in this regard. This presynaptic neurotoxin represents a two-units complex, consisting of a phospholipaseA_2 (component B) less toxic than the complex itself, and an acidic component A, devoid of enzymatic and neurotoxic activity. It has been established that crotapotin prevent component B from non specific binding to membranes, allowing it to reach the nerve terminal and to exert there its enzymatic activity (Chang and Su, 1978; Habermann and Breithaupt, 1978). Our results agree with those findings:component B was found pertaining to the anticoagulant and highly penetrating group I phospholipases. Crotapotin had no effect on clotting. Moreover,when it was added to component B to form the crotoxin complex (group III), the anticoagulant activity disappeared. Along the same lines,ourresults appear consistent with the study concerning the binding of ^{125}I labelled crotoxin, β-bungarotoxin and *Crotalus adamenteus* phospholipases to rabbit erythrocytes and ghosts : Jeng and co-workers (1978) found a much higher binding for crotoxin than for the two others phospholipases. They proved that crotoxin splits in the course of binding into A and B and only the highly penetrating component B was found to be bound to the erythocyte membrane.

These results broaden the concept elaborated from the analysis of the crotoxin complex. It can be suggested that the group I enzymes, once introduced into the blood stream, bind primarily to the nearest membranes (such as red cell membranes) while the group III enzymes because of their low penetrating ability, are able to reach their more distant specific target, such as the nerve end-plate terminal for the neurotoxins, where they exhibit their enzymatic activity.

In conclusion, this classification of phospholipases A_2, primarily settled in regard to their anticoagulant activity, might be useful in the analysis of the numerous biological effects of these lipolytic enzymes.

ACKNOWLEDGEMENTS

This work was supported by grant ATP 33 34 from C.N.R.S. The author wishes to thank C. Millac and M. Baudy for excellent technical assistance.

REFERENCES

Boffa, G.A., M.C. Boffa, M.M. Zakin, and M. Burstein (1971). Role of serum lipoproteins in hemolysis induced by *Vipera aspis* venom phospholipases. *Prot. Biol. Fluids Proc. Colloq.*, 19, 85-88.

Boffa, M.C., P. Delori, and J.P. Soulier (1972). Anticoagulant factors from Viperidae venoms. Platelet phospholipid inhibitor. *Thrombos. Diathes. haemorrh.*, 27, 509-523

Boffa, G.A., M.C. Boffa, and J.J. Winchenne (1976). A phospholipase A_2 with anti-coagulant activity : isolation and properties. *Biochim. Biophys. Acta*, 429, 828-838.

Boffa, M.C., and G.A. Boffa (1976). A phospholipase A_2 with anticoagulant activity. II. Inhibition of the phospholipid activity in coagulation. *Biochim. Biophys. Acta*, 429, 839-852.

Chang, C.C., and M.J.Su (1978). The mechanism of potentiation of the presynaptic effect of phospholipase A_2 by the crotapotin component of the crotoxin complex. *Toxicon*, 16, 402-405.

Chap, H., R.F.A.Zwaal, and L.L.M. Van Deenen (1977). Action of highly purified phospholipases on blood platelet. Evidence for an asymetric distribution of phospholipid in the surface membrane. *Biochim. Biophys. Acta*, 467, 146-164.

Cubero-Robles, E., and D. Van Den Berg (1969). Synthesis of lecithins by acylation of O - (Sn - Glycero - 3 - phosphoryl) choline with fatty acid anhydrides. *Biochim. Biophys. Acta*, 187, 520-526.

Demel, R.A., W.S.M. Geurts Van Dessel, R.F.A. Zwaal, B. Roelofsen and L.L.M. Van Deenen (1975). Relation between various phospholipase actions on human red cell membranes and the interfacial phospholipid pressure in monolayers. *Biochim. Biophys. Acta*, 406, 97- 107.

Dumarey, C., D. Sket, D. Joseph et P. Boquet (1975). Etude d'une phospholipase basique du venin de *Naja nigricollis*. *C.R. Acad. Sc. Paris*, 280, 1633-1636.

Fohlman, J., D. Eaker, E. Karlsson, and S. Thesleff (1976). Taïpoxin, an extremely potent presynaptic neurotoxin from the venom of the Australian snake Taïpan (*Oxyuranus s. scutellatus*). Isolation, characterization, quaternary structure and pharmacological properties. *Eur. J. Biochem.*, 68, 457-469.

Fohlman, J., and D. Eaker (1977). Isolation and characterization of a lethal myotoxin phospholipase A from the venom of the common sea snake *Enhydrina schistosa* causing myoglobinuria in mice. *Toxicon*, 15, 385-393.

Habermann, E. (1954). Untersuchungen über die Hemmung der Blutgerinnung durch Bienengift. *Arch. expl. Path. Pharm.*, 223, 182.

Habermann, E. and H. Breithaupt (1978). The crotoxin complex - an example of biochemical and pharmacological protein complementation. *Toxicon*, 16, 19-30.

Halpert, J., D. Eaker, and E. Karlsson (1976). The role of phospholipase activity in the action of a presynaptic neurotoxin from the venom of *Notechis scutatus scutatus* (Australian Tiger snake). *FEBS Lett.*,61,72-76

Hendon, R.A., and H. Fraenkel-Conrat (1971). Biological roles of the two components of crotoxin. *Proc. Nat. Acad. Sci. U.S.A.*, 68, 1560-1563.

Jeng, T.W., R.A. Hendon, and H. Fraenkel-Conrat (1978). Search for relationship among the hemolytic, phospholipolytic, and neurotoxic activities of snake venoms. *Proc. Nat. Acad. Sci. U.S.A.*, 75, 600-604.
Kruse, I., and H. Dam (1950). Inactivation of thromboplastin by cobra venom. *Biochim. Biophys. Acta*, 5, 268-274.
Lee, C.Y., C.L. Ho, and D. Eaker (1977). Cardiotoxin-like action of a basic phospholipase A isolated from *Naja nigricollis* venom. *Toxicon*, 15, 355-356.
Nieuwenhuizen, W., H. Kunze, and G.H. de Haas (1974). In S. Fleischer, and L. Packer (Ed), *Methods Enzymol. Biomembranes*, Vol. 32 B. Academic Press, New York. Phospholipase A_2 from Porcine pancreas, 147-154.
Ouyang, C., C.M. Teng, Y.C. Chen, and S.C. Lin (1978). Purification and characterization of the anticoagulant principle of *Trimeresurus mucrosquamatus* venom. *Biochim. Biophys. Acta*, 541, 394-407.
Strong, P.N., J. Goerke, S.G. Oberg, and R.B. Kelly (1976). β-bungarotoxin, a pre-synaptic toxin with enzymatic activity. *Proc. Nat. Acad. Sci.*, 73,178-182.
Tu, T.A. (1977). In A.T. Tu (Ed), *Venoms : Chemistry and Molecular biology*. John Wiley and Sons, New York, Phospholipase A_2. 27-46..
Verger, R., and G.H. de Haas (1973). Enzyme reactions in a membrane model. *Chem. Phys. Lipids*, 10, 127-136.
Verger, R., M.C.E. Mieras, and G.H. de Haas (1973). Action of phospholipase A at interfaces. *J. Biol. Chem.*, 248, 4023-4034.
Verger, R., and G.H. de Haas (1976). Interfacial enzyme kinetics of lipolysis. *Ann. Rev. Biophys. Bioeng.*, 5, 77-117.

INTERFERENCE OF ENDOTOXIN WITH BLOOD COAGULATION[1]

G. Müller-Berghaus

Department of Medicine, Justus-Liebig-Universität, Klinikstrasse 36, Giessen, Federal Republic of Germany

ABSTRACT

Intravenous endotoxin can induce generalized intravascular coagulation. The sequence of reactions may be summarized as activation of coagulation, fibrinemia and clot formation. Several mechanisms of coagulation activation are discussed: Hageman factor-, platelet-, leukocyte- and complement-dependent pathways. The result of coagulation activation is an in vivo state of fibrinemia which per se is harmless for the body. The precipitation of soluble fibrin, however, may lead to fibrin-rich microclots causing organ dysfunction.

KEYWORDS

Endotoxin; intravascular coagulation; generalized Schwartzman reaction; platelets; leukocytes; complement; Hageman factor; soluble fibrin; microclots.

INTRODUCTION

Endotoxin from gram-negative bacteria produces multiple biologic effects, one of which is the interference with blood coagulation. The biological effects of endotoxin on blood coagulation are most important in disease states such as bacterial infection, septicemia and endotoxin shock. Some of the pathophysiological changes observed in endotoxin-caused severely ill patients have successfully been imitated in animals. After endotoxin injection, the animal may develop shock, peripheral blood cell changes and generalized intravascular coagulation. Although these biological effects of endotoxin have been recognized for a long time, the precise mechanisms for many of these changes are not well understood at present. This subject has been reviewed several times (for further references see Müller-Berghaus and Lasch, 1975). In this synopsis I shall summarize several sequences of endotoxin-induced reactions which may lead to intravascular coagulation. Direct evidence for a proposed pathophysiological sequence is frequently missing and conclusions are merely drawn by exclusion.

[1]Supported by the Deutsche Forschungsgemeinschaft, Bonn-Bad Godesberg.

GENERALIZED INTRAVASCULAR COAGULATION-CONSUMPTION COAGULOPATHY

The exposure of the circulating blood to endotoxin may result in a hemorrhagic diathesis. The coagulation analysis of patients suffering from endotoxin-induced hemorrhagic diathesis demonstrate low platelet counts, prolongation of the bleeding time, the prothrombin time and the partial thromboplastin time. The concentrations of nearly all coagulation factors in the plasma are generally reduced as well as platelet factor 3 activity. Such coagulation findings may be explained as consequences of intravascular coagulation with consumption of coagulation factors. Therefore, this clinical syndrome is called generalized intravascular coagulation or consumption coagulopathy.

GENERALIZED SCHWARTZMAN REACTION

A few of the mechanisms leading to intravascular coagulation have been elucidated and can best be studied by an examination of the generalized Schwartzman reaction. Two intravenous injections of bacterial endotoxin into rabbits elicit the generalized Schwartzman reaction, which is defined as occlusion of the renal glomerular capillaries with fibrin-rich microclots, resulting in bilateral renal cortical necrosis (McKay, 1963). The microclots occluding the renal glomerular capillaries contain predominantly a fibrinogen-derived material, thus indicating the participation of coagulation in this pathophysiologic event.

The sequence of reactions resulting in microclot formation may be summarized as follows (Fig. 1): endotoxin activates the coagulation system, causing the generation of thrombin. Thrombin converts fibrinogen to fibrin, which polymerizes to microclots. The precise mechanism by which endotoxin activates the coagulation system is not completely understood.

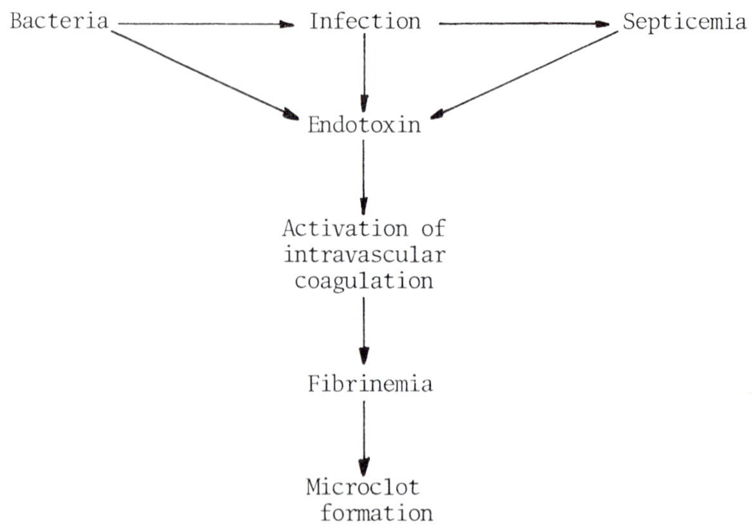

Fig. 1. Schematic representation of the events occurring after the entrance of endotoxin into the circulating blood.

ACTIVATION OF INTRAVASCULAR COAGULATION

Several mechanisms of the activation of coagulation by endotoxin have been proposed, such as the involvement of Hageman factor, platelets, leukocytes, complement and endothelial cells. The validity of the different factors will be critically reviewed.

Hageman Factor Activation

Indirect evidence has indicated that Hageman factor may be activated upon administration of endotoxin. Low Hageman factor activity has been observed in patients in shock from Gram-negative bacteremia as well as in rabbits after endotoxin injection. Thus, the in vitro experiments of Morrison and Cochrane (1974) seemed to be directory, as these authors observed an activation of purified Hageman factor by endotoxin.

Studies in rabbits showed that Hageman factor levels decreased continuously after injection of endotoxin. Hageman factor activity, however, did not decrease if the animals had been pretreated with the vitamin K-antagonist, coumarin (Müller-Berghaus and Schneberger, 1979). A fall in Hageman factor activity similar to that seen in the controls should also have occurred in coumarin-treated animals if endotoxin acted directly on Hageman factor, as vitamin K-antagonists do not affect the first phase of the intrinsic pathway of coagulation. Most likely, the reduction in Hageman factor activity was secondary to other effects of the endotoxin. Furthermore, the activation of intravascular coagulation was not prevented if Hageman factor activation was inhibited by lysozyme infusion (Müller-Berghaus and Schneberger, 1971). Animals continuously infused before and after the injection of endotoxin developed renal glomerular microclots as did control animals not given lysozyme. Thus, the importance of Hageman factor in triggering intravascular coagulation by endotoxin has not been demonstrated, although in vitro purified Hageman factor can be activated by endotoxin.

Platelet-Endotoxin Interaction

In man as well as in different animal species, platelet counts in the circulating blood decrease after endotoxin has entered the circulation. Several studies demonstrate the binding of endotoxin to human as well as to animal platelets (Springer and Adye, 1975; Hawiger and colleagues, 1977). Not surprisingly, platelets clump

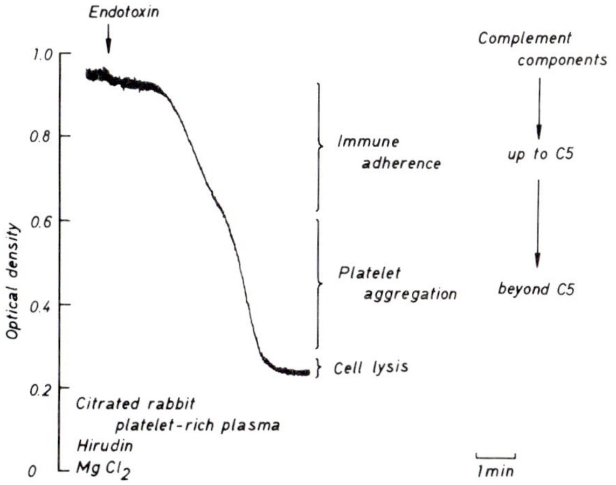

Fig. 2. Endotoxin-induced clumping of rabbit platelets. Two phases of the clumping durve are observed if platelet-rich plasma is stirred after the addition of endotoxin. The postulated mechanisms are: immune adherence for the first phase and complement-dependent platelet aggregation (an active process of platelets) for the second phase. Cell lysis after complete activation on complement occurs at the end of the clumping curve.

upon contact with endotoxin. Recent studies from our laboratory have shown that large amounts of endotoxin induced a two-phase "clumping" curve. Most interestingly, endotoxin also clumped formalin-fixed platelets if plasma and magnesium ions were present (Müller-Berghaus and Heinrich, 1978). Thus, the first part of the clumping curve can be considered as platelet agglutination (Fig. 2). Weber, Malessa and Lasch (1963), and Brown and Lachmann (1973, 1974) observed a release of platelet factor 3 activity into the plasma immediately after addition of endotoxin to the reaction mixture and endotoxin injection, respectively. As platelets are part of the coagulation activation system, and since platelet factor 3 is known to be the most potent accelerator of clotting it was conceivable that platelets are essentially involved in triggering intravascular coagulation. However, the infusion of purified platelet factor 3 could not initiate intravascular coagulation (Müller-Berghaus and colleagues, 1967).

The minor importance of platelets in triggering intravascular coagulation could also be shown by injecting endotoxin into thrombocytopenic rabbits. Thrombocytopenia had been induced by a platelet antiserum. Despite a mean platelet count of 5700/μl rabbits developed the generalized Schwartzman reaction after endotoxin injection, just as did control rabbits pretreated with absorbed platelet antiserum (Kramer and Müller-Berghaus, 1977). From these experiments it can be concluded that platelets participate in endotoxin-induced intravascular coagulation, but are not the principal mediator for triggering the coagulation system.

Leukocyte-Endotoxin Interaction

Similar to platelets, leukocytes have been accused of being involved in the activation of coagulation by endotoxin. Like platelets, the human leukocytes contain endotoxin-binding substances (Springer and Adye, 1975). This *in vitro* observation is consistent with earlier studies by Stetson (1951) and other investigators indicating that intravenous injection of endotoxin leads to a decrease in the number of circulating leukocytes.

Thomas and Good (1952) were the first to demonstrate the significance of leukocytes in the pathogenesis of endotoxin-induced intravascular coagulation. They showed that endotoxin does not initiate intravascular coagulation when animals are rendered leukocytopenic by treatment with nitrogen mustard. Corresponding results were obtained in rabbits pretreated with busulphan to induce leukocytopenia and thrombocytopenia (Müller-Berghaus, Bohn and Höbel, 1976). The experiments indicated that leukocytes - but not platelets - are essential to the activation of endotoxin-induced intravascular coagulation. The aim of the next experiment was to investigate the effects of platelet or leukocyte transfusions into thrombocytopenic as well as leukocytopenic rabbits on the activation of intravascular coagulation by endotoxin (Bohn and Müller-Berghaus, 1976). Busulphan was administered to rabbits in order to cause leukocytopenia and thrombocytopenia. In the control, the mean leukocyte count before the second injection of endotoxin was 1600 and the mean platelet count was 2300/μl (Table 1). Only 3 out of 28 thrombocytopenic and leukocytopenic rabbits developed renal glomerular microclots. If leukocytopenic and thrombocytopenic animals were transfused with platelets before the second dose of endotoxin, platelet counts increased to a mean of 205 000/μl.

Despite this relatively normal platelet count, the second dose of endotoxin did not generate renal glomerular microclots, thus indicating that endotoxin does not activate intravascular coagulation by way of the platelets in the absence of leukocytes. If, however, 1 x 10^9/kg peritoneal leukocytes were transfused into leukocytopenic rabbits the consecutive endotoxin injection caused renal glomerular microclots in 8 out of 12 animals. These experiments allow the conclusion that the activation of coagulation by endotoxin depends on the presence of leukocytes. For a long time it has been known that leukocytes exhibit a procoagulant activity related to the extrinsic coagulation pathway. However, this procoagulant activity is very weak. Niemetz (1969, 1972) and Lerner, Goldstein and Cummings (1971) demonstrated that this weak procoagulant activity of leukocytes can be stimulated by incubation of the cells with endotoxin. This procoagulant activity of leukocytes seems to be similar to tissue thromboplastin. Possibly, the tissue factor activity observed in leukocyte concentrates is mainly derived from monocytes and not from granulocytes (Rivers, Hathaway and Weston, 1975).

Table 1. Effect of Leukocyte or Platelet Transfusion on the Occurrence of Glomerular Microclots after Two Injections of Endotoxin (E_1 & E_2) into Leukocytopenic as well as Thrombocytopenic Rabbits (from Bohn and Müller-Berghaus, 1976).

Treatment	Number of animals	Leukocyte count before E_2 (cells/µl)	Platelet count before E_2 (cells/µl)	Renal glomerular microclots*
Leukocyte transfusion and 2 x endotoxin	12	1 082	4 000	8/12
Platelet transfusion and 2 x endotoxin	11	1 355	204 850	1/11
Saline transfusion and 2 x endotoxin	28	1 581	2 285	3/28

*Expressed as number of positive results over total number of rabbits studied.

From these data a hypothesis can be put forward regarding the manner in which endotoxin activates coagulation (Fig. 3). Endotoxin preferably acts on leukocytes and induces the release of a thromboplastin-like material from these cells. Thus, the coagulation system is activated via the extrinsic pathway. As platelets are normally present in the circulating blood, endotoxin will also attack these cells. In contrast to leukocytes, platelets only accelerate an already activated coagulation system, as platelets in the absence of leukocytes are not capable of inducing intravascular coagulation.

Complement-Endotoxin Interaction

The production of procoagulant activity by leukocytes is dependent on a plasma factor (Fig. 3). There are several indications that this plasma factor is related to the complement system.

Several studies support the concept that endotoxin interacts with the classical as well as the alternate pathway of complement. According to Morrison and Oades (1979) the lipid A region of the endotoxin molecule is responsible primarily for attaching endotoxin to a membrane, whereas the activation of complement is primarily mediated by the polysaccharide region of endotoxin. Obviously, the lipid A region of endotoxin cannot itself initiate complement activation.

The importance of complement in the interaction of endotoxin with cells has best been studied in platelet responses. If endotoxin is added to platelet-rich plasma of rabbits lacking the 6th component of complement, the second phase of the clumping curve does not appear (see Fig. 1). In the same manner, ^{14}C-serotonin is not released from platelets of C_6-deficient rabbits (Müller-Berghaus and Heinrich, 1978). Furthermore, it has been shown by Brown and Lachmann (1974) that platelets of C_6-deficient rabbits do not release platelet factor 3 when mixed with endotoxin. As rabbit platelets have a C3b receptor, it has been concluded that the first phase of the platelet clumping curve represents complement-dependent platelet agglutination, also called immune adherence (Fig. 1).

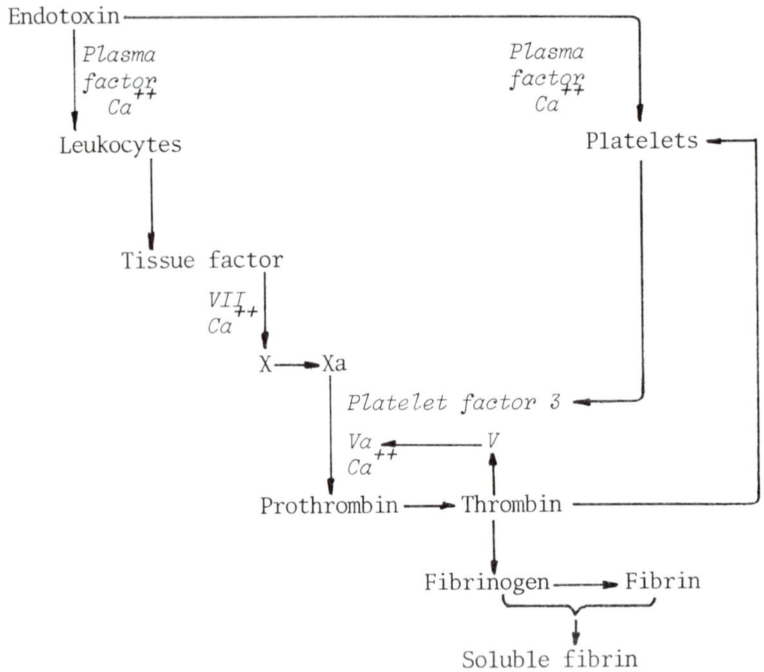

Fig. 3 Activation of intravascular coagulation by endotoxin. Tissue factor (thromboplastin-like material) released from leukocytes activates the extrinsic coagulation system, whereas platelets and their constituents represent amplifiers or modulators of coagulation.

The immune adherence phenomenon has also been demonstrated in vivo. After injection of endotoxin into C6-deficient rabbits, platelet counts decreased to the same degree as in normal rabbits (Müller-Berghaus and Lohmann, 1974). Although platelet factor 3 is not released in these animals (Brown and Lachmann, 1973), intravascular coagulation will occur (Müller-Berghaus and Lohmann, 1974). These experiments indicate again the minor importance of platelets in triggering intravascular coagulation by endotoxin.

The plasma factor necessary for the stimulation of procoagulant activity in leukocytes also seems to be related to the complement system. In recent studies by Muhlfelder and colleagues (1979) it was shown that thromboplastin-like activity does not occur if C5-deficient plasma is used instead of normal plasma in the complement-dependent stimulation of leukocytes. These observations are in agreement with findings in animals. When endotoxin was given to C6-deficient rabbits, leukocytes decreased to the same degree as in normal rabbits (Müller-Berghaus and Lohmann, 1974). In the same manner, the generalized Schwartzman reaction could be induced in C6-deficient rabbits.

The importance of complement in the activation of coagulation by endotoxin can be summarized as follows: The complement system is essential to endotoxin-cell interaction. As platelets do not seem to be involved in triggering intravascular coagulation, the disturbed platelet-endotoxin interaction in C6-deficient rabbits does not interfere with the activation of intravascular coagulation. As the complement system up to C5 is essential to the production of thromboplastin-like material by leukocytes, activation of intravascular coagulation by endotoxin seems to depend on complement and leukocyte interactions. Up to now it has not been decided whether granulocytes or monocytes are the major cells in producing thromboplastin-like material.

PRECIPITATION OF SOLUBLE FIBRIN

Activation of coagulation by endotoxin is the primary event in the coagulation sequence if endotoxin is released into the circulating blood. Generation of thrombin in the course of the activation process leads to the conversion of fibrinogen to fibrin. It has been shown that small amounts of fibrin do not polymerize or precipitate immediately to form visible fibrin clots, but in vivo form so-called soluble fibrin (Müller-Berghaus and colleagues, 1976). The relative harmlessness of soluble fibrin was demonstrated by the following experiments.

Animals were continuously infused with fibrin. In order to exclude side effects caused by the experimental procedure, the animals were given high doses of heparin at the same time. Animals infused with heparin and fibrin did not develop glomerular microclots. If, however, endotoxin was given in addition to fibrin, 3 out of 9 animals showed microclots in the kidneys (Hofmann, Mahn and Müller-Berghaus, 1979). The incidence of microclot formation could even be increased by the addition of aprotinin. Thus, endotoxin stimulated microclot formation independent of the activation of coagulation.

Several observations are consistent with the hypothesis that endotoxin causes precipitation of soluble fibrin in vivo. This effect of endotoxin is again not a direct action of endotoxin on soluble fibrin, but is mediated by an unknown mechanism. One possibility is that endotoxin inhibits fibrinolysis, thereby causing the preservation of fibrin strands and fibrin clots (Bergstein and Michael, 1973).

REFERENCES

Bergstein, J. M., and A. F. Michael. Jr. (1973). Thrombos. Diathes. Haemorrh., 29, 27-32.

Bohn, E., and G. Müller-Berghaus (1976). Am. J. Pathol., 84, 239-258.

Brown, D. L., and P. J. Lachmann (1973). Int. Arch. Allergy Appl. Immunol., 45, 193-205.

Brown, D. L., and P. J. Lachmann (1974). Adv. Biosci., 12, 300-310.

Hawiger, J., A Hawiger, S. Steckley, S. Timmons, and C. Cheng (1977). Br. J. Haematol., 35, 285-299.

Hofmann, H., I Mahn, and G. Müller-Berghaus (1979). Thrombos. Haemostas., 42, 39.

Kramer, W., and G. Müller-Berghaus (1977). Thrombos. Res., 10, 47-70.

Lerner, R. G., R. Goldstein, and G. Cummings (1971). Proc. Soc. Exp. Biol. Med., 138, 145-148.

McKay, D. G. (1963). Fed. Proc., 22, 1373-1379.

Morrison, D. C., and C. G. Cochrane (1974). J. Exp. Med., 140, 797-811.

Morrison, D. C., and Z. G. Oades (1979). J. Immunol., 122, 753-758.

Muhlfelder, T. W., J. Niemetz, D. Kreutzer, D. Beebe, P. A. Ward, and S. I. Rosenfeld (1979). J. Clin. Invest., 63, 147-150.

Müller-Berghaus, G., and D. Heinrich (1978). XVIII Congr. Internat. Soc. Hematol., Abstracts, p. 870.
Müller-Berghaus, G., and H. G. Lasch (1975). Handbook Exp. Pharmacol., XVI/3, 429-514.
Müller-Berghaus, G., and E. Lohmann (1974). Br. J. Haematol., 28, 403-418.
Müller-Berghaus, G., and R. Schneberger (1971). Br. J. Haematol., 21, 513-527.
Müller-Berghaus, G., E. Bohn, and W. Höbel (1976). Br. J. Haematol., 33, 212-220.
Müller-Berghaus, G., D. Goldfinger, W. Margaretten, and D. G. McKay (1967). Thrombos. Diathes. Haemorrh., 18, 726-735.
Müller-Berghaus, G., I. Mahn, G. Köveker, and F.-D. Maul (1976). Br. J. Haematol., 33, 61-79.
Niemetz, J. (1969). Fed. Proc., 28, 442.
Niemetz, J. (1972). J. Clin. Invest., 51, 307-313.
Rivers, R. P. A., W. E. Hathaway, and W. L. Weston (1975). Br. J. Haematol., 30, 311-316.
Springer, G. F., and J. C. Adye (1975). Infect. Immun., 12, 978-986.
Stetson, L. A., Jr. (1951). J. Exp. Med., 93, 489-504.
Thomas, L., and R. A. Good (1952). J. Exp. Med., 96, 605-623.
Weber, E., S. Malessa, and H. G. Lasch (1963). Thrombos. Diathes. Haemorrh., 9, 304-316.

BACTERIAL INFECTION AND DISSEMINATED INTRAVASCULAR COAGULATION

J. J. Corrigan, Jr.

Chief, Section of Pediatric Hematology/Oncology, University of Arizona Health Sciences Center, Tucson, Arizona 85724, USA

ABSTRACT

Humans and rabbits with bacterial infection consistently show a hypercoagulable state. In the human with septicemia and normal blood pressure the most consistent coagulopathy appears to be thrombocytopenia and a reduction in the vitamin K dependent coagulation factors. In those with septic shock the coagulation defect is due to disseminated intravascular coagulation. In rabbits the coagulopathy can be abolished by 2 different methods; by anticoagulation with heparin and by neutralization of the endotoxin effect with polymyxin sulfate. The endotoxin from the gram-negative organism probably activates the coagulation mechanism through platelet injury and/or through the release of tissue factors. It is also conceivable that the endotoxin may activate the clotting mechanism through factor XII activation; although, some studies have not confirmed this. Since gram-negative infections and death from septic shock continue to be a major health problem, continued research into the understanding of endotoxin effects and agents that can neutralize these is indicated.

KEYWORDS

Endotoxin; polymyxin B sulfate; disseminated intravascular coagulation; coagulopathy; heparin.

INTRODUCTION

Bacteria and some of their products such as endotoxin can activate the coagulation mechanism of humans and animals. The mechanism by which these agents induce a coagulopathy is not clearly understood. The data presented will be from three areas of investigation. The first will show the effect of endotoxin on the coagulation mechanism of the rabbit, the second the changes that occur in humans with bacterial infection, and the third the changes induced in a rabbit model for gram-negative septicemia. In addition, data will be presented that demonstrate two means by which the endotoxin effect can be altered; that is, by the use of an anticoagulant (heparin) and by the administration of an endotoxin neutralizing agent (polymyxin B sulfate).

RESULTS

Since the clinical manifestations of gram-negative infections are very similar to the experimental effects of endotoxin, it is presumed that the clinical findings are related to the lipopolysaccharide; therefore, many studies have been performed using the purified endotoxin. In our investigations, we analyzed the role of endotoxin in activating the coagulation mechanism of the rabbit particularly in reference to the generalized Shwartzman reaction (Corrigan, Abildgaard, Vanderheiden, Schulman, 1967). In this reaction, two intravenous injections of endotoxin are given 24 hours apart. Twenty-four hours after the second injection the majority of animals exhibit bilateral renal cortical necrosis. After the first injection, there is a reduction in the white blood cell and platelet counts within four hours and by 24 hours the white blood cell count recovers and exceed baseline, but the platelet count remains low. Following the second injection a second drop in the white blood cell and platelet count occurs with the white cell count recovering 24 hours later. The coagulation factors which are consumed during the process of disseminated intravascular coagulation (factors II, V, VIII, and fibrinogen) show the most significant change 4 hours after the second endotoxin injection. At that time there is a precipitous fall in all of these factors. It is during this period of time that fibrin deposition occurs in the kidneys. If the animals are anticoagulated during this 4 hour period the process can be abolished (Corrigan, 1970).

TABLE 1 Percent Change of Clotting Data Between Zero and Four Hours After Second Dose of Endotoxin

	Percent Change		
	Saline	Heparin	Polymyxin
Platelets	-70	-72	+11
Factor VIII	-54	-52	-20
Factor V	-50	-50	+25
Factor II	-25	-24	-3
Fibrinogen	-40	-5	+8
Renal Cortical Necrosis	+	0	0

Table 1 demonstrates a comparison between saline, heparin and polymyxin treated animals (Corrigan, Bell, 1971). With heparin a significant reduction occurred in the platelets, factors V, VIII, and II. However, fibrinogen did not decrease and the animals did not develop renal cortical necrosis. The polymyxin treated rabbits showed no reduction in the coagulation factors or platelets and renal cortical necrosis also did not develop. The reason for the differences between these two groups had to do with the fact that heparin was acting as an anticoagulant, mainly as an antithrombin, whereas, polymyxin was neutralizing the endotoxin. The timing of the injection of the polymyxin appears to be quite critical as is shown on Table 2.

TABLE 2 Effect of Polymyxin B in Endotoxin Treated Rabbits (Percent Change Between 0 and 4 Hours After Second Endotoxin Dose)

	E + NSS (0 hr)	E + P (0 hr)	E + P (15 min.)	P(no E) (0 hr)
WBC	-75	+4	-63	+12
Platelets	-69	+2	-68	-2
Fibrinogen	-34	+20	-27	+3
Renal Cortical Necrosis (% Positive)	80	0	25	0

E = endotoxin; NSS = saline; P = polymyxin

When the endotoxin and polymyxin were injected simultaneously (0 hour) there was no significant reduction, and the animals did not develop renal cortical necrosis. However, when the polymyxin was delayed 15 minutes the coagulation mechanism was activated and 25% of the animals developed the disease. These data suggested that the polymyxin must neutralize the endotoxin prior to its attachment to membranes. From these studies and data by other investigators, it seemed clear that endotoxin was able to activate the coagulation mechanism to induce disseminated intravascular coagulation. In this particular animal model the effect could be abolished by either anticoagulating the animal or by neutralizing the endotoxin. Therefore, it seems logical to apply the animal data to human disease.

Coagulation studies were performed in over 200 humans with bacterial infections and are summarized on Table 3.

TABLE 3 Bacterial Infections: Effect on Blood Platelets and Certain Coagulation Factors

	Sepsis Absent	Sepsis Present B.P.-Normal	Sepsis Present B.P.-Reduced
Platelets	N to E	N to R	R
Factor II	N	N to R	R
Factor V	E	E	R
Factor VIII	E	E	R
Fibrinogen	E	E	R
FSP	±	±	+

N = normal; E = elevated; R = reduced;
FSP - fibrinolytic split products; + = present

In patients with localized infections without septicemia (such as pneumonia, meningitis, urinary tract infections and so forth), the platelets were normal or elevated and coagulation factors II, V, VIII and fibrinogen were normal or elevated. However, humans with bacterial septicemia demonstrated two different types of coagulopathies (Corrigan, Ray, May, 1968; Corrigan, Jordan, 1970; Goldenfarb, Zucker, Corrigan, Cathey, 1970). Sixty percent of the normotensive septicemic patients had thrombocytopenia. In addition, the vitamin K dependent factors (factors II, VII, IX, X) were found to be reduced in 25%. However, factors V, VIII and fibrinogen were elevated. In the septic shock patients the coagulopathy was clearly due to disseminated intravascular coagulation; these patients demonstrated thrombocytopenia, reduction in factors II, V, VIII and fibrinogen, and fibrinolytic split products in serum.

The data on 10 surviving septicemic patients with shock are shown on Fig. 1. The platelet count, fibrinogen, and factor V are shown although factors II and VIII demonstrated a similar pattern. As can be seen, these individuals had a reduction in the platelets, factors V and fibrinogen with fibrinolytic split products in serum. After 24-48 hours these returned to normal except for the platelets which took 7-14 days before they normalized. The figure also demonstrates that these patients were given heparin. However, more recent data suggest that the coagulation abnormalities may return to normal without the use of heparin and this will be discussed later (Corrigan, Jordan, Bennett, 1973). Since the animal studies suggested that anticoagulation with heparin might be beneficial, the effect of heparin on the survival rate in patients with septic shock was studied. In our own experience with the first 24 patients in whom we heparinized, 16 died, and 14 of the 16 died because of the shock state. Thus, the mortality rate of 58% was no better nor worse than what had been previously reported for gram-negative septic shock. A retrospective review of 222 cases that were recorded in the literature of patients with septic shock is shown on Table 4 (Corrigan, 1977).

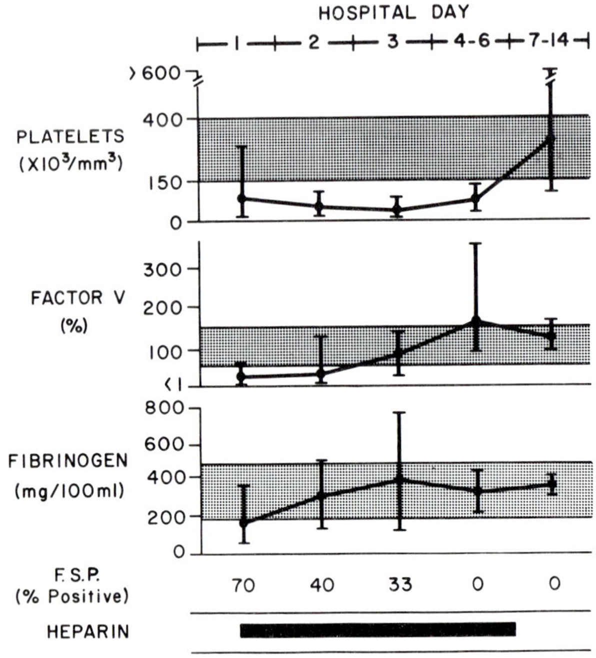

Fig 1. Coagulation data of ten patients with septicemia and hypotension who survived (Corrigan, Jordan, 1970)

TABLE 4 Septic Shock: Survival Data in Patients Treated and Not Treated with Heparin

Organisms	Total	Heparin Survived	Heparin Died	No Heparin Survived	No Heparin Died
Gram-negative					
Meningococcus	167	43	48	35	41
Other (E. coli, Pseudomonas, Pasteurella Klebsiella, H. influenzae, Herellae, etc.)	31	8	8	10	5
Gram-positive					
Pneumococcus, Stephylococcus, Streptococcus, Listeria, etc.	24	3	10	2	9
Grand Total	222	54 (24%)	66 (30%)	47 (21%)	55 (25%)

The mortality rate in the heparin treated group was no different from those in the non-treated group. Thus, these data suggested that heparin did not improve the mortality rate of patients with septic shock. In order to study this effect more carefully, an experimental model for gram-negative septicemia was developed.

Rabbits are naturally infected with Pasturella multocida, a gram-negative organism. This particular organism is sensitive to penicillin but not to the antibacterial ability of polymyxin B sulfate. After the intraperitoneal injection of 10^9 live organisms the animals developed significant numbers of organisms in their blood (Corrigan, Kiernat, 1975). All the animals died within 24 hours. Table 5 shows the changes that occurred in the white blood cell, platelets and factor VIII levels in animals infected with the organisms and compared to heat-killed organisms as the controls.

TABLE 5 Mean Hematologic Data of 50 Rabbits Given Live (LO) or Heat-Killed (DO) Pasteurella Multocida

Hour After Injection	Organism	WBC ($/mm^3$)	Platelets ($x10^3/mm^3$)	Factor VIII (%)
0	-	4018	416	100
8	LO	0810*	196*	72
	DO	7000	579	116
12	LO	0436*	166*	50*
	DO	-	-	-
16	LO	0360*	78*	20*
	DO	10,368	689	122
24	LO	Dead	Dead	Dead
	DO	6543	519	128

*Significant reduction

As can be seen, significant leukopenia, thrombocytopenia, and reduction in factor VIII occurred as the infection progressed. Similar changes also occurred in factors II, V, and fibrinogen. If at the time of the fourth hour the animals are given one injection of penicillin and also treated with either saline or heparin the mortality rates could be compared and are shown on Table 6 (Corrigan, Kiernat, 1975).

TABLE 6 Mortality Rate in Rabbits Treated with Penicillin and Heparin

Time (hrs)	Penicillin (one dose at 4 hours) Saline (20)	Heparin (20)
12	30%	35%
24	50%	85%
36	85%	95%

( ) = number of animals

Thus, the addition of heparin did not improve and might have worsened the survival rate in these animals. Detailed coagulation studies revealed that these animals also developed disseminated intravascular coagulation. When the animals were heparinized the changes in the fibrinogen concentration, platelets, and white cells were compared with saline treated controls and are shown on Table 7.

TABLE 7 Hematological Data in Rabbits Given Live Organisms with and without Heparin (Data Given as Percent Change from Zero Hour)

	Time (Hours) After Injection of Organisms		
	8	12	16
WBC			
With Heparin	-90%	-84%	-82%
Without Heparin	-80%	-89%	-91%
Platelets			
With Heparin	-8%	-60%	-60%
Without Heparin	-53%	-60%	-81%
Fibrinogen			
With Heparin	+33%	+49%	+78%
Without Heparin	0%	+6%	0%

Heparin therapy had no effect on the changes in the white cell or platelet count; however, the fibrinogen consumption stopped. These data indicated that heparinization appeared to control the DIC in the rabbits, however, the mortality rate remained high. Thus, this experimental model simulated the clinical condition.

Using this experimental model the effect of polymyxin B was investigated. Three experiments were performed: polymyxin was given before injection of live organisms after the injection of live organisms, and the effect of therapy on the mortality rate was studied (Corrigan, Kiernat, 1979). In the first experiments the rabbits were treated 90 minutes before the intraperitoneal injection of the pasturella organisms with either normal saline or polymyxin B intravenously, and blood samples were collected 6 hours after the IP injection of live organisms.

Normal rabbits had negative blood cultures and endotoxin levels prior to the start of the experiment. Subsequently, the cultures became positive in 100% of the saline and 80% of the polymyxin treated animals. The endotoxin activity, in micrograms/ml plasma, was measured by the Limulus method. There was a significant reduction in endotoxin activity in the polymyxin treated animals as compared to the saline controls. Significant leukopenia and thrombocytopenia only occurred in the saline treated animals, whereas, there was no difference between baseline and 6 hours in the polymyxin treated rabbits.

In the next experiment, the polymyxin was given 6 hours after the IP injection of live organisms. Blood samples were obtained 1 and 3 hours after the administration of the polymyxin. The blood cultures remained positive in 100% of the animals at both time periods. Endotoxin activity was significantly reduced at both time periods. The animals exhibited leukopenia and thrombocytopenia at the time of the injection of the saline or polymyxin which remained throughout the testing period. The mortality studies showed that the penicillin treated animals had a 70% mortality rate at 24 hours, and the polymyxin treated rabbits were no different than the saline treated controls (100% and 86% respectively). However, the combination of penicillin and polymyxin appeared to have a more favorable effect than either antibiotic alone having a mortality rate of 50%. The data from these experiments using live organisms corroborates the findings in animals given lipopolysaccharide and suggest that once the endotoxin has exerted its effect, the toxic reaction cannot be neutralized by the polymyxin B.

Although the data in animals and humans strongly suggest that endotoxin can activate the coagulation mechanism, the human data also suggest that other criteria must be present in order to develop disseminated intravascular coagulation. As noted earlier, humans without shock did not demonstrate DIC, whereas, those that did have hypotension associated with the septicemic state clearly developed the coagulopathy. In addition, survival in these hypotensive patients was not improved with the use of anticoagulation. However, survival was more closely linked to improvement in the cardiovascular status of the patients as noted on Table 9 (Corrigan, Ray, May, 1968).

TABLE 9 Response of Blood Pressure and Coagulation Defect as Related to Mortality Rate (24 Patients Treated with Heparin)

	Number of Cases	Deaths	Mortality Rate
Blood Pressure Restorable (10)			
Coagulation Defect Improved	10	0	0%
Coagulation Defect Not Improved	0	-	-
Blood Pressure Not Restorable (14)			
Coagulation Defect Improved	3*	3	100%
Coagulation Defect Not Improved	11	11	100%

*Survived >36 hours

In 10 patients in whom their blood pressures were restored to normal, the coagulopathy disappeared and the mortality rate was 0. However, in 14 patients in whom the blood pressure could not be restored, in other words, they remained in shock, the mortality rate was 100% and the coagulopathy continued in the majority of the patients in spite of heparin therapy. These data suggested that the heparin did not improve the mortality rate of patients with septic shock, but may have a role in the treatment of the coagulopathy. They further suggested that improvement of the shock state without the use of anticoagulants may also abolish the DIC. This experience would suggest that the following approach be done in patients with bacterial septicemia (Corrigan, 1977). At the time the diagnosis is suspected, coagulation screening tests, platelet counts and fibrinogen concentration should be obtained. If the patient has a normal blood pressure with normal coagulation data, then no hematologic treatment is necessary. If the patient is normotensive but has abnormal coagulation data and is not bleeding, then again no specific therapy needs to be given. However, if the patient is bleeding then the bleeding is most likely due to the thrombocytopenia, or to a reduction in the vitamin K dependent coagulation factors. Therapy at that time may be directed toward platelet transfusion or the administration of vitamin K. In the hypotensive or shock cases the first aim of therapy is aggressive antishock therapy. If the blood pressure responds to such therapy, then the approach to the hematological management would be the same as in the normotensive patient. If the blood pressure is unresponsive and bleeding is present, then the patient may need to have replacement therapy with platelets or coagulation factors and also may benefit from the use of heparin. Polymyxin B has not been studied in this clinical setting as of this date, but theoretically would be more effective in the initial treatment phase of the septicemia.

REFERENCES

Corrigan, J. J., Jr., C.F. Abildgaard, J. F. Vanderheiden, and I Schulman (1967). Quantitative aspects of blood coagulation in the generalized Shwartzmann reaction. I. Effects of variations of preparative and provocative doses of E. coli endotoxin. Pediat. Res., 1, 39-49.

Corrigan, J. J., Jr., W. L Ray and N. May (1968). Changes in the blood coagulation system associated with septicemia. New England J. Med., 279, 851-856.

Corrigan, J. J., Jr. (1970). Effect of anticoagulating and non-anticoagulating concentrations of heparin on the generalized Shwartzman reaction. Thrombos. et Diath. Haemorrh., 24, 136-145.

Corrigan, J. J., Jr., and C. M. Jordan (1970). Heparin Therapy in septicemia with disseminated intravascular coagulation. New Eng. J. Med., 283, 778-782.

Corrigan, J. J., Jr., and B. M. Bell (1971). Endotoxin-induced intravascular coagulation: prevention with polymyxin B sulfate. J. Lab. Clin. Med., 77, 802-810.

Corrigan, J. J., Jr., C. M. Jordan, and B. B. Bennett (1973). Disseminated intravascular coagulation in septic shock. Report of three cases not treated with heparin. Am. J. Dis. Child., 126, 629-632.

Corrigan, J. J., Jr., and J. F. Kiernat (1975). Effect of heparin in experimental gram-negative septicemia. J. Infect. Dis., 131, 138-143.

Corrigan, J. J., Jr. (1977). Heparin therapy in bacterial septicemia. J. Pediat., 91, 695-700.

Corrigan, J. J., Jr., and J. F. Kiernat (1979). Effect of polymyxin B sulfate on endotoxin activity in a gram-negative septicemic model. Pediat. Res., 13, 48-51.

Goldenfarb, P. B., S Zucker, J. J. Corrigan, Jr., and M. H. Cathey (1979). The coagulation mechanism in acute bacterial infection. Brit. J. Haemat., 18, 643-652.

Cytolytic Toxins

CYTOTOXINS OF SOME MARINE INVERTEBRATES

W. R. Kem*, K. M. Blumenthal and J. W. Doyle***

**Department of Pharmacology and Therapeutics, University of Florida, College of Medicine, Gainesville, Florida 32610, USA*
***Department of Biological Chemistry, University of Cincinnati, College of Medicine, Cincinnati, Ohio 45267, USA*

ABSTRACT

The lower marine invertebrate phyla are a particularly rich source of new cytotoxins. Current investigations by several laboratories aimed at the characterization of these toxins and elucidation of their mechanisms of action upon model lipid and cell membrane systems are reviewed herein. The few toxins which have been purified sufficiently for such studies were found to interact with specific membrane lipids: (1) basic protein cytotoxins from the sea anemone Stoichactis and the nemertine Cerebratulus were inhibited by small amounts of sphingolipids, (2) phospholipase A's and a protein colytic factor from the nematocyst venom of the sea anemone Aiptaisia synergistically promoted cell lysis by attacking glycerophosphatides, and (3) the Metridium (sea anemone) cytotoxin and echinoderm saponins displayed high binding affinities for cholesterol. The cytolytic sequence activated by membrane-active cytotoxins consists of three major steps: (1) toxin binding to the cell membrane, (2) alteration of the membrane by the bound toxin, and (3) the release of cytoplasmic solutes. Techniques permitting concurrent measurement of both toxin binding and efficacy are crucial for analyzing cytolytic mechanisms. A bioassay method was used to measure the relative importance of these two parameters for understanding the large differences in the sensitivities of erythrocytes from six mammalian species to Stoichactis and Cerebratulus toxins. Liposomes prepared with pure lipids were useful for initially determining if a cytotoxin preferentially interacted with specific lipids and also for spectroscopic analyses of cytotoxic protein-membrane lipid interactions.

KEYWORDS

Cytotoxins; membranes; lipids; sphingomyelin; gangliosides; phospholipase A; cholesterol; erythrocytes; nemertines; cnidarians.

INTRODUCTION

Membrane-active cytotoxins possibly are the most common type of toxin elaborated by living organisms. Only a few cytotoxins have so far been purified sufficiently to permit detailed characterization of their chemical and pharmacological properties; they vary over one million-fold in their ability to lyse cells (Table 1). The least potent substances are small amphipathic molecules such as lysolecithin which nonspecifically interact with most membrane lipids and proteins, dispersing them into smaller micellar structures. The most potent cytotoxins are large proteins such as the bacterial exotoxin streptolysin O and the sea anemone (*Stoichactis*) toxin which selectively bind certain membrane lipids and likely cause cell lysis by nondetergent mechanisms such as the formulation of membrane pores. Our own humoral cytotoxin system (complement) certainly belongs at the top of this list, as under favorable conditions one C5-9 complex may be sufficient to lyse an erythrocyte (Rommel and Mayer, 1971)

TABLE 1 Median Hemolytic Concentrations of Lysins for Human Red Cells (Kem and Blumenthal, 1978)

Lysin	Organism	Molecular Weight	HC_{50} ug/ml	HC_{50} umol/l
Streptolysin O	Bacterium	60,000	0.005	0.00008
Stoichactis toxin	Sea Anemone	16,000	0.006	0.0004
Phallolysin	Mushroom	30,000	2	0.07
Staph. α-toxin	Bacterium	44,000	5	0.1
C.1.-A-III	Nemertine	9,600	3	0.3
Holothurin A	Sea Cucumber	1,200	0.4	0.3
Digitonin	Foxglove (plant)	1,200	1	0.8
Melittin	Honey Bee	2,800	4	1.4
Lysolecithin	Chicken	510	4	8
Cardiotoxin	Cobra	7,000	>200	>30
SDS	---	290	30	100

For the sake of simplicity one can conceptualize the cytolytic process triggered by a cytotoxin as consisting of three major steps: (1) binding of the toxin to the membrane, (2) alteration of membrane structure by the bound toxin, and (3) the release of soluble cytoplasmic constituents:

$$\text{FREE TOXIN} \overset{1}{\rightleftarrows} \text{BOUND TOXIN} \overset{2}{\rightleftarrows} \text{MEMBRANE DEFECT} \overset{3}{\rightarrow} \text{CELL LYSIS}$$

Several major questions arise for each of these steps.

Step 1. Does the toxin in solution exist only as the monomeric species, or does it self-associate? Is toxin binding to the membrane saturable? Does the toxin bind to specific membrane molecules? Do the bound toxin molecules aggregate within the membrane? Is the conformation of the bound toxin the same as for the free toxin?

Step 2. Is membrane alteration limited to a small patch surrounding the bound toxin, or does it involve a generalized change in the fluid-mosaic structure? Are there lipid and/or protein lateral phase separations? Are discrete pores of a particular size formed, or do cracks develop from a progressive reduction in cooperative binding between membrane lipids? Are all bound toxin molecules in the same conformational state or is there an equilibrium between several states which may differ in their ability to alter the membrane? Is cytolytic efficacy related to depth of penetration into the nonpolar interior of the bilayer? The initial and final cytolytic steps are experimentally most accessible, thereby making the analysis of the membrane alterations of these toxins a particular challenge for future research. Fortunately many new spectroscopic, calorimetric and electrophysiological techniques capable of yielding important information on Step 2 are becoming available with time.

Step 3. Are there selective permeability increases which lead to an increase in cell volume preceding lysis? Is the functional state of the Na,K-pump a factor determining the extent of lysis? Does lysis occur as readily in the absence of a colloid osmotic gradient? Are micelles removed from the membrane during lysis?

METHODOLOGICAL COMMENTS

We shall consider only two subjects which are especially critical in as they apply to cytotoxin investigations: purification, and analysis of cytotoxin binding to membranes. Mechanistic studies with impure toxins are frequently a waste of time since interpretation of the results is always open to question. Nature generally supplies a complex system of toxins in any venom. Thanks to Pharmacia (a symposium sponsor) and other firms, the biologist can now purify toxins in most cases without undue effort. There are two especially frequent problems involved in purifying cytotoxic proteins. The first one results from the plethora of genetic variants (isotoxins) generally found in venoms which are usually resolved by repetitive low-pressure column chromatographic runs and/or isoelectric focusing. Since isotoxins usually possess similar molecular sizes, it is essential to exploit differences in charge characteristics between isotoxins. Isoelectric focusing is such a powerful method for resolving protein genetic variants that the older chromatographic methods are often not fully exploited. It should be remembered that two proteins with identical pI's may nevertheless possess different net charges in other pH regions. This apparently occurs for both types of sphingolipid-inhibitable toxins discussed below. The very basic Cerebratulus toxins A-III and A-IV were only separable in the pH range 3.5-5.0; although isoelectric focusing of Stoichactis toxin yielded a single peak centered as pH 9.8, CM-cellulose chromatography at pH 6.5 resolved three distinct isotoxin fractions (Kem and Blumenthal, 1978; Bernheimer and Avigad, 1976; Kem and Dunn, in preparation). Although the focusing and ion-exchange column runs require about 24 hr., one worries less about disulfide bond interchange reactions and precipitation at neutral pH than at pH 10. These factors may explain why our Stoichractis isotoxin samples possessed >10 times more hemolytic activity than was previously reported for the focused toxin. SDS-PAGE and analytical molecular sieve chromatography are not very stringent methods for assessing isotoxin separations, so one must rely more heavily upon native toxin PAGE at several pH's, amino acid compositions, and partial sequencing of the N-terminal chain. Another major problem concerning cytotoxin purifications involves separation of other venom components which also affect membranes. Here enzymological (phospholipase A) and neurotoxicity assays become very important. This is a major problem where synergistic venom constituents such as the direct lytic factor-phospholipase A system coexist; recently hydrophobic and immunoaffinity chromatographic methods have successfully separated these synergistic proteins. Most venoms possess neurotoxins as well as cytotoxins; thus electrophysiological investigations of either component must be based upon samples vigorously checked for contamination by the others.

In cytotoxin research it is often desirable to compare the lytic potencies of different toxins, or changes in the potency of the same toxin under different conditions. Two fundamental parameters (affinity and efficacy) determine potency, which by itself possesses little mechanistic significance. These comparisons would be much more informative if these two factors were independently estimated. Thron (1964) has presented a simple method for extracting such estimates from experiments where lysis is measured as a function of the membrane concentration (M) employed. This method assumes that the total toxin concentration required to produce a specified lytic effect(X) increases in direct proportion to the membrane concentration(M) tested:

$$(\text{Toxin})_{\text{Total},X} = a_X(M) + (\text{Toxin})_{\text{Free},X}$$

where a_X = the amount of bound toxin per unit concentration of membrane required to evoke X% lysis

$$\text{Affinity} \ \alpha \ \frac{a_X}{(\text{Toxin})_{\text{Free},X}} \quad ; \quad \text{Efficacy} \ \alpha \ \frac{1}{a_X}$$

Radioisotopic labelling of the cytotoxin may be avoided with this method since binding can be estimated by cytolytic assays. The major disadvantage of the "membrane bioassay" method is that nonspecific membrane binding is not distinguished from binding to specific receptor sites (Thron, 1964).

SPHINGOLIPID-INHIBITABLE TOXINS

Sphingomyelin has been the most neglected of the three major lipid constituents of the outer half of the cell membrane where cytotoxins are generally thought to act. The amounts of this lipid present in membranes varies considerably with the cell type, membrane type, and species. Among red cells, variations in sphingomyelin content are generally compensated for by opposite alterations in phosphatidylcholines (Nelson, 1967). Nevertheless, this lipid differs from lecithin by possessing a greater H-bonding capability (sphingosine moiety) and by generally possessing an N-acyl paraffin chain which is longer than the sphingosine chain or lecithin acyl chains. These two molecular features may be the basis for the much greater viscosity of sphingomyelin bilayers relative to lecithin bilayers (Shinitzky and Barenholz, 1974). Sphingomyelin may also serve as a trans-bilayer coupling agent (Schmidt and colleagues, 1978). Gangliosides are sphingolipids possessing a sialic acid-containing glycoside moiety in place of the phosphorylcholine group; ganglioside GM_1 acts as a membrane receptor for cholera toxin (Bennett and colleagues, 1976). In the past two years cytotoxins from the sea anemones Stoichactis (Bernheimer and Avigad, 1976) and Condylactis (Lebez, Macek and Sedmak, 1979) and the nemertine Cerebratulus have been shown to be specifically inhibited by sphingomyelin; it is hoped that these proteins may serve as useful tools to improve our knowledge of the disposition and functions of this lipid in membranes.

The affinity of Stoichactis toxin for sphingomyelin was first demonstrated by specific inhibition of toxin-mediated hemolysis (Table 2) and subsequently by demonstrating direct binding during isoelectric focusing (Bernheimer and Avigad, 1976; Linder, Bernheimer and Kim, 1977). Preincubation of erythrocytes with sphingomyelin-selective phospholipases C or D also made the cells insensitive to Stoichactis toxin. Bacteria (which lack sphingomyelin) were resistant to high concentrations of the toxin. We have recently obtained spectroscopic evidence for a sphingomyelin-selective change in conformation of Stoichactis toxin. The intrinsic fluorescence emission spectrum possesses a peak at 332nm indicating that the tryptophans are probably in a nonpolar environment when the toxin is in an aqueous medium; adding a sonicated and centrifuged (100,000 g x 1 hr) sphingomyelin dispersion caused a shift in the peak wavelength to 325nm and a maximum intensity increase of approximately 30%. The circular dichroism spectrum of the toxin possessed a single peak ($-8{,}000$ deg-cm^2-dmol^{-1}) at 217nm diagnostic of B-sheet; computer calculations provided the best fit of the spectrum with 55% B-sheet, 15% α-helix, and 30% remainder. In the presence of sonicated sphingomyelin the 217nm CD peak was enhanced almost 40%, suggesting that the toxin undergoes considerable change in its secondary structure with sphingomyelin binding. Dimyristoylphosphatidylcholine and cholesterol dispersions (or an equimolar mixture of the two) failed to cause the fluorescence and CD changes described above (Kem and Doyle, in preparation).

Two recent investigations of the action of the partially purified Stoichactis toxin upon black lipid bilayers and liposomes lacking sphingomyelin suggest that there is no sphingomyelin requirement for the membrane actions of Stoichactis toxin. Conductance fluctuations indicative of the formation of relatively stable ionic channels were observed in the presence of low concentrations of the toxin and the concentration dependence of the conductance increase was considered as evidence that the aggregation of 3 toxin molecules was required to form each channel (Michaels, 1979). Exposure of liposomes containing radioactive lecithin and rubidium to the toxin caused release of both substances as a function of toxin concentration, which was rather high (>1000 times higher than hemolytic concentrations). Although liposomes made with sphingomyelin released the greatest amount of these markers, distearoylphosphatidylcholine and other lecithin liposomes also were disrupted in a similar fashion (Shin, Michaels and Mayer, 1979).

Erythrocytes from different species frequently display large differences in their sensitivities to cytotoxins. We have utilized the membrane bioassay method of Thron to investigate differences in the affinity and efficacy parameters regulating hemolysis for erythrocyte lysis by Stoichactis toxin III (the most abundant isotoxin). Erythrocyte suspensions from six mammalian species were investigated. The affinity of the toxin for erythrocytes from all six species was so high that the free toxin concentration at 50% hemolysis could not be estimated, but efficacy was readily determined and shown to be the major determinant of differences in the sensitivities of the various red cells to the toxin. The a_{50} estimates decreased in the order rat>goat>sheep, horse, human>cat. Cat erythrocytes required about 30 times fewer bound toxin molecules to lyse than did rat erythrocytes (Doyle and Kem, unpublished results). Further analyses of these species differences are in progress using isotopically-labelled toxin III to assess the affinity term as well. Nevertheless it is apparent that the order of sensitivity of the red cells is not a simple function of the membrane sphingomyelin:lecithin ratios (Nelson, 1967).

TABLE 2 Lipid Inhibition Tests

	µg Required for Inhibition		
Substance	Cerebratulus A-IV*	Stoichactis Toxin**	Metrodiolysin***
Phosphatidylcholine	>500	>500	>500
Phosphatidylethanolamine	>500	>500	>500
Phosphatidylserine	>210	>500	>500
Phosphatidylinositol	>170	>500	---
Cerebrosides	>300	>500	---
Sphingomyelin	9	2	>500
Brain Gangliosides	6	>500	> 50
Ceramide	>500	50	---
Sphingosine	>125	>500	---
Cholesterol	>500	>500	1 to 2

*Amount required to inhibit by 1/2 the test amount (30µg), rat erythrocytes (Doyle and Kem, in preparation).

**Amount required to inhibit 2/3 of 3 hemolytic units, rabbit erythrocytes (Bernheimer and Avigad, 1976).

***Amount required to inhibit 2/3 of 3 hemolytic units, sheet erythrocytes (Bernheimer and Avigad, 1979).

The Cerebratulus A toxins are superficially similar to the Stoichactis toxins in that they are small basic proteins which preferentially bind sphingomyelin, but in other respects they appear to be quite different. Inhibition of Cerebratulus toxin A-IV hemolysis (Table 2) required 10-20 molecules of sphingomyelin per molecule of toxin, whereas for Stoichactis toxin the ratio exceeded 1000; these values suggest that these toxins require aggregates of the lipid for binding and may not have an appreciable affinity for monomeric sphingomyelin. Cerebratulus toxin A-IV was also significantly inhibited by three acidic lipids (gangliosides, phosphatidylserine, and phosphatidylinositol). This interaction must be investigated further to ascertain if it is just an ion exchange phenomenon. The covalent structures of both the Cerebratulus and Stoichactis cytotoxins are currently being investigated.

The CD spectrum of A-III possessed the two peaks characteristic of a predominantly α-helical protein; the computer least squares fit was best with 40% α-helix, 10% B-sheet, and 50% remainder. We were unable to detect significant changes in the CD or intrinsic fluorescense spectra when A-III was exposed to sonicated sphingomyelin or ganglioside dispersions. The *Cerebratulus* cytotoxins differ from the *Stoichactis* toxins in several other ways: they are much more highly basic, contain a greater proportion of disulfide bonds, and they apparently lack carbohydrate residues. The a_{50} estimates for A-III decreased in the order goat>sheep, horse>rat>cat, human. Although the hemolytic activities of both groups of toxins do not require calcium ions, raising $(Ca^{++})_o$ to 20mM completely inhibited A-III hemolysis but enhanced *Stoichactis* toxin III hemolysis. Elevated $Ca^{++})_o$ also suppressed the effects of *Cerebratulus* toxin A-III upon cardiac membrane resting and action potentials (Posner and Kem, 1978). Our working hypothesis is that this interaction between *Cerebratulus* cytotoxins (and cobra cardiotoxin) and membranes occurs primarily at the water-lipid interface where electrostatic bonding forces are very important, while *Stoichactis* toxins are able to penetrate further into the nonpolar center of the lipid bilayer where hydrophobic forces are dominant. This hypothesis would also be consistent with the 300 fold greater efficacy (40 molecules bound/μ^2) of *Stoichactis* toxin III relative to A-III (12000 molecules/μ^2).

PHOSPHOLIPASE-MEDIATED LYTIC SYSTEMS

Nematocyst venom obtained from the Caribbean sea anemone *Aiptaisia* possesses a complex cytolytic system consisting of phospholipase A_2, a high molecular weight cofactor which acts synergistically with the phospholipase, and probably one or more additional components. Two basic phospholipase A_2 isoenzymes were recently separated; the most abundant variant (pI of 8.8, size of 43,000 daltons by SDS-PAGE) was more sensitive to urea and high temperature than many previously described forms of this enzyme. The colytic factor (93,000 or 135,000 daltons, depending upon determination method) nonspecifically bound detergents, including fatty acids. Although the pure phospholipases were unable to hydrolyze the phospholipids of intact red cells or cause hemolysis by themselves, addition of a high molecular weight fraction of the venom which includes the colytic factor allowed hydrolysis and hemolysis to occur. Pure colytic factor and pure phospholipase together were still insufficient to permit this sequence to proceed significantly, so that it appears that other constituents of the venom were involved (Hessinger and Lenhoff, 1976; Grotondorst, 1979).

CHOLESTEROL-INHIBITABLE TOXINS

An important step in the purification of the echinoderm sterol glycosides (the first group of marine invertebrate cytotoxins to be purified) was their selective precipitation by cholesterol and certain other 3-B-hydroxy-sterols (Chanley and colleagues, 1959). Although holothurin A was crystallized from the Caribbean sea cucumber *Actinopyga* 20 years ago, elucidation of the structures of the native holothurins and asterosaponins (from starfish) is still incomplete, particularly concerning the localization of the sulfate ester moiety which contributes to the biological activity. Although little evidence presently exists for a membrane 3-B-hydroyl sterol requirement for the cytolytic actions of these saponins, the specificity of their complex formation with certain sterols in the test tube suggests that it may also occur in membranes. Recently a cholesterol-inhibitable cytolytic protein (pI 5, 80,000 daltons) was partially purified from the sea anemone *Metridium*. The activity of the toxin was optimal at pH 5-6 (near its pI), and rapidly decreased as the pH was increased above 6. It at least superficially resembled the bacterial thiol-activated cytoysins in its cholesterol affinity and its activation by thiols. Although variations in cholesterol content among mammalian red cells are very small, the erythrocytes of 10 mammalian species varied over a 100-fold range of sensitivity to Metridiolysin (Bernheimer, Avigad and Kim, 1979).

CONCLUDING COMMENTS

We have focused upon the interactions of purified cytotoxins with specific types of membrane lipids under laboratory conditions. One must also ask how the toxic organisms avoid poisoning themselves! Presumably the integumentary surfaces are protected from cytolytic attack by mucus or are resistant to the cytotoxin. The latter mechanism may be exploited by holothurians and asteroids. These are the only two echinoderm classes which possess saponins. Also the tissue sterols are Δ^7-analogs of cholesterol (Gupta and Scheuer, 1978). The major sterol (lathosterol) stabilizes lipid bilayers as well as cholesterol but has much less tendency to form complexes with asterosaponins (Mackie, Singh and Owen, 1977).

REFERENCES

Bennett, V., S. Craig, M. D. Hollenberg, E. O'Keefe, N. Sahyoun and P. Cuatrecasas 1976). J. Supramol. Str., 4, 99-120.
Bernheimer, A. W. and L. S. Avigad (1976). Proc. Natl. Acad. Sci. USA, 73, 467-471.
Bernheimer, A. W., L. S. Avigad, and K. S. Kim (1979). Toxicon, 17, 69-75.
Chanley, J. D., R. Ledeen, J. Wax, R. F. Nigrelli, and H. Sobotka (1959). J. Am. Chem. Soc., 81, 5180.
Grotondorst, C. (1979). Studies on the Hemolytic Toxins from Sea Anemone Nematocyst Venom. Diss., University of South Florida, Tampa. Florida.
Gupta, K. C. and P. J. Scheuer (1968). Tetrahed., 24, 5831-5837.
Hessinger, D. A. and H. M. Lenhoff (1976). Arch. Biochem. Biophys., 173, 603-613.
Kem, W. R. and K. M. Blumenthal (1978). J. Biol. Chem., 253, 5752-5757.
Lebez, D., P. Macek and B. Sedmak (1979). Toxicon, 17 (Suppl. 1), p. 99.
Linder, R., A. W. Bernheimer and K. S. Kim (1977). Biochim. Biophys. Acta, 467, 290-300.
Mackie, A. M., H. T. Singh and J. M. Owen (1977). Comp. Biochem. Physiol. 56B, 9-14.
Michaels, D. W. (1979). Biochim. Biophys. Acta, 555, 67-78.
Nelson, G. J. (1967). Biochim. Biophys. Acta, 144, 221-232.
Posner, P. and W. R. Kem (1978). Toxicon, 16, 343-349.
Rommel, R. A. and M. M. Mayer (1971). J. Immunol., 107, 319.
Schmidt, D. F., Y. Barenholz, C. Huang and T. E. Thompson (1978). Nature, 271, 775-777.
Shin, M. L., D. W. Michaels and M. M. Mayer (1979). Biochim. Biophys. Acta, 555, 79-88.
Shinitzky, M. and Y. Barenholz (1974). J. Biol. Chem., 249, 2652-2657.
Thron, C. D. (1964). J. Pharm. Exper. Ther., 145, 194-202.

CYTOLYTIC TOXINS OF BASIDIOMYCETES

R. Seeger

Department of Pharmacology and Toxicology, University of Würzburg, Federal Republic of Germany

ABSTRACT

Toxins with cytolytic action are widely distributed in the fungus realm. Five of them, proteins with direct haemolytic activity, have been isolated: Phallolysin (Seeger and co-workers, 1973) from Amanita phalloides, a thermo- and acid-labile, basic protein with a molecular weight of ca. 30 000 daltons, lyzes red cells of various species, bovine and sheep erythrocytes being rather resistant. Besides red cells, a large variety of mammalian cells, normal as well as transformed ones, are affected; however, no therapeutic antitumour effect was observed. The i.v. LD_{50} in rats is ca. 50 μg/kg. Toxicity is mainly due to intravascular haemolysis; direct cardiotoxic effects may occur, too. - Volvatoxin (Lin and co-workers, 1973) from Volvariella volvacea, a thermolabile protein consisting of two non-identical subunits with molecular weights of 50 000 and 23 000 daltons, lyzes human erythrocytes and in laboratory animals exhibits cardiotoxic effects in vitro and in vivo. The i.p. LD_{50} in mice is 1.23 mg/kg. - Flammutoxin (Lin and co-workers, 1974) from Flammulina velutipes, a thermolabile, acid protein with an apparent molecular weight of 22 000 daltons, lyzes red cells from various species, sheep, goat and toad cells being resistant. Furthermore, local irritation, cardiotoxic effects, histamine release and damage of tumour cells are observed. The i.p. LD_{50} in mice is 2.45 mg/kg. - Rubescenslysin (Seeger, 1976) from Amanita rubescens, a thermolabile, acid protein with a molecular weight of ca. 35 000 daltons, lyzes red cells from various species, differences in susceptibility being slight. The i.v. LD_{50} in rats is 1.4 mg/kg, severe obstruction of airways and signs of haemolysis being present. It is considered to act as a detergent. - Pleurotolysin (Bernheimer and Avigad, 1979) from Pleurotus ostreatus, an acid polypeptide of unusual amino acid composition, seems to exist in the form of dimers of 25 000 daltons. In haemolysis, species differences are pronounced, sheep erythrocytes being most susceptible. It probably functions as a detergent and sphingomyelin is involved in its cytolytic action. - The cytolysins so far isolated from mushrooms are labile proteins; hence, these toxins are not likely to be involved in human mushroom poisoning. However, some of them might become useful tools in membrane solubilisation.

KEYWORDS

Cytolysins; haemolysins; proteins; phallolysin; volvatoxin; flammutoxin; rubescenslysin; pleurotolysin; mushrooms.

INTRODUCTION

Towards the end of the last century, Kobert (1891) discovered a thermolabile haemolysin in Amanita phalloides which he considered to be the death cap poison. His work was taken up by Ford in America who proved the existence of a directly acting haemolysin also in fatally poisonous American white Amanitas; this was antigen and Ford was of the opinion that it was similar to the bacterial toxins (Ford, 1906a). The possible chemical nature of this substance remained a point of debate: Kobert (1891) considered his "phallin" to be a protein, Abel and Ford (1907; 1908) maintained that they had proof that their "amanita-haemolysin" was a glycoside; it was also doubtful whether a haemolysin constantly occurs in Amanita phalloides, not surprising in view of the fact that different experimenters worked with different species of fungus - the name "Amanita phalloides" seems to have been used as a collective term for various toxic Amanita species.

These early investigations aimed at the isolation of the poison responsible for the fatal outcome of death cap poisoning. Of course it soon became obvious that a thermolabile haemolysin could not play a part, especially as similar haemolysins were discovered shortly afterwards in edible fungi (Ford, 1907). Since a thermostable toxin was discovered alongside the thermolabile haemolysin in Amanita phalloides and was found to be the cause of death cap poisoning in humans (Kobert, 1899; Ford, 1906b), interest was centered more and more on this component, and the haemolysins of the fungi were forgotten for decades.

The haemolysin which we isolated from the green death cap Amanita phalloides (Vaill. ex Fr.) Secr. was named "phallolysin" (Seeger and co-workers, 1973) to emphasize its conspicuous similarity to some cytolytically acting bacterial toxins - Kobert's name "phallin" meantime had been given to two cyclopeptides from Amanita phalloides (Wieland and de Vries, 1966). To our surprise it became clear that phallolysin is not identical with Kobert's haemolysin (apparently because of work with different mushroom species): it does not haemolyze the bovine erythrocytes he used in his tests.

PHALLOLYSIN

is a basic protein and is electrophoretically heterogeneous. In Ampholine pH 7-9 the main component (phallolysin A) is isoelectric at pH 8.05, a smaller part (phallolysin B) at pH 7.5; in some experiments a third peak was observed with a pI of 6.9. In gel chromatography and in SDS disk electrophoresis phallolysin has a molecular weight of 30 - 33 000 daltons. It contains no cysteine. 70% pure phallolysin A has its u.v. absorption maximum at 278 nm. It is irreversibly denatured by urea (8 M) and SDS (0.1%); it is inactivated by desalting and is unstable on storage in purified form as well as in lyophilized mushrooms. It is thermolabile and at a temperature of 65 $^{\circ}$C it loses 90% of its activity within 10 min. Moreover it is acid-labile and also at pH 2.0 (37 $^{\circ}$C) it becomes inactive within 10 min. On the other hand, it is relatively stable in alkaline buffers, and the haemolytic activity is also resistant to proteases (pepsin, trypsin, α-chymotrypsin, subtilisin, pronase E, bromelin, proteinase K), α-amylase and pancreatin (Seeger, 1975a; 1975b; unpublished; Seeger and co-workers, 1973b).

Phallolysin is a directly acting cytolysin. It haemolyzes erythrocytes of various species. Total haemolysis of rabbit red cells is produced with a concentration of 0.6 µg/ml. A marked species specifity is observed: bovine and sheep erythrocytes are largely resistant. Apart from erythrocytes it affects numerous cell systems and isolated organs (Table 1). This results in a complete destruction of the cells and in irreversible damage to the organs. All the types of tumour cells examined in vitro (Table 2) were destroyed by phallolysin. In vivo phallolysin inhibits the

TABLE 1 in vitro Effects of Phallolysin on Isolated or Cultivated Cells and Isolated Organs

Cells and Organs	Effects	References
Erythrocytes of various species	Direct lysis	Seeger and co-workers, 1973
Human lymphocytes	Stainable with trypan blue	Faulstich and co-workers, 1974
Human amnion cells	Damage observed microscopically	Fiume, 1967
	Stainable with trypan blue	Faulstich and co-workers, 1974
Rat liver cells	Stainable with trypan blue	Faulstich and co-workers, 1974
	Bulky, bursting protrusions expelling cell content	Petzinger and Seeger, 1976
Chinese hamster peritoneum cells	Stainable with trypan blue	Faulstich and co-workers, 1974
Isolated guinea-pig heart	Irreversible decrease of contraction amplitude; cardiac arrest	Odenthal and co-workers, 1975
Isolated rat liver	Outflow of potassium	Odenthal and co-workers, 1975
Isolated guinea-pig ileum	Slow contraction; reduced sensitivity to ACh, histamin, KCL	Mosthaf, 1975
Isolated rat diaphragm	Irreversible contracture	Seeger, unpublished

implantation (Villa and Agostoni, 1967) or at least delayes the development of ascites tumours (Seeger and Lehmann, 1973), however, only when the cytolysin came into direct contact with the hitherto unimplanted tumour cells. No therapeutic antitumour effect was observed (Villa and Agostoni, 1968; Seeger and Lehmann, 1973).

Phallolysin is highly toxic when administered parenterally. In rats, the i.v. LD_{50} is 85 HU/kg b.w., corresponding to about 0.05 mg protein/kg; in mice, it is 200 HU/kg. Death occurs by intravasal haemolysis and cardiotoxic effects; cardiotoxicity partly can be explained by the effects of potassium released in haemolysis (Odenthal and co-workers, 1975).

The mechanism of phallolysin's membrane-damaging effect is still in doubt. It was not apparent from the kinetics of haemolysis (Seeger and Burkhardt, 1976), neither could one prove the existence of a phospholipase C activity (Neeb, 1973). Since phallolysin haemolysis is markedly inhibited by wheat germ lectin, N-acetylglucosamine containing lectin receptors of the cell membrane were assumed to be the site of action (Faulstich and Weckauf, 1975). However, the haemolysis inhibition by lectins was recognized as being non-specific for phallolysin (Avigad and Bernheimer, 1976; Seeger, in press). It is conceivable that phallolysin has a detergent action, although there was no evidence for this in our earlier investigations: it was inhibited neither by cholesterol nor by various naturally occurring phospholipids

TABLE 2 Effects of Phallolysin on Tumour Cells in vitro. Results Obtained with Crude or Partially Purified Preparations, Obviously Due to Phallolysin, are Included

Cells and Organs	Effects	References
KB cells	Damage observed microscopically	Fiume, 1967
Yoshida tumour AH 130 ascites cells	Destruction of cells observed microscopically	Villa and Agostoni, 1969
HeLa (S_3) cells	Stainable with trypan blue	Seeger and Lehmann, 1973
Sarcoma P_{43} ascites cells	Stainable with trypan blue	Faulstich and co-workers, 1974
Transformed human lymphocytes	Stainable with trypan blue	Faulstich and co-workers, 1974
AS 30 D hepatoma cells	Bulky, bursting protrusions expelling cell content; stainable with trypan blue	Petzinger and Seeger, 1976

(Seeger and Burkhardt, 1976). However, recently an inhibition was observed by certain synthetic phosphatidyl cholines (Seeger, unpublished), so that a detergent action with a somewhat more specific attack seems at least a possibility.

VOLVATOXIN

(Table 3) is a thermolabile toxin from the edible fungus Volvariella volvacea. It is composed of two protein components, which are separated on gel chromatography and differ in their molecular weight, their amino acid composition, and their tryptic peptide maps. The individual isolated components proved not to be poisonous for mice; when they were combined again the toxicity was restituted.

Volvatoxin is a directly acting haemolysin. Total haemolysis of human erythrocytes is produced by a concentration of 2 mg/ml. It has a cardiotoxic action in vitro and in vivo and is highly toxic when administered parenterally. Of the two proteins, only the A_2 component has a biological activity, which, however, is modified by the A_1 component: A_2 produces effects which are not even observed with volvatoxin, namely a fall in blood pressure in cats, and swelling and metabolic inhibition of Ehrlich ascites tumour cells. The mechanism of action is unknown (Lin and co-workers, 1973; 1974).

FLAMMUTOXIN

is an acid protein (pI_o 4.2) from the edible fungus Flammulina velutipes. It is thermolabile and at 60 ^oC loses its activity within 30 min. On gel chromatography and SDS disk electrophoresis it shows a molecular weight of 20 000 daltons and it contains neither cysteine nor methionine.

Flammutoxin lyzes erythrocytes of man, rabbit and cat directly. Total haemolysis of human red cells is achieved by 25 µg/ml. Species specifity is very pronounced:

TABLE 3 Physico-chemical Properties and Biological Effects of Volvatoxin from Volvariella volvacea (as Reported by Lin and Co-workers, 1973)

Physico-chemical properties

Inactivated by heating (100°C, 20 min)

Composed of 2 non-identical protein subunits, A_1 and A_2

A_1	Mol. wt. 50 000 daltons Contains the amino acids usually present in proteins except cysteine
A_2	Mol. wt. 23 000 daltons Contains all the usual amino acids

Biological effects

Biological system	Effects
Human red cells	Direct lysis
Mouse, i.p.	Writhing reaction LD_{50} 1.23 mg/kg b.w.
Isolated toad heart	Ventricular systolic arrest
Cat, i.v.	Dose-dependent irreversible ECG changes: depression of ST-segment, inversion of T-wave; AV block with nodal rhythm

sheep, goat and toad erythrocytes are completely resistant. Toxic effects on Ehrlich ascites tumour cells are also observed. When applied locally, flammutoxin causes irritation phenomena, e.g. oedema of rat paw or pain reaction after intraperitoneal administration; the latter occurs together with a release of histamin and can be partially antagonized by antihistamines. Flammutoxin is highly poisonous when administered parenterally. In mice, the i.p. LD_{50} is 2.45 mg/kg b.w.; toxicity cannot be reduced by antihistamines. Cardiotoxic effects are very evident. Intravascular haemolysis also occurs: Haemorrhages of the lungs and respiratory failure were observed prior to death. The mechanism of action is unknown; an enzymatic reaction is discussed (Lin and co-workers, 1974; 1975).

RUBESCENSLYSIN

is an acid protein (pI 4.9) from the edible fungus Amanita rubescens. It is clearly surface active, forms aggregates of varying size in aqueous solution, and has a molecular weight of approx. 35 000 daltons in electrophoresis under conditions of disaggregation in SDS. It has its u.v. absorption maximum at 280 nm and contains no cysteine. It is irreversibly denatured by urea (8 M) and SDS (0.1%), is inactivated by desalting and the purified toxin can only be stored for a very short time; in lyophilized mushrooms the activity also gradually decreases. It is extremely thermolabile and loses its activity almost completely within 10 min at a temperature of 50°C; even at 35°C a slow inactivation within a few hours takes place at pH 7.0. Rubescenslysin is alkali-labile, but is relatively stable in acid buffers, even in diluted hydrochloric acid at room temperature; furthermore, the haemolytic activity is resistant to various proteases (α-chymotrypsin, bromelin,

TABLE 4 In vitro Effects of Rubescenslysin on Isolated Cells and Isolated Organs (as Reported by Seeger, 1976 and by Odenthal and Co-workers, 1977

Cells and organs	Effects
Erythrocytes of various species	Direct lysis
Human leucocytes	Destruction of plasma membrane observed microscopically
Isolated rat and guinea-pig heart	Dose-dependent negative inotropic and negative chronotropic effects; cardiac systolic arrest
Isolated rat liver	Outflow of potassium and cytoplasmatic and lysosomal enzymes
Isolated rat kidney	Loss of enzymes; decrease of K^+, Na^+, and water reabsorption
Isolated guinea-pig ileum	Slow contraction; reduced sensitivity to acetylcholine and KCl
Isolated rat diaphragm	Irreversible contracture

proteinase K)(Seeger, 1976; 1980; unpublished).

Rubescenslysin, too, is a directly acting cytolysin (Table 4). It lyzes erythrocytes, species specifity being small. Total haemolysis of human red cells is produced with a concentration of 1 µg/ml. The plasma membrane of human leucocytes is more sensitive than the erythrocyte membrane, but the nuclear membrane seems to be rather resistant as far as can be judged by light microscopy. In addition, rubescenslysin irreversibly damages all isolated organs examined so far.

Rubescenslysin is highly toxic when administered parenterally. The i.v. LD_{50} is 140 HU/kg b.w. or about 0.14 mg protein/kg for the rat and 310 HU/kg or ca. 0.31 mg/kg for mice. Intravascular haemolysis together with more or less severe cardiovascular depression and very pronounced haemorrhagic oedema of the lung were clinically and electrocardiographically detected and confirmed by autopsy. The alveolar obstruction is the main cause of death in the rat (Seeger, 1976; Odenthal and co-workers, 1976).

Clues to the mode of action of rubescenslysin were obtained from the kinetics of haemolysis and from inhibition experiments: rubescenslysin is expended in haemolysis and its activity is inhibited by both cholesterol and phospholipids, particularly sphingomyelin and phosphatidyl choline; within the naturally occurring phospholipids, the inhibitory capacity is dependent on their origin; with synthetic phosphatidyl cholines it is dependent on the chain length and degree of saturation of the fatty acid residue (Seeger, 1980). Furthermore, rubescenslysin solubilizes phospholipids to a higher degree than does an albumin solution of the same concentration (Bönhof, in preparation) and releases marker substance from liposomes (Wachter, in preparation). On the other hand, phospholipase C activity was not observed (Bönhof, in preparation). These results point to the conclusion, that the cytolytic action of rubescenslysin is due to a detergent action of this protein.

PLEUROTOLYSIN

from the edible fungus Pleurotus ostreatus is a weakly acid protein (pI 6.4) with an unusual amino acid composition: it lacks cysteine, methionine, histidine, arginine, proline, tyrosine, and phenylalanine. On electrophoresis under conditions of dieaggregation in SDS it has a molecular weight of 12 300 daltons; under non-dissociating conditions it apparently forms dimers with a molecular weight of 25 000 daltons in gel chromatography. It seems to become inactive when stored and could be isolated from fresh fungi only.

Also pleurotolysin has a direct cytolytic action. It lyzes erythrocytes with a high degree of specifity, cattle and sheep erythrocytes being particularly sensitive. Pleurotolysin differs from the previously mentioned cytolysins in that it did not damage every tissue examined: morphological changes were observed in human thrombocytes, not, however, in fibroblasts. The lysin also proved to be non-toxic for mice when administered intravenously up to a dosage of 320 HU (1 HU produces 50% haemolysis of sheep erythrocytes).

The sensitivity of erythrocytes of various species correlated to a certain extent to their sphingomyelin content. Pleurotolysin is inhibited by sheep red cell ghosts, but only when they have not been pretreated with sphingomyelin-specific phospholipases. Moreover it is inhibited by sphingomyelin from sheep erythrocytes, provided it is in the form of liposomes. Pleurotolysin is regarded as a detergent, which attacks sphingomyelin (Bernheimer and Avigad, 1979).

OTHER CYTOLYSINS

In higher fungi there are numerous other cytolysins, which have not yet been characterized in detail. In screening we found directly acting haemolysins in 152 out of 306 species examined; extracts of 46 of these species produced agglutination as well as haemolysis; extracts of a further 17 species produced agglutination, but no haemolysis. We found haemolysins in all families, of which a sufficiently large number of species were available, but they were widespread in Hygrophoraceae and Strophariaceae, in the genera Oudemansiella and Mycena of the Tricholomataceae, Hebeloma and Gymnopilus of the Cortinariaceae and in the genus Amanita. On the other hand, they rarely appeared in Boletaceae and in the genus Russula. Evidently the haemolysin content is subject to seasonal influences (Seeger and Wiedmann, 1972; Seeger and co-workers, 1973b). In the case of negative results, which we obtained in 137 species, it must be borne in mind that these cytolysins are labile substances: often no activity was observed in originally active samples which had been in storage for a number of years. When dried fungi have to be examined, the haemolysin originally contained therein could have lost its activity.

CONCLUSIONS

The question on the possible practical significance of these cytolysins touches on several aspects: for one thing, substances which are so commonly found in fungi must be considered as possibly having a function in the metabolism of the fungus. Data on this matter do not seem to be available. - On the other hand, in human mushroom poisoning, these cytolysins seem to play a minor part only, if any: there are many edible fungi among these containing cytolysins, and the cytolysins isolated so far are thermolabile; so they cannot contribute to poisoning from boiled fungi. Phallolysin is also acid-labile, so it would be destroyed in the gastric juice under normal conditions. However, rubescenslysin is rather acid-stable, and both phallolysin and rubescenslysin are resistant to proteases. So far it is not known why raw Amanita phalloides are particularly poisonous and why Amanita rubescens, no doubt an edible fungus, sometimes causes poisoning. Whether local effects of these cytolysins here could be responsible is an open question. Absorptive poisonings can be discounted in view of the symptoms. Non-denaturing detergents play an important role in the isolation of membrane proteins; here one takes advantage of the fact that detergents, though they form micelles with various membrane constituents, have a high affinity for certain membrane components. Fungus cytolysins with a detergent-like action could acquire a significance in this context.

REFERENCES

Abel, J. J., and W. W. Ford (1907). J. Biol. Chem., 2, 273-288.
Abel, J. J., and W. W. Ford (1908). Naunyn-Schmiedebergs Arch. Exp. Path.Pharmak. Suppl. Band Schmiedeberg-Festschrift, 8-15.
Avigad, L. S., and A W. Bernheimer (1976). Infect. Immun., 13, 1378-1381.
Bernheimer, A. W., and L. S. Avigad (1979). Biochim. Biophys. Acta, 585, 451-461.
Faulstich, H., S. Zobeley, and M. Weckauf-Bloching (1974). Hoppe-Seyler's Z. Physiol. Chem., 355, 1495-1498.
Faulstich, H., and M. Weckauf (1975). Hoppe-Seyler's Z. Physiol. Chem., 356, 1187-1189.
Fiume, L. (1967). Arch. Sci. Biol., 51, 85-88.
Ford, W. W. (1906a). J. Infect Dis., 3, 191-224.
Ford, W. W. (1906b). J. Exp. Med., 8, 437-450.
Ford, W. W. (1907). J. Infect. Dis., 4, 434-439.
Kobert, R. (1891). St. Petersb. med Wschr., 16, 471-474.
Kobert, R. (1899). Sitzungsber. Naturforsch. Ges. Rostock, 26, zit. nach Abel, J. J., amd W. W. Ford (1907). J. Biol. Chem.,2, 273-288.
Lin, Y.-J., T.-W. Jeng. C.-C Chen, G.-Y. Shi, and T.-C. Tung (1973). Nature, 246, 524-525.
Lin, J.-Y., Y.-J. Lin, C.-C. Chen, H.-L. Wu, G.-Y. Shi, and T.-W. Jeng (1974). Nature, 252, 235-237.
Lin, J.-y., H.-L. Wu, and G.-Y. Shi (1975). Toxicon, 13, 323-331.
Mosthaf, H. (1975). Die Eirkung von Phallolysin und Rubescens-Hämolysin auf das isolierte Meerschweinchenileum. Zahnmed. Diss., Würzburg.
Neeb, G. (1973). Untersuchungen zur Frage einer Phospholipase-Aktivität von Phallolysin. Zahnmed. Diss., Würzburg.
Odenthal, K. P., R. Seeger, and G. Vogel (1975). Naunyn-Schmiedeberg's Arch. Pharmacol., 290, 133-143.
Odenthal, K. P., U. Mengs, and R. Seeger (1976). Naunyn-Schmiedeberg's Arch. Pharmacol., 294, R 24.
Odenthal, K. P., R. Braatz, R. Seeger, H. Mosthaf, and C. Hehn (1977). Naunyn-Schmiedeberg's Arch. Pharmacol., 297, Suppl. 2, R 17.
Petzinger, E., and R. Seeger (1976). Naunyn-Schmiedeberg's Arch. Physiol., 295, 211-213.
Seeger, R., and R. Wiedmann (1972). Arch. Toxikol., 29, 189-217.
Seeger, R., H. Scharrer, and M. Haupt (1973a). Experientia (Basel), 29, 829.
Seeger, R., H. Kraus, and R. Wiedmann (1973b). Arch. Toxikol., 30, 215-226.
Seeger, R., and D. Lehmann (1973). Naunyn-Schmiedeberg's Arch. Pharmacol., 279, 235-242.
Seeger, R.(1975a). Naunyn-Schmiedeberg's Arch. Pharmacol., 287, 277-287.
Seeger, R. (1975b). Naunyn-Schmiedeberg's Arch. Pharmacol., 288, 155-162.
Seeger, R. (1976). Naunyn-Schmiedeberg's Arch. Pharmacol., 284, R25.
Seeger, R., and M. Burkhardt (1976). Naunyn-Schmiedeberg's Arch Pharmacol., 293, 161-170.
Seeger, R. (1980). Naunyn-Schmiedeberg's Arch. Pharmacol., in press.
Villa, L., and A Agostoni (1969). Experientia (Basel), 25, 1300.
Wieland, T., and J.-X. de Vries (1966). Liebigs Ann. Chem., 700, 174-179.

MELITTIN - STRUCTURE AND ACTIVITY

E. Habermann

Pharmacological Institute, Justus Liebig-Universität, Giessen, Federal Republic of Germany

ABSTRACT

Research on and with melittin has given new incentives to molecular biology and pharmacology:

1. Melittin represents a novel structural principle in the field of biologically active peptides.
2. Melittin is a valuable tool for studying the interaction between polypeptides and lipid micelles or membranes.
3. The pharmacological effects of melittin appear to be due to a membrane disturbance which is nonspecific as to the cells afflicted but specific in terms of physical chemistry.

KEYWORDS

Melittin; membranes; peptides; structure-activity relationship; bee; venom; hemolysis.

1. Primary structure and its modification.

The primary structure of the melittins (review: Habermann, 1972) is characterized by overall hydrophobicity of the larger N-terminal moiety (1-20), and hydrophilic, basic residues concentrated at the C-terminus (21-26). More than one, however closely related arrangements of amino acid residues (Table 1) have been realized in the melittins from four bee subspecies. The exchanges do not alter the general structure mentioned. In any case, the C-terminal part remains hydrophilic and basic, despite of its slight changes in *A. florea* melittin. The crucial proline bend is always found in pos. 14. The variations, however slight, of the N-terminal moiety suggest that the term melittin should no longer be restricted to a single peptide but denotes a structurally related class. Individual melittins to be dealt with should be given an extra mark according to their provenance.
The relative number of exchanges allows some phylogenetic classification. The melittins from *A. mellifera* and *A. ceranea* are identical. They differ by only two minor exchanges from *A. dorsata* melittin, whereas *A. florea* melittin is less related to the others.

TABLE 1. Amino Acid Sequences of Four Melittins

		Sequence (1 … 10 … 20 … 26)	
Mellifera	(I)	G I G A *V* L K V L *T* T G L P *A* L I S W I K *R* K R Q Q	1)
Ceranea	(I)		3)
Dorsata	(II)	G I G A *I* L K V L *S* T G L P *A* L I S W I K *R* K R Q Q	2)
Florea	(III)	G I G A *I* L K V L *A* T G L P *T* L I S W I K *N* K R *K* Q	3)

[1] Habermann and Jentsch, 1967; [2] Kreil, 1975; [3] Kreil, 1973

it. exchanges; □ basic residues; ○ hydrophilic, neutral residues

Number of exchanges

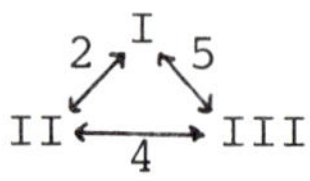

Additional modifications:
The N- terminus of I may be blocked (Habermann and Jentsch, 1967) by N-formylation (Kreil and Kreil-Kiss, 1967); Lübke and others, 1971). The C-terminus is always amidated. A. dorsata melittin ends with isoglutamine. The C-terminus of I is possibly replaced in another melittin (Habermann and Jentsch, 1967) by

21 27
- S R K K R Q Q

In order to understand the relationship between structure and activity, we may compare A. mellifera melittin a) with other natural peptides, b) with its derivatives prepared by substitutions at side-chains and c) with synthetic derivatives.

ad a). So far, information is sparse. Lübke and others (1971) found native N_α-formyl melittin to possess about 80% of the hemolytic activity of melittin. Synthetic melittin (1-26) was equieffective not only with its native prototype but also with synthetic melittin (1-27) (Schröder and others, 1971). Other peptides resemble melittin only superficially. For instance, the membrane-active gramicidin A shares with melittin a large hydrophobic moiety and a hydrophilic end (N-Form - val - gly - ala - (D)leu - ala - (D)val - val - (D)val - trp - (D)leu - trp - (D)leu - trp - (D)leu - trp - NH-CH_2 - CH_2 - OH). However, its lack of basic or proline residues and its large tryptophan content forbid a closer comparison.

ad b) and c). The interpretations of the effects of substitutions on the biological activity of peptides are ambiguous because any substitution will add some group to the peptide, mask an existing group, and may change the secondary structure of even remote parts of the peptide. Consequently, modifications of amino or tryptophan groups (Habermann and Kowallek, 1970) by aid of different reagents lead to products with different properties. For instance, photo-oxidation of the tryptophan decreases the hemolytic power whereas substitution with 2-hydroxy-5-nitro benzyl bromide increases it or leaves it unchanged. Guanidination of the lysines increases the hemolytic power, acetylation slightly and succinylation considerably decreases it. Apparently there is some correlation between hemolysis and electrical charge whereas the parallelism between changes of surface activity and hemolysis is not pronounced (see Table 2).

2. Interactions of melittin with itself.

As expected from its primary structure melittin lowers the surface tension of water which indicates an overall amphiphilic behaviour (Habermann, 1958b). When subjected to preparative gel filtration, its

TABLE 2 Haemolytic activity and action on surface tension of synthetic melittins and their partial sequences

	Haemolytic activity (%)	Surface activity (%)	References
1——————26	100	100	Schröder and others (1971)
1——————27	100	110	
Fo1——————26	80	?	Lübke and others (1971)
7——————27	3	70	Schröder and others (1971)
Boc Boc Boc 7——23–24——27	6	120	" "
15——————26	1	5	" "
Boc Boc 15—21—23——26	5	100	" "
18——————27	inactive	inactive	" "
Boc Boc 18——23–24——27	-	65	" "
Boc Boc 18—21——23——26	1	70	" "
1————20	inactive	110	" "
7———20	inactive	90	" "
1———14	inactive	8	" "
4——14	inactive	50	" "
7—14	inactive	inactive	" "
1————19 Tyr————26	13	?	Miura and others (1972)

molecular weight appeared to be about 4 times larger than calculated from its amino acid content (Habermann and Reiz, 1965). In low concentrations and low ionic strength melittin behaves as a monomer, and its fluorescence shows Trp 19 to be totally exposed to the solvent. Increase of ionic strength and/or melittin concentration gives rise to aggregates of different sizes up to the tetramer (see Table 3). Aggregate formation leads to hydrophobic burying of Trp (Talbot and others, 1979) and profound changes in secondary structure. No ordered structure was found on ORD (Jentsch, 1969) or CD measurements of monomeric melittin in aqueous or ethanolic (77%) solutions (Dawson and others, 1978; Lauterwein and others, 1979).

However, a helical structure becomes visible when the tetramer is formed (Strom and others, 1978; Drake and Hider, 1979; Lauterwein and others, 1979)or in the presence of 2.5% SDS (Dawson and others, 1978). To explain the appearance of the "hidden" order, we have to remind that the probability of the helical arrangement inversely depends on the dielectricity constant. Because the dielectricity constant of membranes and their immediate surroundings (i.e. the Gouy-Chapman-layer)is much lower than that of their environment, it is to be expected that melittin takes its ordered structure when interacting with itself, with lipid micelles, or with membranes. The typical CD-spectrum does not strongly depend on the exact type of lipid but results from the insertion of melittin into a hydrophobic environment, independent of its chemical composition. Possibly (see Strom and others, 1978) the helix formation in lecithin-dicetylphosphate micelles is biphasic, an initial increase of helical content appears to be

TABLE 3 The apparent molecular weight of melittin (MW 2840) depends on the concentrations and buffers used in gel filtration.
Sephadex G 50 column (1.8 x 88 cm), pH 7.4, room temperature. The column was calibrated with ribonuclease (MW 13 680), aprotinin (MW 6512) and glucagon (MW 3483). The elution volumes of the standards did not depend on the buffer used. All melittin peaks are skew (adsorption). The smallest melittin concentration yields a very flat peak.

Amount(mg) of melittin applied	Tris-HCl (0.01M) $MW_{appar.}$	$\frac{\text{MW appar.}}{\text{MW monomer}}$	Na-phosphate (0.15 M) $MW_{appar.}$	$\frac{\text{MW appar.}}{\text{MW monomer}}$
20	I. 8200[1)]	2.89(3)	12 300	4.33(4)
	II. 5100[1)]	1.80(2)		
2	5500	1.95(2)	10 800	3.80(4)
0.2	2100	0.74(1?)	2 000	0.7 (1?)

1) On repeated gel filtration, both fractions yielded the monomer.

followed by a later decrease.

Which parts of the amino acid sequence might contribute to the amphiphilic tendency, the helical tendency, or both? Dawson and others (1978) have calculated the "hydrophobic index", based on the data from Segrest and Feldman (1974), and Nozaki and Tanford (1971). As expected, its average for pos. 1 to 20 is as high as 2.45[x)], well in the range of the value calculated for the intramembranous domain of the MN-glycoprotein (2.6; 23 residues) by Segrest and Feldman (1974). - Chou and Fassman (1974) have evaluated the probability with which an amino acid occurs in the α-helices, ß-sheets or random coils of known protein structures. When applied to melittin four different parts of the molecule can be discerned: (a) A N-terminal helix, covering the segment 2-11. This helix is amphiphilic in itself, because the hydrophilic residues glycine (3), lysine (7), threonine (10) and threonine (11) all are directed towards one side; (b) a "hinge" region containing the proline and its two preceding amino acids; (c) a second, largely hydrophobic helix (pos. 15-21), and (d) the basic, hydrophilic, coiled C-terminal amino acids (pos. 22-26). Dawson and others (1978) have constructed a model how melittin, in contrast to the inactive 8-26 peptide, might interact with membranes (Fig. 1).

3. Interactions with micelles and membranes. May we start with the assumption that melittin interacts with lipid membranes in two consecutive steps. a) In a first step its electrostatic interaction between the C-terminal, positively-charged part of the peptide and negatively charged groups may disturb the bilayer membrane by dislocation of polar head groups (Miller and Bach, 1974) and position the hydrophobic peptide moiety appropriately for the second step. b) In a second step the hydrophobic residues of melittin up to Trp 19 intrude into the hydrophobic region of the bilayer, at the same time taking its ordered structure described in the preceding paragraph. Only a few experimental data deal with the first, binding step. Sessa and others (1969) working with liposomes containing marker CrO_4^{2-} or glucose thought ionic interactions not to be critical for release reactions because liposomes with negative charges (dicetylphosphate)

x) Lysine was not included owing to lack of data.

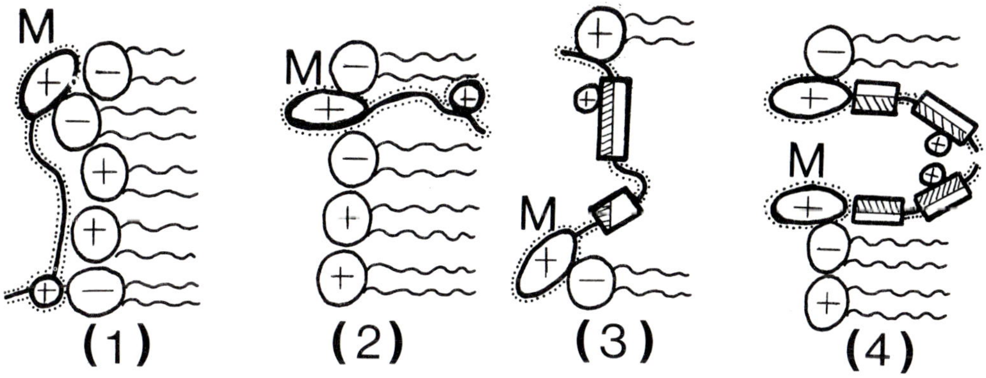

FIG. 1. Four alternatives for the interaction of melittin (M) with lipid bilayers. Alternative (3) according to Dawson and others (1978).

were as sensitive as liposomes with positive charges (stearylamine). However, Dufourcq and Faucon (1977) stated a massive influence of the charge of phospholipid liposomes, as measured by the blue shift of the Trp 19 fluorescence. Phosphatidyl serine vesicles bound up to eight times more melittin than phosphatidyl choline vesicles. Accordingly, binding is also increased by raising the pH value, which results in an increase of the net negative charge of the particles, as is hemolysis increased (Habermann, 1958a). The seeming difference between the findings of the two groups appears to be due to different melittin/lipid ratios. Sessa and others (1969) always used a large excess of phospholipids, thus obscuring quantitative differences depending on charge. - Measuring intrinsic fluorescence polarization, Faucon and others (1979) have found binding of melittin to lipid vesicles even in the presence of 2 M NaCl, which shifts melittin to the tetramer state. Thus tetramers bind to phospholipids as well as monomers. To decide between alternative No. 4 and the other alternatives in Fig. 1, it is important to know the degree of self-aggregation between melittin molecules once in a lipid environment. Equilibrium ultracentrifugation of melittin-dodecylphosphocholine micelles indicates the presence of monomeric melittin (Lauterwein and others, 1979). However, if the melittin/phospholipid ratio is high, melittin monomers might also aggregate with each other, and not only with the lipids.

The second step - <u>insertion into the lipid bilayer</u> - depends on three interdependent factors: The primary structure of melittin, the changes in membrane structure due to melittin, and the changes of the melittin structure due to its membrane environment. Träuble and others (1974) have demonstrated a large increase of helical content of a lipoprotein when added to lipid bilayers. CD-spectra of model peptides polymerized randomly strongly suggest structural changes upon interaction with phospholipid liposomes, resulting in either increased α-helical conformation of polylysine, or transition into ß structure of $(lys, tyr)_n$, or no changes at all $(lys, ser)_n$, (Bach and others, 1975). As discussed before, melittin may yield amphiphilic helices inserted either with their axis parallel to the acyl residues, or in a more complicated manner compatible with the model of Dawson and others (1978) (see Fig. 1).

How deeply does melittin intrude into the membranes or micelles? We may regard this from the side of melittin or of the lipids. At least after insertion (step 2) has taken place, the hydrophilic tail of melittin is not firmly bound. In discussing their NMR data Lauterwein and others (1979) state that the methyl groups of the amino acids in the hydrophobic portion of the melittin molecule (alanines 4 and 15, threonines 10 and 11, one of the isoleucines 17 or 20, valines 5 and 8) change their signals upon binding of melittin to micelles. In contrast, the glutamines 25 and 26, the arginines 22 and 24, and two of the three lysine residues (7, 21, 23) show only small shifts to either direction. These measurements render the alternative (1) in Figure 1 highly improbable. - There is agreement that the Trp 19 residue becomes buried upon interaction with membranes, as indicated by the blue-shift of its fluorescence. This amino acid is also buried in the melittin tetramer in solution (Talbot and others, 1979), which is in accordance with the view (Lauterwein and others, 1979) that melittin reacts with itself in a similar manner as with membranes. As to pos. 1-18, there is ample evidence that they do not pass deeply into, or even traverse the lipid bilayer. For instance, the calculations of Dawson and others (1978) (see. Fig. 1), indicate a flat arrangement, and explain the need of the N-terminus for membrane perturbation. Melittin may "swim" within the lipid lamellae, since evidences from mixtures between distearoyl - and dioleyl-lecithin favor the assumption that melittin preferably interacts with fluid lamellae (Mollay and Kreil, 1973; see also Dufourcq and Faucon, 1977). Accordingly melittin once bound is released by cooling from dipalmitoyl lecithin, in contrast to previous claims.
Quantitative data indicate that one melittin molecule may influence many phospholipid molecules. As measured by intrinsic fluorescence, Trp 19 is immobilized when the lipid to protein ratio is equal to 3 or 4 in the case of phosphatidyl serine and about 25 for phosphatidylcholine (Dufourcq and Faucon, 1977). Differential scanning calorimetry indicates that about 10 lecithin molecules per melittin molecule are prevented from participating in the cooperative temperature-dependent phase transitions. In addition, melittin increases the amount of lipid-bound, i.e. non-freezing water from 10 to 23 moles/mole dipalmitoyl glyceryl phosphoryl choline (Mollay, 1976). As shown by Raman spectroscopy, melittin sharply increases the transition temperature of phospholipid acyl chains. Because the effect occurs already with low ratios of melittin to phospholipid, it has been assumed that the peptide induces constraints extending over larger areas, perhaps a shell surrounding the polypeptide (Verma and Wallach, 1976).

Verma and Wallach's (1976) Raman spectra allow to assess stretch vibrations when melittin is inserted into liposomes of different composition. In the case of dimyristoyl phosphatidyl choline, there is a gradient of structuring perpendicular to the membrane plane because vibrations due to methylene groups are more changed than those involving the terminal methyl groups. Melittin sharply increases the transition temperature of phospholipid acyl chains. - Proton NMR spectroscopy (de Bony and others, 1979) also indicate that lipid perturbation by melittin is maximal in the α- and ß-position from the ester groups, minimal at the methyl terminal, and absent at the polar heads.

4. Sequelae of interactions between melittin and membranes.
As indicated by liposome disruption due to melittin, the physicochemical properties of lipids are heavily changed. This explains why melittin-treated membranes vigorously take up spin-labeled fatty acid

residues from the surrounding solution, a phenomenon which is largely independent from surface charge. In contrast, the mobility of spin label is only slightly diminished by melittin, whereas other peptides which also interact with bilayers hydrophobically, like chlorothicin or polymyxin B, induce cooperative immobilization over large regions of the lipid matrix (Williams and Bell, 1972). - In the presence of melittin, phospholipase A apparently gains a better access to its substrate (Habermann, 1957). Using E. coli membrane-labeled by biosynthesis with ^{14}C-oleic acid, a weak endogenous phospholipase A activity could be measured, which was 6-7 fold enhanced by adding melittin. Accordingly, (exogenous) bee venom enzyme is activated in a similar manner (Mollay et al., 1976).
Melittin is a potent drug on any organ tested so far (for review see Habermann, 1972). Its ability to interact with structures common to many cell membranes has been compiled in this paper and explains why melittin is a potent but non-specific agent at the level of organ pharmacology.
Why does melittin damage membranes? In the light of recent data its surface activity is certainly not a sufficient explanation. Therefore our earlier definition of melittin as an "invert soap on peptide basis" can no longer be held. We now propose that the peptide, once in a hydrophobic environment, takes an ordered, rigid structure where the more flexible membrane lipids have to comply with. By that way, the functional integrity of the membrane will be lost. This hypothesis would also explain why one melittin molecule alters the state of many phospholipid molecules, why melittin is released on cooling, and why it preferably reacts with fluid lamellae. However, it does not take into account the biphasic process described by Strom and others (1978).

REFERENCES

Bach, D., K. Rosenbeck, and I.R. Miller (1975). Interaction of basic polypeptides with phospholipid vesicles: Conformational study. Europ. J. Biochem., 53, 265-269.
Chou, P.Y., and G.D. Fassman (1974). Conformational parameters for amino acids in helical, ß-sheet and random coil regions calculated from proteins. Biochemistry, 13, 211-222.
Dawson, C.R., A.F. Drake, J. Helliwell, and R.C. Hider (1978). The interaction of bee melittin with lipid bilayer membranes. Biochim. Biophys. Acta, 510, 75-86.
de Bony, J., J. Dufourcq, and B. Clin (1979). Lipid-protein interactions: NMR study of melittin and its binding to lysophosphatidyl choline. Biochim. Biophys. Acta, 552, 531-534.
Drake, A.F., and R.C. Hider (1979). The structure of melittin in lipid bilayer membranes. Biochim. Biophys. Acta, 555, 371-373.
Dufourcq, J., and J.-F. Faucon (1977). Intrinsic fluorescence study of lipid-protein interactions in membrane models. Binding of melittin, and amphipathic peptide, to phospholipid vesicles. Biochim. Biophys. Acta, 467, 1-11.
Faucon, J.F., J. Dufourcq, and C. Lussan (1979). The self-association of melittin and its binding to lipids. FEBS Letters, 102, 187-190.
Habermann, E. (1957). Manometrische Bestimmung von Phospholipase A. Biochem. Z., 328, 474-484.
Habermann, E. (1958a). Über die Wirkung tierischer Gifte auf Erythrozyten Z. ges. exper. Med., 129, 436-464.
Habermann, E. (1958b). Zur Wirkung tierischer Gifte und von Lysocithin auf Grenzflächen. Z. ges. exper. Med. 130, 19-23.

Habermann, E. (1972). Bee and wasp venoms. Science, 177, 314-322.
Habermann, E., and J. Jentsch (1967). Sequenzanalyse des Melittins aus seinen tryptischen und peptischen Spaltstücken. Hoppe-Seyler's Z. Physiol. Chem., 348, 37-50.
Habermann, E., and H. Kowallek (1970). Modifikationen der Aminogruppen und des Tryptophans in Melittin als Mittel zur Erkennung von Struktur-Wirkungs-Beziehungen. Hoppe-Seyler's Z. Physiol. Chem., 351, 884-890.
Habermann, E., and K.G. Reiz (1965). Ein neues Verfahren zur Gewinnung der Komponenten von Bienengift, insbesondere des zentralwirksamen Peptids Apamin. Biochem. Z., 341, 451-466.
Jentsch, J. (1969). Weitere Untersuchungen zur Aminosäuresequenz des Melittins. IV. Messung der optischen Rotationsdispersion. Z. Naturforsch., 24b, 33-35.
Kreil, G. (1973). Structure of melittin isolated from two species of honey bees. Febs Letters, 33, 241-244.
Kreil, G. (1975). The structure of Apis dorsata melittin: Phylogenetic relationships between honey bees as deduced from sequence data. Febs Letters, 54, 100-102.
Kreil, G., and G. Kreil-Kiss (1967). The isolation of N-formylglycine from a polypeptide present in bee venom. Biochem. Biophys. Res. Comm., 27, 275-280.
Lauterwein, J., C. Bösch, L.R. Brown, and K. Wüthrich (1979). Physicochemical studies of the protein-lipid interactions in melittin-containing micelles. Biochim. Biophys. Acta, 556, 244-264.
Lübke, K., S. Mathes, and G. Kloss (1971). Isolation and structure of N_α-formyl melittin. Experientia, 27, 765-767.
Miller, I.R., and D. Bach (1974). Interaction of basic polypeptides with phospholipid monolayers. Chem. Phys. Lipids, 13, 453-465.
Miura, Y., H. Sugiyama, Y. Maki, and S. Seto (1972). The solid phase synthesis of 19-tyrosine melittin. Chem. a. Pharmac. Bull., 20, 215-218.
Mollay, C. (1976). Effect of melittin and melittin fragments on the thermotropic phase transition of dipalmitoyllecithin and on the amount of lipid-bound water. FEBS Letters, 64, 65-68.
Mollay, C., and G. Kreil (1973). Fluorometric measurements on the interaction of melittin with lecithin. Biochim. Biophys. Acta, 316, 196-203.
Mollay, C., G. Kreil, and H. Berger (1976). Action of phospholipase on the cytoplasmic membrane of Escherichia coli. Stimulation by melittin. Biochim. Biophys. Acta, 426, 317-324.
Nozaki, Y., and C. Tanford (1971). The solubility of amino acids and two glycine peptides in aqueous ethanol and dioxane solutions. Establishment of a hydrophobicity scale. J. Biol. Chem., 246, 2211-2217.
Schröder, E., K. Lübke, M. Lehmann, and I. Beetz (1971). Haemolytic activity and action on the surface tension of aqueous solutions of synthetic melittins and their derivatives. Experientia, 27, 764-765
Segrest, J.P., and R.J. Feldman (1974). Membrane proteins: Amino acid sequence and membrane penetration. J. Mol. Biol. 87, 853-858.
Sessa, G., J.H. Freer, G. Colacicco, and G. Weissmann (1969). Interaction of a lytic polypeptide, melittin, with lipid membrane systems. J. Biol. Chem., 244, 3575-3582.
Strom, R., C. Crifo, V. Viti, L. Guidoni, and F. Podo (1978). Variations in circular dichroism and proton-NMR relaxation properties of melittin upon interaction with phospholipids. FEBS Letters, 96, 45-50.

Talbot, J.C., J. Dufourcq, J. de Bony, J.F. Faucon, and C. Lussan (1979). Conformational change and self association of monomeric melittin. FEBS Letters, 102, 191-193.

Träuble, H., G. Middelhoff, and V.W. Brown (1974). Interaction of a serum apo-lipoprotein with ordered and fluid lipid bilayers. Correlation between lipid and protein structure. FEBS Letters, 49, 269-275.

Verma, S.P., and D.F.H. Wallach (1976). Effect of melittin on thermotropic lipid state transitions in phosphotidyl choline liposomes. Biochim. Biophys. Acta, 426, 616-623.

Williams, J.C., and R.M. Bell (1972). Membrane matrix disruption by melittin. Biochim. Biophys. Acta, 288, 255-262.

LIPOSOMES AS MODELS FOR THE STUDY OF CYTOLYTIC TOXINS

J. H. Freer

Department of Microbiology, University of Glasgow, Alexander Stone Building, Garscube Estate, Bearsden, Glasgow G64 1RB, UK

ABSTRACT

The preparation of liposomes and assays for permeability changes are described. The utility of the liposome system in morphological, permeability and binding studies of staphylococcal and oxygen-labile haemolysins is discussed.

KEYWORDS

Liposomes; cytolysins; bacteria; Streptolysin O; Staphylococcal α-toxin; Staphylococcal δ-lysin; membranes; model; permeability; toxin.

INTRODUCTION

The preferred arrangement of many biological lipids, when suspended in aqueous media at appropriate temperatures, is the liquid crystal. Its form will depend upon several factors the most dominant of which are the structure and concentration of the lipid(s) and the temperature and ionic composition of the aqueous phase (for reviews see Lee, 1977a, 1977b; Papahadjopoulos & Miller, 1967; Papahadjopoulos & Watkins, 1967).

The most frequently observed form of liquid crystal when phospholipids are resuspended in excess water or buffer is the multilamellar vesicle consisting of concentric sealed lipid bilayers, each bilayer separated from the other by a closed aqueous compartment (Fig 1(a)). The results of structural, osmotic and ion permeability studies on such liposomes were first reported almost fifteen years ago (Bangham, Standish & Watkins, 1965; Bangham, de Gier & Greville, 1967). The general rules regarding selective permeability and osmotic properties of liposomes also apply to biomembranes and the lipid bilayer configuration of the liposomal lipid is a basic feature in the currently accepted model for biomembrane structure (Singer & Nicholson, 1972).

The applicability of the liposome as a useful model for studying certain aspects of the structure and behaviour of biomembranes is evidenced by the vast amount of literature in this field. A useful collection of information on diverse aspects of liposome structure and function is provided in the proceedings of a recent meeting devoted to the use of liposomes in biology and medicine (Papahadjopoulos, 1978).

One of the more attractive features of liposomes is the ease and simplicity with which they can be prepared. The most commonly used preparation method is based on that originally described by Bangham, Standish & Watkins (1965) where lipid or a mixture of lipids in chloroform is dried in vacuo as a thin shell in a suitable flask. The dried lipid is then vigorously resuspended in a suitable aqueous buffer under N_2 by vigorous hand shaking. Alternatively ultrasound can be used to aid dispersion. After a period of time to allow 'swelling' of the lipids (~1 h at room temperature) the liposomes, largely consisting of multilamellar concentric vesicles can be used.

For permeability studies, a suitable marker (eg. CrO_4^-,glucose, ^{14}C-glucose, ^{14}C-arginine, ^{42}K, ^{22}Na etc) is included in the swelling buffer, and the unsequestered marker removed after swelling either by dialysis or by gel filtration. Changes in the release of sequestered marker as a response to treatment with membrane-active agents can be followed in one of two ways. In the "dialysis assay" the liposomes plus agent can be sealed in a dialysis sac and the external dialysis fluid assayed for marker after various time intervals. Where glucose is used as a marker a more convenient assay for its release is that described by Kinsky and colleagues (1968) using a "spectrophotometric assay". Glucose is sequestered and the liposomes are suspended in a buffer system containing hexokinase, ATP, glucose 6-phosphate dehydrogenase and NADP and the rate of reduction of NADP, measured by an increase in E_{340} is a measure of the rate of glucose released from the liposomes, since the enzyme system cannot cross the intact bilayer. One advantage of this assay is the relatively small quantity of lipid used, the kinetic data being obtained without the need to remove liposomes from the assay system. The relative merits of the dialysis and spectrophotometric assays were compared in a study of the effects of cholesterol concentration on the sensitivity of liposomes to the polyene antibiotic filipin by Kinsky and colleagues (1968). In the spectrophotometric assay, kinetic data can be obtained since the concentration of lytic agent is the rate limiting factor, whereas in the dialysis assay, if transfer of marker across the dialysis membrane is rate limiting, interpretation of results may be erroneous.

Liposomes also provide a useful membrane model when morphological effects of cytolysins are thought to occur via interaction with membrane lipids. Since it is usually possible to prepare liposomes from total extractable erythrocyte lipids a comparison between lytic effects on intact membranes in the erythrocyte and in the liposomal membrane formed from erythrocyte lipids alone is possible. It should be borne in mind however that the distribution of constituent lipid species in the intact erythrocyte is not uniform. Cholesterol may be present as two pools in the plane of the membrane (Elias, Goerke & Friend, 1978); also the choline-containing lipids are considerably enriched in the outer lipid leaflet of the erythrocyte membrane (Verklej & colleagues, 1973). The distribution of cholesterol and hence phospholipid in liposomal membranes may also be non-random and influenced by the lipid species present (De Kruyff and colleagues, 1974).

BACTERIAL CYTOLYTIC TOXINS

By definition, bacterial cytolytic toxins are capable of membrane disruption leading to cell lysis. Many of them are also capable of disrupting the membranes of subcellular organelles such as lysosomes and mitochondria. However, the basis for the sensitivity of the membrane to the action of bacterial cytolysins is understood in relatively few cases (Freer & Arbuthnott, 1976). Those toxins which are also enzymes (staphylococcal β-lysin and clostridial α-toxin) capable of hydrolysing membrane phospholipids appear to cause lysis by destruction of structural membrane lipids. Also, the group of toxins known as the oxygen-labile haemolysins appear to perturb membrane structure as a result of their interaction with membrane cholesterol. In the majority of cases however, the precise mode of action of cytolysins still remains to be elucidated.

Staphylococcal α-toxin

The mode of cytolysis induced by α-toxin is unknown, but the primary site of damage is undoubtedly the cell membrane. No enzymic activity has been consistently demonstrated in purified toxin using as substrates either whole cells, erythrocyte ghosts or liposomes made from extractable lipids of rabbit erythrocytes, the most sensitive cell type (Freer, Arbuthnott & Bernheimer, 1968; Freer, Arbuthnott & Billcliffe, 1973).

The first indication that staphylococcal α-toxin is able to interact with lipids came from the work of Weissmann, Sessa & Bernheimer (1966) who demonstrated permeability changes in liposomes composed of egg lecithin, dicetyl phosphate and cholesterol exposed to α-toxin. Freer, Arbuthnott & Bernheimer (1968) confirmed this observation and also showed that the toxin also penetrated mixed lipid monolayers of similar composition. Disruption of both erythrocyte membranes and liposomal membranes was accompanied by polymerisation of the toxin to a higher molecular weight form, although this effect was not considered directly related to the lytic activity of the toxin. The membrane-mediated polymerisation observed in both natural and artificial membranes suggested that it was a lipid-induced phenomenon. Evidence supporting this suggestion came from the work of Arbuthnott, Freer & Billcliffe (1973) who showed that while aqueous dispersion of single lipids such as diglyceride, lecithin, cholesterol or lysolecithin promoted toxin polymerisation, no individual lipid was as effective in promoting polymer formation as was a mixture of lipids in the form of liposomes. No absolute specificity for a single lipid species was observed in contrast with the O-labile haemolysins (see below).

While α-toxin will react with membrane lipids, this interaction does not fully explain the pronounced sensitivity of rabbit erythrocytes for α-toxin. Cassidy, Six & Harshman (1974) used the liposome system to show that α-toxin caused approximately equivalent release of low molecular weight glucose marker from liposomes prepared from either rabbit erythrocyte lipids or from human erythrocyte lipids whereas intact erythrocytes show a 100 fold difference in sensitivity to the toxin, as measured by haemoglobin release. It would be of interest to follow the release of a similarly high molecular weight marker from such liposomes as a response to α-lysin, since rabbit erythrocytes differ in their osmotic stability and in their response to melittin (Freer & Birkbeck, unpublished observations).

Staphylococcal δ-lysin

There is considerable circumstantial evidence that δ-lysin disrupts cell membranes by virtue of its high surface activity (Freer & Arbuthnott, 1976). Mammalian erythrocytes show only a 5-fold difference in sensitivity to the lysin, the specific haemolytic activity being low (∿300 HU/mg protein for human or horse erythrocytes) compared with other cytolytic toxins. Cod erythrocytes show a 4-fold increase in sensitivity over those of horse, the most sensitive mammalian species (Chao & Birkbeck, 1978). The basis for this increased sensitivity may be related to the low free sterol content (∿10% w/w of total lipid) and/or the high content of polyunsaturated fatty acyl residues in the erythrocyte phospholipids (Addison & Ackman, 1971). If erythrocyte sensitivity to δ-lysin is a function of membrane lipid composition (and hence membrane fluidity), then liposomes prepared from different erythrocyte lipids should also display similar differences in sensitivity to disruption by δ-lysin as those seen in intact cells. While electron microscopy showed extensive disruption of cod lipid liposomes after exposure to δ-lysin, the untreated liposomes appeared as small vesicles of irregular outline showing many apparent discontinuities in the bilayers. This apparent instability was confirmed in permeability studies where liposomes prepared from cod erythrocyte lipids had spontaneous leakage rates for sequestered glucose such that the measurement of lysin-induced permeability increases was not feasible. This high permeability of cod lipid liposomes even at temperatures of 0-4°C contrasts with the stability of intact erythrocytes at these temperatures and serves to emphasise the different behaviour of the intact membrane and liposomes derived from membrane lipids. A detailed study of the influence of phospholipid fatty-acyl structure on the sensitivity of liposomes to lysin-induced permeability changes is required. With the availability of synthetic lecithins of different degrees of saturation and chain length, such studies would usefully include the binding characteristics of lysin as a function of temperature in the range above and below the lipid phase transition temperature (Tc). These studies on liposomes would further our understanding of the way in which this interesting lytic peptide disrupts membrane structure in such a wide variety of cells and membrane-bounded structures.

Oxygen-labile haemolysins

The oxygen-labile or thiol(-SH)-activated haemolysins are a group of cytolysins remarkably similar in their biological and physical properties, yet produced by a rather diverse collection of Gram-positive bacteria (Smyth & Duncan, 1978). They differ from staphylococcal toxins in that cholesterol serves as their binding component in the membrane, cells lacking cholesterol being insensitive to these toxins. It is still not clear how the binding to cholesterol brings about membrane damage.

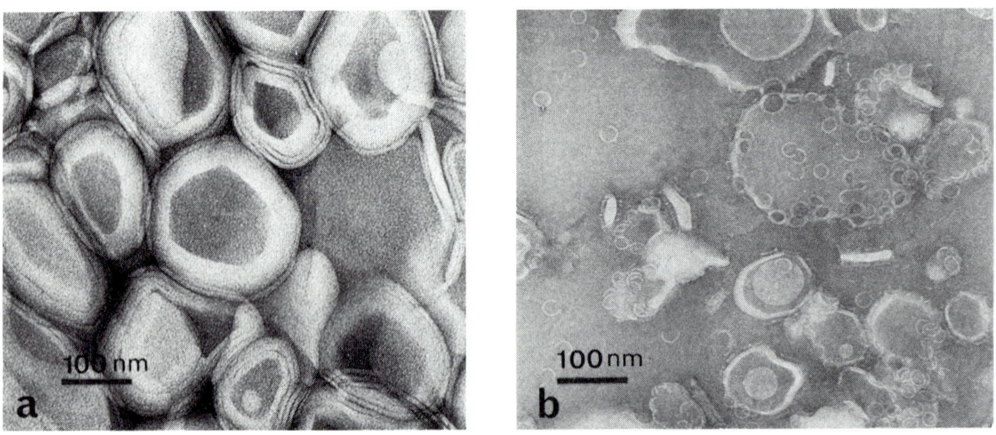

Fig. 1. Electron micrographs of liposomes (lecithin, dicetyl phosphate, cholesterol; molar ratio 70:20:10) negatively stained with ammonium molybdate. (a) Untreated (b) exposed to perfringolysin.

A good deal of effort in recent years has been focused on the study of morphological changes in target membranes which result from the interaction with oxygen-labile haemolysins. This followed from the initial observation that Streptolysin O (SLO, produced by *Streptococcus pyogenes*) caused 'doughnut' or pit-like structures to appear in sensitive membranes, somewhat similar in appearance to those produced by the action of complement, alfalfa saponin and filipin. Bernheimer (1974) suggested that these 'doughnut' structures, seen after Streptolysin O treatment, may represent the coalescence of toxin/cholesterol complexes in the plane of the membrane to form a pore and that lysis may result from leakage through the pores or via an unknown mechanism resulting from the depletion of cholesterol from contiguous areas of the membrane. These interesting suggestions were followed by a number of investigations where attention was focused on the conditions necessary for the formation of the doughnut rings and their involvement in the lytic process. Smyth, Freer & Arbuthnott (1975) showed that perfringolysin (*Clostridium perfringens* θ-toxin) caused the formation of ring or arc shaped structures on erythrocyte membranes and on liposomes containing cholesterol (Fig 1(b)). They also showed that the ring and arc structures formed after addition of the lysin to aqueous dispersions of cholesterol. At the toxin concentrations used no such structures were visible after interaction of toxin with liposomes lacking cholesterol. However, in the purified toxin occasional ring structures were seen. At about the same time Duncan & Schlegel (1975) showed that similar structures occurred after treatment of erythrocytes and liposomes containing cholesterol with SLO. Also, cholesterol dispersions treated with SLO contained abundant rings and arcs. Both these groups of workers exploited the liposome model in an attempt to define precisely which membrane constituents were necessary for ring formation. Both groups concluded that cholesterol was responsible for induction of the ring and arc forms although no information was presented to clarify the precise composition of these structures. The fact that they appeared only after interaction of toxin with cholesterol or cholesterol-containing membranes suggested that they were in some way involved in the process of membrane disruption although Smyth, Freer & Arbuthnott (1975) did note that rings and arcs were very occasionally seen in small numbers in both active and inactive (oxidised) toxin preparations alone. This observation led them to suggest that rather than the rings being sterol-toxin complexes, they may in fact represent toxin polymers, the polymerisation being somehow promoted by the presence of cholesterol.

The significance of the ring and arc shaped structures was made more difficult to assess after a later report by Cowell, Kim & Bernheimer (1978) which showed that in the case of cereolysin (produced by Bacillus cereus), ring and arc structures were formed in purified toxin preparations alone at protein concentrations greater than 6 μg/ml. In addition, low but lytic concentration of cereolysin failed to produce rings or arcs on sensitive erythrocyte ghost membranes.

In the study of Duncan & Schlegel, it was also noted that even though the rings and arcs were present on liposomes containing cholesterol, no increased release of sequestered marker resulted after treatment with the toxin (SLO), which suggested that the rings did not represent transmembrane pores. This finding was at variance with the earlier report by Sessa & Weissmann (1968) that both cereolysin and SLO did induce release of sequestered marker from liposomes containing cholesterol, although the degree of release was only 'modest' compared to that induced by other cytolytic toxins such as Streptolysin S or staphylococcal α-toxin.

More recently the bearing that sterol/phospholipid ratios and phospholipid structure has on the sensitivity of liposomes to SLO has been investigated in detailed studies by Prigent & Alouf (1978), Alouf (unpublished results) and by Delattre, Lebsir, Panouse-Perrin & Badin (1979). With ^{14}C-arginine as a sequestered marker, Prigent & Alouf (1978) utilised liposomes prepared from phosphatidylcholine, sterol and phosphatidic acid to determine the influence of both sterol concentration (i.e. sterol:phospholipid ratio) and sterol type on their sensitivity to lysis by SLO. Maximal sensitivity, as evidenced by degree of leakage of marker, was found in liposomes with a sterol:phospholipid ratio of 0.85, a ratio close to that found in the membranes of sensitive cells. Liposomes containing cholesterol as the sterol species were sensitive to lysis by SLO while substitution of cholesterol by a related sterol (either ergosterol, lanosterol or stigmasterol) rendered them insensitive. As the molar ratio of cholesterol:phosphatidylcholine fell, the degree of leakage and the amount of ^{125}I-labelled toxin bound also declined (Alouf, unpublished observations). Prigent & Alouf (1978) point out that the reason why earlier investigators failed to show SLO-induced leakage of marker from liposomes was probably due to unfavourable sterol:phospholipid ratios. However, the sterol:phospholipid ratio ($\sim$1.0) used in the liposome preparation of Duncan & Schlegel does not account for the absence of increased permeability after SLO treatment. The influence of phospholipid species on the binding of SLO to liposomal cholesterol was investigated by Delattre and colleagues (1979). The fraction of liposome cholesterol available for binding with SLO was assessed by determining the amount of inhibition of SLO after reaction with liposomes. As suggested by the studies of Alouf, the sterol:phospholipid ratio was of critical importance in the process of SLO binding. With either phosphatidylcholine or sphingomyelin as the liposome phospholipid, a cholesterol:phospholipid ratio of less than 0.66 resulted in no inhibition of SLO activity, indicating no liposomal cholesterol available for toxin binding. At a ratio of 1 or more cholesterol appeared to be totally available for binding toxin. This compares reasonably well with the optimal ratio >0.85 for SLO-induced leakage reported by Prigent & Alouf (1978). As might be expected the phospholipid head group structure also influences the degree of binding of SLO to membrane cholesterol. The choline-containing phospholipids (phosphatidylcholine and sphingomyelin) totally inhibited binding at ratios of 0.66 or less, whereas if the sterol content in the liposome was increased to give a ratio >1.0 the cholesterol appeared to be totally available for toxin binding. With phosphatidylserine as the phospholipid species, cholesterol remained almost totally available for binding down to a ratio of 0.33 (lowest tested). Also, phosphatidic acid and phosphatidylethanolamine behaved in a similar manner. In the case of phosphatidylserine and phosphatidic acid, both have a net negative charge at neutral pH and head group repulsion may account for the increased accessibility of sterol to the SLO molecules.

The observation that phospholipase D treatment of phosphatidylcholine:cholesterol liposomes (cholesterol:phospholipid ratio = 0.5) rendered the cholesterol accessible to SLO binding suggests that the choline group may cause steric hindrance to SLO binding; however the removal of the choline group would result in the generation of phosphatidic acid residues, where the net negative charge may be the more important factor.

Anatomical evidence from electron microscopy of SLO-treated liposomes supports the results of the binding studies. Delattre and colleagues showed that at ratios of cholesterol:phosphatidylcholine <0.5, liposomes were unaltered by exposure to SLO whereas the structure of liposomes with a ratio of 1.0 or more was rapidly destroyed upon interaction with toxin. This destruction was accompanied by the appearance of structures thought to be cholesterol:SLO complexes (however see above).

DISCUSSION

In this short article, the utilisation of the liposome model in studies of the mode of action of bacterial cytolytic toxins illustrates some advantages, but also some major limitations of the model. In the case of staphylococcal α-toxin, Cassidy and colleagues (1974) concluded that the liposome system was not useful when studying the selectivity of α-toxin on biomembranes, since liposomes prepared from both rabbit and human erythrocyte lipids showed a similar degree of sensitivity to disruption by the toxin. However, this finding in itself confirms previous observations that α-toxin is surface-active, and also shows that the erythrocyte specificity of the toxin is not likely to be related to specific membrane lipids alone.

While it is usually possible to prepare stable liposomes from erythrocyte lipid extracts, those prepared from cod erythrocyte lipids have a high rate of spontaneous release of sequestered marker even at $0^{o}C$, due to the relatively large amounts of highly unsaturated fatty acyl residues in the membrane lipids. The relatively high sensitivity of cod erythrocytes to lysis by staphylococcal δ-lysin, together with the detergent-like properties of the lysin suggests that the basis for the sensitivity may lie in the structure of the membrane lipids. However the high intrinsic permeability of liposomes containing cod erythrocyte lipids makes them unsuitable for the study of permeability changes induced by δ-lysin. The differences in permeability of the liposomes compared with intact erythrocytes also serve to emphasise the dangers of extrapolating results obtained from liposomes directly to intact erythrocytes.

The liposome experimental system has been fruitfully applied in several studies of the mode of interaction of oxygen-labile haemolysins with membrane lipids, and these serve to illustrate some advantages of this model. Structural features of the sterol molecule necessary for toxin binding and lytic activity against liposomes have been defined for SLO together with the influence phospholipid structure (Delattre and colleagues, 1973, 1975, 1979). In order to gain a clearer picture of the common features of the interaction of oxygen-labile haemolysins with membranes, the studies involving SLO must be applied to other related lysins in this group.

Fruitful areas for future work will also involve the wider application of physical methods in the study of lysin/membrane interactions. As suggested by Smyth & Duncan (1978) the effect of O-labile lysin binding to membrane cholesterol on the temperature dependent phase transition of membrane lipids may provide data which relate to the proposed lytic mechanism involving cholesterol sequestration and consequent membrane destabilisation.

Also the use of spin-labelled fatty acyl residues on liposome phospholipids will provide data relating to the effects of staphylococcal δ-lysin on lipid mobility. Differential scanning calorimetry and fluorescence depolarisation techniques applied to membranes of differing sensitivity to δ-lysin may help to clarify the role of phospholipid structure and influence of membrane fluidity on toxin sensitivity and toxin binding.

The possibility of incorporating toxin receptors such as the protein receptor (130,000 MW) for staphylococcal α-toxin recently discussed by Harshman (1979) provides a further challenge for future workers in this field. A simplified membrane system containing defined lipids and a single protein species as has been produced using the detergent/dialysis procedure for the preparation of liposomes containing proteins in the bilayer (see Tyrell, Heath, Colley & Ryman, 1976) would provide a model in which parameters governing the toxin/receptor binding and subsequent events involved in membrane disruption might be investigated.

ACKNOWLEDGEMENT

I wish to thank The Welcome Trust and Glasgow University for travel grants, Drs. J. Alouf and J. Delattre for providing data prior to publication and Anne Strachan for typing the script.

REFERENCES

Addison, R.F. and R.G. Ackman (1971). Erythrocyte lipids of Atlantic Cod, Gadus morhua. Canad. J. Biochem., 49, 873-876.

Arbuthnott, J.P., J.H. Freer and B. Billcliffe (1973). Lipid-induced polymerisation of staphylococcal α-toxin. J. Gen. Microbiol., 75, 309-319.

Bangham, A.D., J. de Gier and G.D. Greville (1967). Osmotic properties and water permeability of phospholipid liquid crystals. Chem. Phys. Lipids, 1, 225-246.

Bangham, A.D., M.M. Standish and J.C. Watkins (1965). Diffusion of univalent ions across the lamellae of swollen phospholipids. J. Mol. Biol., 13, 238-252.

Bernheimer, A.W. (1974). Interactions between membranes and cytolytic bacterial toxins. Biochim. Biophys. Acta., 344, 27-50.

Cassidy, P., H.R. Six and S. Harshman (1974). Biological properties of staphylococcal α-toxin. Biochim. Biophys. Acta., 332, 413-423.

Chao, L.P. and T.H. Birkbeck (1978). Assay of staphylococcal δ-haemolysin with fish erythrocytes. J. Med. Microbiol., 11, 303-313.

Cowell, J.L., K.S. Kim and A.W. Bernheimer (1978). Alteration by cereolysin of the structure of cholesterol-containing membranes. Biochim. Biophys. Acta., 507, 230-241.

De Kruyff, B., P.W.M. van Dijck, R.A. Demel, A. Schuijff, F. Brants and L.L.M. van Deenen (1974). Non-random distribution of cholesterol in phosphatidyl-choline bilayer. Biochim. Biophys. Acta., 356, 1-7.

Delattre, J., R. Lebsir, J. Panouse-Perrin and J. Badin (1979). A cholesterol fraction for streptolysin O binding in cell membranes and lipoproteins. II. Interaction of streptolysin O with phospholipid-cholesterol liposomes of different nature and molar ratios. Cell. Mol. Biol. 24, 157-166.

Delattre, J., J. Badin, J. Canal and M.L. Girard (1975). Rôle du groupement phosphorylcholine sur le pouvoir inhibiteur des liposomes lécithines-cholestérol vis-à-vis de la streptolysine O. C.r.Acad. Sci. Paris. Série D. 280, 1165-1168.

Delattre, J., J. Badin, J. Canal and M.L. Girard (1973). Influence des lécithines sur le pouvoir inhibiteur du cholestérol vis-à-vis de la streptolysine O. C.r. Acad. Sci. Paris. Série D. 277, 441-443.

Duncan, J.L. and R. Schlegel (1975). Effect of streptolysin O on erythrocyte membranes, liposomes and lipid dispersions. J. Cell. Biol., 67, 160-173.

Elias, P.M., J. Goerke and D.S. Friend (1978). Freeze fracture identification of sterol-digitonin complexes in the cell and liposome membranes. J. Cell. Biol., 78, 577-596.

Freer, J.H. and J.P. Arbuthnott (1976). Biochemical and morphological alterations of membranes by bacterial toxins. In A.W. Bernheimer (Ed.), Mechanisms of Bacterial Toxinology, J. Wiley & Sons, New York. pp. 170-193.

Freer, J.H., J.P. Arbuthnott and A.W. Bernheimer (1968). The interaction of staphylococcal α-toxin with natural and artificial membranes. J. Bact., 95, 1153-1168.

Freer, J.H., J.P. Arbuthnott and B. Billcliffe (1973). Effects of staphylococcal α-toxin on the structure of erythrocyte membranes: a biochemical and morphological study. J. Gen. Microbiol., 75, 321-332.

Harshman, S. (1979). Action of staphylococcal α-toxin on membranes: some recent advances. Mol. Cell. Biochem., 23, 143-152.

Kinsky, S.C., J. Haxby, C.B. Kinsky, R.A. Demel and L.L.M. van Deenen (1968). Effect of cholesterol incorporation on the sensitivity of liposomes to the polyene antibiotic, Filipin. Biochim. Biophys. Acta., 152, 174-185.

Lee, A.G. (1977a). Lipid phase transitions and phase diagrams. I. Lipid phase transitions. Biochim. Biophys. Acta., 472, 237-281.

Lee, A.G. (1977b). Lipid phase transitions and phase diagrams. II. Mixtures involving lipids. Biochim. Biophys. Acta., 472, 285-344.

Papahadjopoulos, D. (1978). Liposomes and their uses in biology and medicine. Ann. N.Y. Acad. Sci., Vol. 308, 1-462.

Papahadjopoulos, D. and N. Miller (1967). Phospholipid model membranes. I. Structural characteristics of hydrated liquid crystals. Biochim. Biophys. Acta., 135, 624-638.

Pendleton, I.R., K.S. Kim and A.W. Bernheimer (1972). Detection of cholesterol in cell membranes by use of bacterial toxins. J. Bact., 110, 722-730.

Prigent, D. and J.E. Alouf (1978). Interaction de la streptolysine O avec les liposomes. Labo-Pharma-Problemes et Techniques, 281, 910-913.

Singer, S.J. and G.L. Nicolson (1972). The fluid mosaic model of the structure of cell membranes. Science (N.Y.), 175, 720-731.

Smyth, C.J. and J.L. Duncan (1978). Thiol-activated (oxygen-labile) cytolysins. In J. Jeljaszewicz and T. Wadstrom (Ed.), Bacterial Toxins and Cell Membranes, Academic Press, New York. pp. 129-178.

Smyth, C.J., J.H. Freer and J.P. Arbuthnott (1975). Interaction of Clostridium perfringens θ-haemolysin, a contaminant of commercial phospholipase C, with erythrocyte ghost membranes and lipid dispersions. A morphological study. Biochim. Biophys. Acta., 382, 479-493.

Tyrell, D.A., T.D. Heath, C.M. Colley and B.E. Ryman (1976). New aspects of liposomes. Biochim. Biophys. Acta., 457, 259-302.

Verkleij, A.J., R.F.A. Zwaal, B. Roelofsen, P. Comfurius, D. Kastelijn and L.L.M. van Deenen (1977). The asymetric distribution of phospholipids in the human red cell membrane. Biochim. Biophys. Acta., 465, 1-10.

Weissmann, G., G. Sessa and A.W. Bernheimer (1966). Staphylococcal α-toxin: effects on artificial lipid spherules. Science (N.Y.), 154, 772-774.

ACTIVATION OF SELF-DESTRUCTION AS A MECHANISM OF ACTION FOR CYTOLYTIC TOXINS

W. T. Shier

Cell Biology Laboratory, The Salk Institute, Post Office Box 85800, San Diego, CA 92138, USA

ABSTRACT

Many of the hydrolytic enzymes in a cell, whether they play a degradation/salvage role or a regulatory role, could in principle be subverted by toxins to induce self-destruction. Of these, only the activation of cellular phospholipase A_2 by toxins has as yet been demonstrated. Transient activation of cellular phospholipase A_2 plays a widely recognized role in the regulation of prostaglandin biosynthesis, and it has been proposed to regulate membrane function by alteration of membrane lipid composition. A series of toxins have been identified which in 3T3 mouse fibroblasts appear to function by prolonged activation of phospholipase A_2 activity. These agents include melittin, the major cytolytic polypeptide from bee venom; phallolysin, a cytolytic glycoprotein from the poisonous mushroom *Amanita phalloides*; delta toxin, produced by the skin bacterium *Staphylococcus aureus*; direct lytic factor from the venom of *Hemachatus hemachatus*; prymnesin, produced by the phytoflagellate *Prymnesium parvum*; and a hemolytic protein from the nematocyst venom of Portuguese Man-O-War, *Physalia physalis*. Analysis of the calcium ion requirement of the toxin-activated phospholipases suggests that those activated by phallolysin and melittin are cell surface, Ca^{2+}-requiring enzymes whereas direct lytic factor activates a Ca^{2+}-inhibited phospholipase of possible lysosomal origin.

KEYWORDS

Phospholipase A_2; cell surface; calcium dependence; melittin, phallolysin; staphylococcal delta toxin; direct lytic factor; prymnesin; *Physalia physalis* toxin.

INTRODUCTION

The life of a cell is dependent on the integrity of macromolecules and macromolecular structures. In principle, a cell could be induced to destroy itself by prolonged activation of high levels of any of several possible hydrolytic enzymes, including proteases, nucleases, and phospholipases. In practice, most of a cell's hydrolytic activity is sequestered in lysosomes, and coordinate activation of these enzymes is usually observed. If a toxin could stimulate autophagy (i.e. stimulate lysosomes to fuse with and destroy other organelles, or lyse and attack the entire host cell), it would constitute a very effective toxic mechanism. Toxins acting by this mechanism have yet to be adequately described, but if they could be identified, they would provide very useful and much needed experimental tools for the study of autophagy and possible roles of lysosomal processing in cellular regulation. Non-lysosomal hydrolases (neutral proteases, nucleases and phospholipases) are presumed to play regulatory and turnover roles that cannot be effectively performed by lysosomes. Neutral proteases and phospholipases are believed to function following transient activation, whereas the activities of nucleases involved in turnover and nucleic acid processing appear to be controlled primarily by substrate availability. Neutral proteases play well defined roles in blood coagulation and other processes important to the whole body, but at the cellular level their role in regulation remains largely speculative. Cellular phospholipases play a poorly defined but clearly important role in the first and probably rate controlling step in prostaglandin biosynthesis (Kunze and Vogt,1971; Samuelsson, 1972). They have also been proposed to play a role in the regulating membrane function by altering membrane lipid composition (Shier and co-workers, 1976; Shier, 1977a, 1977b). Of the non-lysosomal hydrolases, only activatable cellular phospholipase A_2 appears to provide a widely utilized mechanism for cytolytic toxins. This may be because cells are particularly vulnerable to phospholipases, because only a lipid bilayer encloses the contents of a mammalian cell.

We have recently identified a variety of toxins that appear to function, at least in their lower concentration ranges, by activation of cellular phospholipase A_2. These toxins were identified as a result of a search for non-physiological agents capable of activating high levels of cellular phospholipase A_2 in cultured cells. The existence of the target enzymes was predicted by a regulatory model being evaluated in this laboratory. In this model cell surface phospholipase A_2 is stimulated directly or indirectly by a hormone or mitogen so that it converts lecithin, the major phospholipid of mammalian membranes, to lysolecithin and free fatty acids (Fig. 1). These two lipids exhibit membrane-active detergent

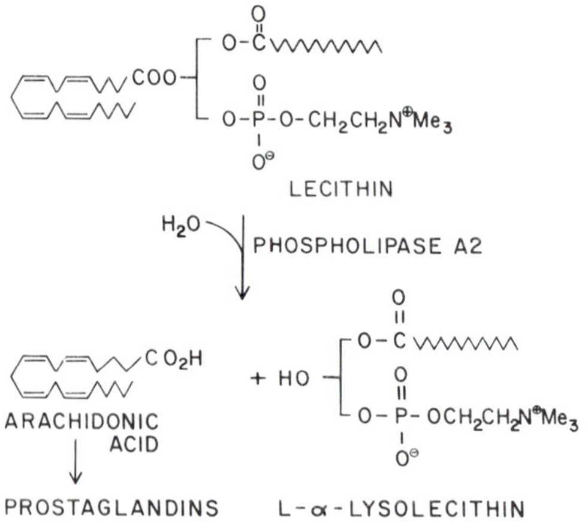

Fig. 1. The reaction catalyzed by phospholipase A_2.

properties, and they are capable of rapid and unrestricted lateral mobility which brings them into contact with membrane-associated enzymes. We have studied a variety of membrane-associated enzymes, including guanylate and adenylate cyclases, glycosyltransferases and fatty acid cyclooygenase, and we have observed that they are stimulated or inhibited by similar amounts of lysolecithin and free fatty acids. The amounts of these lipids that are required to alter enzyme activity would be produced by hydrolysis of 10-12% of the membrane lecithin. For a useful regulatory mechanism this degree of hydrolysis would have to be achieved in a short period of time by transient activation of high levels of cellular phospholipase A_2. Transient activation of high levels of phospholipase A_2 is also involved in the regulation of prostaglandin synthesis. Prostaglandins are a group of highly active short range hormones or intracellular regulatory agents derived primarily from arachidonic acid. Prolonged activation of cellular phospholipase A_2 at levels required for short periods in these two regulatory mechanisms should lead to lysis of the cell membrane both by loss of membrane-forming phospholipids and by the generation of detergent lipid products. Since this would constitute a very effective toxic mechanism we sought activators of high levels of cellular phospholipase A_2 by screening agents that have been reported to be hemolytic by unknown mechanisms. This approach has provided evidence for activation of cellular phospholipase A_2 as the mechanism of action of a variety of toxins from a wide range of biological sources.

Methodology

Activatable cellular phospholipase A_2 activity is readily measured in intact viable cultured cells (3T3 Swiss mouse fibroblasts in these studies) growing as monolayers on the bottom of plastic dishes (Fig. 2). These cells can be

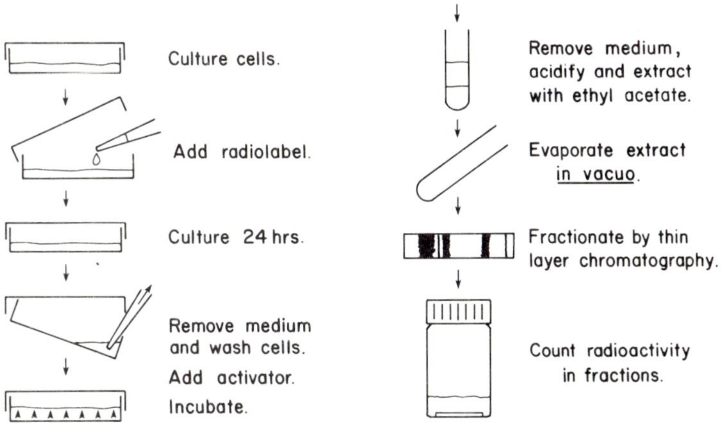

Fig. 2. The experimental procedure for assaying phospholipase A_2 in cultured 3T3 fibroblasts.

biosynthetically labeled (Shier, 1979) with ^{3}H-arachidonic acid under conditions which permit incorporation of label almost exclusively into phospholipids (1-3% of label as free fatty acid and as little as 3% of label in triglycerides) in the C-2 position of the glycerol moiety. The cells are washed on the dish to remove unincorporated radioactivity, then treated with a toxin preparation in culture medium for varying periods of time. When a phospholipase A_2 is activated in these cells the free fatty acids and prostaglandins formed (Fig. 1) exchange rapidly into the culture medium (Hong and Levine, 1976). Removal of the medium, extraction, and analysis of radioactivity co-chromatographing with authentic fatty acid and prostaglandin standards in thin layer chromatography provides a measure of the activation of phospholipase A_2 and prostaglandin synthesis. These activities can be conveniently expressed as a percentage of total incorporated ^{3}H-arachidonate radioactivity. For unknown reasons attempts to detect toxin-activated phospholipase A_2 activity in microsomal preparations have been unsuccessful, in parallel with a similar inability by others to demonstrate thrombin-activated phospholipase A_2 in subcellular preparations from platelets. Despite the limitation of the assay to intact cells numerable characteristics of the phospholipase A_2 activated can be elucidated, including (1) fatty acid specificity, (2) phospholipid (polar head group) specificity, (3) rate of activation, (4) prostaglandin yield from released arachidonic acid, (5) inhibitor specificity, (6) divalent cation specificity, and (7) an indication of subcellular location.

The most useful characteristic for classification of these toxins has been the subcellular location of the calcium-binding site of the activated phospholipase A_2. Its location is implied from measurements of the phospholipase A_2 activity stimulated under a series of conditions designed to alter the Ca^{2+} concentration in different parts of the cell (Fig. 3). Investigations of phospholipases from

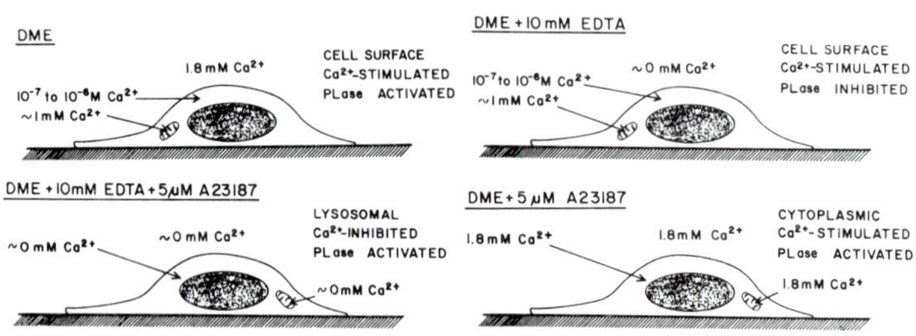

Fig. 3. Experimental conditions designed to alter calcium ion concentrations in various parts of a cell. DME = Dulbecco modified Eagle's medium.

venoms, pancreas and wide variety of tissue sources have shown that virtually all are activated by Ca^{2+} in a millimolar concentration range (van den Bosch, 1974). Exceptions to this generalization are soluble lysosomal phospholipases with low pH optima, which are inhibited by Ca^{2+} and activated by EDTA (Waite et al., 1969). Under normal culture conditions (Fig. 3, upper left panel) a cell in Dulbecco modified Eagle's medium (DME) is exposed to 1.8 mM Ca^{2+} on its cell surface but it maintains a low (0.1 to 1 μM) Ca^{2+} concentration inside the cell, except in the mitochondria (Borle, 1973). Addition of 10 mM EDTA to the medium rapidly reduces the free Ca^{2+} at the cell surface to below 0.1 μM by chelation, whereas a second pool of exchangeable Ca^{2+}, presumed to be cytoplasmic (Borle, 1973), is slowly lost from the cell (half-time to equilibrium in 3T3 cells biosynthetically labeled with ^{45}Ca was 28.9 min under the conditions of the phospholipase A_2 assay). Addition of the divalent cation ionophore A23187 reduces the half-time for loss of exchangeable Ca^{2+} to 1.3 min by shuttling Ca^{2+} out through cell membranes. If there is no EDTA in the medium the ionophore can shuttle Ca^{2+} into the cell raising the intracellular Ca^{2+} concentration to 1.8 mM. Examination of the extent of stimulation of phospholipase A_2 under these different conditions may suggest a possible subcellular location of the Ca^{2+}-binding site of any Ca^{2+}-dependent phospholipase A_2 activated by a toxin. For example, a cell surface Ca^{2+}-requiring phospholipase A_2 will be inhibited by addition of 10 mM EDTA to the medium with or without the ionophore, whereas a lysosomal phospholipase of the type described by

Waite et al. (1969) will be activated by 10 mM EDTA plus the ionophore. Alternately, a cytoplasmic, Ca^{2+}-requiring phospholipase will be activated in the presence of both ionophore and 1.8 mM Ca^{2+} in the medium. If the phospholipase A_2 activated in 3T3 cells by a toxin under the different conditions fits one of these patterns, it suggests a subcellular location for the Ca^{2+}-binding site of the enzyme. Even though this type of study does not provide definitive evidence for subcellular location, it does differentiate various types of phospholipases.

Toxins Which Activate Cell Surface-Type Phospholipase A_2

Cytolytic toxins which activate cellular phospholipase A_2 possessing an apparent cell surface Ca^{2+}-binding site represent the largest group of toxins identified as acting by this mechanism. Each of these toxins activate significant but low levels of phospholipase A_2 activity in the presence of 10 mM EDTA, consistent with some lysosomal involvement in their action. In contrast, poly-L-lysine (a polycation capable of activating a cell surface phospholipase A_2 which does not appear to be involved in the mechanism of cytotoxicity) induces no detectable phospholipase A_2 activity in 3T3 cells assayed in the presence of 10 mM EDTA. With each of these three toxins evidence that activation of cellular phospholipase A_2 is responsible for cytolysis is provided by a close correlation in the dose-response curves for activation of phospholipase A_2 in 30 min and for cytotoxicity assessed at the same time by failure to exclude trypan blue dye.

Phallolysin

Phallolysin, described in more detail elsewhere in these proceedings, is a heat-labile, water soluble, toxic glycoprotein from the poisonous mushroom *Amanita phalloides*. It exhibits no detectable phospholipase A_2 activity and no more surface activity than a typical protein. It is hemolytic and cytolytic, but extensive studies by Seeger and Burkhardt (1976) have failed to identify the mechanism of hemolysis.

In 3T3 cells biosynthetically labeled with ^{3}H-arachidonate phallolysin induced the hydrolysis of up to 40% of labeled lipids in 30 min with half maximal activation occurring at 50 μg/ml. Concomitant synthesis and release of labeled prostaglandins occurred. In cells biosynthetically labeled with ^{14}C-choline phallolysin induced a similar degree of conversion of labeled lecithin to labeled lysolecithin, but no hydrolysis of sphingomyelin. The results are consistent with the activation of a phospholipase A_2 with little or no significant specificity for either fatty acid residue or polar head group of phospholipids and with no significant activation of phospholipases B, C, or D or sphingomyelinases. Activation of phospholipase A_2 by phallolysin was biphasic consisting of an initial rapid release of hydrolysis products followed by a slower release phase. The phospholipase A_2 activated in 3T3 was inhibited by 0.1 mM p-bromophenacylbromide but not by 5 mM diisopropylfluorophosphate or 5 mM *N*-ethylmaleimide.

Faulstich and Weckauf (1975) showed that phallolysin-induced hemolysis is inhibited by wheat germ agglutinin. Similarly, phallolysin-induced activation of phospholipase A_2 in 3T3 cells was inhibited by wheat germ agglutinin at > 10 μg/ml but not by soybean agglutinin, a lectin with a different saccharide specificity. Phallolysin-induced activation of phospholipase A_2 in 3T3 was also inhibited by a series of oligosaccharides that inhibit wheat germ agglutinin hemagglutination of sheep red blood cells. Taken together these results suggest a model for cytolysis in which toxin binding occurs at a glycoprotein receptor site which also binds wheat germ agglutinin. The bound toxin activates a cell surface phospholipase A_2 which destroys the cell membrane by hydrolysis of membrane lipids.

Melittin

Melittin, as described elsewhere in these proceedings, is the major cytolytic component of honey bee (*Apis mellifera*) venom (Habermann, 1972). It is a 26-amino acid polypeptide consisting of predominantly basic and hydrophobic amino acids with most of the basic amino acids clustered at one end of the molecule. As a result melittin exhibits pronounced surface activity and other properties characteristic of amphipathic molecules.

Melittin activated high levels of phospholipase A_2 in 3T3 cells biosynthetically labeled with ^{3}H-arachidonic acid, hydrolysing up to 60% of the labeled lipids in 30 min with half maximal activation occurring at a concentration of 3 μg/ml (Shier, 1979). Detectable levels of hydrolysis products and prostaglandins appeared in the culture medium within one minute after treatment with melittin. As was observed with phallolysin, the phospholipase activated by melittin exhibited little or no specificity for fatty acid residues or polar head groups on phospholipids, and no detectable phospholipase B, C, or D or sphingomyelinases were activated. However, the phospholipase A_2 activated by melittin could be clearly distinguished from that activated by phallolysin, because it was not inhibited by 0.1 mM p-bromophenacylbromide, 5 mM diisopropylfluorophosphate or 5 mM *N*-ethylmaleimide.

Staphylococcal Delta Toxin

Staphylococcal delta toxin (Bernheimer, 1974) exhibits numerous similarities to melittin. It is also a polypeptide with a high percentage of hydrophobic and basic amino acids; it is soluble in organic and aqueous solvents; and it exhibits significant surface activity, although less than melittin. The phospholipase A_2 activated in 3T3 cells biosynthetically labeled with ^{3}H-arachidonate is similar if not identical to that activated by melittin, although higher concentrations of toxin are required (half maximal activation at 20 μg/ml) and the level of maximal activation is less (maximum of 35% hydrolysis in 30 min). As was observed with melittin, the phospholipase A_2 activated by delta toxin was not inhibited by 5 mM diisopropylfluorophosphate, 0.1 mM p-bromophenacylbromide or 5 mM *N*-ethylmaleimide. Unlike with melittin, the rate of activation of phospholipase A_2 by delta toxin exhibits a distinct lag of about 5 min, but this lag may merely reflect slower transfer of the toxin into the cell membrane as a result of the higher state of aggregation of delta toxin in solution.

Toxins Which Activate Lysosomal-Type Phospholipase

Two toxins have been identified which activate cellular phospholipase A_2 in 3T3 cells in the presence of culture medium (1.8 mM $CaCl_2$), but the level of activation is significantly higher when assayed in the presence of 10 mM EDTA and 5 μM divalent cation ionophore A23187.

Direct Lytic Factor

The direct lytic factor purified (Fryklund and Eaker, 1973) from the venom of African Ringhals cobra (*Hemachatus hemachatus*) is a 61-amino acid basic polypeptide with hemolytic, cardiotoxic and hypotensive activities but with no neurotoxic activity. In the presence of 1.8 mM $CaCl_2$ it activates moderate levels of phospholipase activity and prostaglandin synthesis in 3T3 cells biosynthetically labeled with ^{3}H-arachidonic acid (20% of labeled lipids hydrolyzed in one hour) with half maximal activation at 50 μg/ml (Shier, 1979). In the presence of

10 mM EDTA and 5 μM A23187 the phospholipase activity was increased 19-fold for a 30 min incubation at 10 μg/ml toxin. The activation of phospholipase by direct lytic factor exhibits a distinct lag of about 20 min duration.

A structurally similar cardiotoxin from the venom of *Naja naja atra* (Narita and Lee, 1970) activates phospholipase in 3T3 cells with a similar Ca^{2+} dependence.

Other Toxins Which Activate Cellular Phospholipase A_2

Two other toxins have been shown to activate cellular phospholipase A_2 in 3T3 cells, but the phospholipase A_2 activated by them has not yet been characterized with respect to Ca^{2+} dependence.

Prymnesin

Prymnesin is a hemolytic, cytolytic toxin produced by the phytoflagellate *Prymnesium parvum*. It has been reported (Ulitzur and Shilo, 1970) to be a proteoglycolipid with greater solubility in organic solvents than in water. It activates substantial levels of phospholipase A_2 in 3T3 cells biosynthetically labeled with ^3H-arachidonate (up to 20% hydrolysis of labeled lipids in 30 min) at low toxin concentrations (half maximal activation at 16 ng/ml).

Portuguese Man-O-War Toxin

The tenacles of Portuguese Man-O-War (*Physalia physalis*) contain specialized stinging cells, nematocysts, which discharge a venom. Tamkun and Hessinger (1979) have purified the major hemolytic toxin from this venom and shown it to be a high molecular weight water-soluble glycoprotein, the action of which is inhibited by the red cell glycoprotein glycophorin. The venom activates high levels of phospholipase A_2 in 3T3 cells biosynthetically labeled with ^3H-arachidonate (up to 35% hydrolysis of labeled lipids in 30 min) and it is active at relatively low concentrations (half-maximal activation at 0.5 μg/ml).

CONCLUSIONS

The cytolytic toxins which appear to function by activation of cellular phospholipase A_2 are derived from a wide range of biological sources. This observation suggests that activatable cellular phospholipases are present in a similarly wide range of organisms that constitute the predators or prey of the toxin-producing organisms. Examination of the characteristics of the phospholipase A_2 activities induced by the various toxins in 3T3 cells indicates that even a cloned cell line (3T3) contains high levels of activatable phospholipase A_2. Examination of the characteristics of the phospholipase A_2 activated by the individual toxins suggests that there are probably multiple, independently activated phospholipases, although the possibility that there are various mechanisms for activating the same enzyme has not been excluded. Obviously these cells do not elaborate high levels of activatable phospholipase A_2 in order to provide targets for cytolytic toxins no matter how interesting their mechanism of action. The multiplicity and probable ubiquity of these enzymes argues for an important role for them in the normal metabolic processes of the cell.

ACKNOWLEDGEMENT

I gratefully acknowledge the assistance of Mr. J. T. Trotter and Dr. J. P. Durkin, and the generous gifts of purified toxins which made this work possible: Drs. R. Seeger and H. Faulstich (phallolysin), A. W. Bernheimer (staphylococcal delta toxin), D. Eaker, C. Y. Lee (direct lytic factors), and D. A. Hessinger (*Physalia physalis* venom). The work described was supported in part by U. S. National Cancer Institute Grants CA16123 and CA20636 and a grant from the Cystic Fibrosis Foundation.

REFERENCES

Bernheimer, A. W. (1974). Interactions between membranes and cytolytic bacterial toxins. *Biochim. Biophys. Acta, 344,* 27-50.

Borle, A. B. (1973). Calcium metabolism at the cellular level. *Fed. Proc. Fed. Am. Soc. Exp. Biol., 32,* 1944-1950.

van den Bosch, H. (1974). Phosphoglyceride metabolism. *Annu. Rev. Biochem. 43,* 243-277.

Faulstich, H., and M. Weckauf (1975). Cytolysis of red cells by phallolysin, a toxin binding to N-acetylglucosamine on the cell surface. *Z. Physiol. Chem., 356,* 1187-1189.

Fryklund, L., and D. Eaker (1973). Complete amino acid sequence of a nonneurotoxic hemolytic protein from the venom of *Haemachatus haemachatus* (African Ringhals Cobra). *Biochemistry, 12,* 661-667.

Habermann, E. (1972). Bee and wasp venoms. *Science, 177,* 314-322.

Hong, S. L., and L. Levine (1976). Inhibition of arachidonic acid release from cells as the biochemical action of anti-inflammatory corticosteroids. *Proc. Natl. Acad. Sci. USA, 73,* 1730-1734.

Kunze, H., and W. Vogt (1971). Significance of phospholipase A for prostaglandin formation. *Ann. N. Y. Acad. Sci., 180,* 123-125.

Narita, K., and C. Y. Lee (1970). The amino acid sequence of cardiotoxin from Formosan cobra (*Naja naja atra)* venom. *Biochem. Biophys. Res. Commun., 41,* 339-343.

Samuelsson, B. (1972). Biosynthesis of prostaglandins. *Fed. Proc. Fed. Am. Soc. Exp. Biol., 31,* 1442-1450.

Seeger, R., and M. Burkhardt (1976). The hemolytic effect of phallolysin. *Naunyn-Schmiedeberg's Arch. Pharmakol., 293,* 163-170.

Shier, W. T. (1977a). Inhibition of acyl coenzyme A: lysolecithin acyltransferases by local anesthetics, detergents, and inhibitors of cyclic nucleotide phosphodiesterases. *Biochem. Biophys. Res. Commun., 75,* 186-193.

Shier, W. T. (1977b). Inhibition of prostaglandin biosynthesis by lysolecithin. *Biochem. Biophys. Res. Commun., 78,* 1168-1174.

Shier, W. T. (1979). Activation of high levels of endogenous phospholipase A_2 in cultured cells. *Proc. Natl. Acad. Sci. USA, 76.* 195-199.

Shier, W. T., J. H. Baldwin, M. Nilsen-Hamilton, R. T. Hamilton and N. M. Thanassi (1976). Regulation of guanylate and adenylate cyclase activities by lysolecithin. *Proc. Natl. Acad. Sci. USA, 73,* 1586-1590.

Tamkun, M. M., and D. A. Hessinger (1979). Isolation of a hemolytic and lethal protein from *Physalia physalis* (Portuguese Man-O-War) nematocyst venom. *Fed. Proc. Fed. Am. Soc. Exp. Biol., 38,* 824.

Ulitzur, S., and M. Shilo (1970). Procedure for purification and separation of *Prymnesium parvum* toxins. *Biochim. Biophys. Acta, 201,* 350-363.

Waite, M., G. L. Scherphof, F. M. G. Boshouwers and L. L. M. van Deenen (1969). Differentiation of phospholipases A in mitochondria and lysosomes of rat liver. *J. Lipid Res., 10,* 411-420.

MECHANISMS OF ACTION OF CYTOLYTIC TOXINS ON HUMAN FIBROBLASTS

M. Thelestam* and R. Möllby**

**Dept. Bact., Karolinska Institutet, S-104 01 Stockholm, Sweden*
***Dept. Bact., National Bacteriological Laboratory, S-105 21 Stockholm, Sweden*

ABSTRACT

A classification system for cytolytic toxins is described, which is based on one of their main functions, i.e. ability to induce different size functional "holes" in plasma membranes of cultured fibroblasts. Using leakage of three different size cytoplasmic markers to indicate altered plasma membrane permeability, leakage patterns were established for a number of membrane damaging agents of animal, plant and microbial origin. These agents were classified into five groups on basis of five distinct types of leakage patterns. Interaction of two SH-activated bacterial cytolysins (streptolysin O and theta-toxin from Clostridium perfringens) with fibroblasts was studied in more detail. Despite the fact that these toxins caused similar leakage patterns the initial stages in their membrane damaging actions differed with regard to temperature dependency, binding to the fibroblast membrane and effect on uptake of neutral amino acids.

KEYWORDS

Cytolysin, haemolysin, toxin, fibroblasts, plasma membrane, membrane damage, leakage pattern.

INTRODUCTION

The following main stages are involved in the action of cytolytic toxins on metabolizing fibroblasts: (a) cytolysin interaction with receptors on the cell membrane, (b) disorganization of the plasma membrane structure and (c) counteracting processes such as repair activities in the membrane. A final outcome of these events is either a destruction of the membrane organization or an increased membrane permeability to various intracellular molecules such as K^+, trace elements, amino acids etc. Such cytoplasmic leakage will lead to secondary intracellular effects, possibly causing cell death (Ledbetter and Lubin, 1977; Thelestam and Möllby, 1976).

Bacterial cytolysins have traditionally been grouped as follows according to their modes of action on red blood cells (Bernheimer, 1974; Alouf, 1976): (1) Phospholipases, (2) surface active, (3) SH-activated and (4) toxins with unknown mode of action. Also animal- and plant-derived cytolysins roughly fall into these four categories. The molecular basis for the membrane damaging action is comprehensible in the case of phospholipases and the surface active cytolysins. As regards the SH-activated toxins the target molecules in the membrane have been identified but the exact molecular mechanisms of the membrane damaging process have not been clarified. This work was undertaken to investigate the relation between mechanisms of action of cytolysins and the relative size of the functional "holes" they induce in cytoplasmic membranes of human fibroblasts.

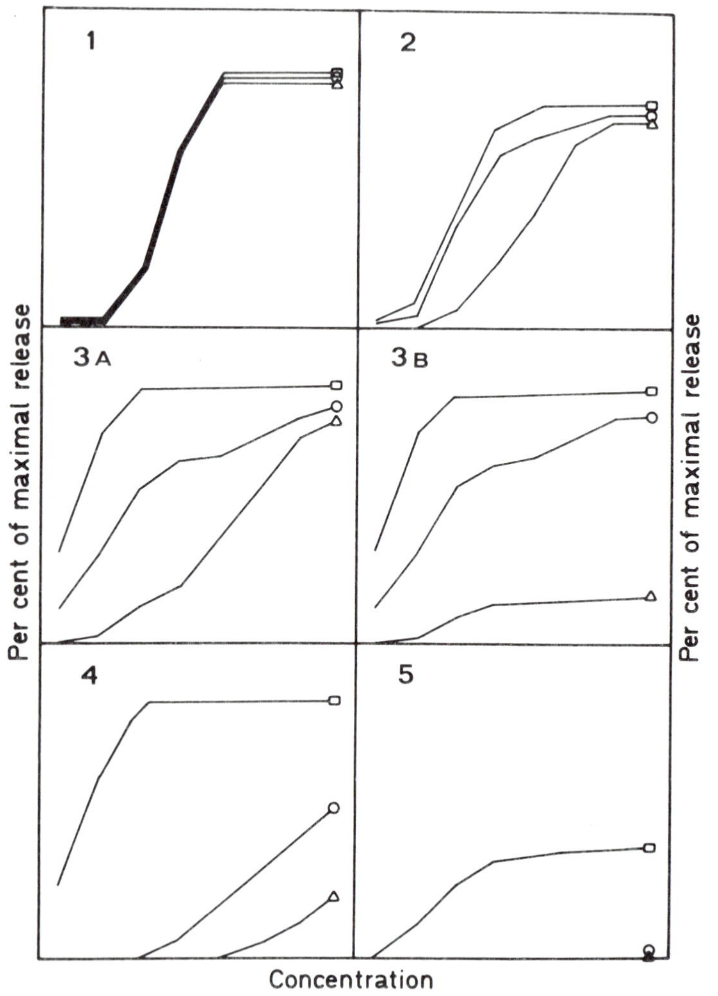

Fig. 1. Schematic leakage patterns representative of the five groups. △——△ RNA, o——o uridine nucleotides, □——□ AIB.

TABLE 1. Main characteristics of the five groups.

Group No.	Type of leakage pattern	Range of ED_{50}-ratios Nucleotide/AIB RNA/AIB	Examples of cytolytic agents	Implicated type of membrane interaction
1.	Equal release of all three markers	0.6-1.6 0.9-1.9	True detergents (Tritons, SDS etc). Fucidin Crude phospholipase A Haemolysin (P.aeruginosa)	Detergent-like (solubilization of both proteins and lipids).
2.	Restricted release of RNA	1.5-4.8	Phospholipase C (C.perfringens) Surfactin (B.natto) Melittin (Apis mellifera) Alfalfa saponin	Solubilization or degradation of only certain membrane constituents.
3.	Restricted release of nucleotide and low release of RNA	1 - 38 26 - >200	3A Delta-toxin (S.aureus) Alpha-toxin (A.hydrophila) 3B Filipin SH-activated toxins Vibriolysin (V.parahaemolyticus) Direct lytic factor (Naja naja)	Interaction with specific receptors in the cell membrane (such as glycoproteins, gangliosides, cholesterol) leading to membrane destabilization.
4.	Release of nucleotide and RNA only at elevated concentrations	>4-2500 >200	Amphotericin B Nystatin Alpha-toxin (S.aureus)	Formation of narrow transverse pores (<5 Å) in the cell membrane (by interaction with specific receptors).
5.	Only AIB released		Polymyxin B Sphingomyelinase C (S.aureus) Sphingomyelinase D (Cor. ovis) Phospholipase C (B.cereus) Gamma-toxin (S.aureus) Streptolysin S (S.pyogenes) Delta-toxin (S.aureus)	Induction of only slight increase in membrane permeability (possibly by attack on specific phospholipids).

CLASSIFICATION OF CYTOLYSINS ON FUNCTIONAL BASIS.

Cultured human fibroblasts (MRC-5) were exposed for 30 min to various concentrations of cytolysins of animal, plant and microbial origin. Leakage from prelabelled fibroblasts of three different sized cytoplasmic markers, i.e. radiolabelled RNA, uridine nucleotides and alpha-aminoisobutyric acid (AIB), was measured and expressed as per cent of a maximal release (Thelestam and Möllby, 1975). Leakage patterns were established from dose-response curves with the three markers. The relative sizes of cytolysin-induced holes were estimated from ED_{50}-ratios, i.e. the ratios between the amounts of agent needed to release 50% of the respective markers. Five main groups were established on basis of character of leakage patterns and ED_{50}-ratios (Fig. 1 and Table I).

The types of membrane interaction proposed for each group were based on the known mechanisms for one or several reference substances assigned to these groups. Further details regarding this classification were published elsewhere (Thelestam and Möllby, 1979).

STREPTOLYSIN O AND CLOSTRIDIUM PERFRINGENS THETA TOXIN

By comparison with reference substances the character of leakage patterns may give some clue to the mechanism of action of cytolytic agents. However, the leakage patterns reflect the final stage of the membrane damage, the resulting increased permeability or "functional hole", whereas the first steps leading to these effects may still remain obscure. The interactions with membrane receptors and the membrane damaging process may indeed be different in spite of similar final effects. Thus, two SH-activated bacterial cytolysins producing identical leakage patterns (group 3 B) were investigated in more detail with regard to their initial interactions with the fibroblast membrane.

Streptolysin O and theta-toxin from C.perfringens are closely related toxins believed to cause haemolysis by identical mechanisms via binding to membrane cholesterol (Smyth and Duncan, 1978). However, the action of these cytolysins on fibroblasts differed as follows: In terms of haemolytic units ten times lower amounts of theta-toxin than of SLO were needed to damage the fibroblast membrane. Furthermore, theta-toxin was membrane damaging at $0^{o}C$ while SLO did not induce any significant membrane damage at low temperature (Table II).

TABLE II Membrane damaging effects of SLO and theta-toxin at different tempeatures.

Concentration haemolytic units/ml	Per cent nucleotide release +) 0°C	37°C
SLO		
15	15	63
7.5	0	50
5.0	0	38
2.5	0	17
Theta-toxin		
2.0	71	73
1.0	58	67
0.5	40	55
0.1	4	21

+) Expressed as per cent of maximal release (Thelestam and Möllby, 1975). Incubation time: 30 min.

Theta-toxin did not bind to the fibroblast membrane while SLO bound in a temperature independent step (Table III).

TABLE III Binding of SLO and theta-toxin to fibroblasts +)

Concentration haemolytic units/ml	PER CENT NUCLEOTIDE RELEASE A toxins 15 min 0°C	B "adsorbed" solutions from A. 30 min, 37°C	C Fresh toxins 30 min, 37°C	D TBS after A. 30 min, 37°C
SLO				
12	1	12	65	67
6.2	0	4	52	56
2.5	0	3	34	29
Theta-toxin				
1.0	40	70	73	66
0.5	0	55	56	57
0.1	0	32	36	34

+) Nucleotide labelled cells were treated at 0°C for 15 min, with the concentrations indicated of SLO and theta-toxin, to allow for adsorption of the toxins to the cells (A). These "adsorbed" solutions were then transferred to another set of nucleotide labelled cells now incubated for 30 min at 37°C (B). As controls fresh toxin solutions, that had not been in contact with cells, were used for treatment (30 min at 37°C) of a parallel set of nucleotide labelled cultures (C). The cultures initially incubated at 0°C were rinsed twice and then incubated in tris-buffered saline for 30 min at 37°C (D).

Theta-toxin inhibited the uptake of a model amino acid (AIB) at concentrations causing no structural membrane damage, measured as leakage of the nucleotide marker. By contrast, SLO exerted a very limited effect on the AIB uptake even at concentrations clearly causing structural membrane damage (Fig. 2).

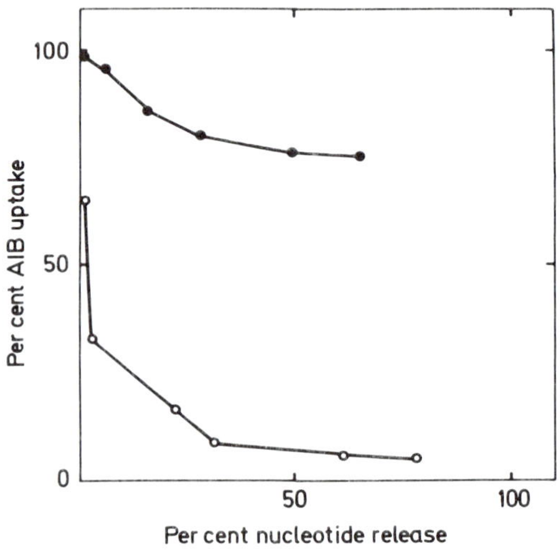

Fig. 2. Effect of various concentrations of SLO (1-15 HU/ml; •—•) and theta-toxin (0.01 - 2 HU/ml; o—o) on uptake of AIB in relation to induced structural membrane damage, i.e. nucleotide release.

Thus, SLO seems to act on fibroblasts as could be expected from earlier reports on red blood cells (Smyth and Duncan, 1978). Since theta-toxin did not bind to the fibroblasts it is supposed to act by a "hit-and-run" mechanism but further details of its mechanism of action are not known. However, theta-toxin apparently differs from SLO, which has hitherto been regarded as the prototype of SH-activated cytolysins.

ACKNOWLEDGEMENTS

Expert technical assistance by Greger Blomquist, Eva Brännkärr, Lena Norenius and Gunnel Sigstam is gratefully acknowledged. This work was supported by the Medical Research Council, grant No. 16X-2562 and by Karolinska institutets fonder.

REFERENCES

Alouf, J.E. (1976). Cell membranes and cytolytic bacterial toxins. In P.Cuatrecasas, Ed. Receptors and recognition, series B. vol. 1. The specificity and action of animal, bacterial and plant toxins. Chapman and Hall, London. p.p. 219-270.

Bernheimer, A.W. (1974). Interactions between membranes and cytolytic toxins. Biochim. Biophys. Acta, 344, 27-50.

Ledbetter, M.L.S. and Lubin, M. (1977). Control of protein synthesis in human fibroblasts by intracellular potassium. Exptl. Cell Res. 105, 223-236.

Smyth, C.J. and Duncan, J.L. (1978). Thiol-activated (oxygen labile) cytolysins. In. J. Jeljaszewicz and T. Wadström, Ed., Bacterial toxins and cell membranes. Academic Press/London. p.p. 129-183.

Thelestam, M. and Möllby, R. (1975). Determination of toxin-induced leakage of different size nucleotides through the plasma membrane of human diploid fibroblasts. Infect. Immunity, 11, 640-648.

Thelestam, M. and Möllby, R. (1976). Cytotoxic effects on the plasma membrane of human diploid fibroblasts - a comparative study of leakage tests. Medical Biology, 54, 39-49.

Thelestam, M. and Möllby, R. (1979). Classification of microbial, plant and animal cytolysins based on their membrane-damaging effects on human fibroblasts. Biochim. Biophys. Acta, in press.

Phospholipases and Cell Membranes

HEMOLYTIC EFFECTS OF SNAKE VENOMS

E. Condrea

School of Pharmacology and Toxicology, The University of Connecticut, School of Pharmacy, Storrs, Ct., USA
On leave of absence from the Rogoff-Wellcome Medical Research Institute, Tel Aviv University Medical School, Tel Aviv, Israel

ABSTRACT

Red cell lysis which may develop following snake bite does not play a prominent role in the overall venom lethality. In vitro, all snake venoms hemolyze red cells indirectly, i.e. in the presence of an exogenous phospholipid which is hydrolyzed by the venom phospholipase A_2 with formation of lytic products. Only those snake venoms possessing direct lytic factor (DLF) in addition to phospholipases A_2, hemolize washed erythrocytes directly. Purified venom phospholipases A_2 (PLA_2) induce a non-lytic hydrolysis of exposed phospholipids in the outer layer of human erythrocytes. However, a basic PLA_2 from Naja nigricollis venom directly hemolyzes and completely hydrolyzes phospholipids in ATP-depleted human erythrocytes and fresh guinea pig erythrocytes. The sensitivity of erythrocyt from various species to whole venom results from their sensitivity to DLF as well as from their susceptibility to the direct action of lytic PLA_2. The lytic PLA_2 might play a role in hemolysis following envenomation.

KEYWORDS

Hemolysis, direct and indirect; direct lytic factor; lytic phospholipases; basic phospholipases; erythrocyte sensitivities.

INTRODUCTION

Studies on snake venom components including phospholipases and direct lytic factors have been frequently reviewed with special emphasis on their chemistry and pharmacology (Meldrum, 1965; Jimenez-Porras, 1968, 1970; Lee, 1971, 1972; Tu, 1973). On the other hand, reviews on red cell membrane structure deal with the action of venom phospholipases as tools in localizing membrane phospholipids (Zwaal, Roelofsen and Colley, 1973; Singer, 1974). The purpose of the present survey is to integrate clinical observations with pharmacologic and biochemical data as well as with recent studies on the direct effects of phospholipases on red cells.

HEMOLYSIS IN ENVENOMATION

Elapid venoms are predominantly neurotoxic and, when administered in lethal doses, no evidence of hemolysis was found (Condrea, Barzilay and de Vries, 1969). However the occurence of hemolysis following bites by various elapids has been confirmed by numerous observations. (Campbell, 1969; Trethewie, 1971; Reid, 1968). Viperid or crotalid venoms are predominantly hemorrhagic and evidence for intravascular hemolysis is difficult to obtain. Although lysis *in vivo* is seldom observed, when it does occur, the process involved seems to be the sensitization of the erythrocytes by the action of lytic factors, followed by trapping of the fragile erythrocytes within the clots of fibrin promoted by the procoagulant venom factors (Klibansky and co-workers, 1966).

VENOM FACTORS INVOLVED IN HEMOLYSIS

The main venom factors involved in hemolysis are the phospholipase A_2 (PLA_2) and the direct lytic factor (DLF). While PLA_2 is an esterolytic enzyme catalizing the hydrolysis of the ester bond at the C_2 position in 1,2-diacyl-sn-glycerophophatides forming lysophospholipids and releasing fatty acids (Van Deenen and de Haas, 1963), the DLF is a basic polypeptide devoid of enzymatic activity and moderately lytic *per se* (Condrea, 1974). While phospholipases have been identified in all snake venoms tested, DLF is found mainly in elapid venoms. The ubiquitous presence of PLA_2 explains why all venoms are able to lyse human or various animal erythrocytes indirectly, i.e. in the presence of exogenous phospholipid, by a two-step process in which the evolved lytic lyso-products act on the red blood cell. However, only venoms which contain DLF in addition to PLA_2, such as of the elapids, are able to hemolyze washed human erythrocytes directly without added substrate. This was found to be due to a synergistic action between the two venom factors, DLF inducing full exposure of erythrocyte membrane phospholipids to the PLA_2 (Condrea, 1979).

ERYTHROCYTE SENSITIVITES TO VENOM HEMOLYSIS

When washed red blood cells from various animal species are subjected to the action of direct lytic venoms, a range of sensitivites emerges which is, in decreasing order: guinea pig, dog, cat, human, rabbit, horse, sheep, camel. The sequence of red cell sensitivites roughly parallels that of decreasing lecithin/sphingomyelin ratios in the membrane, (Zwaal and co-workers, 1973; Livne and Kuiper, 1973), although with a few exceptions. Recognition of the direct hemolysis as a synergistic effect between PLA_2 and DLF (Condrea, de Vries and Mager, 1964a) raised the question which the two factors determines the sensitivity to whole venom. We previously argued (Condrea and co-workers, 1964b) that the red cell sensitivites are primarily a reflection of their susceptibility to DLF. This concept is now revised as shown in the following chapter.

EFFECTS OF PURIFIED PHOSPHOLIPASES ON RED CELL MEMBRANES

Non-Lytic Phospholipid Degradation

Purified PLA_2 from various snake venoms differ in their ability to hydrolyze phospholipids in washed erythrocytes. *Naja naja* and *Hemachatus haemachatus* PLA_2 hydrolyze, in various conditions, up to 70% of phosphatidycholine and 20% of phosphatidylethanolamine of human erythrocytes (Zwaal and co-workers, 1975); Barzilay, Kaminsky and Condrea, 1977a). In contradistinction, PLA_2 from *Crotalus adamanteus* (Zwaal and co-workers, 1975) and *Vipera palestinae* (Barzilay, de Vries and Condrea, 1977b) are inactive. Since degradation of phospholipids in the human erythrocyte is limited to the outer half of the membrane bilayer, it does not result in hemolysis (Verkleij and co-workers, 1973).

Lytic Phospholipid Degradation

If human erythrocytes are subjected to certain treatments producing little or no hemolysis, such as hypotonic swelling (Barzilay, Kaminsky and Condrea, 19772) or sublytic concentrations of detergents (Lankish, Jacobi and Schoner, 1972) phospholipases become able to hydrolyze extensively membrane phospholipids and induce hemolysis.

While most venom phospholipases A_2 are acidic or neutral, a number of basic PLA_2 have recently been isolated and characterized (Eaker, 1978). The basic PLA_2 from N. nigricollis venom has been reported to hemolyze directly horse erythrocytes preheated at 45° (Dumarey and co-workers, 1975) and guinea pig erythrocytes at 37° (Lee, Ho and Eaker, 1977). Another basic PLA_2 from Agkistrodon halys blomhofii venom hemolyzes directly human and guinea pig erythrocytes depleted of ATP (Martin and co-workers, 1975). We compared the effects of the basic N. Nigricollis PLA_2 and of the neutral H. haemachatus PLA_2 on ATP- depleted human erythrocytes and on fresh guinea pig erythrocytes, the results being illustrated in Figs. 1 and 2.

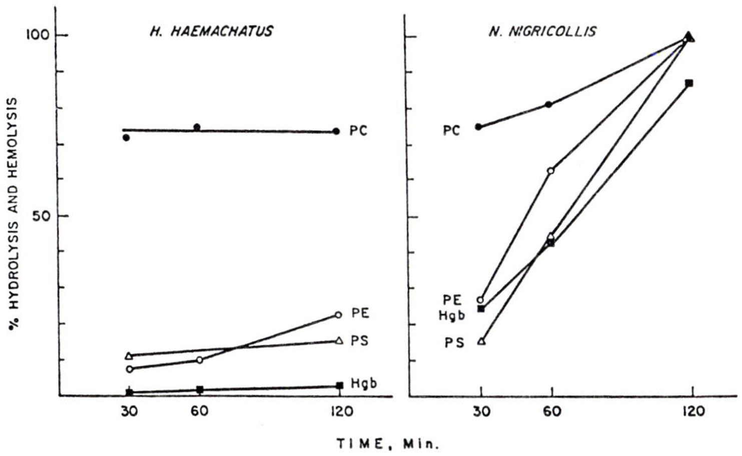

Fig. 1. Phospholipid hydrolysis and hemolysis induced by phospholipases A_2 in human erythocytes separated from stored blood.

Assay conditions: 1 ml red cells suspensions in isotonic saline, containing 10 mM Tris-HCl (pH 7.4) and 1 mM $CaCl_2$ were incubated at 37° with 120 µg of either H. haemachatus or N. nigricollis phospholipase A_2, for the time indicated. Phospholipids were extracted and separated by thin-layer chromatography. Symbols: •, phosphatidylcholine; o, phosphatidylethanolamine; △, phosphatidylserine and ■, hemoglobin.

It can be seen that, while the H. haemachatus enzyme is non-lytic and induces limited phospholipid hydrolysis, the basic N. nigricollis enzyme hemolyzes and fully hydrolyzes red cell phospholipids.

It is noteworthy that the enzymatic activity of the lytic N. nigricollis PLA_2 is about one-fourth that of the non-lytic H. haemachatus PLA_2 when compared on purified egg lecithin.

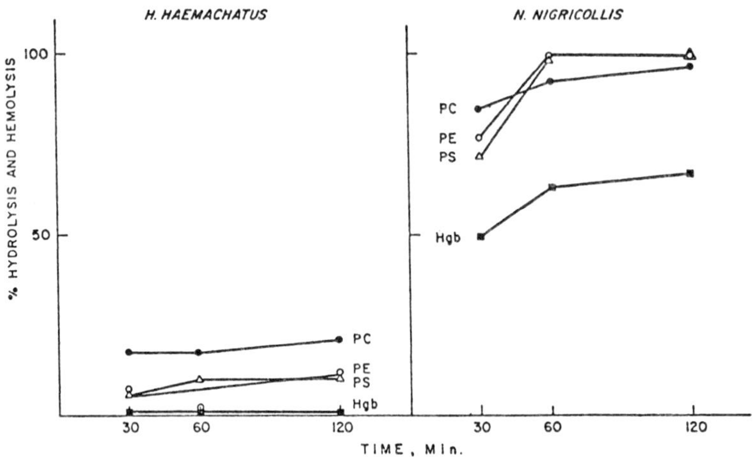

Fig. 2. Phospholipid hydrolysis and hemolysis induced by phospholipase A_2 in guinea pig erythrocytes.

Assay conditions as in Fig. 1 except for the enzymes being in a concentration of 30 µg/ml. Symbols as in Fig. 1.

It seemed an attractive speculation that the basic N. nigricollis PLA_2 combines the properties of DLF and enzymatic activity in the same molecule. However, an acidic PLA_2 from N. naja venom was also reported to hemolyze ATP-depleted human erythrocytes (Martin and co-workers, 1975; Haest and Deuticke, 1976). In contrast, acidic PLA_2 from C. adamanteus and from A. h. blomhofii do not lyse ATP-depleted human red cells (Martin and co-workers, 1975). We tested the ability of a number of purified PLA_2 to hemolyze fresh guinea pig erythrocytes and the results are given in Table 1.

TABLE 1 Direct Hemolysis of Guinea Pig Erythrocytes by Various Phospholipases A_2.

Phospholipases (30 µg)	LD_{50}	Hemolysis % 30 min.	60 min.	120 min.
B. caudalis	200	0	1	54
N. nigricollis (basic)	250	49	90	--
N. melanoleuca I	1600	0	1	62
N. melanoleuca III	1800	0	1	57
H. haemachatus	4500	0	0	0
B. gabonica	10,000	0	0	2

A 50% washed erythrocytes suspension in Tris-buffered saline (pH 7.4) and 1mM Ca^{2+} was incubated with PLA_2 in 1 ml final volume at 37°C. Hemoglobin in supernatants was assayed as $O.D_{540}$.

From our results and those reported by others it appears that not only basic PLA_2 are directly lytic to erythrocytes of a sensitive species, or to ATP-depleted human erythrocytes. Among the directly lytic enzymes there is however a great variability in hemolytic potency. It also results that erythrocytes from various species exhibit different sensitivities to direct lytic phospholipases. Thus, red cell sensitivity to whole venom is reflecting both their susceptibility to DLF and to PLA_2.

An attempt was made to dissociate between the contribution of the phospholipase activity and that of the electropositive charge of the protein in the direct lytic effect. As seen in Table 2, inhibition of PLA_2 activity by EDTA completely prevented hemolysis, while addition of heparin had no effect.

TABLE 2 Effects of EDTA and Heparin on Hemolysis Induced by N. nigricollis Phospholipase in ATP-depleted Human Erythrocytes

		HEMOLYSIS, %		
			ADDITIONS	
PLA_2	Time, min.	NONE	EDTA	HEPARIN
60 µg	60	86	1	87
	120	86	2	--
120 µg	60	92	1	--

Incubation conditions as in Table 1. EDTA, 50 mM heparin, 60 µg.

In conclusion, the direct lytic action of the basic and certain acidic phospholipases on red cells from sensitive animal species might contribute to the appearance of hemolysis in envenomation. This is borne out by our results on mice injected intravenously with lethal doses of N. nigricollis basic PLA_2 (20 µg) or H. haemachatus PLA_2 (250 µg), the first inducing moderate hemolysis (~10%) while the latter being practically non-lytic (2% hemolysis).

REFERENCES

Barzilay, M., A. de Vries, and E. Condrea (1977b). Toxicon, 16, 145-152.
Barzilay, M., E. Kaminsky, and E. Condrea (1977a). Toxicon, 16, 153-161.
Campbell, C. H. (1969). Toxicon, 7, 25-28.
Condrea, E. (1974). Experientia, 3, 121-129.
Condrea, E. (1979). In C.-Y Lee (Ed.). Handbook of Experimental Pharmacology, Vol. 52, Springer-Verlag, Berlin, Chap. 13, pp. 448-479.
Condrea, E., M. Barzilay, and A. de Vries. (1969). Toxicon, 7, 95-98.
Condrea, E., A. de Vries, and J. Mager. (1964a). Biochim. biophys. Acta, 84, 60-73.
Condrea, E., Z. Mammon, S. Aloof, and A. de Vries. (1964b). Biochim. biophys. Acta, 84, 365-375.
Dumarey, C., D. Sket, D. Joseph, and P. Boquet. (1975). C. R. Acad. Sci. (Paris), 280, 1633-1635.
Eaker, D. (1978). In C. H. Li (Ed.), Versatility of Proteins, Academic Press, New York, pp. 413-431.
Haest, C. W. M., and B. Deuticke. (1976). Biochim. biophys. Acta, 436, 353-365.
Jimenez-Porras, J. M. (1968). Ann. Rev. Pharmacol., 8, 299-318.
Jimenez-Porras, J. M. (1970). Clin. Toxicol., 3, 389-431
Klibansky, C., E. Ozcan, H. Joshua, M. Djaldetti, H. Bessler, and A. de Vries (1966). Toxicon, 3, 213-221.
Lankish, P. G., C. Jacobi, and K. Schoner. (1972). FEBS Letters, 23, 61-64.
Lee, C. Y. (1971). In L. L. Simpson (Ed.), Neuropoisons, Vol. 1., Plenum Press, New York-London, Chap. 2, pp. 21-63.

Lee, C. Y. (1972). Ann. Rev. Pharmacol., 12, 265-286.
Lee, C. Y., C. L. Ho, and D. Eaker. (1977). Toxicon, 15, 355-356.
Livne, A. and P. J. C. Kuiper. (1973). Biochim. biophys. Acta, 318, 41-49.
Martin, J. K., M. G. Luthra, M. A. Wells, R. P. Watts, and D. J. Hanahan (1975). Biochemistry, 14, 5400-5408.
Meldrum, B. S. (1965). Pharmacol. Rev., 17, 393-445.
Reid, A. H. (1968). In E. E. Buckley and W. Blicherl (Eds.), Venomous animals and their venoms, Vol. 1, Academic Press, New York-London, Chap. 20, pp. 611-641.
Singer, S. J. (1974). Ann. Rev. Biochem., 43, 805-833.
Trethewie, E. R. (1971). In E. E. Buckley and W. Blicherl (Eds.), Venomous animals and their venoms, Vol. 2, Academic Press, New York-London, Chap. 24, pp. 80-99.
Tu, A. T. (1973). Ann. Rev. Biochem., 42, 235-258.
Van Deenen, L. L. M. and G. H. de Haas. (1963). Biochim. biophys. Acta, 70, 538-553.
Verkleij, A. J., R. F. A. Zwaal, B. Roelofsen, P. Comfurius, D. Kastelijnn, and L. L. M. Van Deenen (1973). Biochim. biophys. Acta, 323, 178-193.
Zwaal, R. F. A., B. Roelofsen, and M. Colley (1973). Biochim. biophys. Acta, 300, 159-182.
Zwaal, R. F. A., B. Roelofsen, P. Confurius, and L. L. M. Van Deenen (1975). Biochim. biophys. Acta, 406, 83-96.

THE ACTIONS OF BACTERIAL PHOSPHOLIPASES C ON PLASMA MEMBRANE

H. Ikezawa

Fac. Pharma. Sci., Nagoya City Univ., Mizuhoku, Nagoya, Japan

ABSTRACT

In this study, the actions of bacterial phospholipases C were extensively investigated in their hemolytic, ectoenzyme-releasing, and growth-inhibiting activities against the cell of several eucaryotes including mammals, Sarcoma 180, and yeast. Also in this report, it was revealed that invagination or deformation of cell surfaces was brought about by the action of these phospholipases. It was concluded that most of these phospholipases C must be produced for the purpose of attack against plasma membranes of eucaryotes.

KEYWORDS

Bacterial phospholipases C; the action of phospholipase C; hot-cold and hot hemolysis; sphingomyelinase adsorption; ectoenzyme-releasing activity; invagination of erythrocytes; invagination of Sarcoma 180 cells; growth inhibition of Sarcoma 180 cells.

INTRODUCTION

Bacterial phospholipases C are known to act on biological membranes, although biological roles of these enzymes have not been realized exactly. As shown at first by Slein and Logan(1965), three kinds of bacterial phospholipases C have been reported; phosphatidylcholine-hydrolyzing phospholipase C(PCase), sphingomyelinase C(SMase) and phosphatidylinositol-specific phospholipase C(PIase). Among these phospholipases, PCases have been known to hemolyze memmalian erythrocytes in the presence of divalent metal ions(Macfarlane and Knight, 1941; Ikezawa, 1963; Taguchi and Ikezawa, 1976a, 1976b), with some exceptions such as PCase from Bacillus cereus which was shown to be different from the hemolysin produced by this microorganism(Johnson and Bonventre, 1967). Also, SMase of staphylococcus aureus has been reported to be a "hot-cold hemolysin", in that SMase-treated sheep erythrocytes are susceptible to cold shock(Walbum, 1921; Bigger, Boland and O'Meara, 1927; Doery and others, 1963). This enzyme was extensively purified by Maheswaran and Lindorfer(1967), Gow and Robinson(1969), Wadström and Möllby(1971), and Bernheimer, Avigad and Kim(1974). PIase of <u>Bacillus cereus</u> was at first discovered by Slein and Logan(1965), who

proposed this enzyme to be responsible for the phosphatase release from kidney and bone slices in vitro, and for the increase in blood alkaline phosphatase in vivo.
Recently, several bacterial phospholipases including PCases, SMase and PIases were purified in my laboratory, and were investigated in details on their actions toward plasma membranes of eucaryotic cells. The purpose of this article is to describe the recent results and to discuss the physiological roles of bacterial phospholipases C in relation to host-parasite interaction.

HEMOLYTIC ACTION OF PHOSPHATIDYLCHOLINE-HYDROLYZING PHOSPHOLIPASE C

Most of bacterial PCases hemolyzed mammalian erythrocytes in the presence of divalent metal ions such as Ca^{2+} and Mg^{2+}, with exception of *Bacillus cereus* PCase which is non-hemolytic(Roelofsen and others, 1971; Zwaal and others, 1971; Woodward and Zwaal, 1972). In the cases of PCases from *C. perfringens*, *C. novyi* and *P. aureofaciens*, hot-cold hemolysis of rat, human, horse, rabit and sheep erythrocytes by these enzymes occurred more intensely in the presence of Ca^{2+} than of Mg^{2+}. In the absence of metal ions, no appreciable hemolysis was observed in each case. The maximal stimulation of hot-cold hemolysis by Ca^{2+} was brought about at approx. 10^{-2}M, reagardless of species of erythrocytes. As previously reported by Taguchi and Ikezawa(1976a, 1976b), hydrolysis of phosphatidylcholine proved to be a key step in the hemolysis of horse erythrocytes by PCases from *C. perfringens*, *C. novyi* and *P. aureofaciens*, while, in the hemolysis of sheep erythrocytes by *C. perfringens* PCase, breakdown of sphingomyelin corresponded to that step.

MODE OF HEMOLYTIC ACTION OF SPHINGOMYELINASE OF *BACILLUS CEREUS*

Recently, Ikezawa and his colleagues have reported the purification and properties of *Bacillus cereus* SMase(Ikezawa and others, 1978). This enzyme also proved to hemolyze mammalian erythrocytes. The hemolytic sensitivity to SMase of various erythrocytes paralleled with their sphingomyelin contents in the following oder; sheep > human > rabit > horse > rat. The order of sensitivity to *B. cereus*

SMase was also consistent with that to staphylococcal enzyme, which was reported by Wiseman and Caird(1967). However, a striking difference between these two SMases exists in their hemolytic activities: As reported by several authors, staphylococcal SMase causes hot-cold hemolysis of sheep erythrocytes(Glenny and Stevens, 1935; Walbum, 1921) but does not lyze these cells directly at 37°C. On the other hand, SMase from Bacillus cereus induces not only hot-cold hemolysis of sheep erythrocytes, but also lyses these cells at 37°C(so-called "hot-hemolysis"). Even in the absence of divalent metal ions, sphingomyelin in sheep erythrocytes was extensively hydrolyzed during incubation with B. cereus SMase at 37°C(Ikezawa and others, in press). When the incubated cells were cooled in ice bath, hot-cold hemolysis occurred. Hemolysis without cooling, i.e., hot hemolysis, took place a little later than initiation of hot-cold lysis. As observed in the reaction with purified brain sphingomyelin(Ikezawa and others, 1978), both substrate breakdown and hemolysis were stimulated by 10mM Mg^{2+}, but inhibited by 10mM Ca^{2+}. In the presence of both Ca^{2+} and Mg^{2+}, however, both hydrolysis of sphingomyelin in sheep erythrocytes and hemolysis of these cells proceeded more rapidly than in the presence of Mg^{2+} alone. Thus Ca^{2+} did not compete with Mg^{2+}, but enhanced its stimulatory effect. Another interesting information was obtained on the mode of action of B. cereus SMase toward sheep erythrocytes. When SMase was incubated withe these cells, the significant amount of SMase was adsorbed onto the surfaces of erythrocytes. Fig. 1 shows the time course of adsorption, which proceeded either in the presence or absence of divalent metal ions such as Mg^{2+}.

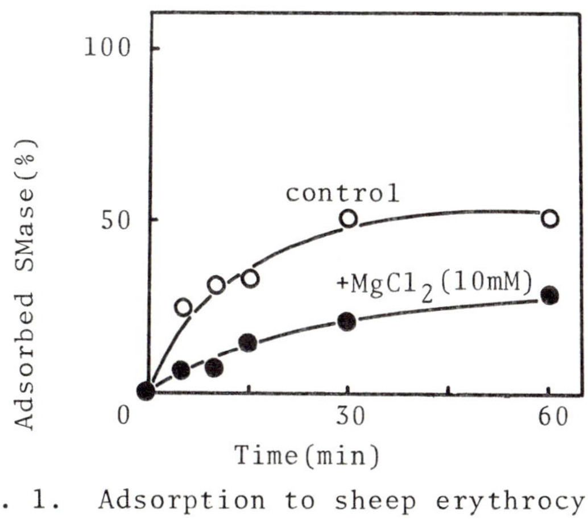

Fig. 1. Adsorption to sheep erythrocyte membrane of SMase.

The phenomenon of enzyme adsorption may be partly responsible for the increase in temperature-sensitivity of erythrocytes and for hot lysis of these cells.

The scanning electronmicrograph of sheep erythrocytes disclosed that the morphological changes were brought about in these cells by the action of B. cereus SMase; invagination appeared at first on the cell surface, then the cells were transformed into spherocytes(Ikezawa, Mori and Taguchi, in press).

ECTOENZYME RELEASE FROM PLASMA MEMBRANE BY PHOSPHATIDYLINOSITOL-SPECIFIC PHOSPHOLIPASE C

Purified preparations of PIase were obtained from the culture broth of B. cereus and Bacillus thuringiensis to homogeneity, according to polyacrylamide gel electrophoresis(Ikezawa and others, 1976; Taguchi, Asahi and Ikezawa, to be published). When the purified PIase of B. cereus was incubated with slices from rat kidney, alkaline phosphatase was released linearly with time, as shown in Fig. 2. Phosphatase release was proportinal to the concentration of PIase and the amount of slices(Ikezawa and others, 1976;1977).

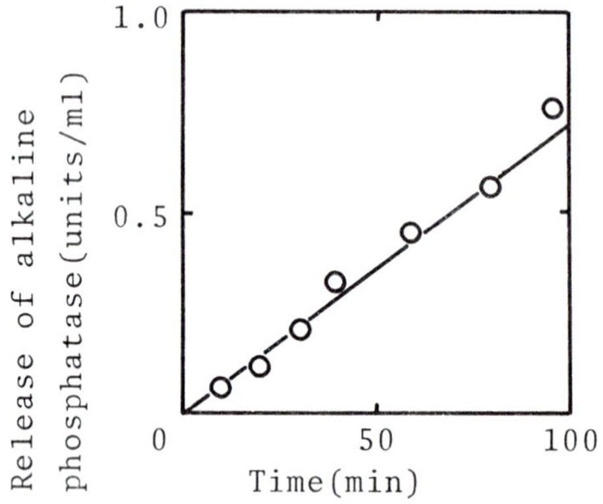

Fig. 2. Time course of phosphatase release by PIase from rat kidney slices.

The molecular weight of alkaline phosphatase liberated was determined by gel-filtration to be 100,000 to 110,000 daltons(Ohyabu, Taguchi and Ikezawa, 1978). Both phosphatidylinositol-hydrolyzing and phosphatase-releasing activities of B. cereus proved to be due to the same protein, in that these activities were completely neutralized by the same amount of anti-PIase IgG which was purified from antiserum of PIase-immunized rabbits. When the purified PIase of *B. cereus* was injected into the tail veins of rats, the activity of alkaline phosphatase in rat blood plasma increased with time in proportion to the enzyme units injected. Also this *in vivo* release of alkaline phosphatase was reduced by neutralization with purified anti-PIase IgG. The inhibition studies using sodium deoxycholate and L-phenylalanine showed that the molecular form of alkaline phosphatase liberated *in vivo* was similar to the isozyme from kidney or liver but was different from that of intestine. Likewise alkaline phosphatase, 5'-nucleotidase was released linearly by increasing amount of PIase of *B. cereus*. Purified PIase of *B. thuringiensis* also liberated alkaline phosphatase from yeast protoplast and the slices of several organs such as kidney, liver, intestine and pancreas. Also, *Clostridium novyi* PIase was established as the separate entity from PCase (γ-toxin) of the same origin(Taguchi and Ikezawa, 1978). This PIase also liberated alkaline phosphatase as well as 5'-nucleotidase from rat liver slices. Recently, Low and Finean(1977a, 1978) reported that PIase of *Staphylococcus aureus* exhibited the similar enzyme-releasing activity. Furthermore, they also reported the release of acetylcholinesterase from erythrocyte membrane by PIase(Low and Finean, 1977b). In my laboratory, acetylcholinesterase release by *B. thuringiensis* PIase was also confirmed with horse, sheep and bovine erythrocytes, and with their ghosts. Generally, the release was much easier from ghosts than from intact cells. By the attack of PIase, acetylcholinesterase was released without hemolysis of erythrocytes. Alkaline phosphatase, 5'-nucleotidase and acylcholinesterase are known to be ectoenzymes associated with plasma membranes of eucaryotic cells. Thus phosphatidylinositol may play a special role for binding of these enzymes to plasma membranes, and the ecto-enzyme-releasing activity must be one of the common, specific properties of bacterial PIase. In addition to these findings, PIase from *B. cereus* or *B. thuringiensis* proved to inhibit the growth of Sarcoma 180 cells by intraperitoneous injection into mice of ICR-SLC strain which had been transplanted with the cells of this ascites tumour(Ikezawa, Asahi and Taguchi, to be published). At the same time, invagination of cell surfaces was brought about by the action of PIase, according to scanning electronmicroscopy. When PIase of *B. thuringiensis* was incubated with Sarcoma 180 cells, alkaline phosphatase and 5'-nucleotidase were also released without cell lysis.

THE ROLE OF BACTERIAL PHOSPHOLIPASES C AS TOXINS

The actions of bacterial phospholipases C on plasma membranes of eucaryotic cells are summarized in Table I. PCase and SMase hydrolyze choline-containing phospholipids such as phosphatidylcholine and sphingomyelin. These phospholipids are the major constituents of outer leaflet of membrane bilayer. Therefore, as the result of hydrolytic actions, these enzymes make plasma membranes sensitive to cold or osmotic shock and cause hot-cold hemolysis, with exception of *B. cereus* PCase.

TABLE I THE ACTIONS OF PHOSPHOLIPASES C ON PLASMA MEMBRANES

			Hemolysis		ecto-enzyme
			hot-cold	hot	release
(1)	PCase	*C. perfringens*	(+)	(+)	(-)
		C. novyi	(+)	(+)	(-)
		P. aureofaciens	(+)	(+)	(-)
		B. cereus	(-)	(-)	(-)
(2)	SMase	*B. cereus*	(+)	(+)	(-)
		S. aureus	(+)	(-)	
(3)	PIase	*B. cereus*	(-)	(-)	(+)
		B. thuringiensis	(-)	(-)	(+)
		C. novyi	(-)	(-)	(+)
		S. aureus		(-)	(+)

Of two bacterial SMases, the staphylococcal enzyme does not cause hemolysis of erythrocytes during incubation at 37°C. On the other hand, SMase of *B. cereus* can cause hot hemolysis, probably due to specific adsorption and to subsequent hydrolysis of sphingomyelin. Bacterial PIases liberate several ectoenzymes such as alkaline phosphatase, 5'-nucleotidase and acetylcholinesterase from plasma membranes in vitro or in vivo. Also the growth of transplanted Sarcoma 180 cells was inhibited by PIases. Phospholipases C remove the polar head groups from membrane phospholipids, and phospholipase C-producing bacteria(*Bacillus* sp., *Clostridium* sp., *Staphylococcus* sp., and so forth) are mostly parasites of eucaryotes. Therefore, most of these enzymes must be produced primarily for the purpose of attack against plasma membranes of eucaryotic cells. When the enzymes hydrolyze major constituent phospholipids such as phosphatidylcholine and sphingomyelin, the lysis of cells occurs; when the enzymes hydrolyze minor, functional phospholipid such as phosphatidylinositol, the release of ectoenzymes or inhibition of cell growth takes place.

ACKNOWLEDGEMENT

The author is greatly indebted to his colleagues, Dr. Taguchi and others.

REFERENCES

Bernheimer, A. W., L. S. Avigad, and K. S. Kim (1974). Ann. N. Y. Acad. Sci., 236, 292-306.

Bigger, J. W., C. R. Boland, and R. A. Q. O'Meara (1927). J. Path. Bact., 30, 271-277.

Doery, H. M., B. J. Magnusson, I. M. Cheyne, and J. Gulasekharam (1963). Nature (London), 198, 1091-1092.

Glenny, A. T., and M. F. Stevens (1935). J. Path. Bact., 40, 201-210.

Gow, J. A., and J. Robinson (1969). J. Bacteriol., 97, 1026-1032.

Ikezawa, H. (1963). J. Biochem., 54, 301-311.

Ikezawa, H., M. Yamanegi, R. Taguchi, T. Miyashita, and T. Ohyabu (1976). Biochim. Biophys. Acta, 450, 154-164.

Ikezawa, H., M. Yamanegi, R. Taguchi, T. Miyashita, and T. Ohyabu (1977). Jap. J. med. Sci. Biol., 30, 81-82.

Ikezawa, H., M. Mori, T. Ohyabu, and R. Taguchi (1978). Biochim. Biophys. Acta, 528, 247-256.

Ikezawa, H., M. Mori, and R. Taguchi (1980). Arch. Biochem. Biophys., in press.

Ikezawa, H., Y. Asahi, and R. Taguchi, to be published.

Johnson, C. E., and P. F. Bonventre (1967). J. Bacteriol., 94, 306-316.

Low, M. G., and J. B. Finean (1977a). Biochem. J., 167, 281-284.

Low, M. G., and J. B. Finean (1977b). FEBS Lett., 82, 143-146.

Low, M. G., and J. B. Finean (1978). Biochim. Biophys. Acta, 508, 565-570.

Macfarlane, M. G., and B. C. J. G. Knight (1941). Biochem. J., 35, 884-902

Maheswaran, S. K., and R. K. Lindorfer (1967). J. Bacteriol., 94, 1313-1319.

Ohyabu, T., R. Taguchi, and H. Ikezawa (1978) Arch. Biochem. Biophys., 190, 1-7.

Roelofsen, B., R. F. A. Zwaal, P. Comfurious, C. B. Woodward, and L. L. M. Van Deenen (1971). Biochim. Biophys. Acta, 241, 925-929.

Slein, M. W., and G. F. Logan, Jr. (1965). J. Bacteriol., 90, 69-81.

Taguchi, R., and H. Ikezawa (1976a). Arch. Biochem. Biophys., 173, 538-545.

Taguchi, R., and H. Ikezawa (1976b). In A. Ohsaka, K. Hayashi, and Y. Sawai (Ed.), Animal, Plant and Microbial Toxins, Vol. I. Prenum Press, New York and London. pp 429-436.

Taguchi, R., and Ikezawa (1978). Arch. Biochem. Biophys., 186, 196-201.

Taguchi, R., Y. Asahi, and H. Ikezawa, to be published.

Wadström, T., and R. Möllby (1971). Biochim Biophys. Acta, 242, 288-307.

Walbum, L. E. (1921). C. R. Seanc. Soc. Biol., 85, 1205-1206.

Wiseman, G. M., and J. D. Caird (1967) Can. J. Microbiol., 13, 369-376.

Woodward, C. B., and R. F. A. Zwaal (1972). Biochim. Biophys. Acta, 274, 272-278.

Zwaal, R. F. A., B. Roelofsen, P. Comfurious, and L. L. M. Van Deenen (1971). Biochim. Biophys. Acta, 233, 474-479.

DIFFERENTIAL PHOSPHOLIPID HYDROLYSIS BY PHOSPHOLIPASE C IN SARCOLEMMA OF MUSCLES WITH CALCIUM OR SODIUM GENERATED ACTION POTENTIALS*

P. Rosenberg and R. G. Knickelbein**

Section of Pharmacology and Toxicology, The University of Connecticut, School of Pharmacy, Storrs, CT. 06268, USA

ABSTRACT

Phospholipase C (PhC) and tetrodotoxin (TTX) block conduction in muscles with sodium generated action potentials, but do not alter conduction in muscles with calcium generated action potentials (Johansson and Thesleff, 1968). The hypothesis that intact phospholipids may be essential for functioning of the sodium channel was tested by isolating sarcolemma from sodium spike (rat extensor digitorum longus and frog sartorius) and calcium spike (guinea pig taenia coli and lobster walking leg) muscles. The highly purified and membrane enriched preparations were incubated for one hr with 0.008 to 0.8 units of PhC per ml. At the highest dose of PhC, sphingomyelin, phosphatidylcholine and phosphatidylethanolamine were extensively (50% or greater) hydrolyzed in all of the sarcolemmal preparations. In contrast, approximately 50% of phosphatidylinositol (PI) and phosphatidylserine (PS) were hydrolyzed in sarcolemma from sodium spike muscles whereas no hydrolysis was seen in sarcolemma from calcium spike muscles. In the presence of 100 nM TTX, less PI and PS were hydrolyzed in the sodium spike sarcolemma. These results suggest that PI and PS may be associated with the sodium and calcium channels, however, only in the sodium channels are the phospholipids accessible to PhC.

KEYWORDS

Phospholipase C; phospholipids; tetrodotoxin; muscle; sodium channel; calcium channel; sarcolemma.

---

*A full report on these studies will appear in TOXICON.

**Submitted in partial fulfillment of the requirements for a PhD. degree. Present address: Dept. of Pharmacology, Medical Univ. of South Carolina, Charleston, South Carolina 29403, U.S.A.

INTRODUCTION

Johansson and Thesleff (1968) utilized two naturally occurring toxins (tetrodotoxin and phospholipase C) to study muscle bioelectricity. They found that tetrodotoxin (TTX) which specifically blocks the sodium channels, prevented electrical activity only in muscles which depend on sodium for genesis of bioelectricity. Similarly, they found that small concentrations of phospholipase C (PhC; E.C. 3.1.4.3) an enzyme which breaks down phospholipids, also terminated electrical activity only in muscles with sodium generated electrical activity. Their results suggested that intact phospholipids may be required for sodium channel function. We tested the ability of PhC to hydrolyze phospholipids in sarcolemma isolated from the same muscles which Johansson and Thesleff had used. We also studied whether TTX altered the extent of hydrolysis produced by PhC.

MATERIALS AND METHODS

PhC (89 units per mg; 0.65 mg/ml in 30% glycerol), prepared from <u>Clostridium</u> <u>perfringens</u> and chromatographically purified, obtained from Worthington Biochemical Corporation (Freehold, New Jersey U.S.A.) was used in all the studies with muscle sarcolemma. TTX (in pH 4.8 citrate buffer) was purchased from Sankyo Chemical Co. Japan.

Sarcolemma were isolated from two muscles with sodium generated action potentials (rat extensor digitorum longus and frog sartorius) and two with calcium generated action potentials (lobster walking leg muscle and guinea pig taenia coli), according to a modification of the method described by Rosenthal and co-workers (1965). Na, K-ATPase (E.C. 3.6.1.3) was assayed by a modification of the method of Shirachi, Allard, and Trevor (1970). Fumarase (E.C. 4.2.1.2) was assayed by the procedure described by Racker (1950). Lactate dehydrogenase (E.C. 1.1.1.27) was monitored by a modification of the method described by Kornberg (1955). Protein content was assayed by the procedure of Lowry and co-workers (1951).

Sarcolemmal suspensions in Ringer's solution (8 mg protein per ml) were incubated with PhC (0.008, 0.08 or 0.8 units/ml) for one hr at room temperature with continuous shaking. Some suspensions were supplemented with 100 nM TTX and pre-incubated for 15 min prior to the enzyme treatment. Following incubation lipids were extracted by the method of Folch, Lees, and Sloane Stanley (1957) and phospholipids separated using a micro-modification of the thin-layer chromatographic method described by Condrea, Rosenberg, and Dettbarn (1967). Phospholipids were quantified by phosphorus analyses using modifications of previously described methods (Bartlett, 1959; Kleinig and Lempert, 1970).

RESULTS

The sarcolemma appeared as transparent empty tubules, in marked contrast to the unemptied muscle cells which are dense, and in which myofibrillae and other intracellular structures are readily seen (Fig. 1). Frog sartorius, rat extensor digitorum longus and lobster walking leg muscle sarcolemma (not shown) were similar. The purity of the sarcolemma were further studied using marker enzymes. The sarcolemma had little or no lactate dehydrogenase or fumarase activity indicating little cytoplasmic or mitochondrial contamination.

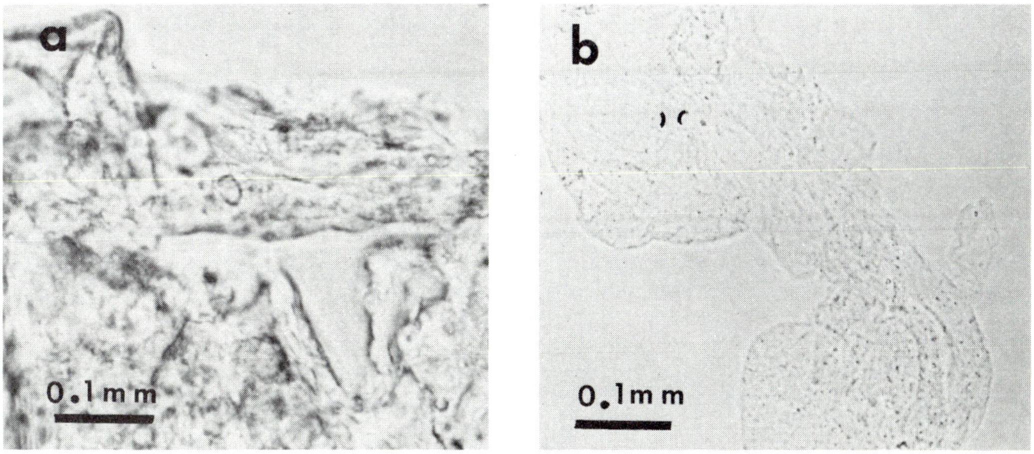

Fig. 1. Phase contrast photomicrographs of guinea pig taenia coli muscle. a) partially emptied muscle cells. b) relatively pure sarcolemmal tubule.

In contrast Na, K-ATPase was at least twice as active in the sarcolemma as in the whole muscle, indicating an enrichment in plasma membrane (Fig. 2).

The phospholipid content of the four sarcolemmal preparations used in this study as well as the % distribution of the individual phospholipids are shown in Table 1. The calcium spike sarcolemma are about three to six fold richer in phospholipids than sarcolemma from the sodium spike muscles, however, the distribution of the individual phospholipids is similar with phosphatidylcholine and -ethanolamine being present in largest amounts. The overall extent of phospholipid hydrolysis was similar in the four sarcolemmal preparations (Table 1).

Sphingomyelin, phosphatidylcholine and phosphatidylethanolamine were extensively hydrolyzed in all of the sarcolemmal preparations and the presence of TTX did not markedly alter the extent of their hydrolysis (Table 2). In marked contrast phosphatidylinositol and phosphatidylserine of the calcium spike sarcolemma were not hydrolyzed even by the highest concentration of PhC, whereas they were hydrolyzed in the

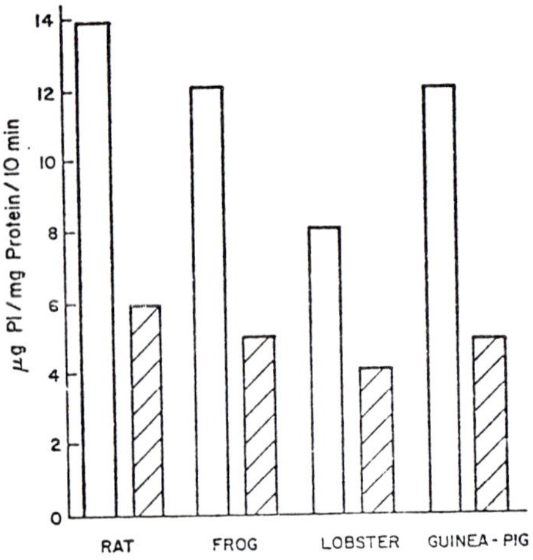

Fig. 2. Na^{+}-K^{+}-ATPase activity of rat extensor digitorum longus, frog sartorius, guinea pig taenia coli, and lobster walking leg muscle whole homogenate (hatched bars) and sarcolemma (open bars).

TABLE 1 Phospholipid Content of Sarcolemma and % Hydrolysis of Total Phospholipids By PhC

		Lobster W.L.M.	Guinea Pig T.C.	Rat E.D.L.	Frog Sartorius
A.	TLP (ug Pi/mg protein)				
		3.2±0.4	4.4±0.02	0.73±0.03	1.09±0.2
B.	% DISTRIBUTION				
	SM	4±0.2	19±0.3	3±0.2	3±0.2
	PC	62±2	39±2	61±2	57±2
	PE	28±0.2	25±2	24±1	25±0.8
	PI	4±0.3	8±0.5	8±0.4	11±1
	PS	2±0.1	10±0.2	5±0.3	4±0.3
C.	% HYDROLYSIS				
	PhC (U/ml)				
	0.008	0, 3	1, 2	4, 5	8
	0.08	35, 36	21	36, 40	31, 34
	0.8	73, 74	43, 44	55, 58	54, 56

The results in A and B are means ± standard deviation (four determinations); individual values are shown in C. In C the sarcolemmal preparations were incubated at room temperature for one hr with PhC. W.L.M.=walking leg muscle; T.C.=taenia coli; E.D.L.=extensor digitorum longus; SM=sphingomyelin; PC=phosphatidylcholine; PE=phosphatidylethanolamine; PS=phosphatidylserine; PI=phosphatidylinositol; Pi=inorganic phosphorus; TLP=total lipid phosphorus; PhC=phospholipase C.

TABLE 2 Percent Hydrolysis of Sarcolemmal Phospholipids By PhC

PL	PhC units/ml	Taenia Coli No TTX	Taenia Coli TTX	Walking Leg No TTX	Walking Leg TTX	E.D.L. No TTX	E.D.L. TTX	Sartorius No TTX	Sartorius TTX
		% Hydrolysis							
SM	.008	9	5	9	18	0	6	18	20
		4	5	22	13	9	12	12	
	.08	14	11	48	54	63	50	76	34
		15	14	54	48	75	62		41
	.8	70	72	73	83	87	62		91
		66	70	82	74	75	75		
PC	.008	5	16	0	2	5	16	0	8
		5	16	5	1	12	13	0	6
	.08	35	22	50	56	70	68	43	34
		40	35	53	54	61	68	41	41
	.8	72	84	94	93	88	87	68	79
		69	78	94	92	88	85	70	82
PE	.008	4	5	1	6	0	0	9	16
		4	10	7	4	8	5	12	16
	.08	10	18	51	51	29	36	37	69
		12	7	43	46	25	35	41	66
	.8	54	68	84	80	49	61	60	72
		46	67	85	80	50	57	56	72
PI	.008	5	3	14	22	0	0	0	0
		20	17		20	0	5	0	0
	.08	26	6	36	30	0	4	8	0
		37	11	35	36	0	3	11	4
	.8	40	8	38	34	4	3	2	0
		42	14	42	32	8	6	0	4
PS	.008	30	48	20	6	0	2	7	0
		50	24	16		0	0	0	0
	.08	25	38	43	8	0	13	0	0
			29	55	0	0	0	0	0
	.8	50	38	50	33	0	4	0	0
		55		57	44	8	4	7	0

The % hydrolysis of each of the major phospholipids is shown after incubating at room temperature for one hr with the indicated concentrations of PhC. The sarcolemma were incubated both with and without the addition of 100 nM TTX. Abbreviations as in Table 1.

sodium spike sarcolemma (Table 2). The addition of TTX decreased the hydrolysis of phosphatidylinositol in the extensor digitorum longus sarcolemma and decreased the hydrolysis of phosphatidylserine in the sartorius sarcolemma (Table 2).

DISCUSSION

While phosphatidylcholine, phosphatidylethanolamine and sphingomyelin were hydrolyzed to a similar extent in all sarcolemmal preparations,

tissues. J. Biol. Chem., 226, 497-509.

Jacobson, K., and Papahadjopoules, D. (1975). Phase transitions and phase separations in phospholipid membranes induced by changes in temperature, pH, and concentration of bivalent cations. Biochemistry 14, 152-161.

Johansson, P., and Thesleff, S. (1968). A comparison of the effects of phospholipase C and tetrodotoxin on spike generation in muscle. Eur. J. Pharmacol., 4, 347-348.

Kleinig, H., and Lempert, U. (1970). Phospholipid analysis on a micro scale. J. Chromatogr., 53, 595-597.

Kornberg, A. (1955). Lactic dehydrogenase of muscle. In S.P. Colowick, and N.O. Kaplan (Eds.), Methods in Enzymology, Vol. 1 Academic Press, New York. pp. 441-443.

Lee, A.G. (1977). Local anesthesia: the interaction between phospholipids and chlorpromazine, propranolol, and practolol. Mol. Pharmacol., 13, 474-487.

Lowry, D.H., Rosebrough, N.J., Farr, A.L. and Randall, R.J. (1951). Protein measurement with the folin phenol reagent. J. Biol. Chem., 193, 265-275.

Michell, R.H. (1975). Inositol phospholipids and cell surface receptor function. Biochim. Biophys. Acta 415, 81-147.

Ottolenghi, A.C. (1969). Phospholipase C. In J.M. Lowenstein (Ed.) Methods in Enzymology, Vol. 14, Lipids. Academic Press, New York. pp. 188-197.

Racker, E. (1950). Spectrophotometric measurements of the enzymatic formation of fumaric and cis-aconitic acids. Biochim. Biophys. Acta 4, 211-214.

Rosenthal, S.L., Edelman, P.M., and Schwartz, I.L. (1965). A method for the preparation of skeletal muscle sarcolemma. Biochim. Biophys. Acta 109, 512-517.

Shirachi, D.Y., Allard, A.A., and Trevor, A.J. (1970). Partial purification and ouabain sensitivity of lubrol-extracted Na^+-K^+-transport adenosine triphosphatases from brain and cardiac tissues. Biochem. Pharmacol., 19, 1-14.

Stahl, W.L. (1973). Phospholipase C purification and specificity with respect to individual phospholipids and brain microsomal membrane phospholipids. Arch. Biochem. Biophys., 153, 47-55.

Trudell, J.R. (1977). A unitary theory of anesthesia based on lateral phase separations in nerve membranes. Anesthesiology, 16, 5-10.

COOPERATIVE ACTION OF PURIFIED BACTERICIDAL/PERMEABILITY INCREASING PROTEIN AND PHOSPHOLIPASE A_2 FROM RABBIT POLYMORPHONUCLEAR LEUKOCYTES

P. Elsbach and J. Weiss

Department of Medicine, New York, University School of Medicine, New York, N.Y., USA

ABSTRACT

We have purified from rabbit and human polymorphonuclear leukocytes a potent bactericidal cationic membrane-active protein. These two proteins kill gram-negative bacteria only and are closely similar in molecular and biological properties. Leukocytes also contain a phospholipase A_2 which we have purified to near homogeneity from rabbit leukocytes. This phospholipase A_2 only degrades the phospholipids of susceptible bacteria when in combination with the rabbit leukocyte bactericidal protein. The very similar human leukocyte bactericidal protein cannot substitute in this cooperative action, nor can four other purified phospholipases A_2.

KEYWORDS

Polymorphonuclear leukocytes; bactericidal protein; membrane-active protein; phospholipase A_2; cooperative action.

Polymorphonuclear leukocytes (PMN) play a cardinal role in defense against bacterial infection. The leukocyte's ability to kill microorganisms rests on a complex antimicrobial arsenal, consisting of O_2-dependent and O_2-independent bactericidal systems. Among the O_2-independent antimicrobial substances are an incompletely resolved group of granule-associated cationic proteins (Spitznagel, 1975; Olsson and colleagues, 1978).

Our studies concern the properties of a toxin-like protein purified to near homogeneity from both human and rabbit PMN granules. The purification of these two proteins and their biological properties have been described very recently. To avoid duplication of reporting the interested reader is therefore referred to these recent publications for details (Weiss and colleagues, 1978, 1979; Elsbach and coworkers, 1979). Only a summary of our findings follows: The purified human PMN protein (M_r approx. 60,000) and rabbit PMN protein (M_r approx. 50,000) are closely similar in amino acid composition and isoelectric point (> 9.6). Both proteins appear devoid of catalytic activity. The potency and antibacterial specificity of the human and rabbit PMN proteins are practically identical. Only gram-negative bacteria are sensitive to their action, apparently because binding of the proteins to constituents of the outer membrane, that are specific for the gram-negative bacterial envelope, is a requisite for antibacterial action (Weiss and co-workers, 1978). Rapid loss of bacterial colony-forming ability occurs without appreciable structural or functional impairment. However, two almost immediate envelope alterations accompany loss of viability: 1) a discrete increase in permeability of the outer membrane, recognizable as entry of the normally impermeant antibiotic Actinomycin D (Beckerdite and co-workers, 1974; Weiss and co-workers, 1975), and 2) net degradation of outer membrane phospholipids caused by activation of bacterial phospholipase A which resides in the outer membrane (Weiss and co-workers, 1976, 1977; Vos and co-workers, 1978). This degradation of bacterial phospholipid is not part of a generalized autolysis, because no catabolism of bacterial protein or nucleic acids is evident. By using an Escherichia coli K12 mutant strain [1] that lacks the usual phospholipase A activity of E.coli we have been able to demonstrate, unequivocally (Weiss and Elsbach, 1977) that the leukocyte phospholipase A_2 (Franson and co-workers, 1974, 1977; Elsbach and co-workers, 1979) also contributes to bacterial phospholipid degradation, but only in combination with the bactericidal protein. In this study we examined the specificity of this cooperativity. To this end we compared the ability of three bactericidal polypeptides with surface-active properties on gram-negative bacterial envelopes (human PMN bactericidal protein; rabbit PMN bactericidal protein; the cationic peptide antibiotic polymixin B) to facilitate the action of five purified phospholipases A_2(from rabbit PMN, pig pancreas, cow pancreas, Naja naja snake venom, bee venom[2]) on the phospholipids of the phospholipase A deficient E.coli mutant.

Incubation mixtures contained an amount of each bactericidal protein that produces greater than 95% loss of bacterial colony forming ability. Of each phospholipase A_2 the same number of units of activity was added.

None of the purified phospholipases A_2, when added alone, had an effect on bacterial viability or degraded bacterial phospholipids.

Recombination of the purified rabbit PMN phospholipase A_2 and the purified rabbit PMN bactericidal protein restores the net hydrolysis of the phospholipids of the phospholipase A deficient E.coli mutant, during bacterial killing, to the same levels produced by cruder fractions. This facilitating effect of the rabbit bactericidal protein appears specific for the rabbit PMN phospholipase A_2. It is not seen with purified phospholipase A_2 from snake venom, pig or cow pancreas and is 4-fold less with bee venom phospholipase A_2. Furthermore, neither the rabbit leukocyte phospholipase A_2 nor the other four phospholipases A_2 are activated by human PMN bactericidal protein. In contrast, in the presence of bactericidal concentrations of the cationic membrane-active antibiotic polymixin B all five phospholipases A_2 degrade almost all of the E.coli phospholipids, indicating that no intrinsic differences exist in the catalytic activities of these phospholipases A_2 towards the bacterial phospholipids.

The fact that bacterial phospholipid degradation is nearly complete further implies that polymixin B renders both outer and inner membrane phospholipids accessible to hydrolysis by these added phospholipases A_2. Net phospholipid hydrolysis generated by the combination of the rabbit PMN phospholipase A_2 and bactericidal protein, however, does not exceed 25% of total E.coli phospholipids. The difference in the extent of phospholipid hydrolysis produced by the facilitating action of polymixin B and the rabbit bactericidal protein appears to reflect differences in the site of action and in the magnitude of the membrane-perturbing effects of the two bactericidal proteins. Polymixin B passes through outer and inner mem-

---

[1] Kindly donated by Dr. S. Nojima, Faculty of Pharmaceutical Sciences, University of Tokyo.

[2] The latter four phospholipases A_2 were gifts from Drs. G.H. de Haas, C. Dutilh and R.F.A. Zwaal, Department of Biochemistry, University of Utrecht.

brane of the gram-negative envelope, affecting structural and functional properties of both phospholipid-containing envelope layers. In contrast, our evidence suggests that the PMN bactericidal proteins attach to surface sites and do not penetrate the envelope, leaving the inner (cytoplasmic) membrane intact and its phospholipids inaccessible to enzymatic attack (Weiss and co-workers, 1976, 1977, 1978, 1979).

A remarkable feature of the activation by polymixin B or rabbit PMN bactericidal protein of the action of the five phospholipases A_2 studied on the E.coli envelope phospholipids is that it occurs in the absence of added Ca^{2+} (Weiss and co-workers, 1979). Since all phospholipases A_2 examined absolutely require Ca^{2+} for catalytic activity we propose that intramembrane Ca^{2+} provides this essential cofactor.

Comparison of the fates of wild type E.coli and of an E.coli mutant that is unable to degrade its own phospholipids, when exposed to the rabbit PMN bactericidal protein in the absence or presence of rabbit PMN phospholipase A_2, has shown that neither bacterial killing nor the envelope permeability changes require net hydrolysis of phospholipid (Elsbach and co-workers, 1979). It seems likely, however, that an attack on bacterial phospholipids, coincident with rapid killing is an important step in the overall destruction and digestion by the leukocyte of ingested bacteria. In fact, the highly specific cooperativity between the rabbit PMN bactericidal protein and the rabbit PMN phospholipase A_2 suggests that, within the antimicrobial arsenal of the leukocyte, these two membrane-active proteins are destined to act in concert.

Substantial evidence indicates that phospholipases A_2 contribute prominently to the cytotoxic effects of a number of venoms (Howard and Truog, 1977; Eaker, these proceedings). The nature of the cooperative effects between venom phospholipases A_2 and other constituents has not been clearly established. It does appear, however, that facilitating effects of venom components such as melittin and direct lytic factor (Habermann, 1972; Mollay and Kreil, 1974; Mollay and co-workers, 1976; Shier, 1979), on hydrolysis by exogenous and endogenous phospholipases A_2 of phospholipids of natural and artificial membranes are quite non-specific, i.e. peptides from different sources stimulate multiple phospholipases A_2.

Thus, our findings do not only reveal the first instance of facilitation by a mammalian protein of the action of a phospholipase A_2 on an intact (bacterial) cell, but also a degree of specificity of this cooperative effect that has not been observed before. This cooperativity between two proteins of a mammalian cell is of particular interest because it is manifest in a physiological event, namely the destruction of a gram-negative bacterium by a phagocytic cell.

REFERENCES

Beckerdite, S., C. Mooney, J. Weiss, R.C. Franson, and P. Elsbach (1974). Early and discrete changes in permeability of E.coli and certain other gram-negative microorganisms during killing by granulocytes. J. Exp. Med., 140, 396-409.

Eaker, D. (1980). Structural features of neuro- and myotoxic phospholipases A_2. (These proceedings).

Elsbach, P., J. Weiss, R.C. Franson, S. Beckerdite-Quagliata, A. Schneider, and L. Harris (1979). Separation and purification of a potent bactericidal/permeability increasing protein and a closely associated phospholipase A_2 from rabbit polymorphonuclear leukocytes. Observations on their relationship. J. Biol. Chem., 254 11000-11009.

Franson, R.C., P. Patriarca and P. Elsbach (1974). Phospholipid metabolism by phagocytic cells. Phospholipases A_2 associated with rabbit polymorphonuclear leukocyte granules. J. Lipid Res., 15, 380-388.

Franson, R.C., J. Weiss, L. Martin, J.K. Spitznagel and P. Elsbach (1977). Phospholipase A activity associated with the membranes of human polymorphonuclear leukocytes. Biochem. J. 167, 839-841.

Habermann, E. (1972). Bee and wasp venoms. Science, 177, 314-322.

Howard, B.D. and R. Truog (1977). Relationship between the neurotoxicity and phospholipase A activity of β-bungarotoxin. Biochemistry, 16, 122-125.

Mollay, C., and G. Kreil (1974). Enhancement of bee venom phospholipase A_2 activity by melittin, direct lytic factor from cobra venom and polymixin B. FEBS Letters, 46, 141-144.

Mollay, C., G. Kreil and H. Berger (1976). Action of phospholipases on the cytoplasmic membrane of Escherichia coli. Stimulation by melittin. Biochim. Biophys. Acta, 426, 317-324.

Olsson, I., H. Odeberg, J. Weiss and P. Elsbach (1978). Bactericidal cationic proteins of human granulocytes. In K. Havemann and A. Janoff (Ed.), Neutral Proteases of Human PolymorphonucLear Leukocytes. Urban & Schwarzenberg, Baltimore, pp. 18-32.

Shier, W.T. (1979). Activation of high levels of endogenous phospholipase A_2 in cultured cells. Proc. Natl. Acad. Sci. USA, 76, 195-199.

Spitznagel, J.K. (1975). Advances in the study of cytoplasmic granules of human neutrophilic leukocytes. In J.A. Bellanti and D.H. Dayton (Ed.). The Phagocytic Cell in Host Resistance. Raven Press, New York, pp. 77-85.

Vos, M.M., J.A.F. Op den Kamp, S. Beckerdite-Quagliata and P. Elsbach (1978). Acylation of monoacylglycerophosphoethanolamine in the inner and outer membranes of the envelope of an Escherichia coli K12 strain and its phospholipase A-deficient mutant. Biochim. Biophys. Acta, 508, 165-173.

Weiss, J., R. Franson, S. Beckerdite, K. Schmeidler and P. Elsbach (1975). Partial characterization and purification of a rabbit granulocyte factor that increases permeability of E.coli. J. Clin. Invest., 55, 33-42.

Weiss, J., K. Schmeidler, S. Beckerdite-Quagliata, R. Franson and P. Elsbach (1976). Reversible envelope effects during and after killing by a highly purified granulocyte preparation. Biochim. Biophys. Acta, 436, 154-169.

Weiss, J., and P. Elsbach (1977). The use of a phospholipase A-less Escherichia coli mutant to establish the action of granulocyte phospholipase A on bacterial phospholipids during killing by a highly purified granulocyte fraction. Biochim. Biophys. Acta, 466, 23-33.

Weiss, J., P. Elsbach, I. Olsson, and H. Odeberg (1978) Purification and characterization of a potent bactericidal and membrane active protein from the granules of human polymorphonuclear leukocytes. J. Biol. Chem. 253, 2664-2672.

Weiss, J., S. Beckerdite-Quagliata and P. Elsbach (1979). Determinants of the action of phospholipases A on the envelope phospholipids of Escherichia coli. J. Biol. Chem. 254, (in press).

Enterotoxins

ESCHERICHIA COLI HEAT LABILE ENTEROTOXIN: DNA DIRECTED *IN VITRO* SYNTHESIS AND STRUCTURE

F. Dorner*, C. Hughes, G. Nahler** and G. Högenauer****

**Department of Bacteriology, Swiss Serum and Vaccine Institute, Berne, Switzerland*
***Department of Experimental Chemotherapy, Sandoz Research Institute, Vienna, Austria*

ABSTRACT

Escherichia coli heat labile enterotoxin was synthesized in a cell-free system directed by DNA of the plasmid P307. Synthesis of the toxin, assayed by the elongation induced in Chinese hamster ovary cells, was strongly stimulated by cyclic AMP and occurred at physiological levels of Mg^{2+} only when the polyamine spermidine was present. Activity was abolished by heat and antisera prepared against the enterotoxins of both E. coli P263 and Vibrio Cholera. Tritium labelled enterotoxin was purified by immunoprecipitation and examined by sodium dodecyl sulphate / polyacrylamide gel electrophoresis. When gel slices were assayed for the ability to stimulate adenylate cyclase activity in erythrocyte ghosts, two peaks were found, one at molecular weight 26,000 and frequently, but not always, another at 23,000. Detection of radiolabelled protein by fluorography and scintillation counting of gel slices revealed three prominent polypeptides, two corresponding to the peaks having adenylate cyclase stimulating activity and a further one of molecular weight 11,500, identical to that of the cholera subunit B. The data suggest that the E. coli heat labile enterotoxin synthesized in the cell-free system has a subunit structure.

KEYWORDS

Immunoprecipitation; subunit; cyclic AMP; adenylate cyclase;

INTRODUCTION

Enteropahtogenic Escherichia coli produce two classes of enterotoxin, heat stable (ST) and heat labile (LT), which cause diarrhoeal disease in man and domestic animals. Interest in the latter has been intensified by reports of its biological and immunological resemblance to the well-characterized enterotoxin of Vibro cholera (Dorner, Jaksche, Stöckl, 1976; Smith and Sack, 1973;), but structural relationships have not yet been demonstrated as comparisons at the molecular level have proved difficult, primarily because of the heterogeneity of E. coli enterotoxin preparations.

While the plasmid-mediated nature of enterotoxigenicity and other characteristics of medically-important enterobacteria is well established (Falkow, 1975;), little data is available on the regulation of expression of the plasmid genes involved. Furthermore, although coupled transcription-translation systems have been extensively used to study the expression of bacterial and viral genomes, only the syntheses of β-lactamase and bacteriocins have been investigated in plasmid DNA-directed systems (Grindley, Blumberg, Nakada, 1976; Konings and colleagues, 1976; Sidikaro and Nomura, 1975;).

As part of a study of plasmid gene expression, we report on the cell-free synthesis of *E. coli* LT toxin, directed by the *ent*$^+$ plasmid P307, and demonstrate the probable subunit structure of the gene product.

MATERIALS AND METHODS

PLASMID DNA

The plasmid P307 (molecular weight 65.10^6) determines the production of both LT and ST toxins and was first described in *E. coli* P307 isolated from an outbreak of porcine diarrhoea. The plasmid was transferred to *E. coli* 711, a plasmid-free laboratory strain, and Ent$^+$ 711 (obtained from Dr. S. Falkow of the University of Washington Medical School) was used as the source of *ent*$^+$ plasmid DNA. DNA of the drug resistance (R) plasmid NR1, isolated from *E. coli* CR34/R12 (supplied by Dr. R. Rownd, University of Wisconsin), was used as a control template.

Cleared lysates were prepared by the method of Clewell and Helsinki (1969) and DNA was concentrated by overnight centrifugation (20,000 rpm in a Beckman SW27 rotor) onto a caesium chloride "shelf". Plasmid DNA was then isolated by two dyebuoyant density equilibrium centrifugations (40 - 60 h x 120,000 g) and purity was confirmed by gel electrophoresis in 0.7 % agarose (Green and co-workers, 1974).

CELL-FREE PROTEIN SYNTHESIS (Zubay, Chambers and Cheong, 1970)

Reaction mixtures, in a final volume of 50 or 100 µl, contained 30,000 x g cell-free extract (S30), prepared from the plasmid-free strain *E. coli* CSH 73 (final protein concentration 5 - 7 mg/ml), plasmid DNA (20 - 240 µg/ml), 40 mM Tris-acetate, (pH 8.2), 55 mM potassium acetate, magnesium acetate (17 mM unless stated), 1.4 mM dithioethreitol, 27 mM ammonium acetate, 0.25 mM each of 20 amino acids, 2.2 mM trisodium phosphoenolpyruvate, 7.5 mM calcium chloride, 100 µg/ml *E. coli* tRNA, 27 µg/ml folinic acid, flavine adenine dinucleotide, triphosphopyridine nucleotide, pyridoxine-HCl, 11 µg/ml p-aminobenzoic acid. Spermidine hydrochloride (0.8 mM) was added where indicated. To synthesize radioactively-labelled proteins tritiated amino acids (Leu, Lys, Phe, Pro, Tyr, 76 - 119 Ci/mmol; Amersham TRK 550) were added to a concentration of 150 µCi/ml. In these incubations unlabelled amino acids were added to 100 µM instead of 250 µM.

CHINESE HAMSTER OVARY CELL ASSAY

Details of the preparation of the Chinese hamster ovary (CHO) cell line CHO-K1 for studies of morphological changes have been described (Guerrant and colleagues, 1974)

ANTISERA

Antiserum against purified cholera toxin (anticholeragen) was provided by Dr. Carl E. Miller (National Institute of Health, Bethesda, Md., U.S.A.). Heterologous antitoxin was prepared in rabbits against semipurified toxin from enterotoxigenic E. coli strain P263 (Dorner, Jaksche and Stöckl, 1975).

AFFINITY CHROMATOGRAPHY

Semipurified cyclic AMP binding protein from bovine muscle was obtained from Boehringer Mannheim and further purified as described by Gilman (1970). The major peak of kinase and binding activity (peak II of Gilman) was subjected to gel filtration on Sephadex G-200 and coupled to the N-hydroxysuccinimide ester of succinylated amino alkyl agarose (Cuatrecasas and Parikh, 1972). 50 µl aliquots of the reaction mixture were diluted to 1 ml with 50 mM sodium acetate/acetic acid, pH 4.0 and applied to a 0.4 x 2 cm column containing the adsorbent. The column was washed with the sodium acetate buffer. 3 ml fractions were collected and immediately neutralized. The first three fractions which contain all the proteinaceous materials, were pooled and concentrated to the initial volume by ultrafiltration in a minicon B15 macrosolute concentrator (Amicon Corp., Lexington, Mass., U.S.A.).

ADENYLATE CYCLASE ASSAY

Adenylate cyclase activity was measured by a pigeon erythrocyte assay developed from Gill and King (1975). Adenylate cyclase activity was then assayed using a modification of the radioisotope dilution test described by Gilman (1970).

PROTEIN A - ANTIBODY ADSORBENT

The preparation of the bacterial adsorbent has been described by Kessler (1975).

ISOLATION OF IN VITRO TRITIATED ENTEROTOXIN

100 µl of monospecific anticholeragen were added to 500 µl of cell-free sample in 12 x 75 mm polystyrene test tubes; after 30 min 2000 µl (v/v) of a suspension of the bacterial adsorbent were added. After a further 30 min the reaction mixture was carefully layered on a 1 ml 1M sucrose solution (PBS, 1 % Triton X-100, 5 mM EDTA) in a test tube and centrifuged (2000 x g, 15 min). The top phase was removed and after a final wash the supernatant was drawn off and replaced with 200 µl of 10 % glycerol, 0.01 % bromophenol blue, 5 % 2-mercapto ethanol, 3 % SDS in 6.25 mM Tris-HCl, pH 8.0. Resuspension was performed with a siliconized Pasteur pipette or on a vortex mixer. Complete elution followed incubation in a boiling water bath for 3 min and the eluate was carefully collected after centrifugation. Aliquots of the eluate were either loaded directly onto a polyacrylamide gel or following removal of the bacterial cells by filtration.

POLYACRYLAMIDE GEL ELECTROPHORESIS IN SODIUM DODECYL SULFATE

Polyacrylamide gel electrophoresis in 0.1 % sodium dodecyl sulfate was performed at pH 7.2 in 7.5 % acrylamide (Weber and Osborn 1969). For fluorography, gels were equilibrated with dimethylsulphoxide, impregnated with PPO by immersion in 4 vol. 20 % (w/w) PPO in dimethylsulphoxide, soaked in water, dried and exposed to Kodak RP Royal X-O mat film (RP/R) at -70°C. The distribution of radioactivity within the gel was confirmed by scintillation counting of dissolved gel slices.

RESULTS

The amount of in vitro synthesized heat labile enterotoxin is quantified by the CHO cell assay, which measures the morphological change in the cells associated with increased intracellular concentrations of cAMP. The gradation of the morphological response of CHO cells to increasing dosage of highly purified enterotoxin is shown in Fig. 1. The amount of heat labile enterotoxin synthesized in the cell-free system was proportional to the concentration of P307 plasmid DNA (Fig. 2).

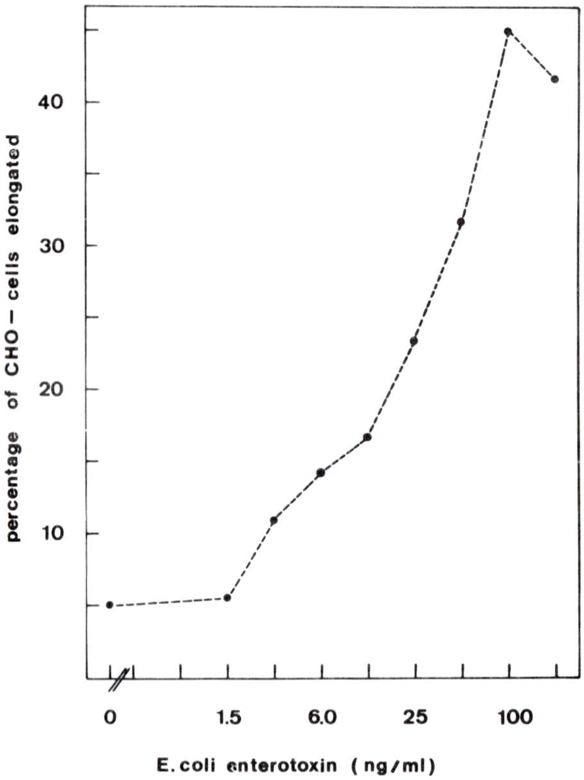

Fig. 1. Effect of purified Escherichia coli P263 toxin on morphology of Chinese hamster (CHO) cells.

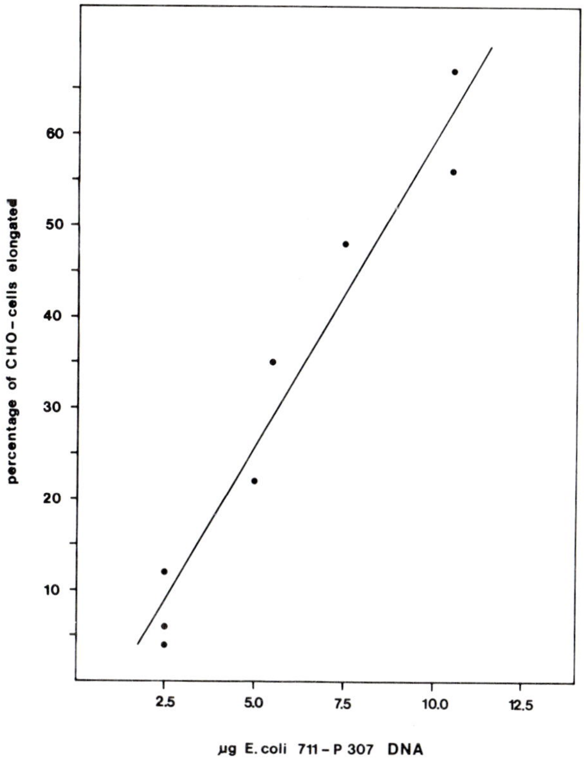

Fig. 2. Amount of heat labile enterotoxin synthesized in the cell-free system as a function of the concentration of P307 plasmid DNA.

No activity was observed when plasmid DNA was omitted or when DNA of the plasmid NR1 was introduced as template. Cyclic AMP controls a number of functions in E. coli (Pastan and Perlman, 1970) and its role in regulating the synthesis of the inducible enzymes involved in sugar utilization has been well documented for both *in vivo* and *in vitro* systems. Reports that cAMP also regulates the levels of plasmid-determined antibiotic inactivating enzymes, chloramphenicol-acetyltransferase (Harwood and Smith, 1971) and kanamycin-phosphotransferase (Tsukada and colleagues, 1972) prompted us to examine its effect on the synthesis of enterotoxin.

As the CHO cell assay measures the response to cAMP resulting from addition of enterotoxin, endogenous cAMP was removed from cell-free samples by affinity chromatography.

Synthesis of enterotoxin was observed in the absence of cAMP (when background activity was eliminated) and was stimulated up to 10-fold in its presence. The dependence of enterotoxin synthesis on the concentration of cAMP (Fig. 3) showed a saturation plateau above 0.5 mM, so in all subsequent cell-free incubations cAMP was added to a final concentration of 1 mM.

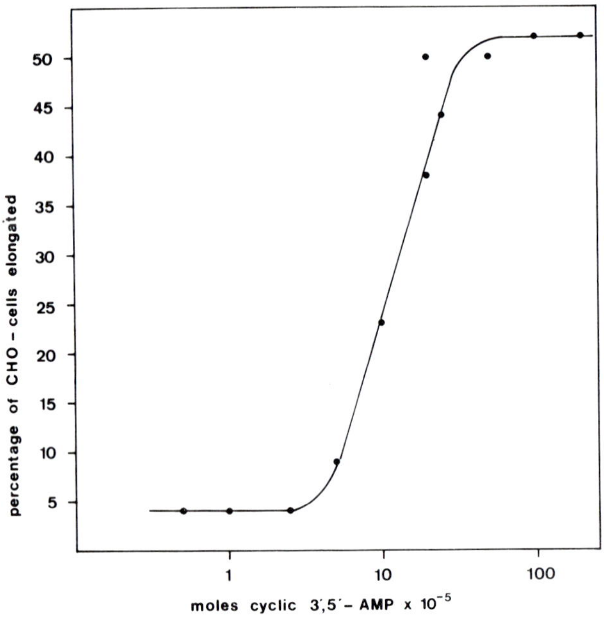

Fig. 3. Enterotoxigenic activity of the in vitro synthesized material as a function of cyclic AMP concentration.

Investigations by other workers (Cohen, 1971; Nathans and Lipmann, 1961;) have demonstrated that polyamines, such as spermidine, lower the concentration of Mg^{2+} required for optimal protein synthesis in both eucaryotic and procaryotic systems. In addition, polyamines have been reported to stimulate DNA-directed cell-free protein synthesis (Abraham, 1968; Nuss and Herbst, 1975). We observed that the addition of spermidine (Table 1) lowered the Mg^{2+} concentration required for optimal enterotoxin synthesis from 17 mM to 4 mM and gave a 1.5-fold stimulation of the amount of enterotoxin produced. At 4 mM Mg^{2+}, in the absence of spermidine, there was no enterotoxin synthesis. As with LT enterotoxin released into culture supernatant, the activity of the cell-free preparation was abolished by heating to 65°C for 30 minutes and neutralized by antisera prepared against both partially purified E. coli enterotoxin (from porcine enteropathogen P263) and purified Vibria cholera enterotoxin.

Table 1. INFLUENCE OF SPERMIDINE ON ENTEROTOXIN SYNTHESES

plasmid DNA ug/ml	spermidine* mM	Mg^{++} mM	CHO assay %
0	0.8	17	5
220	-	17	32
0	-	4	5
220	0.8	4	46

* 0.8 mM spermidine hydrochloride was observed, in preliminary experiments, to give optimal stimulation.

In view of the established immunological relationship between the LT enterotoxin of E. coli and V. cholera, we applied the technique of specific immune precipitation to purify synthesized toxin from the cell-free system. The toxin, labelled with tritiated amino acids, was complexed with anticholeragen and absorbed to the Cowan I strain of Staphylococcus aureus. With a combination of sodium dodecyl sulphate (SDS) and high temperature almost all of the enterotoxin was eluted from the inert adsorbent and run on polyacrylamide gels containing 0.1 % SDS. After electrophoresis, gels were sliced, extracted and assayed for ability to activate adenylate cyclase (Fig. 4). Two active peaks were observed, one at about molecular weight 26,000 and frequently but not always, another at about 23,000. Separation of immunoprecipitated proteins by SDS-acrylamide gel electrophoresis and examination by fluorography revealed three prominent polypeptide bands, two corresponding to the peak which activated adenylate cyclase and a third indicating a protein of molecular weight 11,500 (Fig. 5). This was confirmed in separate experiments where the distribution of radioactivity within the gel was calculated by scintillation counts of dissolved gel slices (Fig. 6). The number of counts associated with the 11,500 molecular weight species was observed to be 1.5 - 1.7 times greater than that corresponding to the active peaks (23,000 - 26,000).

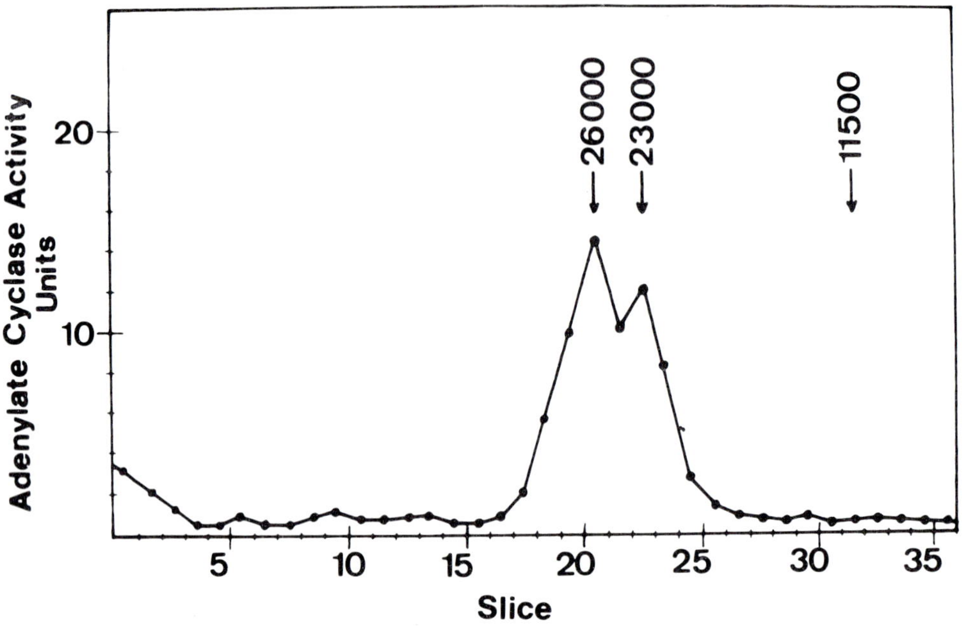

Fig. 4. Adenylate cyclase activity of in vitro synthesized proteins, extracted following electrophoresis in polyacrylamide gels

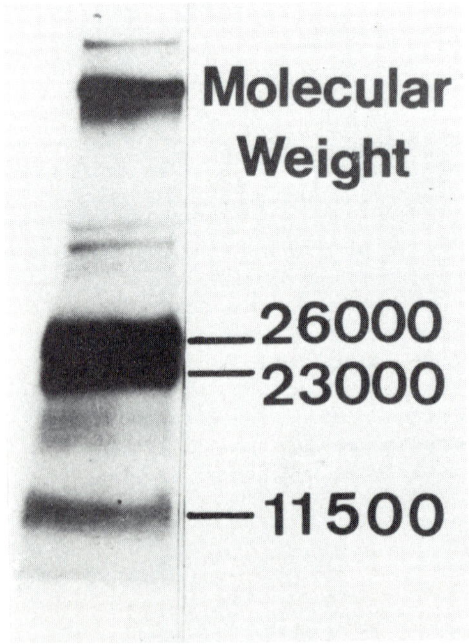

Fig. 5.

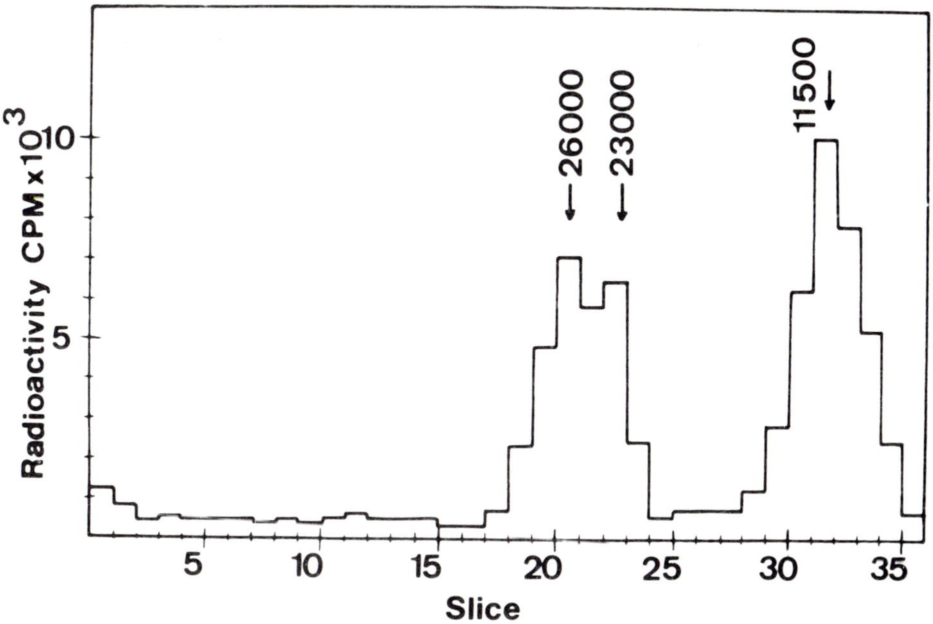

Fig. 5. and 6. Analysis of SDS-polyacrylamide gels containing ^{3}H-labelled immunoprecipitate. Samples were reduced and electrophoresed in 9 mm slots in slab gels containing 7.5 % acrylamide and 0.1 % SDS. The distribution of radioactivity was ascertained by fluorography (Fig. 5) and scintillation counts on dissolved gel slices (Fig. 6).

DISCUSSION

Molecular weight estimations for purified E. coli enterotoxin range from 20,000 (for LT released from the periplasmic space by polymysin B treatment) to 200,000 (for LT from culture supernatants) (Dorner, Jaksche, Stöckl, 1976; Evans and Gorbach, 1974; Finkelstein and colleagues, 1976). The isoelectric point has been quoted variously as being between 4.5 and 7 (Söderlind, Möllby and Wadström, 1974) and it is still unclear whether its structure comprises a single polypeptide chain or a number of subunits (Schenkein and co-workers, 1976). In addition, confusion arises from the lack of immunological identity observed between toxins from different serotypes and host specificity and more remarkably, between toxins produced by the same strain grown in different culture media.

Although some of the differences between the various enterotoxin preparations may be attributed, in part, to differences in strains and/or methodology, a complete explanation of the differences between E. coli enterotoxin is likely to include a fundamental difference in their mechanism of release. Evidence (Rappaport 1977) supports the view that enterotoxin is not an extracellular product of E. coli, at least under normal growth conditions. Rather, the majority of molecules appear in the growth medium only after the bacterial population begins to decline, and they seem to be released in association with surface components of the cell. As there is only scarce information available on the structure of E. coli enterotoxin synthesized in the periplastic space and its proposed structural changes during its release into the supernatant, it would seem profitable to study these processes in vitro.

When P307 plasmid DNA was added to the cell-free system a substance with CHO cell morphology changing activity was synthesized. That this substance was E. coli heat labile enterotoxin was confirmed by the following observations:

1. The amount of substance produced was dependent on the concentration of P307 plasmid DNA in the system and increased linearly in the range of 20 - 240 µg DNA per ml of incubation mixture. No activity was detected with NR1 plasmid as template or when DNA was omitted.
2. Antisera prepared against both semipurified E. coli enterotoxin (from the culture supernatant of a different strain) and cholera toxin abolished the activity synthesized in the cell-free system.
3. Activity of the cell-free synthesized material, was not expressed in mixtures heated for 30 min at 65°C. This behaviour is typical of the heat labile E. coli enterotoxin.

The in vitro synthesis of the enterotoxin, which has no catabolic function, was strongly stimulated by cyclic AMP, the internal messenger substance of catabolite repression. This phenomenon agrees with the reduction in enterotoxin yield observed in toxigenic cultures when glucose, the inducer of catabolite repression, is present in the growth medium. Also of interest is the stimulatory effect of spermidine on in vitro synthesis of enterotoxin. This polyamine, present in all living cells, is known to spare the magnesium concentration required for optimal protein synthesis. In the presence of spermidine, enterotoxin synthesis occurs at a magnesium concentration which is similar to that prevailing in whole cells.

Techniques using antibodies for the specific isolation of radiolabelled antigens have been widely used but difficulties are presented by the high background of non-specifically precipitated material, the difficulty of determining equivalent points and proteolytic degradation occurring during processing. The protein A-antibody technique used here provides a partial solution as it exploits the high adsorption capacity of IgG by protein A molecules on the surface of certain staphylococcal strains, and also the sedimentation properties of these bacteria. Analyses of the immunoprecipitated gene products by SDS-polyacrylamide electrophoresis revealed three prominent bands, two of molecular weight 23,000 - 26,000 (A) having adenylate cyclase stimulating activity and a third, molecular weight 11,500 (B), migrating at an identical rate to cholera B. As the band of molecular weight 23,000 was observed with varying prominence, but always with adenylate cyclase stimulating activity, we suggest that this is either a breakdown product of the 26,000 species or that a precursor product relationship exists between the two. We are at present investigating these possibilities in addition to studying the ratio in which active protein and that of the other polypeptide, which may have a binding function similar to the B subunit of cholera toxin, are synthesized. The data presented on ^{3}H incorporation (Fig. 6) suggest a possible enterotoxin structure of one active subunit (A; molecular weight 11,500) but this ratio may not be constant in our cell-free system and may even be a reflection of the specificity of the immunoprecipitation procedure. The data do, however, indicate that the LT toxins of E. coli and V. cholera, possessing related biological and immunological properties, may also have a similar structure.

REFERENCES

Abraham, K.A. (1968) Eur. J. Biochem. 5, 143-146.

Clewell, D.B. and Helinski, D.R. (1969) Proc. Natl. Acad. Sci. USA 62, 1159-1166.

Cohen, S.S. (1971) in Introduction to the Polyamines, ed. S.S. Cohen (Prentice Hall, Englewood Cliffs, New Jersey) p. 137.

Cuatrecasas, P. and Parikh I. (1972) Biochemistry 11, 2291-2299.

Dorner, F., Jaksche, H. and Stöckl, W. (1976) J. Infect. Dis. 133, 142-156.

Evans, D.J., Evans, D.G. and Gorbach, S.L. (1974) Infect. Immun. 10, 1010-1017.

Falkow, S. (1975) Infectious multiple drug resistance Pion Ltd., London.

Finkelstein, R.A., LaRue, M.K., Johnston, D.W., Vasil, M.L. Cho, G.J. and Jones, J.R. (1976) J. Infect. Dis. 133, 120-137.

Gill, D.M. and King, C.A. (1975) J. Biol. Chem. 250, 6424-6432.

Gilman, A.G. (1970) Proc. Natl. Acad. Sci. USA 67, 305-312.

Greene, P.M., Betlack, M.C., Goodman, H.M. and Boyer, H.W. (1974) in Methods in Molecular Biology, DNA replication and biosynthesis, ed. Wickner, R.B. (Marcel-Dekker Inc. New York) 302-322.

Grindley, J.N., Blumberg, R. and Nakada, D. (1976) J. Bact. 130, 852-859.

Guerrant, R.L., Brunton, L.L., Schnaitman, T.C., Rebhun, L.I. and Gilman, A.G. (1974) Infect. Immun. 10, 320-327.

Harwood, J. and Smith, D.H. (1971) Biochem. Biophys. Res. Comm. 42, 57-61.

Kessler, S.W. (1975) J. Immun. 115, 1617-1624.

Konings, R.N.H., Andreoli, P.M., Veltkamp, E. and Nikamp, H.J.H. (1976) J. Bact. 126, 861-868.

Nathans, D. and Lipmann, F. (1961) Proc. Natl. Acad. Sci. USA 47, 497-504.

Nuss, D.L. and Herbst, E.J. (1975) Arch. Biochem. Biophys. 169, 513-521.

Pastan, I. and Perlman, R. (1970) Science 169, 339-344.

Rappaport, R.S. (1977) in Proc. XIII Joint Conf. on Cholera USA - Japan Coop. Med. Sci. Program, 443-474.

Schenkein, I., Green, R.F., Santos, D.S. and Maas, W.K. (1976) Infect. Immun. 13, 1710-1720.

Sidikaro, J. and Nomura, M. (1975) J. Biol. Chem. 250, 1123-1131.

Smith, N.W. and Sack, R.B. (1973) J. Infect. Dis. 127, 164-170.

Söderlind, O., Möllby, R. and Wadström, T. (1974) Zentralbl. Bakteriol. 229, 190-204.

Tsukada, I., Yagisawa, M., Umezawa, M., Hori, M. and Umezawa, H. (1972) J. Antibiot. 25, 144-146.

Weber, K. and Osborn, M. (1969) J. Biol. Chem. 244, 4406-4412.

Zubay, G., Chambers, D.A. and Cheong, L.C. (1970) The Lactase Operon, Cold Spring Harbor Laboratory, 375 ff.

PATHOGENESIS OF *VIBRIO PARAHAEMOLYTICUS*

T. Takeda, T. Honda, Y. Takeda and T. Miwatani

Department of Bacteriology and Serology, Research Institute for Microbial Diseases, Osaka University, Yamada-Kami, Suita, Osaka 565, Japan

ABSTRACT

Vibrio parahaemolyticus, a causative bacterium of food poisoning or acute gastroenteritis, is divided into two groups based on hemolytic activity on a special blood agar. The hemolytic strains are called Kanagawa-phenomenon positive and they are closely associated with human disease. A thermostable direct hemolysin is responsible for the Kanagawa-phenomenon. Highly purified thermostable direct hemolysin shows hemolytic activity, cytotoxic activity in various cultured cells and lethal toxicity in mice and rats. Death is due to cardiotoxicity of the hemolysin. The roles of cytotoxicity and cardiotoxicity of the hemolysin in the clinical manifestations of V. parahaemolyticus infection are discussed.

KEY WORDS

Vibrio parahaemolyticus, pathogenesis, thermostable direct hemolysin, Kanagawa-phenomenon, cytotoxicity, lethal toxicity, cardiotoxicity.

Vibrio parahaemolyticus was isolated by Fujino and his coworkers (1953) from a victim of food poisoning in 1950. In Japan, V. parahaemolyticus is the organism most frequently isolated from cases of food poisoning or acute gastroenteritis (Table 1). Several outbreaks of food poisoning associated with V. parahaemolyticus have also been reported from United States of America (Miwatani and Takeda, 1976).

The main symptoms of V. parahaemolyticus infection are diarrhea and abdominal pain. Diarrhea is usually watery but sometimes bloody discharges are observed.

In this paper, we discuss the pathogenesis of V. parahaemolyticus infection, and especially the possible role(s) of the thermostable direct hemolysin in the clinical manifestations of the disease.

Kanagawa-phenomenon

In epidemiological studies on V. parahaemolyticus, Kato and his coworkers (1965) at the Kanagawa Prefectural Public Health Laboratory discovered that strains from the feces of patients caused hemolysis on a special blood-agar, whereas strains isolated from vehicles of food poisoning were not hemolytic. Sakazaki and his coworkers (1968) confirmed this by examining 3,370 cultures from various sources (Table 2). The special blood-agar medium for measuring the hemolytic

TABLE 1. Bacterial food poisoning in Japan.

Causative bacteria	Number of outbreaks					
	1973	1974	1975	1976	1977	1978
Total bacterial food poisoning	670	654	1059	524	857	818
Vibrio parahaemolyticus	356	368	667	195	461	382
Staphylococcus aureus	212	184	275	207	226	277
Salmonella	62	66	73	81	114	110
pathogenic *Escherichia coli*	20	16	22	26	23	23
Botulinus	3	1	1	2	5	4
others	17	9	21	13	28	22

TABLE 2. Hemolytic activity of 3,370 cultures of *V. parahaemolyticus* on Wagatsuma's medium.

Source	Hemolytic activity		Total
	+	-	
Human patients	2,655 (96.5%)	75 (3.5%)	2720
Sea fish and sea water	7 (1.0%)	643 (99.0%)	650

character of *V. parahaemolyticus* was developed by Wagatsuma (1968), and the hemolysis produced by *V. parahaemolyticus* on Wagatsuma's medium has been called the Kanagawa-phenomenon.

Purification of thermostable direct hemolysin

Among several hemolysins produced by *V. parahaemolyticus*, a thermostable direct hemolysin was found to be responsible for the Kanagawa-phenomenon. This hemolysin was isolated and purified by several workers (Nikkawa and others, 1972; Sakurai, Matsuzaki and Miwatani, 1973; Miwatani and others, 1974; Zen-Yoji and others, 1976; Honda and others, 1976c). Table 3 summarizes typical purification data from our laboratory. From 42 liters of culture supernatant of a Kanagawa-phenomenon positive strain, *V. parahaemolyticus* WP-1, about 43 mg of the purified hemolysin were obtained with a yield of about 30%.

TABLE 3. Purification of thermostable direct hemolysin from *V. parahaemolyticus*.

Fraction	Total volume (ml)	Total protein (mg)	Total activity (HU)	Specific activity	Relative activity	Yield of HU (%)
Culture supernatant	42000	22500	23400	1.04	(1.0)	100
Alumina C_γ treatment	63	724	19900	27.49	26.43	85.0
DEAE-cellulose column	745	150	9780	65.20	62.69	41.8
Hydroxylapatite column	151	58	8530	147.07	141.41	36.5
Sephadex G-200 column	2.4	43.5	7165	164.71	158.38	30.6

Physico-chemical properties of the thermostable direct hemolysin

The purified thermostable direct hemolysin gave one band on SDS-polyacrylamide gel disc electrophoresis and a single symmetric peak in analytical ultracentrifugation. The hemolysin was a pure protein free from lipids and carbohydrates. The isoelectric point was found to be about 4.2. The amino acid composition was also determined (Zen-Yoji and others, 1976; Honda and others, 1976c). Partial sequence of the N-terminal area of the hemolysin has been reported by Zen-Yoji and his coworkers (1976).

The molecular weight of the purified hemolysin determined by gel filtration was about 42,000 (Zen-Yoji and others, 1976; Honda and others, 1976c). We further examined the molecular structure of this direct hemolysin by Triton X-100- and SDS-polyacrylamide gel disc electrophoresis. Although SDS-polyacrylamide gel disc electrophoresis showed that the molecular weight of the hemolysin was 21,000, Triton X-100-polyacrylamide gel disc electrophoresis yielded a value of 42,000. Moreover, when cross-linked with glutaraldehyde, it gave several bands of 21,000, 41,000, 63,000, 87,000, 108,000 and 130,000 on SDS-polyacrylamide gel disc electrophoresis (Takeda, Taga and Miwatani, 1978). Thus, it is concluded that the thermostable direct hemolysin is composed of two subunit molecules of approximately 21,000 daltons.

Biological activities of the thermostable direct hemolysin

The hemolytic activity of the thermostable direct hemolysin on different kinds of erythrocytes varied significantly. Zen-Yoji and his coworkers (1971) found that it showed high hemolytic activity with erythrocytes from rat, dog, mouse, monkey, man, rabbit and guinae pig, but no activity with horse erythrocytes. The activity was not enhanced by adding lecithin and was distinguishable from the activity of indirect hemolysins, such as phospholipases.

The thermostable direct hemolysin is cytotoxic for various cultured cells, such as HeLa cell (Sakazaki and others, 1974), L cells (Sakazaki and others, 1974), FL cells (Sakurai and others, 1975), neuroblastoma cells, primary cultures of foetal mouse heart cells and CCL 6 cells derived from human intestine. Figure 1 shows the cytotoxic effect of the hemolysin on human intestinal cells CCL 6. It was shown that 10 μg/ml of the hemolysin killed almost all cells as determined by uptake of trypan blue.

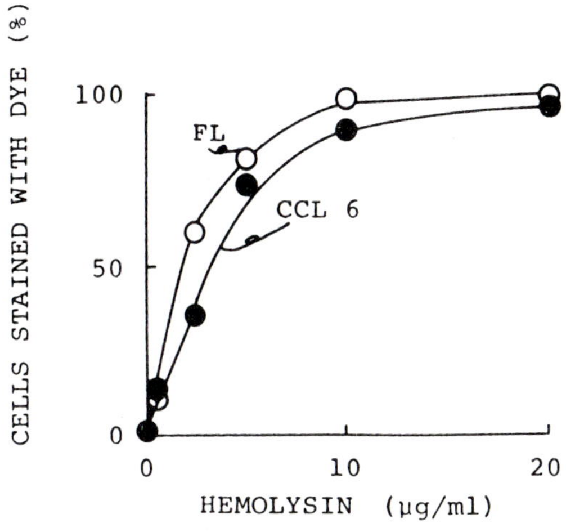

Fig. 1. Lethal effect of the purified thermostable direct hemolysin on human intestinal cells (CCL 6) and FL cells. 6.6×10^5 cells were treated with various amounts of the hemolysin indicated in 1 ml of Eagle MEM medium for 60 min and then cells were stained with trypan blue.

Lethal activity of the purified thermostable direct hemolysin in small experimental animals, such as mice and rats was reported by Honda and his coworkers (1976c). Intravenous administration of 5 μg of the purified hemolysin in 6-week-old mice killed all animals within 1 minute. Even 1 μg of the hemolysin killed the animals within 20 minutes. Intravenous injection of 10 μg of the purified hemolysin in 12- to 15-week-old rats killed them after about 2 minutes.

Since rapid death of mice and rats injected with small doses of the hemolysin suggests that the hemolysin affects some vital organs of the animals, it is assumed that possible target organs of the hemolysin might be either the central nervous system or the heart. Thus an attempt was made to record both electroencephalograms and electrocardiograms of rats injected with the purified hemolysin. The results showed that after intravenous injection of the hemolysin the electroencephalogram remained normal for quite a long time after the heart of the animals had stopped beating (Honda and others, 1976a). The hemolysin was also found to be toxic to cultured mouse heart cells (Honda and others, 1976a; Goshima and others, 1977). When the purified hemolysin was added to the medium, the beating of the cultured heart cells stopped abruptly. Spontaneous beating of isolated adult rat atrial preparations also stopped on addition of the hemolysin (Goshima and others, 1977; Seyama and others, 1977). Thus, it is concluded that the thermostable direct hemolysin had cardiotoxicity, and rapid death of the animals injected with the hemolysin is due to the cardiotoxic activity of the hemolysin.

Role of the thermostable direct hemolysin in V. parahaemolyticus infection

Zen-Yoji and his coworkers (1974) injected the purified hemolysin into ligated rabbit ileal loops and found that injection of 500 μg of the hemolysin caused turbid, bloody fluid accumulation in the loops. Histopathological examination showed significant erosive lesions and desquamation of necrotic mucosa accompanied by marked neutrophil-infiltration into the intestinal wall.

Obara and his coworkers (1974) studied the histopathological changes in the small intestine of suckling mice after oral administration of hemolysin. After administration of 50 μg of the purified hemolysin into the stomach of 5 to 6 day old suckling mice, almost all the animals developed diarrhea and soon died. With doses of 12.5 and 2.0 μg, only some animals died while others developed diarrhea

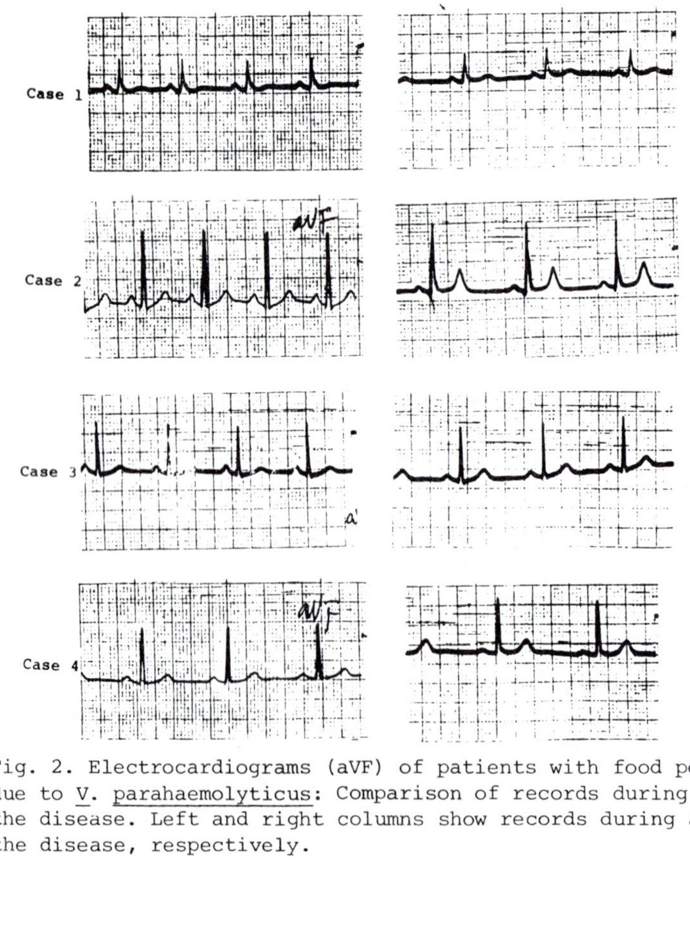

Fig. 2. Electrocardiograms (aVF) of patients with food poisoning due to V. parahaemolyticus: Comparison of records during and after the disease. Left and right columns show records during and after the disease, respectively.

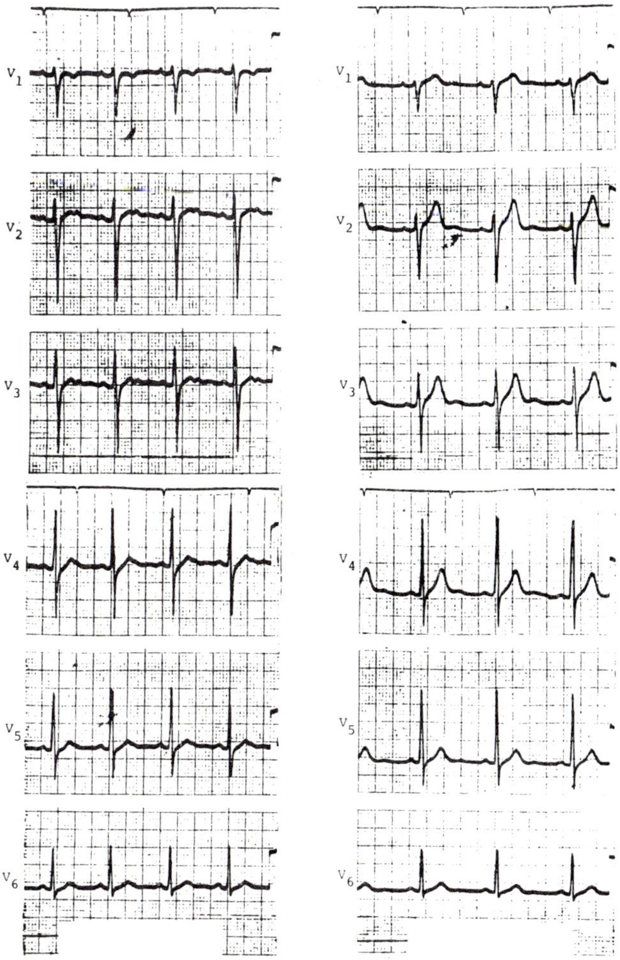

Fig. 3. Electrocardiograms (chest leads) of a patient suffering from severe diarrhea due to V. parahaemolyticus infection. Anti-hemolysin titer was very high after the disease. Left and right columns show records during and after the disease, respectively.

temporarily and then recovered. With a relatively small dose of the hemolysin the lamina propria was edematous. In ultrathin sections, intercellular junctions at interdigitations were observed to have become very loose, and the spaces between cells were greatly enlarged, suggesting fluid accumulation. From these results, they concluded that the hemolysin is an important agent in causing gastroenteritis.

As described in the preceding section, the thermostable direct hemolysin showed cytotoxicity. Thus, it is probable that the hemolysin damages the intestinal cells resulting in diarrhea.

We have reported the isolation and purification of a toxic factor from the culture filtrates of V. parahaemolyticus, which causes morphological changes in Chinese hamster ovary cells (Honda and others, 1976b). However, further study is necessary to determine whether this factor is an enterotoxin and whether it plays an important role in causing diarrhea in V. parahaemolyticus infection.

Figure 2 shows electrocardiograms of four patients with V. parahaemolyticus food poisoning (Honda and others, 1976d). The P waves were wider and higher and the T waves lower during the disease as compared to convalescense. Typical changes in electrocardiograms of the chest leads of one of these patients are shown in Fig. 3. Changes in T waves are very clear. During the disease, the T waves not only became lower but also became biphasic in V_2 and V_3 leads.

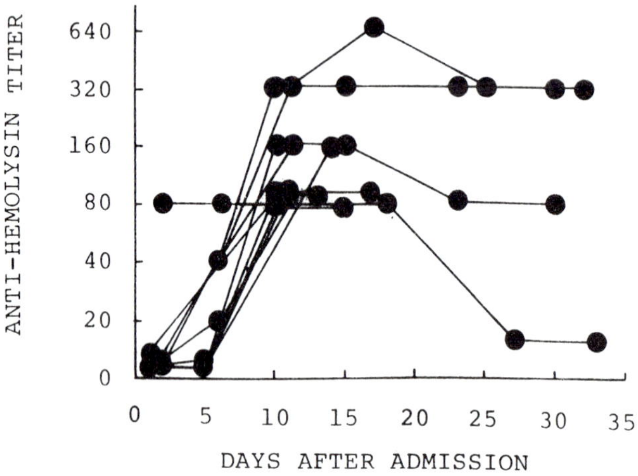

Fig. 4. Change of anti-hemolysin titers in the serum during food poisoning due to V. parahaemolyticus. Eleven typical cases which showed increase of anti-hemolysin titer are shown. A total of 33 cases were examined and 16 cases showed no increase of anti-hemolysin titer.

Anti-hemolysin titers in sera of patitents with V. parahaemolyticus infection were determined (Miwatani and others, 1976), and the data are shown in Fig. 4. In about 33% of the patients studied we observed an increase of anti-hemolysin titers during the course of disease. The increase in titer began about 5 days after admission and reached a maximal value after 10 to 15 days. These data suggest that the thermostable direct hemolysin produced by V. parahaemolyticus is absorbed during disease and could therefore affect the heart, and cause electrocariographic changes.

ACKNOWLEDGEMENT

We thank to Dr. J. P. Craig for his help in preparing this manuscript.

REFERENCES

Fujino, T., Y. Okuno, D. Nakada, A. Aoyama, K. Fukai, T. Mukai, and T. Ueho (1953). On the bacteriological examination of shirasu food poisoning. Med. J. Osaka Univ., 4, 299-304.

Goshima, K., T. Honda, M. Hirata, K. Kikuchi, Y. Takeda, and T. Miwatani (1977). Stopping of the spontaneous beating of mouse and rat myocardial cells in vitro by a toxin from Vibrio parahaemolyticus. J. Molecul. Cellul. Cardiol., 9, 191-213.

Honda, T., K. Goshima, Y. Takeda, Y. Sugino, and T. Miwatani (1976a). Demonstration of the cardiotoxicity of the thermostable direct hemolysin (lethal toxin) produced by Vibrio parahaemolyticus. Infect. Immun., 13, 163-171.

Honda, T., M. Shimizu, Y. Takeda, and T. Miwatani (1976b). Isolation of a factor causing morphological changes of Chinese hamster ovary cells from the culture filtrate of Vibrio parahaemolyticus. Infect. Immun., 14, 1028-1033.

Honda, T., S. Taga, T. Takeda, M. A. Hashibuan, Y. Takeda, and T. Miwatani (1976c). Identification of lethal toxin with the thermostable direct hemolysin produced by Vibrio parahaemolyticus, and some physicochemical properties of the purified toxin. Infect. Immun., 13, 133-139.

Honda, T., Y. Takeda, T. Miwatani, K. Kato, and Y. Nimura (1976d). Clinical features of patients suffering from food poisoning due to Vibrio parahaemolyticus -- especially on changes in electrocardiograms (in Japanese with English summary). J. Japan. Assoc. Infect. Dis., 50, 216-223.

Kato, T., Y. Obara, H. Ichinoe, K. Nagashima, S. Akiyama, K. Takizawa, A. Matsushima, S. Yamai, and Y. Miyamoto (1965). Grouping of Vibrio parahaemolyticus (biotype 1) by hemolytic reaction (in Japanese). Shokuhin Eisei Kenkyu, 15(8), 83-86.

Miwatani, T., J. Sakurai, Y. Takeda, and S. Shinoda (1974). Studies on direct hemolysins of Vibrio parahaemolyticus. p. 245-251. In T. Fujino, G. Sakaguchi, R. Sakazaki and Y. Takeda (eds.). International Symposium on Vibrio parahaemolyticus. Saikon Publishing Co., Tokyo.

Miwatani, T., and Y. Takeda (1976). Vibrio parahaemolyticus -- A causative bacterium of food poisoning. Saikon Publishing Co., Tokyo.

Miwatani, T., J. Sakurai, Y. Takeda, S. Sugiyama, and T. Adachi (1976). Antibody titers against the thermostable direct hemolysin in sera of patients suffering from gastroenteritis due to Vibrio parahaemolyticus (in Japanese with English summary). J. Japan. Assoc. Infect. Dis., 50, 46-51.

Nikkawa, T., Y. Obara, S. Yamai, and Y. Miyamoto (1972). Purification of a hemolysin from Vibrio parahaemolyticus. Jap. J. Med. Sci. Biol., 25, 197-200.

Obara, Y., S. Yamai, T. Nikkawa, Y. Miyamoto, M. Ohashi, and T. Shimada (1974). Histopathological changes in the small intestine of suckling mice challenged orally with purified hemolysin from Vibrio parahaemolyticus. p. 253-257. In T. Fujino, G. Sakaguchi, R. Sakazaki and Y. Takeda (eds.). International Symposium on Vibrio parahaemolyticus. Saikon Publishing Co., Tokyo.

Sakazaki, R., K. Tamura, T. Kato, Y. Obara, S. Yamai, and K. Hobo (1968). Studies on the enteropathogenic, facultatively halophilic bacteria, Vibrio parahaemolyticus. III. Enteropathogenicity. Jap. J. Med. Sci. Biol., 21, 325-331.

Sakazaki, R., K. Tamura, A. Nakamura, T. Kurata, A. Ghoda, and Y. Kazuno (1974). Enteropathogenic activity of Vibrio parahaemolyticus. p. 231-235. In T. Fujino, G. Sakaguchi, R. Sakazaki and Y. Takeda (eds.). International Symposium on Vibrio parahaemolyticus. Saikon Publishing Co., Tokyo.

Sakurai, J., A. Matsuzaki, and T. Miwatani (1973). Purification and characterization of thermostable direct hemolysin of Vibrio parahaemolyticus. Infect. Immun., 8, 775-780.

Sakurai, J., T. Honda, Y. Jinguji, M. Arita, and T. Miwatani (1975). Cytotoxic effect of the thermostable direct hemolysin produced by Vibrio parahaemolyticus on FL cells. Infect. Immun., 13, 876-883.

Seyama, J., H. Irisawa, T. Honda, Y. Takeda, and T. Miwatani (1977). Effect of hemolysin produced by Vibrio parahaemolyticus on membrane conduction and mechanical tension of rabbit myocardium. Jap. J. Physiol., 27, 43-56.

Takeda, Y., S. Taga, and T. Miwatani (1978). Evidence that thermostable direct hemolysin of Vibrio parahaemolyticus is composed of two subunits. FEMS Microbiol. Lett., 4, 271-274.

Wagatsuma, S. (1968). On a medium for hemolytic reaction (in Japanese). Media Circle, 13, 159-162.

Zen-Yoji, H., H. Hitokoto, S. Morozumi, and R. A. LeClair (1971). Purification and characterization of a hemolysin produced by Vibrio parahaemolyticus. J. Infect. Dis., 123, 665-667.

Zen-Yoji, H., Y. Kudoh, H. Igarashi, K. Ohta, and K. Fukai (1974). Purification and identification of enteropathogenic toxins "a" and "a'" produced by Vibrio parahaemolyticus and their biological and pathological activities. p. 237-243. In T. Fujino, G. Sakaguchi, R. Sakazaki and Y. Takeda (eds.). International Symposium on Vibrio parahaemolyticus. Saikon Publishing Co., Tokyo.

Zen-Yoji, H., Y. Kudoh, H. Igarashi, K. Ohta, K. Fukai, and T. Hoshino (1976). Further studies on characterization and biological activities of an enteropathogenic toxin of Vibrio parahaemolyticus. p. 479-498. In A. Ohsaka, K. Hayashi and Y. Sawai (eds.). Animal, Plant and Microbial Toxins. Vol. 1., Plenumn, New York.

PURIFICATION OF *AEROMONAS HYDROPHILA* ENTEROTOXIN AND ITS MODE OF ACTION IN EXPERIMENTAL MODEL

R. S. Dubey, S. C. Sanyal and O. P. Malhotra

Enteric Infection Unit, Departments of Microbiology and Chemistry, Banaras Hindu University, Varanasi 221005, India

ABSTRACT

The present study was undertaken (a) to purify the enterotoxin and skin permeability factor of *Aeromonas hydrophila* using acetone fractionation, DEAE Sephadex A50 chromatography, ammonium sulphate precipitation and CM cellulose chromatography and (b) to study the mode of action of the enterotoxin in the rabbit ileal loop model. The enterotoxic factor for rabbit gut loop and the skin permeability factor were obtained as two separate protein fractions. Each gave a single band on polyacrylamide gel electrophoresis. An inoculum of 4 μg of the *A. hydrophila* enterotoxin caused fluid accumulation in the range of 1-2 ml in rabbit ileal loops. The skin permeability factor when injected in doses of 1.5 μg elicited a positive blueing response as well as induration in rabbit skin. There was a 3-fold increase in the level of total 3'5' adenosine monophosphate (cyclic AMP) per mg protein in epithelial cells of rabbit ileal loops treated with culture filtrates and crude enterotoxin preparations of *A. hydrophila* for 6-8 h as compared to the level in normal intestinal epithelial cells. By analogy with *Vibrio cholerae* enterotoxin and *Escherichia coli* heat-labile enterotoxin, this is indicative of cyclic AMP mediation in the enterotoxic activity of *A. hydrophila* enterotoxin in rabbit gut loops.

KEYWORDS

Aeromonas hydrophila ; enterotoxin ; skin permeability factor ; purification ; cyclic AMP; mode of action in rabbit ileal loop.

INTRODUCTION

Strains and culture filtrates of *Aeromonas hydrophila* isolated from man, domestic animals and the environment have been shown to cause fluid accumulation in rabbit gut loops (Annapurna and Sanyal, 1975, 1977; Gurwith and co-workers, 1977; Sanyal, Singh and Sen, 1975; Wadström, Ljungh and Wretlind, 1976). The culture filtrates also increase permeability in rabbit skin (Dubey and Sanyal, 1978). Preliminary characterization and *in vivo* neutralization of these two biological properties have also been described (Dubey and Sanyal, 1978, 1979). The latter studies indicated that two factors were involved which were both heat- and acid-labile, non-dialysable antigenic proteins. These factors appear to be similar to the heat-labile enterotoxins of *Vibrio cholerae* and enterotoxigenic *Escherichia coli*. Cholera enterotoxin and *E. coli* heat-labile enterotoxin (LT) have been shown to activate adenylate cyclase, leading to an increased intracellular concentration of cyclic AMP and fluid transport into the intestinal lumen.

The heat-labile enterotoxins of *V. cholerae* and *E. coli* have been purified to homogeneity using conventional biochemical purification techniques (Dorner, 1975; Finkelstein and LoSpalluto, 1969, 1972; Finkelstein and co-workers, 1976; Richardson, Evans and Feeley, 1970) which has enabled understanding of their mechanism of action. It seems evident that purification of *A. hydrophila* enterotoxin is necessary to fully evaluate its role in disease. The present study was, therefore, undertaken with an enterotoxigenic strain of *A. hydrophila* (a) to purify the enterotoxic and skin permeability factors using conventional purification techniques and (b) to study the mode of action of the enterotoxin in the rabbit ileal loop model.

MATERIALS AND METHODS

Organism

The strain of *A. hydrophila* 20571 used in the present study was isolated in our laboratory from an adult suffering from diarrhoea. *V. cholerae* strain 569B was used as a positive control for enterotoxicity tests.

Preparation of Culture Supernate

The strain of *A. hydrophila* was streaked onto 12 Trypticase Soy Agar (BBL) plates and after incubation at $37^{0}C$ for 24 h, cells from surface growth were transferred to each of thirty 500 ml conical flasks containing 100 ml of chemically defined medium of Finkelstein and Lankford (Craig, 1966). The flasks were incubated at $37^{0}C$ for 16-18 h with constant shaking at 120 oscillations per min. Cells were harvested by centrifugation at 22,000 *g* for 30 min at $4^{0}C$. Supernates were pooled together, passed through a Seitz filter and checked for sterility. Sterile culture supernates were concentrated by lyophilization at $-20^{0}C$ to 1/20 of the original volume and dialysed at $4^{0}C$ against phosphate buffered saline (PBS; 0.04 M sodium phosphate buffer in 0.145 M NaCl, pH 7.2).

Acetone Fractionation

This was done at $-15^{0}C$ in an alcohol bath. Three hundred ml of double distilled pre-cooled acetone (BDH) was added dropwise with constant shaking to 150 ml of concentrated dialysate contained in a 1 litre conical flask. The dialysate was saturated to 66.6 % v/v with acetone and the precipitate harvested by centrifugation at 22,000 *g* for 30 min at $4^{0}C$. Traces of acetone were removed from the precipitate under a stream of nitrogen for 2 h. The precipitate was dissolved in 3 ml PBS at $4^{0}C$.

DEAE Sephadex A50 Chromatography

This was performed at $4^{0}C$ using DEAE Sephadex A50 (Pharmacia, capacity 3.5 ± 0.5 m-equiv. g^{-1}, particle size 40-120 μ). A column (1.25 x 26.5 cm) was packed with DEAE Sephadex in 0.02 M sodium phosphate buffer following the method of Andrews (1964). The crude preparation obtained after acetone precipitation was applied to the column and eluted with the same buffer. Fractions of 5 ml were collected. After nearly 60 ml of elution volume when the A_{280} was zero , stepwise elution was done first with 0.02 M sodium phosphate buffer, pH 7.2 containing 0.1 M KCl and fractions for a further 60 ml elution volume collected. A further stepwise elution was performed with 1 M sodium phosphate buffer, pH 7.2. All the fractions were tested for gut loop reactivity and skin permeability factor (PF) activity.

Ammonium Sulphate Precipitation

The fractions showing fluid accumulation in ileal loops and skin PF activity were pooled and saturated to 100 % with recrystallized ammonium sulphate at 4^0C maintaining the pH at 7.2. After continuous stirring for 2 h, the suspension was kept overnight at 4^0C and then centrifuged at 22,000 *g* for 30 min at 4^0C. The precipitate was dissolved in 1 ml of 0.04 M sodium phosphate buffer, pH 7.2, centrifuged at 22,000 *g* for 30 min at 4^0C and the supernate was dialysed against 0.04 M phosphate buffer.

CM Cellulose Chromatography

The dialysate obtained as above was applied onto a carboxymethyl cellulose (Sigma) column (1.25 x 6 cm) equilibrated with 0.02 M sodium phosphate buffer, pH 7.0 at 4^0C and eluted with about 32 ml of the same buffer. Fractions of 4 ml were collected. Stepwise elutions were done with about 24 ml of 0.02 M sodium phosphate buffer, pH 7.2 containing 0.1 M KCl and with 20 ml of the same buffer containing 1 M KCl. Again fractions of 4 ml were collected. After dialysis of the fractions, protein contents were determined and the ileal reactivity and skin PF activity were tested.

Polyacrylamide Gel Electrophoresis

After each stage of purification polyacrylamide gel electrophoresis was done with each toxin sample as described by Davis (1964). Samples of 0.1 ml were mixed with sucrose (BDH) and placed on top of the gels (60 x 6 mm). Electrophoresis was run at constant current of 2 mA per tube for about 4 h at 4^0C until the marker dye (bromophenol blue) had run about 50 mm. Gels were stained with Coomassie brilliant blue and destained for 2-3 days in 10 % acetic acid.

Determination of Protein

Protein contents of the various fractions were determined by calculation from the A_{280} and A_{260} values (Layne, 1957) and by the method of Lowry and co-workers (1951) using bovine serum albumin as the standard protein.

Determination of Enterotoxic and Skin PF Activities

Enterotoxic activity of the toxin preparations at each stage of purification was assayed in ligated rabbit ileal loops and in rabbit skin following methods described earlier (Dubey and Sanyal, 1978, 1979). At all stages of purification, toxin samples were titrated to a 50 % dose end-point using serial dilutions. In titration of skin PF activity, the dose giving a 4 mm blueing zone was considered as 1 unit, i.e. 1 $BD_{4\ mm}$.

Measurement of Cyclic 3'5' Adenosine Monophosphate (cyclic AMP) in Toxin-treated Epithelial Cells

Culture filtrates and crude enterotoxin, i.e. dialysed ammonium sulphate precipitate of culture supernate from chemically defined medium (Dubey and Sanyal, 1978), were inoculated into rabbit gut loops. The animals were killed after 6-8 h and the levels of cyclic AMP in toxin-treated as well as untreated epithelial cells of gut loops were determined following the method of Gilman (1970). To observe the dose response relationship, various amounts of crude enterotoxin preparations with protein contents varying between 32.5 µg (1 ED_{50}) and 325 µg (10 ED_{50}) were inoculated into loops and the animals killed after 6-8 h. Cyclic AMP levels were determined as above in both enterotoxin-treated and untreated epithelial cells of loops.

RESULTS

Purification of Enterotoxin

Table 1 outlines the purification steps and the enterotoxin activities of sequential fractions of *A. hydrophila* 20571 culture filtrate.

TABLE 1 Purification of *Aeromonas hydrophila* Enterotoxin

Fraction	Volume (ml)	Protein (mg)	Activity (Total units)[†]	Specific activity (U mg^{-1})	Recovery (%)	Fold purification
I. Culture supernatant	3,000	15	333.3	22.2	100	-
II. Concentrated culture supernatant	150	15	333.3	22.2	100	-
III. Acetone fractionation (66.6%)	3	8.5	283.3	33.3	85.0	1.5
IV. DEAE-Sephadex A50 chromatography	30	2.3	176.9	76.9	53.0	2.9
V. $(NH_4)_2SO_4$ precipitation	1	2.15	172.0	80.0	51.6	3.6
VI. CM cellulose chromatography	16	0.64	162.5	254.0	48.7	11.3

† 1 unit of enterotoxin is equivalent to the ED_{50} in rabbit ileal loops as determined according to Dubey and Sanyal (1979).

The culture supernate retained its enterotoxic activity after lyophilization and 85 % in the acetone-fractionated precipitate with 1.5 fold purification. When 8.5 mg of acetone-fractionated material was eluted from a DEAE Sephadex A50 column, five major peaks were obtained (Fig. 1). The enterotoxin fraction eluted in the fifth peak (F_5) retaining 53 % of the total activity with 2.9 fold purification. When this active fraction was precipitated with ammonium sulphate and then applied onto to a CM cellulose column, two major peaks were obtained (Fig. 2). The fraction which eluted with buffer containing 0.1 M KCl retained 48.7 % of total enterotoxic

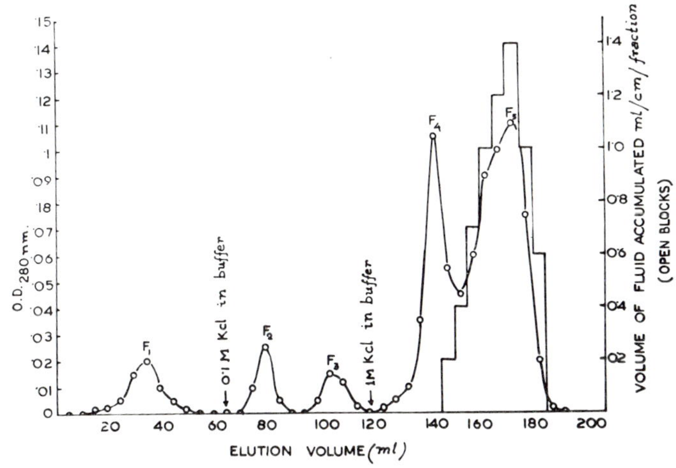

Fig. 1. Elution profile of *A. hydrophila* 20571 enterotoxin in DEAE Sephadex A50 chromatography.

activity with 11.3 fold purification. The ED_{50} of enterotoxic activity was 45 µg, 30 µg, 13 µg, 12.5 µg and 4 µg protein at stages I and II, III, IV, V and VI, respectively (Table 1).

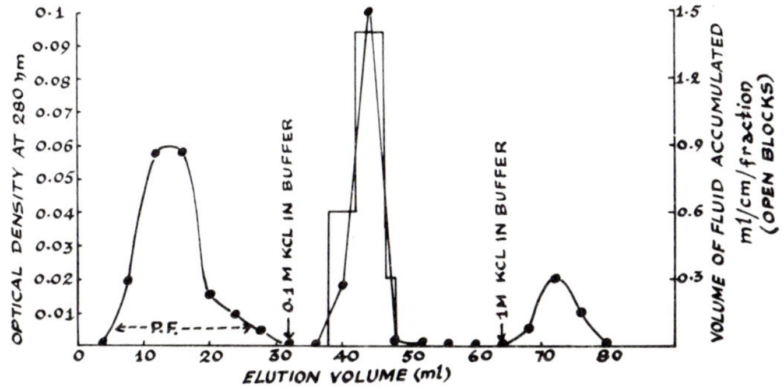

Fig. 2. Elution profile of skin permeability factor and enterotoxin (Fraction F_5) from DEAE Sephadex chromatography in CM cellulose chromatography.

Purification of Skin Permeability Factor

The skin PF activity was also purified (Table 2). This activity was retained completely after lyophilization and 88.2 % of the activity in the precipitate after acetone fractionation with a 1.6 fold purification.

TABLE 2 Purification of *Aeromonas hydrophila* Skin Permeability Factor (PF)

Fraction	Volume (ml)	Protein (mg)	Activity (Total units)†	Specific activity (U mg^{-1})	Recovery (%)	Fold purification
I. Culture supernatant	3,000	15	1071.4	71.4	100	-
II. Concentrated culture supernatant	150	15	1071.4	71.4	100	-
III. Acetone fractionation (66.6%)	3	8.5	944.4	111.1	88.2	1.6
IV. DEAE Sephadex A50 chromatography	30	2.3	920	400	85.9	5.6
V. $(NH_4)_2SO_4$ precipitation	1	2.15	860	400	80.3	5.6
VI. CM cellulose chromatography	24	1.10	733.3	666.6	68.5	9.3

† 1 unit of skin PF activity is equivalent to the dose giving a blueing zone of 4 mm diameter, i.e. $BD_{4\ mm}$.

Fraction F_5 from DEAE Sephadex A50 chromatography (Fig. 1) contained both enterotoxic and skin PF activities showing a recovery of 85.9 % of the latter with 5.6 fold purification. The skin PF activity was retained in the first fraction after elution from the CM cellulose column (Fig. 2) with 68.5 % recovery and about 9 fold purification. The BD_{4mm} was equivalent to 14 µg, 9 µg, 2.5 µg, 2.5 µg and 1.5 µg protein at steps I and II, III, IV, V and VI, respectively.

Tests for Purity of Enterotoxic and Skin Permeability Factors

Purity of enterotoxic factor and skin PF factor obtained after CM cellulose chromatography was tested by polyacrylamide gel electrophoresis. Figure 3 show the electrophoretic patterns at various stages of purification. The partially purified preparation showed 5 bands after fractionation with 66.6 % acetone (Fig. 3A). F_5 obtained after DEAE Sephadex A50 chromatography which contained both enterotoxic and skin PF activities showed 2 bands (Fig. 3B). After CM cellulose chromatography these two components were separated, the band with higher electrophoretic mobility (Fig. 3C) corresponding to the skin PF and the slower band (Fig. 3D), to enterotoxin. The enterotoxic factor was free from skin PF activity and *vice versa*.

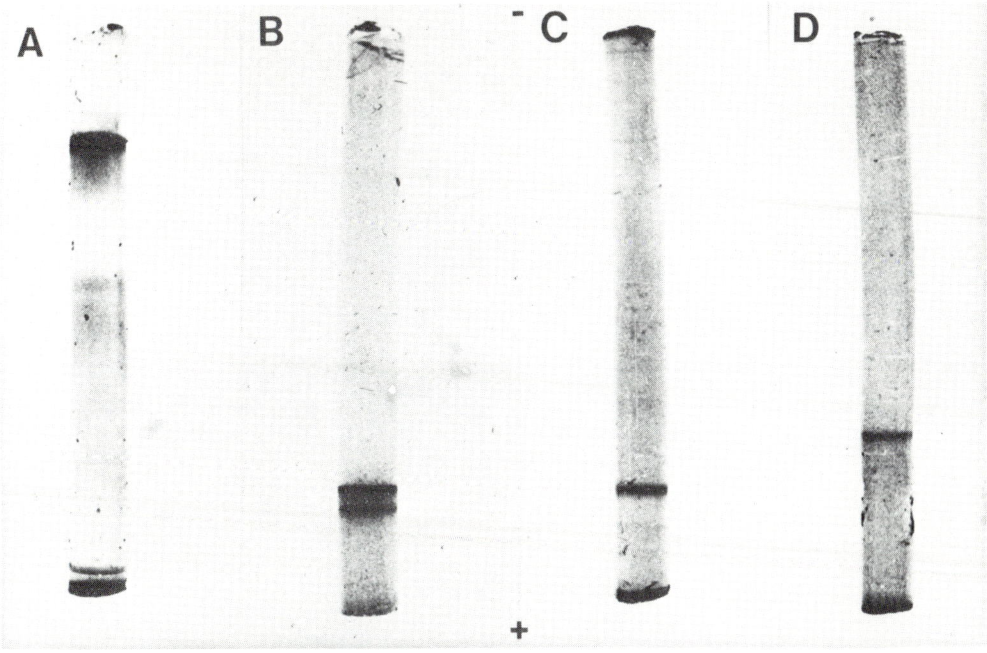

Fig. 3. Polyacrylamide gel electrophoresis of skin permeability factor and enterotoxin from *A. hydrophila*. (A) Acetone-precipitated culture filtrate from step III of purification; (B) Fraction F_5 from DEAE Sephadex A50 chromatography, 8 µg protein; (C) Skin permeability factor obtained after CM cellulose chromatography, 5 µg; (D) Enterotoxin obtained after CM cellulose chromatography, 4 µg protein.

Levels of Cyclic 3'5' Adenosine Monophosphate in Toxin-treated Epithelial Cells

When culture filtrates prepared in Brain Heart Infusion Broth or crude enterotoxins prepared by ammonium sulphate precipitation from defined medium were inoculated into rabbit ileal loops and the epithelial cells were examined for cyclic AMP content, it was observed that toxin-treated epithelial cells showed about 3-times higher levels of cyclic AMP as compared to the levels of normal rabbit intestinal epithelial cells in the same sets of experiments (Table 3). Epithelial cells treated with partially purified enterotoxin showed a lower cyclic AMP increase than cells treated with culture filtrate. When various doses of partially purified enterotoxin containing 1 ED_{50} to 10 ED_{50} were inoculated into ileal loops, the observed levels of cyclic AMP in the enterotoxin-treated epithelial cells were very similar. The cyclic AMP values ranged from 105-138 pmol mg^{-1} compared with a control value of 47 pmol mg^{-1} ($P < 0.01$). These data possibly indicate saturation of receptors for *A. hydrophila* enterotoxin.

DISCUSSION

Ljungh, Wretlind and Wadström (1978) obtained the enterotoxic protein of *A. hydrophila* by isoelectric focusing of concentrated culture filtrates. However, no report is available on the purification of the enterotoxic and skin permeability factors. The present study reports the purification of these two factors using conventional

TABLE 3 Levels of Cyclic AMP in Epithelial Cells Treated with Culture Filtrate or Crude Enterotoxin Preparations

Normal epithelial cells	Culture filtrate treated cells		Crude enterotoxin treated cells	
cyclic AMP[†]	cyclic AMP[†]	Fluid accumulation (ml cm^{-1})	cyclic AMP[†]	Fluid accumulation (ml cm^{-1})
40.0 ± 1.83	122.7 ± 2.7[§]	1.6	85.1 ± 1.1[§]	1.4

† pmol mg^{-1} protein of epithelial cells, mean ± SD of four determinations

§ Student's t-test, $P < 0.001$

purification methods. Each gave one band in polyacrylamide gel electrophoresis at the protein loads examined.

Our earlier experiments on purification of *A. hydrophila* enterotoxin were started with the first step as ammonium sulphate precipitation after concentration of culture supernate from cultivations in defined medium. However, it was observed that ammonium sulphate did not precipitate all of the enterotoxic factor as gauged by titration in ileal loops. Moreover, some other substances (probably lipid or lipid complexes) were precipitated which always interfered with subsequent purification steps. It was further noted that the ammonium sulphate precipitate when dissolved in buffer did not migrate into polyacrylamide gels. This problem was later solved by acetone fractionation instead of ammonium sulphate precipitation.

Only 4 μg of the purified enterotoxin of *A. hydrophila* was required to give rise to a positive ileal loop reaction (1 - 2 ml cm^{-1}). Results with purified *V. cholerae* and *E. coli* LT enterotoxins showed that in a given loop positive results were obtained with doses of 0.2 μg and 20 μg protein, respectively (Finkelstein and co-workers, 1976). However, Dorner (1975) determined the ED_{50} for rabbit ileal loops to be 1.45 μg for choleragen and 4.7 μg for *E. coli* LT. Thus, the activity of our purified *A. hydrophila* enterotoxin is comparable to those of *V. cholerae* and *E. coli*.

Among the various bioassay systems for enterotoxin, the skin permeability test, i.e. PF test, has been used in the case of *V. cholerae* enterotoxin (Finkelstein, 1973) and *C. perfringens* enterotoxin (Sakaguchi, Uemura and Reimann, 1973).The purified skin PF of *A. hydrophila* elicited a blueing response in rabbit skin with erythemic induration in as small a dose as 1.5 μg. The results of the present study indicate that the PF responsible for erythemic induration and increased capillary permeability when injected intracutaneously in rabbit skin is a distinct protein which could be separated by CM cellulose chromatography from the enterotoxic factor causing the rabbit gut loop reactions. Enterotoxin and skin PF thus appear to be separate factors unlike those of *V. cholerae* and *E. coli*. Both the enterotoxic and PF activities in *V. cholerae* are present in a single complex which may be dissociated under appropriate conditions (Barua and Burrows, 1974). PF activity has been associated with *E. coli* LT preparations and it has been suggested that both the enterotoxic and PF activities are different manifestations of the same molecule (Finkelstein and co-workers, 1976; Rappaport and co-workers, 1976). The purified *A. hydrophila* enterotoxin did not produce a blueing response in rabbit skin. It thus resembles *V. parahaemolyticus* enteropathogenic toxin which hardly induced erythema or a blueing response even in 10-25 μg doses (Zen-Yoji and co-workers, 1976). Both the enterotoxic and the PF factors were free from haemolytic activity (unpublished data).

The cyclic AMP findings by direct measurement of the cyclic AMP concentration in ileal mucosa 6-8 h after inoculation of ileal loops with *A. hydrophila* enterotoxin, showing about a 3-fold increase over controls, are similar to those reported by Schafer and co-workers (1970) for canine intestinal mucosa after incubation with cholera toxin *in vivo*. The increase in the concentration of cyclic AMP in epithelial cells by *A. hydrophila* enterotoxin could occur either through the stimulation of the membrane-bound adenylate cyclase, as in the case of choleragen and *E. coli* LT, which catalyses the synthesis of cyclic 3'5' adenosine monophosphate from adenosine triphosphate or through the inhibition of cyclic nucleotide phosphodiesterase, the enzyme that catalyses the breakdown of cyclic 3'5' AMP to 5' AMP. The results of this study indicate that the mode of action of *A. hydrophila* enterotoxin is mediated through intracellular increase in cyclic AMP. However, to elucidate the full pathway of the enterotoxic action it will be necessary to define the potential roles played by *A. hydrophila* enterotoxin, adenylate cyclase and phosphodiesterase.

ACKNOWLEDGEMENTS

The authors express their thanks to C. J. Smyth for helpful criticism of the manuscript, to A. K. Bhattacharya for help with cyclic AMP determinations, and to P. C. Sen for his interest in our studies. R.S.D. was in receipt of a Junior Research Fellowship from the Council of Scientific and Industrial Research.

REFERENCES

Andrews, P. 1964. Estimation of the molecular weights of proteins by Sephadex gel filtration. *Biochem. J.*, 91, 922-923.

Annapurna, E. and S. C. Sanyal. 1975. Studies on enteropathogenicity of *Aeromonas hydrophila* in an experimental model. *Indian J. Prev. Soc. Med.*, 6, 234-237.

Annapurna, E. and S. C. Sanyal. 1977. Enterotoxicity of *Aeromonas hydrophila*. *J. Med. Microbiol.*, 10, 317-323.

Barua, D. and W. Burrows. 1974. *Cholera*. Saunders, Philadelphia. p. 163.

Craig, J. P. 1966. Preparation of the vascular permeability factor of *Vibrio cholerae*. *J. Bacteriol.*, 92, 793-795.

Davis, B. J. 1964. Disc electrophoresis. II. Method and application to human serum proteins. *Ann. N. Y. Acad. Sci.*, 121, 404-427.

Dorner, F. 1975. *Escherichia coli* enterotoxin. Purification and partial characterisation. *J. Biol. Chem.*, 250, 8712-8719.

Dubey, R. S. and S. C. Sanyal. 1978. Enterotoxicity of *Aeromonas hydrophila*: Skin responses and in vivo neutralisation. *Zbl. Bakt. Hyg., I. Abt. Orig. A*, 242, 487-499.

Dubey, R. S. and S. C. Sanyal. 1979. Studies on the characterisation and neutralisation of *Aeromonas hydrophila* enterotoxin in the rabbit ileal loop model. *J. Med. Microbiol.*, 12, 345-352.

Finkelstein, R. A. 1973. Cholera. *CRC Crit. Rev. Microbiol.*, 2, 553-623.

Finkelstein, R. A. and J. J. LoSpalluto. 1969. Pathogenesis of experimental cholera. Preparation and isolation of choleragen and choleragenoid. *J. Exp. Med.*, 130, 185-202.

Finkelstein, R. A. and J. J. LoSpalluto. 1972. Crystalline cholera toxin and toxoid. *Science*, 175, 529-530.

Finkelstein, R. A., M. K. LaRue, D. W. Johnston, M. L. Vasil, G. J. Cho and J. R. Jones. 1976. Isolation and properties of heat labile enterotoxin(s) from enterotoxigenic *E. coli*. *J. Infect. Dis.*, 133, S120-S137.

Gilman, A. G. 1970. A protein binding assay of adenosine 3',5'-cyclic monophosphate. *Proc. Natl. Acad. Sci., U.S.A.*, 67, 305-312.

Gurwith, M., C. Bourque, E. Cameron, G. Forrest, and M. Green. 1977. Cholera like diarrhoea in Canada: Report of a case associated with enterotoxigenic *E. coli* and toxin producing *A. hydrophila*. *Arch. Intern Med.*, 137, 1461-1464.

Layne, E. 1957. Spectrophotometric and turbidimetric methods for measuring protein. *Methods Enzymol.*, 3, 447-457.

Ljungh, Å., B. Wretlind and T. Wadström. 1978. Evidence for enterotoxin and two cytolytic toxins in human isolates of *Aeromonas hydrophila*. In P. Rosenberg (Ed.), *Toxins: Animal, Plant and Microbial*. Pergamon Press, Oxford and New York. pp. 947-960.

Lowry, O. H., N. J. Rosebrough, A. L. Farr and R. J. Randall. 1951. Protein measurement with the Folin phenol reagent. *J. Biol. Chem.*, 193, 265-275.

Rappaport, R. S., J. F. Sagin, W. A. Pierzchala, G. Bonde, B. A. Rubin and H. Tint. 1976. Activation of heat labile *Escherichia coli* enterotoxin by trypsin. *J. Infect. Dis.*, 133, S41-S54.

Richardson, S. H., D. G. Evans and J. C. Feeley. 1970. Biochemistry of *Vibrio cholerae* virulence. I. Purification and biochemical properties of cholera enterotoxin. *Infect. Immun.*, 1, 546-554.

Sakaguchi, G., T. Uemura and H. P. Reimann. 1973. Simplified method for purification of *Clostridium perfringens* type A enterotoxin. *Appl. Microbiol.*, 26, 762-767.

Sanyal, S.C., S. J. Singh and P. C. Sen. 1975. Enteropathogenicity of *Aeromonas hydrophila* and *Plesiomonas shigelloides*. *J. Med. Microbiol.*, 8, 195-198.

Schafer, D. E., W. D. Lust, B. Sircar, and N. D. Goldberg. 1970. Elevation of adenosine 3',5' cyclic monophosphate concentration in intestinal mucosa after treatment with cholera toxin. *Proc. Natl.Acad. Sci., U.S.A.*, 67, 851-853.

Wadström, T., Å. Ljungh and B. Wretlind. 1976. Enterotoxin, haemolysin and cytotoxic protein in *Aeromonas hydrophila* from human infections. *Acta Pathol. Microbiol. Scand.*, *Sect.* B, 84, 112-114.

Zen-Yoji, H., Y. Kudoh, H. Igarashi, K. Ohta, K. Fukai and T. Hoshino. 1976. Further studies on characterization and biological activities of an enteropathogenic toxin of *Vibrio parahaemolyticus*. In A. Ohsaka, K. Hayashi and N. Sawai (Eds.), *Animal, Plant and Microbial Toxins*, Vol. 1. Plenum Press, New York. pp. 479-498.

Lipid A and Endotoxin

DIFFERENCES IN LIPOPOLYSACCHARIDE-INDUCED PROSTAGLANDIN-RELEASE AND PHAGOCYTIC ACTIVITY OF PERITONEAL MACROPHAGES FROM LPS-HYPERREACTIVE AND TOLERANT MICE

U. Schade and E. Th. Rietschel

Max-Planck-Institut für Immunbiologie, Freiburg im Breisgau, Federal Republic of Germany

ABSTRACT

Peritoneal macrophages from mice rendered hyperreactive or tolerant to LPS lethality were tested for their ability to release prostaglandins (PG) E_2 and $F_2\alpha$ on exposure to bacterial lipopolysaccharide (endotoxin). It was found that cells from hyperreactive mice release, as compared to controls, larger amounts of PGE_2 and $PGF_2\alpha$. In contrast, macrophages from tolerant mice could not be stimulated by LPS to produce increased levels ofPGE_2 and $PGF_2\alpha$. Macrophages from hyperreactive mice showed suppressed phagocytic activity while the cells from tolerant animals exhibited activated phagocytosis as compared to controls. Therefore, the ability of peritoneal macrophages to release PGE_2 and $PGF_2\alpha$ on exposure to LPS does not parallel their phagocytic activity. Our findings also indicate that in the mediation of LPS-hyperreactivity enhanced PG-release by macrophages may play a role. Likewise, impaired PG-production by macrophages could be involved in the mechanism underlying LPS-tolerance.

KEYWORDS

Lipopolysaccharide (LPS); endotoxin; LPS-hyperreactivity; LPS-tolerance; macrophages; prostaglandin.

INTRODUCTION

Bacterial lipopolysaccharides cause in experimental animals and humans a variety of endotoxic effects. The susceptibility of the host to LPS-activities such as lethality can be altered by prior exposure of the host to endotoxin. For example, it was previously shown that mice treated (day 0) with sublethal doses of LPS become hyperreactive to LPS lethality 24 hours later (day 1), as evident from a decreased LD_{50}-value, while mice tested 4 days after LPS-pretreatment were found to be highly tolerant to LPS-lethality as indicated by a 5-fold increase in LD_{50} (Greer and Rietschel, 1978).

Certain biological effects of endotoxins including fever, hypotension and also lethality can be prevented or their onset be delayed by acetylsalicylic acid and indomethacin, drugs which are known to be potent inhibitors of prostaglandin biosynthesis (Vane, 1971). Prostaglandins represent a family of biologically highly active molecules and as a potential physiological source of LPS-induced prostaglandins several groups have recently identified the macrophage (Kurland and Bockman, 1978; Wahl and coworkers, 1979; Rietschel and colleagues, 1980).

This paper is dedicated to Dr.Otto Lüderitz on the occasion of his 60th birthday (March 2, 1980)

From these studies the concept emerged that macrophages and the prostaglandins derived thereof are involved in the mediation of certain endotoxin activities.

In the present study it was tested whether the ability of peritoneal macrophages of mice to release prostaglandin-like material on exposure to LPS would be altered during the phases of LPS-hyperreactivity and tolerance. In addition, these macrophages were tested for their phagocytic activity.

The results show that the two properties of macrophages tested are drastically altered during the phases of LPS-hyperreactivity and tolerance.

MATERIALS AND METHODS

Microbial Stimulants of PG-release, Sera, and Mice

The triethylamine-salt of electrodialyzed lipopolysacchride (LPS) of the *Salmonella minnesota* Re mutant R595 was used (Galanos and colleagues, 1977). Zymosan was from ICN Pharmaceuticals Inc. (Plainview, N.Y.). Fluorescent zymosan was a gift of R.L. Rendon-Orpeza (MPI für Immunbiologie, Freiburg). Antisera against PGE_2 and $PGF_{2\alpha}$ were kindly donated by Dr.B.A.Peskar (Institut für Pharmakologie, Universität Freiburg). The preparation and characterisation of these sera has been described (Peskar and coworkers, 1979). (^{3}H)PGE_2 and (^{3}H)$PGF_{2\alpha}$ (specific activity of E_2 and $F_{2\alpha}$: 120 000 -170 000 mCi/mmol) were purchased from Amersham-Buchler. Female NMRI mice (6 - 8 weeks, Hannover) were used in all experiments. Fetal calf serum (FCS) was from Seromed (München).

Induction and Determination of LPS-Hyperreactivity and Tolerance

Essentially, the procedure described previously was followed (Greer and Rietschel, 1978). Briefly, groups of mice were injected with LPS (i.v., 10 ug/mouse) on day 0. LD_{50} determinations using graded doses of LPS were carried out 24 h later (day 1) and on day 4, respectively.

Preparations of Peritoneal Macrophages

Peritoneal cells were obtained from control animals (day 0), as well as from LPS-hyperreactive (day 1) and LPS-tolerant (day 4) mice (pretreated with LPS (10 ug/mouse) on day 0). Cells were harvested by washing the peritoneal cavity with Eagles medium (5 ml) supplemented with Hepes (50 mmol) and fetal calf serum (FCS, 10%). Portions of the outwash containing 1×10^6 cells were placed into wells of a culture cluster (Costar, Technorama, Hüttenberg), macrophages allowed to adhere (3 h, 37°C) and washed (3x) with PBS (37°C). To each well Eagles Medium (1 ml), supplemented with Hepes (50 mmol), was added and the cells allowed to rest for 1 h (37°C).

Induction of PG-Release and PG-Determination

Macrophages were incubated with different concentrations of LPS for 24 h (37°C), the cells centrifuged, and prostaglandin-like activity (PGE_2, $PGF_{2\alpha}$) determined in the supernatant by radioimmunoassay (Jobke and colleagues, 1973).The identity of PGE_2 and $PGF_{2\alpha}$ was confirmed by gas liquid chromatography (Rietschel and coworkers, 1980).

Phagocytic Activity (Zymosan)

Determinations of macrophage phagocytic activity were performed as previously described (Oropeza-Rendon and coworkers, 1979). Briefly, peritoneal cells (2×10^5), in Eagles Medium (100 ul), were transferred to sterile coverslips in petri dishes and the macrophages allowed to adhere (4 h, 37°C). After washing (3x) with PBS, Eagles Medium (2 ml, 50 mmol Hepes, 10% FCS) was added and the cells allowed to rest for 12 h (37°C). Fluorescent zymosan (100 mg) was then added and incubated with the cells for 20 min (37°C). The coverslips were carefully washed (PBS, 37°C) and, after fixation of cells in methanol (15 min), mounted to microscope slides. Ingested particles and phagocytosing cells were counted with a Zeiss fluorescent microscope equipped for simultaneous visible and fluorescent microscopy. The phagocytosis index (PI) was calculated as:

$$PI = \frac{\text{no. of phagocytosing cells x no. of phagocytized particles}}{\text{no. of counted cells}}$$

Determinations of PI were carried out with two different preparations, counting two distinct sites of each coverslip.

RESULTS

Induction of Hyperreactivity and Tolerance to LPS-Lethality

Two groups of mice received LPS (i.v., 10 ug/mouse) on day 0. In one group the LD_{50} was determined 24 h later (day 1); in the other group on day 4. As Fig. 1 shows, animals tested

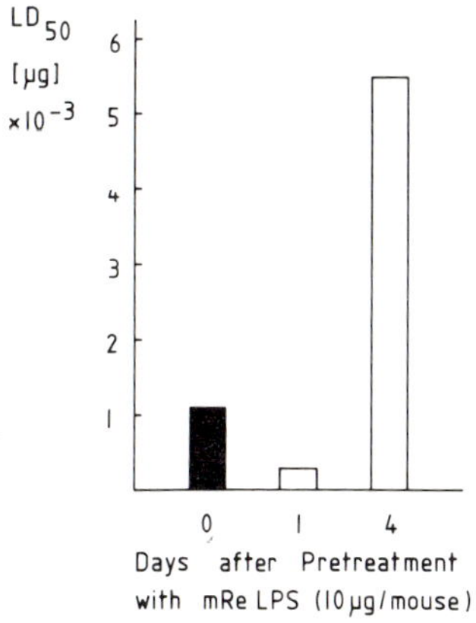

Fig. 1. LPS-induced lethality (LD_{50}) in control (day 0) and LPS-pretreated mice. LPS-hyperreactivity is seen on day 1, LPS-tolerance on day 4.

on day 1 were hyperreactive to LPS-lethality (LD_{50} = 300 ug) while mice challenged on day 4 were tolerant to LPS-lethality (LD_{50} = 5 500 ug) as compared to controls (day 0; LD_{50} = 1 200 ug).

LPS-Induced Prostaglandin-Release

Macrophages obtained from control mice (day 0) were treated with different concentrations of LPS (1 to 100 ug) and prostaglandins released into the medium estimated by radio-immunoassay. It was found that macrophages responded to incubation with LPS with a dose-dependent release of PGE_2 and $PGF_{2}\alpha$. Macrophages from hyperreactive mice (day 1), released in a dose dependent manner higher amounts of PGE_2 and $PGF_{2}\alpha$ on exposure to LPS as compared to controls (day 0). In contrast, macrophages from tolerant animals (day 4) were completely refractory to LPS with no enhanced release of PGE_2 and $PGF_{2}\alpha$ (Fig. 2). This was also true when larger amounts (200 ug/ml) of LPS were used (data not shown).

This refractoriness could not be overcome by preincubation of day 4-cells for 24 or 48 h in medium supplemented with 10% FCS (Fig. 3). With the different LPS-concentrations used (1 to 100 ug/ml) levels of $PGF_{2}\alpha$ did not differ from basal levels. As Fig. 3 shows, tolerant macrophages seemed, after exposure to the higher LPS-doses (50 to 100 ug/ml), to produce even less PGE_2 than non-treated cells. Whether this difference, however, is significant, remains to be elucidated.

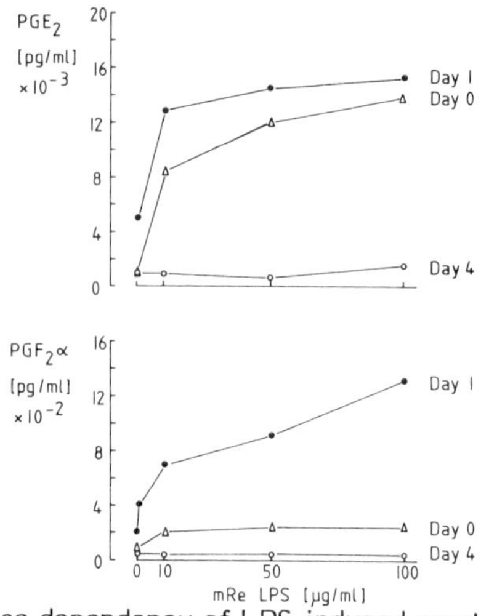

Fig. 2. Dose dependency of LPS-induced prostaglandin-release by macrophages from control (day 0), LPS-hyperreactive (day 1), and LPS-tolerant (day 4) mice.

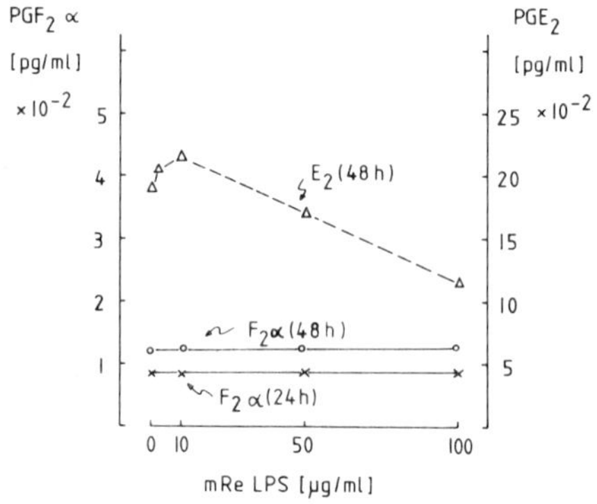

Fig. 3. Refractoriness of macrophages from LPS-tolerant mice to LPS-induced prostaglandin release is not overcome by preincubation of cells for 24 or 48 h in medium

Zymosan-Induced Prostaglandin Synthesis

Macrophages of normal (day 0), hyperreactive (day 1) and tolerant (day 4) mice were incubated (1 h) with zymosan (0.5 mg/ml), a known stimulant of prostaglandin synthesis in phagocytic cells (Weidemann and coworkers, 1978). In this experiment the release of $PGF_{2\alpha}$ was estimated. As shown in Fig. 4, macrophages of non-treated mice released $PGF_{2\alpha}$ (1.8 ng/ml) into the medium. Cells of hyperreactive animals (day 1) appeared to be suppressed in their capacity to produce $PGF_{2\alpha}$ on exposure to zymosan (0.4 ng/ml). Most significantly, however, macrophages obtained from tolerant mice (day 4), released amounts of $PGF_{2\alpha}$ (2.2 ng/ml) comparable to those released by cells from non-treated control mice (Fig. 4).

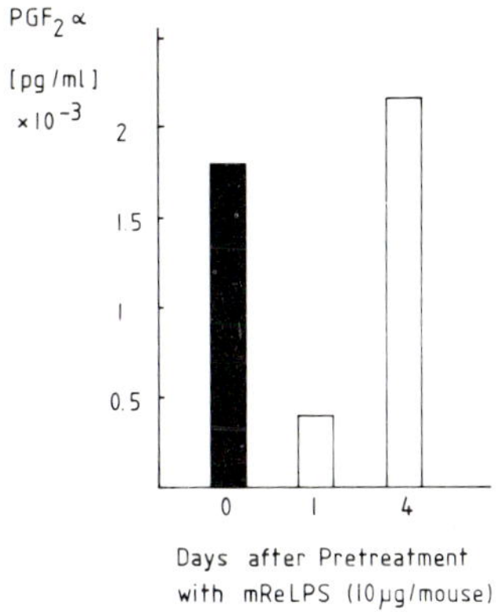

Fig. 4. Zymosan-induced $PGF_2\alpha$-release by macrophages from control (day 0), LPS-hyperreactive (day 1), and LPS-tolerant (day 4) mice.

Phagocytic Activity

The phagocytic activity of peritoneal macrophages was tested by determining the uptake of fluorescent zymosan (incubation for 20 min at 37^oC) and the phagocytosis index (PI) was calculated (Fig. 5). PI values were with macrophages from untreated (day 0)

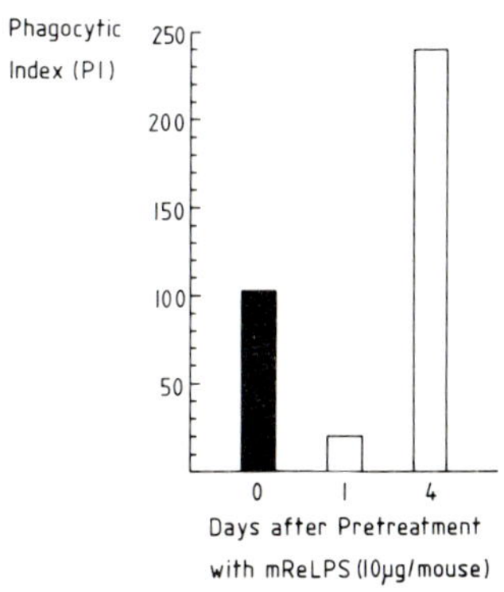

Fig. 5. Phagocytic activity (PI) of macrophages from control (day 0), LPS-hyperreactive (day 1), and LPS-tolerant (day 4) mice.

mice 105, of cells obtained on day 1, 20 and of cells from day 4, 240 (Fig. 5). Thus, phagocytosis of macrophages from hyperreactive mice was suppressed, and that of macrophages from tolerant animals stimulated, as compared to controls.

DISCUSSION

The results presented show that mouse peritoneal macrophages can be stimulated by LPS *in vitro* to release postaglandins E_2 and $F_2\alpha$. This is in agreement with previous findings of other laboratories (Kurland and Bockman, 1978; Wahl and coworkers, 1979; Rietschel and colleagues, 1980). It was further shown that macrophages of mice rendered hyperreactive to LPS-lethality release, on exposure to LPS, larger amounts of PGE_2 and $PGF_2\alpha$ than cells from mice not treated with LPS. In contrast, macrophages from LPS-tolerant mice did not increase their production of PGE_2 and $PGF_2\alpha$ on incubation with LPS. It was also found that the phagocytic activity of macrophages from hyperreactive mice was suppressed, but that of tolerant mice greatly stimulated. Therefore, the ability of peritoneal macrophages to release prostaglandins PGE_2 and $PGF_2\alpha$ on incubation with LPS does not parallel their phagocytic activity.

The failure of macrophages from LPS-resistant mice to elaborate PG on incubation with LPS indicates that LPS-tolerance is expressed on a cellular level. This refractoriness appears to be LPS-specific since, on exposure to zymosan, tolerant macrophages release $PGF_2\alpha$ in amounts comparable to cells from control (not LPS-pretreated) mice. The refractoriness of macrophages from tolerant animals could not be overcome with higher LPS-doses or preincubation in medium. In preliminary experiments, however, it was found that tolerant macrophages released PG on exposure to LPS, if L-conditioned medium containing colony stimulating factor (CSF) was added. In this connection the finding is of interest that macrophages from the LPS-non-responder mouse strain C3H/HeJ require the presence of external CSF to release PG on incubation with LPS (cited in Broxmeyer and Moore, 1978).

The present findings suggest that enhanced PG-release may be involved in the mediation of LPS-hyperreactivity and impaired PG-release of macrophages may play a role in the mechanism underlying LPS-tolerance. Thus, our results are consistent with the hypothesis that macrophage-derived prostaglandins play a role in the mediation of endotoxin activity. They do not, however, prove such a role. Additional studies are obviously needed to elucidate the mechanisms underlying altered prostaglandin production during the phases of hyper-reactivity and tolerance, and to establish the etiologic and regulatory significance of prostaglandins in endotoxicosis.

ACKNOWLEDGEMENT

This investigation was supported by a grant of the Stiftung Volkswagenwerk.

REFERENCES

Broxmeyer, H.E., and M.A.S.Moore (1978). Biochem. Biophys. Acta, 516, 129-166.

Galanos, C., O. Lüderitz, E.Th. Rietschel, and O. Westphal (1977). In: International Review of Biochemistry, Biochemistry of Lipids II (Goodwin, T.W, ed) Vol 14, pp.239-335, University Park Press Baltimore.

Greer, G.G., and E.Th. Rietschel (1978). Infect. Immun., 20, 366-374.

Jobke, A., B.A. Peskar, and B.M. Peskar (1973). FEBS Letters, 37, 192-196.

Kurland, J.I., and R. Bockman (1978). J. Exptl. Med., 147, 952-957.

Oropeza-Rendon, R.L., V. Speth, G. Hiller, K. Weber, and H. Fischer (1979). Exp. Cell Res., 119, 365-371.

Peskar, B.A., H. Anhut, E.E. Kröner, and B.M. Peskar (1979). In: Advances in Pharmacology and Therapeutics, Vol.7, Biochemical Clinical Pharmacology. (J.P.Tillement, ed), Pergamon Press, Oxford, N.Y.

Rietschel, E.Th., U. Schade, O. Lüderitz, H. Fischer, and B.A. Peskar (1980). Prostaglandins in Endotoxicosis. In: Microbiology-1980 (D.Schlessinger, ed). Am. Soc. Microbiol., Washington, D.C.

Vane, J.R. (1971). Nature New Biol. 231, 232-235.

Wahl, L.M., D.L. Rosenstreich, L.M. Glode, A.L. Sandberg, and S.E. Mergenhagen (1979). Infect. Immun. 23, 8-13.

Weidemann, M.J., B.A. Peskar, K. Wrogemann, E.Th. Rietschel, Hj. Staudinger, and H. Fischer (1978). FEBS Letters 89, 136-139.

LPS REGULATION OF THE IMMUNE RESPONSE: CELLULAR AND MOLECULAR BASIS OF ADJUVANTICITY AND THE ROLE OF SUPPRESSOR T CELLS ON HOST RESPONSES

J. R. McGhee*, S. M. Michalek*, H. Kiyono*, J. J. Farrar, D. L. Rosenstreich**, and S. E. Mergenhagen****

**Dept. Micro., Comp. Can. Ctr., Inst. Dent. Res., UAB, Birmingham, AL 35294, USA*
***L. M. I., NIDR, Bldg. 30, NIH, Bethesda, MD 20205, USA*

ABSTRACT

LPS exerts several effects on lymphoid cells and the time of exposure is critical in determining whether augmentation or suppression of the host's immune response will be manifested. If appropriate doses of endotoxin are administered with antigen the well characterized adjuvant response is seen. We have evaluated the contribution of macrophages (MØ) and T cells and certain of their mediators to adjuvanticity by utilizing LPS responsive (C3H/HeN and C57BL/10 Sn) and nonresponsive (C3H/HeJ and C57BL/10 ScN) mice. Purified T and B spleen cells were obtained by glass and nylon wool column chromatography, while MØ were obtained from irradiated (1000 R) spleen cells. Appropriate mixtures of either LPS responsive or nonresponsive cells were cultured with either haptenated or normal heterologous erythrocytes and LPS. Adjuvanticity was obtained only when LPS responsive MØ and T cells (from either C3H/HeN or C57BL/10 Sn spleen) were cultured with B cells from either responder or nonresponder animals. Lymphocyte activating factor (LAF) (Interleukin 1, IL 1) plus LPS gave higher anti-SRC plaque forming cell (PFC) responses only in the presence of T cells from LPS responsive mice. Further, antigen-induced and LPS augmented PFC helper factor gave anti-SRC PFC responses in nonresponsive nude (C57BL/10 ScN) spleen cell cultures, suggesting that LPS induced adjuvanticity may be mediated by increasing the production of LAF (IL 1) and PFC helper factor. We have also investigated the role of suppressor T cells on immunogenic and mitogenic responses to LPS. Evidence is provided that significant suppression of lipid A effects is manifested by gut-associated-lymphoid tissue T cells, indicating that the normal Gram negative gut flora induces a cell population which can regulate B cell responses to bacterial endotoxin.

KEYWORDS

Adjuvanticity; endotoxin; lipopolysaccharide (LPS); TNP-LPS; macrophage (MØ); T and B lymphocytes; suppression; plaque forming cell (PFC); lymphocyte activating factor (LAF); Interleukin 1, (IL 1); PFC helper factor; LPS responsive and nonresponsive mice.

INTRODUCTION

Several host effects of bacterial endotoxin result from its interaction with cells of the lymphoreticular system (Michalek, 1979). In this regard, recent evidence has suggested that both T cells and macrophages (MØ) are important for the well characterized adjuvant property of LPS on the immune response (McGhee, 1979a). In addition, Farrar and coworkers (1977) and Hoffmann and Watson (1979) have suggested that two synergistically-acting factors, one from MØ and the other from T cells can enhance immune responses in vitro. Jacobs (1979) has presented evidence that the T cell lymphokine, T cell replacing factor (TRF) acts synergistically with endotoxin toward enhancement of B cell responses. Finally, the interaction of LPS with T cells has been extended to other effects since Goodman and Weigle (1979) recently reported that T cells enhance polyclonal B cell activation by LPS. The route and time of introduction of LPS into the host can markedly influence the responsiveness of that animal's lymphoid cells. In this regard, Uchiyama and Jacobs (1978a, b) have shown that parenteral administration of LPS prior to antigen results in suppression of the immune response and this suppression is likely T cell derived. In this report evidence is provided that LPS exhibits adjuvant properties by interaction with the MØ and T lymphocytes and together promote greater B cell responsiveness to antigen. Evidence is also provided that LPS can induce a T suppressor cell population which normally occurs in the gut.

MATERIALS AND METHODS

Animals. LPS nonresponder C3H/HeJ and C57BL/10 ScN nude (nu/nu) and nu/+ and responder C3H/HeN (nu/nu, nu/+, +/+) and C57BL/10 Sn mice as well as germfree (GF) and conventional (Conv) Balb/c mice (maintained in the Core Facility for Immunocompromised mice in the Comprehensive Cancer Center at the UAB) were utilized in these studies.

Endotoxin. Escherichia coli K235 LPS was prepared by phenol-water (Ph) extraction method. TNP conjugated Ph-LPS was prepared and used as previously described (McGhee, 1979a). Lipid A from E. coli 055:B5 and lipid A associated protein (LAP) from E. coli 0111:B4 were a kind gift from Dr. D.C. Morrison (Scripps Clinic and Research Foundation, La Jolla, Calif.).

Culture methods. Mouse spleen cultures were prepared by the method of Mishell and Dutton (1967) with modifications. The conditions including concentration of SRC or TNP-SRC immunogens were used as previously described (McGhee, 1979a). In certain studies culture supernatants were added to cell cultures at the same time as immunogen and/or LPS. Cultures were assayed for anti-SRC and anti-TNP PFC on day 5. TNP-LPS immunizations utilized either 0.2 or 2 μg/culture as previously described (McGhee, 1979a). Anti-TNP PFC responses were measured on day 4.

Mitogenesis assay. Proliferative responses of spleen cell cultures (8×10^5) to LPS and various lectins (PHA, Con A and PWM) were determined by tritiated thymidine incorporation (Rosenstreich and Glode, 1975). Cultures were harvested at 48 hr following a pulse with 0.5 μCi tritiated thymidine for the last 6 hr.

Cell purification. T and B cell preparations were obtained by MØ depleted splenocyte preparations resulting from two consecutive passages of spleen cells through Sephadex G-10 columns. Purified T and B cell populations were prepared by first passage of spleen cells through glass wool columns followed by fractionation of the eluant cells on nylon wool. Nonadherent cells were treated with anti-immunoglobulin serum and complement to remove contaminating B cells while the adherent population was treated with anti-Θ serum and complement and used as a source of B cells.

Splenic MØ-rich populations were prepared by irradiation of single spleen cell suspensions followed by addition of aliquots to culture wells. Nonadherent cells were removed by repeated addition and aspiration of media (4 times). The adherent cells served as the source of MØ.

Plaque assay. Following incubation, nonadherent cells were removed from culture plates, washed once with medium and resuspended to the desired volume for assay. Either anti-SRC or anti-TNP PFC was determined by a slide modification of the Jerne and Nordin technique.

Statistics. Results are expressed as mean PFC or proliferative response per culture ± 1 standard error. Significance of differences among means was determined by Student's T-test.

RESULTS

Cells and mediators involved in LPS adjuvanticity. Optimal *in vitro* immune responses of spleen cells from both C3H/HeN LPS responsive (R) and C3H/HeJ LPS nonresponsive (NR) mice to heterologous erythrocytes were obtained utilizing 5×10^6 spleen cells per 0.5 ml medium and adjuvant responses with the addition of either 0.1 or 1.0 µg Ph-LPS per culture (McGhee, 1979a). From Table 1 it is clear that MØ must be derived from LPS responsive mice in order to obtain enhancement of *in vitro* immune responses. Lymphocytes from NR mice did not exhibit adjuvant responses with LPS in the presence of R MØ, implying that R lymphocytes were also required for enhancement *in vitro*. To test the contribution of T cells for adjuvanticity, both R and NR T lymphocytes were mixed with either R or NR B cells and R MØ and anti-TNP PFC responses measured and the results are expressed in Table 2. Only R T cells (in the presence of R MØ) promoted enhanced responses; it was interesting that R T cells and MØ were able to increase responses of C3H/HeJ (NR) B cells. In order to insure that the B cell preparations did not contain contaminating T helper cells, the next series of experiments employed purified B cells from C3H/HeN (R) nude mice. As can be seen in Table 3, when T cells and MØ from R mice were assessed, significant adjuvant responses occurred. A similar study was performed taking advantage of the C57BL/10 ScN nude mouse which, like the C3H/HeJ is nonresponsive to LPS. B cells from C57BL/10 ScN nudes (NR) were mixed with fully histocompatible T cells and MØ from either R (C57BL/10 Sn) or NR (C57BL/10 ScN) mice and enhanced anti-TNP PFC responses measured. The results summarized in Table 4 clearly suggest that R T cells and R MØ enhance NR B cell responses to this immunogen.

TABLE 1. Macrophage Requirement for LPS Augmentation of the Immune Response to Heterologous Erythrocytes

MØ Source*	T and B Lymphocyte Source†	Anti-SRC PFC Response: SRC Only	SRC + Ph-LPS	Percent Increase
C3H/HeN (R)	C3H/HeN (R)	1088 ± 55	1915 ± 110	76%
	C3H/HeJ (NR)	1172 ± 25	1160 ± 30	(-1%)
C3H/HeJ (NR)	C3H/HeN (R)	1135 ± 30	1170 ± 55	3%
	C3H/HeJ (NR)	1110 ± 60	1130 ± 50	2%

*Splenic MØ were obtained from either LPS responsive (R) C3H/HeN or nonresponsive (NR) C3H/HeJ spleen cell preparations given 1000 R of irradiation (5×10^6 cells/culture).

†Splenic lymphocytes were obtained following consecutive passage of spleen cell preparations over G-10 Sephadex columns.

TABLE 2. T Cell Requirement for LPS Augmentation of the Immune Response to TNP-SRC Antigen *in vitro*

Cell Source (C3H)*		Anti-SRC PFC Response		
B Cell	T Cell	SRC Only	SRC + Ph-LPS	Percent Increase
R	R	920 ± 60	1505 ± 75	64%
NR	R	695 ± 35	1035 ± 46	50%
R	NR	1101 ± 60	1185 ± 84	8%
NR	NR	806 ± 85	747 ± 62	(-7%)

*Purified splenic T or B cells (1 x 10^6 cells/culture) prepared by column purification were derived from either LPS responsive (R) C3H/HeN or nonresponsive (NR) C3H/HeJ mice. Splenic MØ were obtained from C3H/HeN nude (nu/nu) spleen cell preparations given 1000 R of irradiation (5 x 10^6 cells/culture).

TABLE 3. Requirement for Endotoxin Sensitive T Cells and Macrophages for LPS Adjuvanticity: Enhancement of Responder B Cells

Cell Source (C3H)			Anti-TNP PFC Response		
B Cell*	T Cell†	MØ#	TNP-SRC Only	TNP-SRC + Ph-LPS	Percent Increase
R	R	R	681 ± 20	1470 ± 50	116%
R	NR	R	819 ± 22	1015 ± 24	24%
R	R	NR	716 ± 35	680 ± 22	(-5%)
R	NR	NR	882 ± 37	750 ± 50	(-15%)

*The responsive (R) B cells were derived by column purification of C3H/HeN nude (nu/nu) mouse spleen cells.
†Splenic T cells from LPS nonresponsive (NR) C3H/HeJ or C3H/HeN (R) mice were column purified and cultured at 1 x 10^6 cells/culture.
#Splenic MØ were obtained from C3H/HeJ (NR) or C3H/HeN (R) spleen cell preparations given 1000 R of irradiation (5 x 10^6 cells/culture).

TABLE 4. Requirement for Endotoxin Sensitive T Cells and Macrophages for LPS Adjuvanticity: Enhancement of Nonresponder B Cells

Cell Source (C57BL)			Anti-TNP PFC Response		
B Cell*	T Cell†	MØ#	TNP-SRC Only	TNP-SRC + Ph-LPS	Percent Increase
NR	R	R	875 ± 45	1435 ± 44	64%
NR	NR	R	941 ± 110	997 ± 20	6%
NR	R	NR	838 ± 80	771 ± 45	(-8%)
NR	NR	NR	710 ± 40	750 ± 30	6%

*The nonresponsive (NR) B cells were obtained by column purification of C57BL/10 ScN nude (nu/nu) mouse spleen cells.
†Splenic T cells from C57BL/10 ScN (NR) or LPS responsive (R) C57BL/10 Sn were obtained by column purification and cultured at 1 x 10^6 cells/ culture.
#Splenic MØ were obtained from C57BL/10 ScN (NR) or C57BL/10 Sn (R) spleen cell preparations given 1000 R of irradiation (5 x 10^6 cells/ culture).

In order to assess whether enhancement of immune responses was correlated with production of factors from either MØ or T cells, e.g., lymphocyte activating factor (LAF) (Interleukin 1, IL 1) or PFC helper factor, respectively, these mediators were studied. When LAF (IL 1) was derived from thioglycolate stimulated peritoneal MØ from C3H/HeN mice and added to cultures of either R (C57BL/10

Sn) or NR (C57BL/10 ScN) spleen cells with antigen, enhanced responses occurred (Table 5). In the R cultures Ph-LPS and LAF (IL 1) yielded very high adjuvant responses, perhaps suggesting that these two substances could act synergistically. For assessment of PFC helper factor production either R (C3H/HeN) or NR (C3H/HeJ) spleen cultures were incubated with either antigen or antigen and LPS and 72 hr culture supernatants were tested for PFC helper factor activity (Table 6). As can be seen, supernatants from immunized R or NR spleens supported immune responses in NR (C57BL/10 ScN) nude cultures. Significantly higher responses were observed in supernatants from R cultures given endotoxin, suggesting enhanced production of PFC helper factor. That this was factor mediated was indicated by the study where aliquots of supernatant were fractionated over G-75 Sephadex columns and 30,000 dalton fraction assessed. These data suggest that LPS induced adjuvanticity is perhaps mediated by enhanced production of LAF (IL 1) (MØ) and PFC helper factor (TRF?) (T cell).

TABLE 5. Macrophage-derived Lymphocyte Activating Factor (LAF; Interleukin 1, IL 1) and LPS Enhanced Immune Responses to Heterologous Erythrocytes

Splenic T Cell Source*	Anti-SRC PFC Response + Culture Additions† SRC Only	LAF (IL 1)	Ph-LPS	LAF (IL 1) + Ph-LPS
C57BL/10 Sn (R)	765 ± 59 (100%)	1342 ± 87 (175%)	1958 ± 79 (256%)	3873 ± 384 (506%)
C57BL/10 ScN (NR)	880 ± 109 (100%)	2670 ± 109 (303%)	798 ± 145 (91%)	2755 ± 398 (313%)

*MØ-depleted spleen cells from LPS nonresponsive (NR) C57BL/10 ScN nude mice were cultured (2 x 10^6 cells/culture) in the presence of column purified splenic T cells (2 x 10^6 cells/culture) from either LPS responsive (R) C57BL/10 Sn or C57BL/10 ScN (NR) mice and incubated with SRC (1-2 x 10^6 cells/culture).
†Estimated biological activity of LAF preparation = 27,024 cpm as determined on C3H/HeJ thymocytes. 1 μg Ph-LPS added to culture.

TABLE 6. LPS Enhancement of PFC Helper Factor Production

Source of Factor*	Anti-SRC PFC Response† Supernatant of Culture with SRC Only	SRC + Ph-LPS Crude	SRC + Ph-LPS Partially-Purified#
C3H/HeN (R)	981 ± 12 (100%)	1614 ± 42 (165%)	1385 ± 26 (141%)
C3H/HeJ (NR)	732 ± 18 (100%)	786 ± 57 (107%)	692 ± 42 (86%)

*Splenic cultures (5 x 10^6 cells/0.5 ml) from either LPS responsive (R) C3H/HeN or C3H/HeJ mice immunized with SRC or SRC + 1 μg Ph-LPS. Supernatants derived from a 72 hr culture.
†MØ-depleted spleen cells from C57BL/10 ScN (NR) nude mice (2 x 10^6 cells) were incubated with helper-factor-containing preparations and SRC.
#Helper-factor was obtained by fractionation of culture supernatants over a G-75 Sephadex column (0.6 x 30 cm) in Tris buffer (pH 7.5). Fractions were concentrated by Amicon filtration to the original volume and dialyzed against incomplete medium.

Role of Suppressor T Cells on LPS Response. Recent work has suggested that injection of mice with LPS prior to immunization of their spleen cells *in vitro* leads to suppression of the immune response (Uchiyama and Jacobs, 1978a,b). Therefore, we have compared mitogenic and immunogenic responses to endotoxin in GF and Conv mice to determine if the normal Gram negative gut flora induces, via LPS, a suppressor cell population. Significantly higher responses to Ph-LPS and to lipid A were found with GF spleen cells (Table 7). Although LAP stimulated high responses in GF spleen cultures, the difference was less than that seen with either Ph-LPS or lipid A. Since a major difference between GF and Conv mice is the presence of an indigenous flora, we next determined whether ex-GF mice conventionalized with Balb/c gut flora would lead to lower LPS responses. Three weeks following conventionalization of GF mice (Cot) their splenic response was similar to that observed in normal Conv animals (Fig. 1), suggesting that the indigenous gut flora may account for the lower Ph-LPS responses obtained. In order to determine the cells responsible for the diminution in responses to Ph-LPS, MØ and T cells were prepared from either GF or Conv mice as described above. In data not shown, MØ from either GF or Conv mice did not affect B cell proliferation. However, as shown in Fig. 2, splenic T cells from Conv mice diminished B cell responses to Ph-LPS, suggesting that normal mice harbor a T suppressor cell population which regulate B cell responses to endotoxin. In order to assess the possible origin of this T cell population, T cells were derived from either Peyer's patches (PP) or spleen from either GF or Conv mice and tested for their ability to suppress TNP-LPS responses in nude mouse spleen cell cultures (Fig. 3). Addition of either Conv splenic or PP T cells to TNP-LPS immunized nude spleen cell cultures dramatically reduced the anti-TNP PFC responses obtained. In other experiments (data not shown), this suppression could be abrogated with anti-Θ serum plus complement.

TABLE 7. LPS-Induced Mitogenesis of Splenic B Cells from Germfree and Conventional Balb/c Mice

Endotoxin Preparation (10 μg/ml)	Proliferative Response* (E/C)	
	Germfree	Conventional
Ph-LPS	46.1	15.3
Lipid A	9.6	3.1
LAP	66.2	52.0

*Represents mean stimulation ratio of 3 separate experiments (quadruplicate cultures/experiment), where E/C = cpm ^{3}HTdR incorporated with endotoxin/cpm ^{3}H-TdR incorporated in medium only.

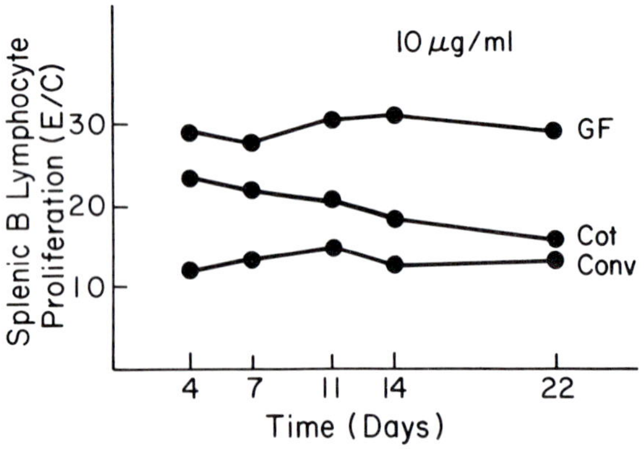

Fig. 1. Comparison of germfree (GF), conventional (Conv) and conventionalized mouse splenocytes at intervals following contamination (Cot) to stimulation with Ph-LPS (10 μg).

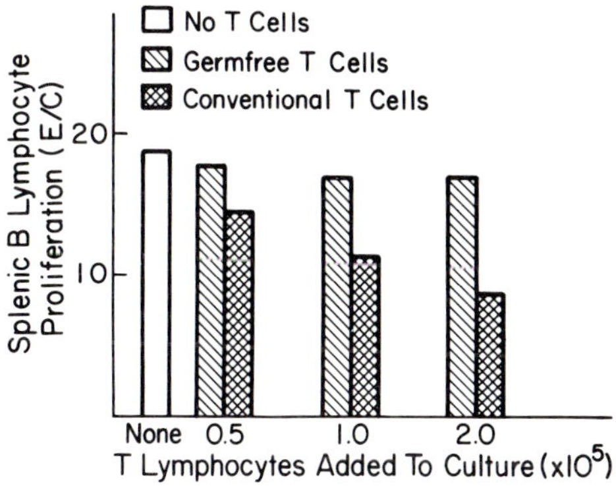

Fig. 2. Effect of germfree (GF) (single hatched bar) or conventional (Conv) (double hatched bar) splenic T cells toward proliferation of GF B cells (open bar) stimulated with Ph-LPS (10 μg).

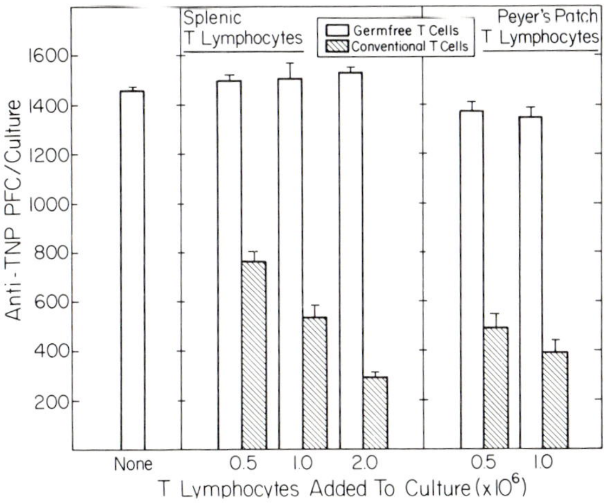

Fig. 3. Effect of germfree (open bar) or conventional (hatched bar) splenic or Peyer's patch (PP) T lymphocytes on the TNP-LPS (1.0 μg) response of GF nude mouse spleen cells (5 x 10^6 cells/0.5 ml culture).

DISCUSSION

Our studies clearly indicate that both T lymphocytes and MØ contribute to LPS potentiation of in vitro immune responses. Earlier work had suggested that the MØ or the T cell might be involved in adjuvanticity, however, this work has clearly shown that all three of the major lymphoid cell types are involved. The data with LAF (IL 1) suggest one mode by which endotoxin acts via the MØ and this could occur in several ways. The first might involve enhancement of LAF (IL 1) production during the immune response. A second possibility would be that LAF (IL 1) acts together with LPS toward the induction of a T helper cell population (McGhee, 1979a). The present work suggests that LPS is also acting on T helper cells because T cells from carrier primed, responder mouse spleen enhanced immune responses to the hapten TNP. Furthermore, the evidence that greater PFC helper factor production may occur in responder cultures treated with endotoxin, offers the possibility that LPS effects on the T cell result in higher levels of factor which influence the immune response of B cells. In this regard, Jacobs (1979) has provided evidence that TRF rich fractions can act synergistically with LPS toward boosting the *in vitro* response to heterologous erythrocytes. In addition to providing evidence that both T cells and MØ are required for adjuvanticity, we have also observed that B cells which are responsive to LPS are not required. Thus, NR B cells from either C3H/HeJ or from nude C57BL/10 ScN animals exhibit enhanced responses when mixed with R T cells and R MØ.

Since T cells are required for IgA immune responses to most antigens and precursor cells for such responses occur in GALT, the potential influence of the Gram negative gut flora bearing endotoxin must be assessed in light of the evidence that LPS acts on the T cell. Studies have been initiated which compare T and B cells and MØ from either GF or Conv mice in terms of their ability to respond to LPS. GF mice yield much higher responses to LPS than their Conv counterparts and we have presented evidence here that a naturally occurring T suppressor cell population can account for lower responses to LPS in the normal mouse. Experiments with purified T cells from PP of Conv mice indicated that GALT could serve as a reservoir for these suppressor cells. If this cell type is first generated in GALT by bacterial cell wall stimulation, e.g., LPS, we know from numerous other studies that GALT T cells can repopulate distant mucosa. This homing pattern could also account for the presence of these cells in spleen. This might represent one means by which the host controls potential toxic manifestations when LPS manages to pass the gut mucosal barrier.

ACKNOWLEDGMENTS

This work was supported in part by US Public Health Service grants DE 04217, DE 02670 and CA 13148.

REFERENCES

Farrar, J.J., W.J. Koopman, and J. Fuller-Bonar (1977). J. Immunol., 119, 47-54.
Goodman, M.G. and W.O. Weigle (1979). J. Immunol., 122, 2548-2553.
Hoffmann, M.K. and J. Watson (1979). J. Immunol., 122, 1371-1375.
Jacobs, D.M. (1979). J. Immunol., 122, 1421-1426.
McGhee, J.R., J.J. Farrar, S.M. Michalek, S.E. Mergenhagen and D.L. Rosenstreich (1979a). J. Exp. Med., 149, 793-807.
McGhee, J.R., S.M. Michalek, R.N. Moore, S.E. Mergenhagen and D.L. Rosenstreich (1979b). J. Immunol., 122, 2052-2058.
Michalek, S.M., R.N. Moore, J.R. McGhee, D.L. Rosenstreich and S.E. Mergenhagen 1979). J. Infect. Dis., (in press).
Mishell, R.I. and R.W. Dutton (1967). J. Exp. Med., 126, 423-442.
Rosenstreich, D.L. and L.M. Glode (1975). J. Immunol., 115, 777-780.
Uchiyama, T. and D.M. Jacobs (1978). J. Immunol., 121, 2340-2346.
Uchiyama, T. and D.M. Jacobs (1978). J. Immunol., 121, 2347-2351.

THE ROLE OF LIPID A AND LIPID A-ASSOCIATED PROTEIN IN CELL DEGRANULATION MECHANISMS

D. C. Morrison, Z. G. Oades and S. J. Betz

Department of Immunopathology, Research Institute of Scripps Clinic, La Jolla, CA 92037, USA

ABSTRACT

The mechanisms by which bacterial endotoxins bring about the release of vasoactive amines from inflammatory mediator cells have been examined. Particular attention has focused upon stimulation of rat peritoneal mast cells and rabbit platelets. In the former experimental system, the protein component of endotoxin (LAP-lipid A associated protein) has been demonstrated to initiate secretion of granule-localized histamine and serotonin from mast cells. The release of similar constituents from rabbit platelets may be accomplished either by endotoxin-mediated, serum complement-dependent platelet lysis or by lipid A-induced calcium dependent platelet secretion. The former platelet response is dependent upon the alternative complement pathway and is enhanced significantly by LAP. The latter secretory response is elicited only by endotoxins from rough mutants and does not require the presence of serum. The relative contribution of these mechanisms to the hypotension characteristic of gram negative sepsis is assessed.

KEYWORDS

Endotoxin; lipid A; lipid A-associated protein; platelets; mast cells; secretion; complement lysis.

INTRODUCTION

The biological effects of bacterial endotoxins following their interaction with host cells and tissues are protean. The consequences of such interactions may in some instances prove to be highly beneficial to the host, as in the case of enhancement of tumor rejection (Coley, 1891) or antibody formation to foreign antigens (Johnson, Gaines and Landy, 1956). In contrast, these same endotoxins may initiate profound hypotensive changes, disseminated intravascular coagulation and bilateral renal necrosis, often resulting in the death of the host (Sanarelli, 1926; Shwartzman, 1928). Yet in spite of intensive investigations into the various factors which may contribute to the total host response to these potent bacterial products, the precise mechanisms which contribute to their profound deleterious effects in vivo remain to be totally defined. This is particularly true in the case of the hypotensive changes brought about by endotoxins, which clinical studies have documented to be a major contributing factor to the more than 100,000 annual deaths resulting from gram negative bacteremia (McCabe, 1976).

It is clear that both humoral and cellular mediation systems offer themselves as potential targets for bacterial endotoxins in the generation of agents capable of bringing about vascular hypotension. With regard to the former mediation systems both the serum complement and the plasma coagulation pathways contain precursor molecules which, when activated, serve as potent vasoactive agents. Activation of serum complement by endotoxins, which may be accomplished by either the classical or the alternative pathway (Morrison and Kline, 1977) leads to the generation of the vasoactive anaphylatoxins C3a and C5a. Alternatively, initiation of the intrinsic coagulation system by Factor XII bound to endotoxin (Morrison and Cochrane, 1974) generates bradykinin from both high and low molecular weight kininogen. However, although there is some evidence to suggest a role for these pathways in endotoxin mediated hypotensive changes, there is equally compelling evidence to suggest that these systems play but a minimal role (reviewed in Morrison and Ulevitch, 1978).

Cellular mediation systems would appear to offer an equally attractive target for endotoxins in the initiation of vascular hypotension. Such cells would include platelets, basophils and mast cells. Each of these cell types contain the potent vasoactive amine histamine (and often serotonin) packaged within intracellular storage granules. Activation or lysis of these cells results in the release of these vasodilators to the external environment, primarily the vasculature. The critical contribution of these cells to the hypotension resulting from anaphylactic shock is well documented. However, the participation of these cells in endotoxin shock is less well understood, even though there is considerable evidence to suggest that, at least, platelets may be altered by an interaction with endotoxins. It is the purpose of this communication to describe the results of a number of in vitro experiments which characterize three distinct mechanisms for the release of vasoactive amines from these mediator cells elicited by endotoxins or endotoxin components. The first demonstrates that the LAP component of endotoxin will initiate secretion from rat peritoneal mast cells. The second system defines the mechanism by which endotoxins and serum complement interact to bring about lysis of rabbit platelets. Finally, we describe a new secretory response of washed rabbit (and more recently mouse) platelets following treatment with either lipid A or endotoxins from rough mutants.

For these experiments we have utilized a number of different preparations of endotoxins and endotoxin components prepared from the following gram negative bacteria: E. coli 0111:B4 (ATCC 12015), and its galactose epimerase deficient J5 mutant (the gift of Dr. L. Leive, NIH, Bethesda, MD), E. coli 055:B5 (ATCC 12014), Freiburg, W. Germany) and S. minnesota R595 (the gift of Dr. A. Nowotny, U. of Penn., Phil. PA). Most bacteria were extracted and purified with phenol-water (Westphal, Lüderitz and Bister, 1954) to prepare protein-free lipopolysaccharide (LPS) or with aqueous butanol (Morrison and Leive, 1975) to prepare endotoxins consisting of LAP-LPS complexes. Purified LAP free of LPS was prepared by subsequent extraction of LAP-LPS with phenol and purification of the phenol phase (Morrison, Betz and Jacobs, 1976). Purified protein free LPS from the J-5 and R595 organisms were prepared by extraction with phenol-chloroform-petroleum ether as described by Galanos and others, (1969). Isolated lipid A was prepared by mild acid hydrolysis of E. coli 055:B5 protein free LPS essentially as described earlier (Morrison and Verroust, 1973). Both the J5 and R595 LPS preparations as well as lipid A, were solubilized in 0.1% triethylamine, sonicated and extensively dialyzed against distilled water prior to use.

RESULTS

1. The Initiation of Mast Cell Secretion by Lipid A-Associated Protein

Preparations of rat peritoneal mast cells were obtained by peritoneal lavage of 300-350 gm male Wistar Rats (Charles River, Boston, MA) essentially as described previously (Morrison and others, 1974). The cells were then labelled with ^{3}H-serotonin (2.2 Ci/mMole, New England Nuclear, Boston, MA) and maintained in tris-tyrodes buffer at room temperature in plastic tubes until used for experiments. (We have previously documented that the release of exogenously supplied ^{3}H-serotonin parallels the release of endogenous histamine and thus serves as a convenient measure of mast cell release of vasoactive amines (Morrison and others, 1974). Following stimulation at 37°C with endotoxin preparations, mast cells were sedimented by centrifugation at 1000 rpm for 5 minutes and aliquots of supernatants assayed for release of ^{3}H-serotonin by liquid scintillation spectrometry. Detailed experimental conditions have been published earlier (Morrison and Betz, 1977).

The data shown in Fig. 1 indicate the response of mast cells, as assessed by the release of ^{3}H-serotonin, to increasing concentrations of protein free LPS, LPS-LAP complexes and LPS-free LAP (all from E. coli 0111:B4).

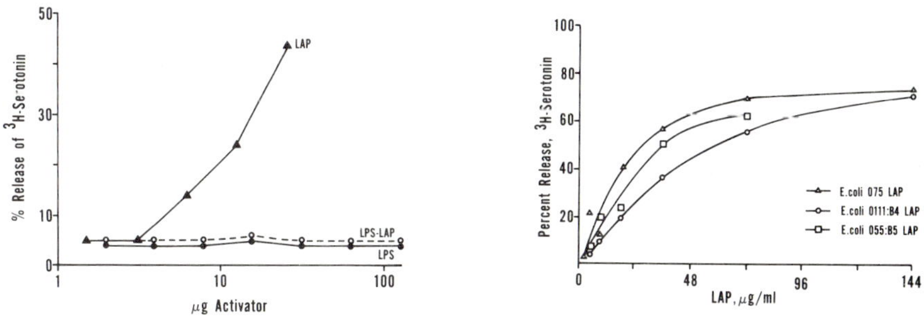

Figs. 1,2: LAP-INITIATED RELEASE OF SEROTONIN FROM MAST CELLS

Neither of the preparations containing LPS initiated any release of serotonin above background at any concentration tested. In contrast, the isolated LAP was highly active with amounts as low as 1-2 μg (in a final volume of 150 μl) initiating significant release of serotonin. The data shown in Fig. 2 confirm that the release of serotonin observed with the LAP isolated from the E. coli 0111:B4 LPS does not represent a unique property of this strain of bacteria. Virtually identical dose response profiles are obtained with LAP from two additional strains of bacteria, E. coli 055:B5 and E. coli 075. These combined data, therefore, support the concept that the isolated LAP component of LAP-LPS endotoxin complexes will initiate release of vasoactive amines from mast cells.

There exist two primary mechanisms by which the release of granule constituents from mast cells might be accomplished; non-cytolytic secretion and degranulation or cell death and subsequent lysis. To distinguish between these two possibilities we utilize the observations that the secretory mechanism for release of granule constituents requires both calcium and cellular energy. We therefore examined the effect of these variables on the release initiated by LAP. Calcium depletion was accomplished by the omission of this ion from the incubation buffer. Mast cells depleted of cellular energy (ATP) were prepared by incubation of cells for 30 minutes in the presence of 10 mM azide with 2-deoxyglucose substituted for glucose. As shown in Fig. 3 each of these procedures reduced significantly the mast cell response to LAP although relatively high concentrations of this stimulus did cause release independent of these variables, probably due to cytolysis. (Equally high concentrations of LAP have also been shown to be cytotoxic to lymphoid cells).

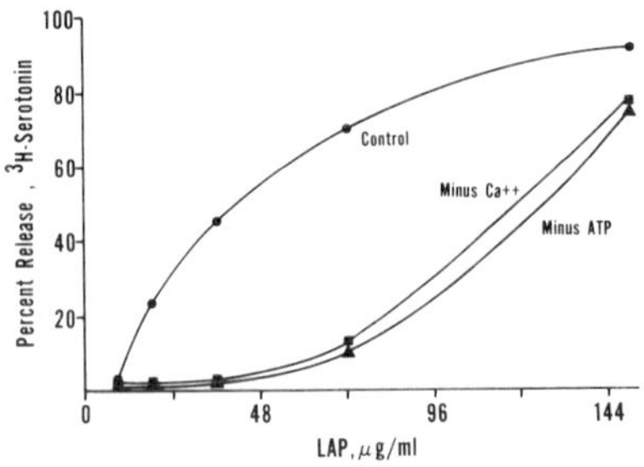

Fig. 3: EFFECT OF CALCIUM AND CELLULAR ENERGY (ATP) ON LAP-INITIATED RELEASE OF SEROTONIN FROM MAST CELLS

We have also demonstrated (data not shown) that mast cells, inactivated by treatment for 10 min at 47°, also do not respond to LAP until relatively high concentrations are achieved. Similarly, in other experiments not shown here, we have demonstrated that removal of macrophages and lymphocytes, both of which are known to respond to LAP (Betz and Morrison, 1977; Doe and others, 1978), had no effect on the mast cell response, thus suggesting that the LAP response is mediated by a direct interaction with the mast cell. At low concentrations of LAP, this interaction leads to mast cell secretion; at higher concentrations it is cytolytic. It may be postulated that the hydrophobic nature of LAP, which allows it to bind firmly to lipid A (Morrison and Betz, unpublished observations) may disrupt cell membranes at high concentrations, leading to release of intracellular granule constituents and lysis. Nevertheless these data would indicate that LAP has the capacity to initiate mast cell release of vasoactive amines by both a secretory and a cytolytic mechanism.

2. Endotoxin Initiated Complement Dependent Rabbit Platelet Lysis

The clinical development of pronounced thrombocytopenia in the bacteremic patient is recognized as one of the primary manifestations of gram negative sepsis (Cohen and Gardner, 1966). Equally profound platelet responses have been observed in experimental animals <u>in vivo</u> and <u>in vitro</u> following treatment with endotoxins (reviewed in Morrison and Ulevitch, 1978). The majority of these and other studies have indicated a prominent role for serum complement in these endotoxin induced platelet responses. The recent recognition of the several mechanisms by which endotoxins may initiate complement activation (Morrison and Kline, 1977) prompted us to explore the relationship between endotoxin initiated complement activation and resultant platelet damage.

For these experiments we utilized platelets obtained from New Zealand White rabbits, about 3-4 kg, which were prepared as described earlier (Morrison and others, 1978). Platelet responses were measured by the release of ^{3}H-serotonin, as a measure of the release of granule constituents, and lactic dehydrogenase (LDH) as a measure of the release of cytoplasmic constituents. For all of the experiments described in this Section the release of ^{3}H-serotonin and LDH were identical, indicating that the platelet responses obtained were the result of platelet lysis and not secretion. The rabbit plasma used in these experiments was anticoagulated with acid citrate dextrose, although essentially equivalent results were obtained with heparinized plasma. Complete experimental details have been published previously (Morrison and Oades, 1979; Morrison and others, 1978).

The results of our experiments have provided evidence that only preparations of endotoxins which activate the alternative complement pathway (e.g. those which have significant amounts of polysaccharide, Morrison and Kline, 1977) will initiate rabbit platelet lysis. In this respect neither isolated lipid A nor LPS from the rough J5 or R595 mutants will induce platelet lysis. Nevertheless our data indicate that the lipid A portion of LPS serves a critical role in attaching the LPS to the platelet. One piece of evidence in support of this hypothesis is presented in Table 1.

1° Incubation			2° Incubation			% Release
Platelets	LPS	PB	Platelets	LPS	Plasma	^3H Serotonin
+	-	-	-	-	+	5.3 ± 0.2
-	+	-	+	-	+	5.9 ± 0.1
+	+	-	-	-	+	28.0 ± 1.6
+	+	+	-	-	+	8.3 ± 0.2
+	-	-	-	+	+	70.5 ± 0.5

TABLE I

These data indicate first that LPS bound to the platelet will initiate lysis upon the subsequent addition of complement (plasma). Importantly, polymyxin B (PB) which we earlier have demonstrated binds to the lipid A portion of LPS (Morrison and Jacobs, 1977) but does not inhibit alternative pathway activation (Morrison and Kline, 1977) inhibits binding of LPS to the platelet. In other studies we have also shown that R595 LPS and lipid A will also inhibit platelet lysis initiated by 0111:B4 LPS, presumably by competing for binding sites on the platelet membrane.

We have also explored the role of LAP in mediating endotoxin induced platelet lysis. The presence of LAP has little detectable effect on alternative pathway complement activation (Morrison and Curry, unpublished observations) but inhibits the binding of complement component C1 to lipid A (Cooper and Morrison, 1978). Somewhat surprizingly the presence of LAP enhanced markedly the capacity of endotoxins to induce complement dependent platelet lysis (Fig. 4).

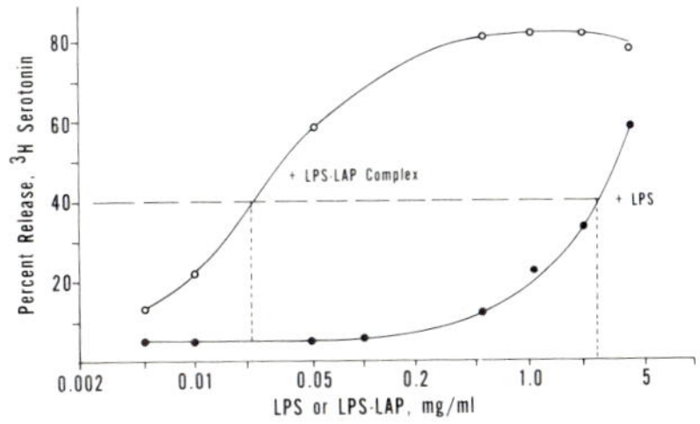

Fig. 4: THE EFFECT OF LAP ON ENDOTOXIN-MEDIATED PLATELET LYSIS BY COMPLEMENT

These combined data, therefore, as well as other experiments not described here, indicate that platelet lysis by endotoxins and complement requires attachment of the endotoxin to the platelet membrane via either the lipid A or LAP. Lysis then proceeds by activation of the alternative complement pathway, resulting in the release of the vasoactive amines histamine and serotonin.

3. Lipid A-Dependent Initiation of Rabbit Platelet Secretion

Although the primary mechanism for the release of platelet granule constituents results from platelet stimulation leading to noncytolytic secretion, such a response to endotoxins has not generally been observed (reviewed in Morrison and Ulevitch, 1978). However, a secretory response from human platelets to at least one endotoxin preparation (from S. enteriditis) has been reported (Hawiger and others, 1977). In the course of our studies to define the mechanism of endotoxin induced platelet lysis (summarized in Section 2) we observed that the LPS from

from S. minnesota R595 could induce platelet release of ^{3}H-serotonin. Equivalent responses were obtained with the J5 LPS and lipid A; however, LPS preparations containing large amounts of polysaccharide (e.g. 055:B5; 0111:B4) were inactive. The response required the preincubation of platelets with R595 LPS for 30-60 minutes prior to the addition of plasma. Subsequent experiments documented that the active component in plasma responsible for the release reaction was calcium. (A preliminary report of these results has been published [Oades, DiPietro and Morrison, 1979]).

Of significance in these experiments, the requirement for calcium in the secretory response was highly specific. As demonstrated by the data shown in Fig. 5, platelets preincubated for 60 min. with R595 LPS responded to the subsequent addition of calcium but not other divalent cations such as magnesium or barium.

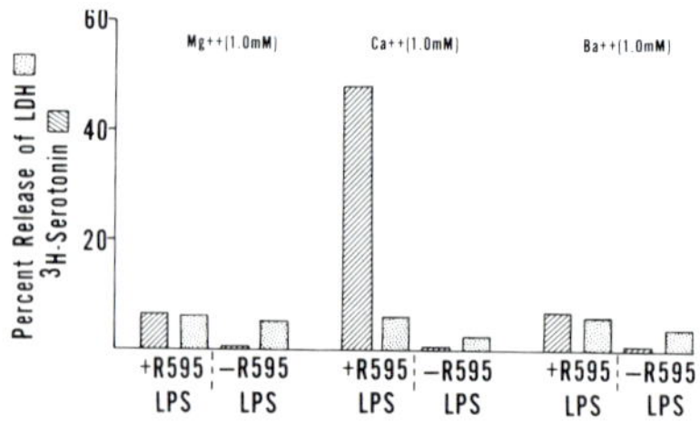

Fig. 5: THE DEPENDENCE OF PLATELET SECRETION UPON CALCIUM

In data not shown we have documented that concentrations of these ions tenfold higher were equally inactive; further, such concentrations did not block the calcium-induced secretion. Fig. 5 also illustrates the secretory nature of the platelet response in that granule-localized serotonin but not cytoplasmic LDH is released.

As indicated above, the platelet response requires that the cells be preincubated with the LPS prior to the addition of calcium. To examine this requirement in more detail, platelets were incubated with radiolabelled R595 LPS (Ulevitch, 1978) for various lengths of time at 37°, 33° and 23°, warmed to 37° and the secretory response to calcium subsequently assessed. In addition, the amount of LPS bound to the platelets was also determined. As shown in Fig. 6, whereas the association of LPS with the platelet was completely independent of time and temperature of incubation, the subsequent secretory response was critically dependent upon both of these variables.

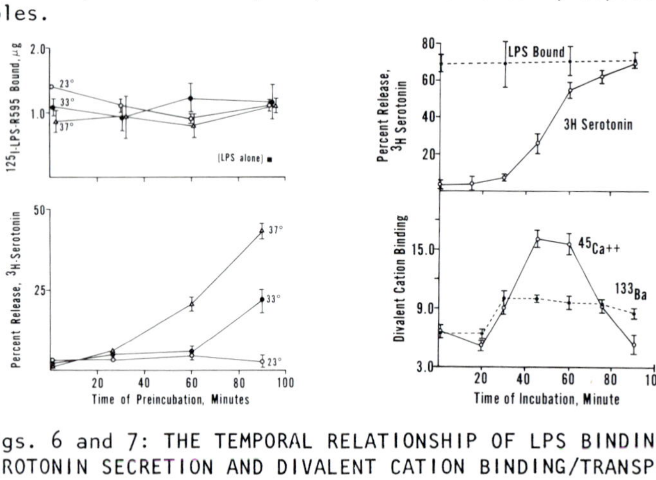

Figs. 6 and 7: THE TEMPORAL RELATIONSHIP OF LPS BINDING, ^{3}H-SEROTONIN SECRETION AND DIVALENT CATION BINDING/TRANSPORT

These data suggest that, following binding, the LPS-platelet association is somehow altered such that the platelet can then respond to the subsequent addition of calcium.

Experiments were also performed to determine whether calcium is preferentially associated with the platelet following incubation with LPS. Platelets were incubated with R595 LPS for various times after which the capacity of the cells to bind ^{45}Ca (as a marker of specific binding) or ^{133}Ba (as a marker of nonspecific binding) was assessed. Parallel samples were assessed for release of ^{3}H serotonin as well as ^{125}I-LPS binding. As shown in Fig. 7, there was a preferential association of ^{45}Ca with the platelet which accompanied the acquisition of the ability of the platelet to degranulate.

These data are consistant with the concept that the LPS can preferentially bind and/or transport calcium in the initiation of platelet secretion.

We have also assessed morphologically the effect of R595 LPS on rabbit platelets. Fig. 8a shows a scanning electron micrograph of a platelet prior to incubation with LPS and Fig. 8b a platelet 60 min. following incubation with LPS at 37°C.

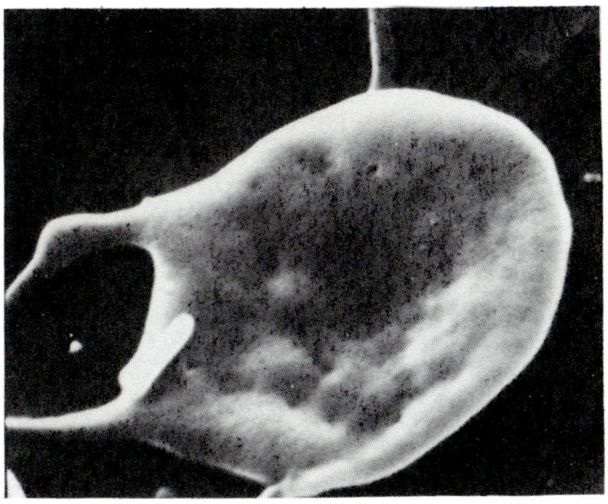

Fig. 8a

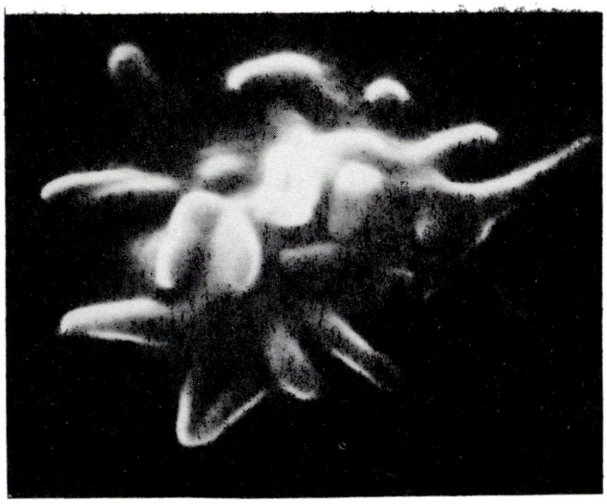

Fig. 8b

The striking morphological changes are readily apparent with the appearance of numerous pseudopods. Transmission electron micrographs confirm that these morphological alterations are not the result of an artifact of preparation.

These combined data demonstrate that lipid A-rich preparations of LPS induce both morphological and functional changes in rabbit platelets. These changes result in the selective capacity of the platelet to bind and/or translocate calcium in the initiation of secretion of vasoactive amines by rabbit platelets.

CONCLUSIONS

We have demonstrated three distinct mechanisms by which endotoxins or endotoxin components bring about the release of vasoactive amines <u>in vitro</u>. The ability of LAP to induce mast cell secretion and/or lysis <u>in vivo</u> would be dependent upon the dissociation of LAP from the LPS following release from the bacterium. Information relevant to this point is, however, currently not available. Complement mediated platelet lysis has been documented in <u>in vivo</u> experimental models of endotoxin shock. Its contribution to human disease is less clear. The lipid A-induced rabbit platelet secretory response, while probably of limited importance as a mechanism for the production of vasoactive amines *in vivo*, nevertheless offers a potentially exciting model system to examine biophysically and biochemically the mechanism of interaction between lipid A and cell membranes in general.

ACKNOWLEDGEMENTS

This research was supported by research grants AI-13187, AI-16411 and AI-07007. DCM is the recipient of a Research Career Development Award AI-00081. This is publication #1885 from the Research Institute of Scripps Clinic. Current address of DCM is Department of Microbiology, Emory University, Atlanta, GA. Current address of SJB is Universite de Lausanne, CH-1066 Epalinges, Switzerland.

REFERENCES

Betz, S. J., and D. C. Morrison (1977). J. Immunol., 119, 1475-1481.
Cohen, P., and F. H. Gardner (1966). Arch. Internal Med., 117, 113-124.
Coley, W. B. (1891). Ann. Surg., 14, 199-220.
Cooper, N. R., and D. C. Morrison (1978). J. Immunol., 120, 1862-1868.
Doe, W. F., D. T. Yang, D. C. Morrison, S.J. Betz, and P. M. Henson (1978). J. Exp. Med., 148, 557-568.
Galanos, C., O. Lüderitz, and O. Westphal (1969). Eur. J. Biochem., 9, 245-249.
Hawiger, J., A. Hawiger, S. Steckley, S. Timmons, and C. Chang (1977). Brit. J. Hematol., 35, 285-299.
Johnson, A. G., S. Gaines, and M. Landy (1956). J. Exp. Med., 103, 225-246.
McCabe, W. R. (1976). Ann. Rev. Med., 27, 335-341.
Morrison, D. C., and P. Verroust (1973). Proc. Soc. Exp. Biol. Med., 143, 1025-1030
Morrison, D. C., and C. G. Cochrane (1974). J. Exp. Med., 140, 797-811.
Morrison, D. C., J. F. Roser, P. M. Henson, and C. G. Cochrane (1974). J. Immunol. 112, 573-582.
Morrison, D. C., and L. Leive (1975). J. Biol. Chem., 250, 2911-2919.
Morrison, D. C., S. J. Betz, and D. M. Jacobs (1976). J. Exp. Med., 114, 840-846.
Morrison, D. C., and S. J. Betz (1977). J. Immunol., 119, 1790-1795.
Morrison, D. C., and D. M. Jacobs (1977). Immunochem., 113, 813-818.
Morrison, D. C., and L. F. Kline (1977). J. Immunol., 118, 362-368.
Morrison, D. C., L. F. Kline, Z. G. Oades, and P. M. Henson (1978). Infect. Immun. 20, 744-751.
Morrison, D. C., and R. J. Ulevitch (1978). Am. J. Path., 93, 527-618.
Morrison, D. C., and Z. G. Oades (1979). J. Immunol., 122, 753-758.
Oades, Z. G., D. DiPietro, and D. C. Morrison (1979). Fed. Proc., 38, 1431.
Sanarelli, G. (1924). Ann. Inst. Pasteur, 38, 11-72.
Schwartzman, G. (1928). J. Exp. Med., 48, 247-268.
Ulevitch, R. J. (1978). Immunochem., 15, 157-164.
Westphal, O., O. Lüderitz, and F. Bister (1954). Z. Naturforsch., 7B, 148-155.

PLATELET-ENDOTOXIN INTERACTIONS IN NORMAL AND RESISTANT ANIMALS

R. I. Walker

Microbiology Dept., Naval Medical Research Institute, Bethesda, Maryland 22014, USA

ABSTRACT

Platelet damage in the microcirculation may be a critical event during endotoxemia. Evidence for this problem was seen in pulmonary capillaries of sensitive (C3Heb/FeJ) mice challenged ip with a lethal (1 mg) dose of Salmonella typhi endotoxin. Leukopenia and thrombocytopenia similar to that in sensitive mice was obtained in endotoxin-resistant C3H/HeJ mice given 1 mg of toxin, but resistant animals resolved the pulmonary congestion which persisted in sensitive animals.

Circulating dog platelets respond to endotoxin in a dose-dependent manner and leukocytes phagocytize the aggregates which result. During phagocytosis hydrogen peroxide which reduces aggregation due to ADP and collagen, but not endotoxin, is released. Plasma factors may reduce endotoxin-induced platelet damage in the microcirculation and induction of tolerance can increase this protection. Tolerance accelerates aggregation in rabbit platelet rich plasma (PRP) exposed to endotoxin as well as reversal of this process. Tolerant characteristics are transferrable to normal PRP with tolerant plasma. The humoral factor is O antibody because it was heat stable, did not affect ADP or collagen induced aggregation, and was associated with appearance of O antibodies, but not lipid A antibodies. In fact, lipid A did not induce aggregation in PRP unless its specific antibody was added.

KEYWORDS

Platelet; endotoxin tolerance; endotoxemia; leukocyte; reticuloendothelial; microcirculation; lipid A; antibody

INTRODUCTION

Platelets are among the first cells to interact with endotoxin in the bloodstream and the nature of this interaction may determine survial. For example, in C_6 deficient rabbits the amount of initial platelet destruction correlated inversely with survival (Brown and Lachman, 1973), and increased binding indices of rabbit platelets for endotoxin is associated with increased mortality following challenge (Washida, 1978).

Platelets are important elements in the clearance of endotoxin (Das, Schwartz, and Folkman, 1973) and other particles (Donald, 1972; Noyes, McInturf and Blahuta, 1959; van Aken and Vreeken, 1969) from the bloodstream. During this process these inflammatory cells attach to particles and undergo dose-dependent (J.R. Fletcher and P.W. Ramwell, Circ. Shock, in press) aggregation and disaggregation until they reach reticuloendothelial (RE) organs (van Aken and Vreeken, 1969). However, lethal amounts of endotoxin may disturb the balance between the aggregation and disaggregation of platelets in non RE organs. The importance of such aberrations of normal platelet function is indicated by the correlation between the toxicity of different endotoxin preparations and their ability to aggregate washed human platelets (Ream and others, 1965) as well as the essential role of platelets in the generalized Shwartzman reaction (Margaretten and McKay, 1969).

The idea that accumulation of damaged platelets in the microcirculation of non RE organs could be a critical event during endotoxemia is consistent with the observation that some agents which protect against endotoxin shock also block aggregation of platelets induced by endotoxin and other substances (Evans, Lewis and Mustard, 1969; Packham and Mustard, 1977). Platelet aggregation induced by ADP (Evans, Lewis and Mustard, 1969) or antigen-antibody complexes (Evans, 1971) can also induce shock. Transient platelet aggregates induce vascular lesions (Jorgensen and others, 1970) which are among the first observable changes in the initial phase of endotoxemia besides leukopenia and thrombocytopenia (Urbaschek, Urbaschek and Neuhof, 1979).

MICROCIRCULATORY CONGESTION

Evidence for the importance of microcirculatory congestion in determining the outcome of endotoxemia was obtained by study of the deposition of platelets and leukocytes in genetically resistant (C3H/HeJ) and sensitive (C3Heb/FeJ) mice challenged ip with 1 mg of *Salmonella typhi* endotoxin. At this dose most of the sensitive animals died, but all of the C3H/HeJ mice survived. In both strains of mice the decreases in numbers of circulating leukocytes and platelets were comparable over a 24h period after challenge. However, in the resistant strain, deposition of cells changed with time. When the number of polymorphonuclear leukocytes (PMN) in pulmonary capillaries was determined, both strains were found to have equal degrees of capillary congestion at the end of the first hour after challenge. At 6h after challenge the resistant animals had resolved the congestion seen in the pulmonary capillaries, but congestion was continuing to increase the capillaries of the sensitive mice.

PLATELET-LEUKOCYTE INTERACTIONS

Platelets have a strong affinity for the endotoxin component of gram negative bacteria (Das, Schwartz and Folkman, 1974; Springer and Adye, 1975). Platelets interact with this component and promote uptake and destruction of bacteria by phagocytes (Smith, 1972). In this way platelets may determine the extent of the leukocyte response to endotoxin.

Evidence for this hypothesis was obtained by observing changes in the number of circulating leukocytes and platelets in dogs challenged iv with 4 ug/kg (no clincal symptoms) or 2 mg/kg (severe clinical symptoms) of endotoxin (Fig. 1). Dogs challenged with either the high dose of endotoxin or the low dose had similar degrees of leukopenia, but thrombocytopenia was only obtained with the high dose of endotoxin. Leukopenia is probably due largely to complement activity (O'Flaherty, Craddock and Jacob, 1977), but thrombocytopenia can be due to direct platelet-endotoxin interactions. This concept is consistent with increased *in vitro* aggregation of dog platelets seen with increasing doses of endotoxin (J.R. Fletcher, and P.W. Ramwell, Circ. Shock, in press).

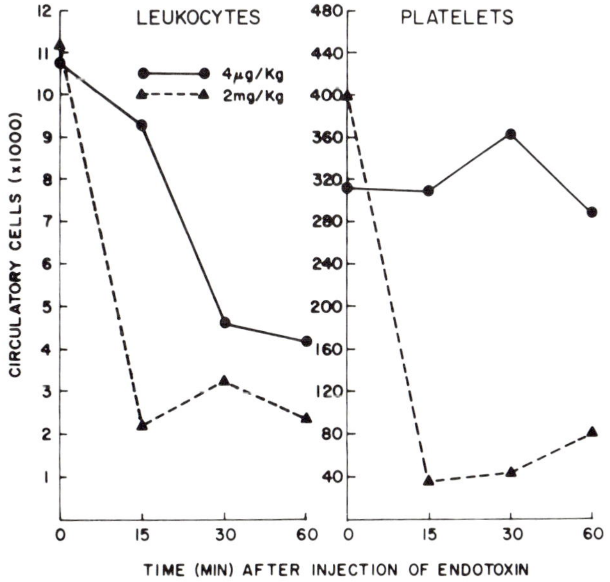

Fig. 1. Comparison of canine platelet and leukocyte responses to high and low doses of S. typhi endotoxin.

Leukocytes migrate towards and efficiently phagocytize platelet aggregates (Shirasawa and Chandler, 1971). If aggregation is too extensive, clearance of the microcirculation will not be achieved and continued phagocytosis with release of inflammatory mediators by the leukocytes will occur (Balis and others, 1978).

Although PMNs phagocytize platelet aggregates and kill bacteria which the aggregates may contain, they do not have the enzymatic capability to degrade endotoxin, a capability which macrophages do have (Filkins, 1971). The PMNs may be important, however, in clearance of the microcirculation and reduction of the formation of potentially harmful platelet aggregates. During the physical removal of cellular aggregates induced by endotoxin in the microcirculation, phagocytizing PMNs release hydrogen peroxide (Canoso and others, 1974; Levine and others, 1976) which can limit additional aggregation induced by ADP or collagen, but not endotoxin (R.I. Walker, J.R. Fletcher and D.A. Walden, Experienta, in press). This type of system would be well suited for elimination of microorganisms with simultaneous reduction of the dangerous additional aggregation induced by exposed collagen, ADP and other host factors (Jabs, Ferrell, and Robb, 1979).

In short, resistance to endotoxin requires development of means to reduce and resolve microcirculatory inflammation. Enhanced mobilization of leukocytes is one adaptation to achieve this goal. Another type of adaptation involves increased resistance of platelets to the damaging effects of endotoxin. This latter type of resistance seems to depend on levels of certain humoral factors in the plasma.

HUMORAL FACTORS AND THE PLATELET-ENDOTOXIN INTERACTION

Dogs (R.I. Walker, G.A. Parker, and T.J. MacVittie, Toxicon, in press; T.J. MacVittie and R.I. Walker, Exp. Hemat., in press) and guinea pigs (B. Urbaschek, personal communication) made tolerant to endotoxin display in vivo resistance to platelet damage in the microcirculation upon subsequent challenge. Platelet aggregation in vitro has also been studied with cells from normal and tolerant rabbits (Walker, Shields, and Fletcher, 1978). This was accomplished by spectrophotometric measurements of increases in transmitted light (aggregation) through platelet rich plasma (PRP) exposed to endotoxin. Normal PRP began to aggregate 1-2 min. after addition of endotoxin, and this aggregation was only slowly reversible (Fig. 2). In contrast, platelet aggregation was accelerated in PRP from tolerant rabbits and was quickly reversible.

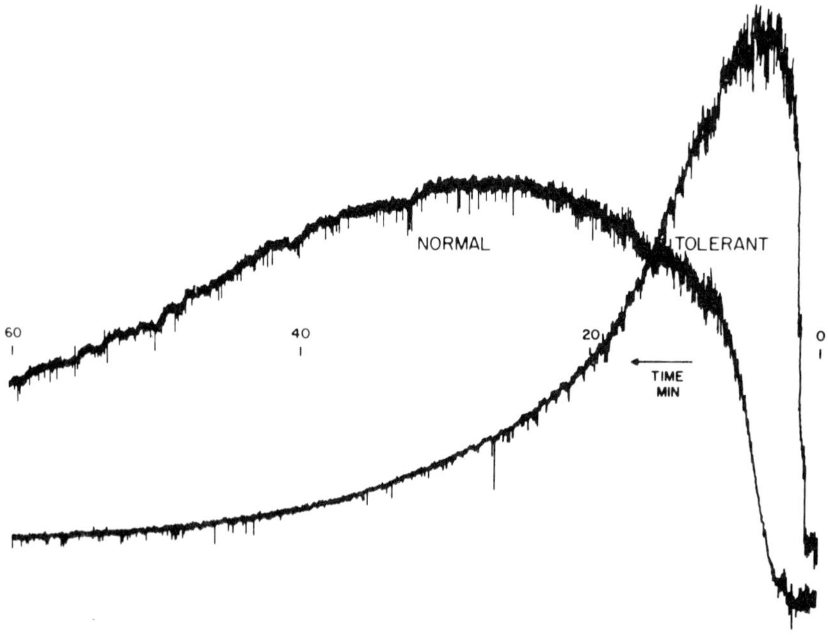

Fig. 2. Endotoxin-induced aggregation of platelets from normal and tolerant rabbits

Further studies were conducted to determine the mechanism responsible for this altered platelet reactivity in tolerant rabbits. Tolerant characteristics were transferable to normal PRP with plasma from tolerant rabbits. This humoral factor is probably antibody rather than a detoxifying enzyme or other non specific factor because it is heat stable (56°C for 1h), its presence correlated with the detection of antibodies, and it did not affect aggregation induced by ADP or collagen.

Antibody in rabbits made tolerant to endotoxin is directed against the O side chains rather than the lipid A moiety. Plasma used in the platelet experiments did not interact with purified lipid A in immunodiffusion plates, nor did antisera against lipid A interact with the smooth endotoxin.

Lipid A alone did not initiate platelet aggregation unless its specific antibody was also present. This could mean that complement activation at the platelet membrane surface is necessary for the aggregation response to occur (Morrison and Oades, 1979).

Although antibodies may alter platelet damage in the microcirculation, thereby facilitating delivery of toxic particles to the RE organs for subsequent detoxification, they are not essential for survival. In fact, tolerance can be achieved in animals incapable of forming antibodies (Zaldivar and Scher, 1979). Nonspecific factors are present in normal plasma which can modify endotoxin and, possibly, thereby alter its interaction with platelets (Ausprunk and Das, 1978; Johnson and others, 1977). Titers of at least some of these factors rise quickly after challenge with endotoxin (Moreau and Skarnes, 1973). The importance of these nonspecific plasma factors is indicated by the fact that transfusion of dogs with adequate amounts a heat-labile factor in normal dog plasma protects the animals against endotoxin-induced death, but not without considerable cellular injury (Walker and others, Adv. Shock Res., in press). Protection with normal plasma has also been observed in rabbits and mice challenged with endotoxin (unpublished data).

Nonspecific plasma factors provided a degree of protection to the host, and later appearance of antibody would enhance the efficiency of the protection obtained. Reduction of mediator release by macrophages (S.L. Snyder, S.K. Eklund and R.I. Walker, Canad. J. Micr., in press) and enhanced leukocyte mobilization (Fruhman, 1972; T.J. MacVittie and R.I. Walker, Exp. Hemat., in press; Walker and others, 1978), are also associated with development of resistance to endotoxin. All of these adaptations can contribute to reduction of endotoxin-induced damage to platelets and other cells in the microcirculation.

OVERVIEW

The studies of platelet interactions with endotoxin described above can be used to construct the model presented in Fig. 3. As shown, platelet membranes have specific receptors for endotoxin. Some plasma factors present in normal animals may modify endotoxin so that less damage follows the toxin-membrane interaction. Also, these factors could reduce toxin interactions with platelet membranes and facilitate direct toxin uptake by macrophages.

Lipid A can bind to platelet membranes, but does not cause aggregation. However, smooth endotoxin has O antigenic side chains which interact with the platelet membrane through activation of the alternative complement pathway, thereby causing aggregation when present in sufficient dose. In tolerant animals, antibody to the O side chains triggers a different aggregation pattern, probably via membrane effects of the classic complement pathway. Under optimal conditions platelets bind to endotoxin and undergo reactions to facilitate delivery of toxin to the RE system, where it is subsequently degraded. A vulnerable stage of this process is failure to resolve inflammatory foci in the microcirculation. Platelet aggregates induced by endotoxin and secondarily by other substances (i.e. collagen, ADP), persist in the capillaries, thereby permitting a continuation of the inflammatory response. Here mast cells degranulate, endothelial barriers are damaged and various inflammatory mediators are generated by leukocytes phagocytizing aggregates. Some mediators (i.e. histamine) can disrupt permeability barriers in the intestine and thereby permit additional toxin to enter the circulation (Walker and Porvaznik, 1978). The subsequent stasis and continued release of mediators contribute to death by interrupting normal function of vital organs.

Resistance to endotoxin involves adaptations to minimize and resolve damage to platelets and subsequent microvascular injury. These adaptations include elevated

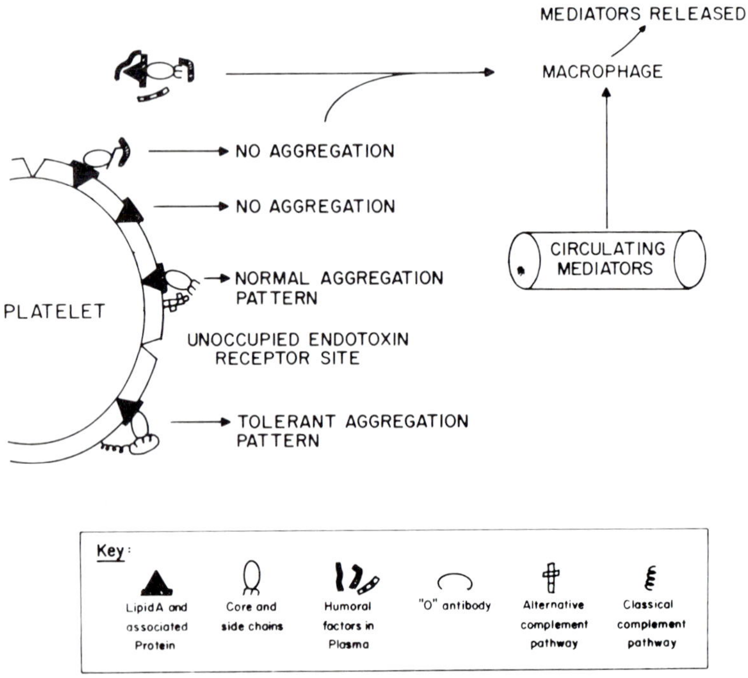

Fig. 3. Summary of types of platelet-endotoxin interaction.

titers of humoral substances which increase resistance of platelets to the effects of endotoxin, increased granulocyte reserves in the marrow which enable leukocytes to be mobilized rapidly to the microcirculation to facilitate clearance and attenuation of macrophage release of toxic amounts of mediators in response to stimulation by phagocytized particles and other mediators.

REFERENCES

Ausprunk, D.H. and J. Das (1978) Endotoxin-induced changes in human platelet membranes: morphologic evidence. Blood, 51,487-495.

Balis, J.U., E.S. Rappaport, L. Gerber, J. Fareed, F. Buddingh, and H.L. Messmore (1978) A primate model for prolonged endotoxin shock. Blood-vascular reactions and effects of glucorticoid treatment. Lab. Invest., 38,511-523.

Brown, D.L., and P.J. Lachmann (1973) The behavior of co4plement and platelets in lethal endotoxin shock in rabbits. Int. Arch. Allergy, 45,193-205.

Das, J., A.A. Schwartz, and J. Folkman (1973) Clearance of endotoxin by platelets: role in increasing the accuracy of the limulus gelation test in combating experimental endotoxemia. Surgery, 74,235-240.

Donald, K.J. (1972) The role of platelets in the clearance of collodial carbon from blood in rabbits: a light and electron microscope study. Pathology, 4, 295-301.

Evans, G., A.F. Lewis, and J.F. Mustard (1969) The role of platelet aggregation in the development of endotoxin shock. Brit. J. Surg., 56, 624.
Evans, G. (1971) Fate of endotoxin in the circulation. Adv Exp. Med. and Biol., 23,81-85.
Filkins, J.P. (1971) Comparison of endotoxin detoxification by leukocytes and macrophages. Proc. Soc. Exp. Biol. Med., 137,1396-1400.
Fruhman, G.J. (1972) Endotoxins and leukocyte mobilization. J. Reticuloendoth. Soc. 12,62-79.
Jabs, C.M., W.J. Ferrell, and H.J. Robb (1979) Plasma changes in endotoxin and anaphylactic shock (ATP, ADP and creatine phosphorus). Ann. Clin. Lab Sci., 9,121-132.
Johnson, K.J., P.A. Ward, S. Goralnik, and M.J. Osborn (1977) Isolation from human serum of an inactivator of bacterial lipopolysaccharide. Am. J. Path., 88,559-574.
Jorgensen, L., T. Hovig, H.C. Rowsell, and J.F. Mustard (1970) Adenosine diphosphate-induced platelet aggregation and vascular injury in swine and rabbits. Am. J. Pathol., 61,161-170.
Levine, P.H., R.S. Weinger, J. Simon, K.L. Scoon, and N.I. Krinsky (1976) Leukocyte-platelet interaction. Release of hydrogen peroxide by granulocytes as a modulator of platelet reactions. J. Clin. Invest. 57,955-963.
Margaretten, W. and D.G. McKay 1969). The role of the platelet in the generalized Shwartzman reaction. J. Exp. Med., 129,585-590.
Moreau, S.C. and R.C. Skarnes (1973) Host resistance to bacterial endotoxemia: mechanisms in endotoxin-tolerant animals. J. Inf. Dis., 128(s),122-133.
Morrison, D.C. and Z.G. Oades (1979) Mechanisms of lipopolysaccharide-initiated rabbit platelet responses II. Evidence that lipid A is responsible for binding of lipopolysaccharide to the platelet. J. Immunol., 122,753-758.
Nelson, W.R., and G.A. Taylor (1975) In vitro inhibition of endotoxin induced platelet aggregation with hydrocortisone sodium succinate (Solu-Cortef) Scand. J. Haematol., 15,35-44.
Noyes, H.E., C.R. McInturf, and G.J. Blahuta (1959) Studies on distribution of Escherichia coli endotoxin in mice. Proc. Soc. Exp. Biol. Med., 100,65-68.
O'Flaherty, J.T., P.R. Craddock, and H.S. Jacob (1977) Mechanism of anti-complementary activity of corticosteroids in vitro: Possible relevance in endotoxin shock. Proc. Soc. Exp. Biol. Med.154,206-209.
Packham, M.A., and J.F. Mustard (1977) Clinical pharmacology of platelets. Blood 50,535-573.
Ream, V.J., D. Deykin, V. Gurewich, and S. Wessler (1965) The aggregation of human platelets by bacterial endotoxin. J. Lab. Clin. Med., 66,245-252.
Shirasawa, K., and A.B. Chandler (1971) Phagocytosis of platelets by leukocytes in artificial thrombi and in platelet aggregates induced by adenosine diphosphate. Am. J. Path., 63,215-230.
Smith, S.B. (1972) Platelets in host resistance: In vitro interaction of platelets, bacteria and polymorphonuclear leukocytes. Blut, 25,104-107.
Springer, G.F., and J.C. Adye (1975) Endotoxin-binding substances from human leukocytes and platelets. Infect. Immun., 12,978-986.
Urbaschek, B., R. Urbaschek, and H. Neuhof (1979) Hemodynamic and metabolic changes in endotoxic shock in the minature pig. Circ. Shock, 6,197.
vanAken, W.G., and J. Vreeken (1969) Accumulation of macromolecular particles in the reticuloendothelial system (RES) mediated by platelet aggregation and disaggregation. Thromb. Diath. Haemorrh., 22,496-507.
Walker, R.I., and M.J. Porvaznik (1978) Disruption of the permeability barrier (zonula occludens) between intestinal epithelial cells by lethal doses of endotoxin. Infect. Immun., 21,655-658.
Walker, R.I., L.J. Shields, and J.R. Fletcher (1978) Platelet aggregation in rabbits made tolerant to endotoxin. Infect. Immun., 19,919-922.
Walker, R.I., S.L. Snyder, P.Z. Sobocinski, K.F. McCarthy and J.E. Egan (1978) Possible association of granulocyte mobilization to the peritoneal cavity with $ZnCl_2$-induced protection against endotoxin. Can. J. Micro., 24,834-838.

Washida, S. (1978) Endotoxin receptor site. II. Specificity of endotoxin receptor of platelets and sensitivity to endotoxin *in vivo*. *Acta. Med. Okayama*, *32*, 217-223.

Zaldivar, N.M., and I. Scher (1979) Endotoxin lethality and tolerance in mice: analysis with the B-lymphocyte-defective CBA/N strain. *Infect. Immun.*, *24*,127-134.

CELL GROWTH AND CANDIDACIDAL ACTIVITY OF MOUSE PERITONEAL MACROPHAGES IN RESPONSE TO GLUCOCORTICOID, CHOLERAGEN AND LIPOPOLYSACCHARIDE

R. T. Nozawa, N. Yanaki, R. Sekiguchi and T. Yokota

Department of Bacteriology, Juntendo University School of Medicine, Hongo, Tokyo 113, Japan

ABSTRACT

Normal, thioglycolate (TG)-stimulated and BCG-activated mouse peritoneal macrophages were cultivated *in vitro* with the conditioned medium of mouse L-929 cells (L-CM). The TG- and BCG-macrophages rapidly proliferated, whereas normal macrophages grew much more slowly. Certain immunomodulators, glucocorticoids at physiological concentrations, choleragen at 10 pg/ml, and *Escherichia coli* lipopolysaccharide (LPS) at 10 ng/ml inhibited the growth of the TG-macrophages. We devised a simple, quantitative assay method for candidacidal activity of macrophages. The normal mouse macrophage monolayers formed in 96-multiwell tissue culture plates were infected with serially diluted *Candida parapsilosis*, and an end-point of dilution, whereby candida cells added were found to be completely destroyed, was determined after a 48 hr incubation period. An addition of the L-CM to 20% of the culture medium, stimulated the killing activity more than 128-fold, compared with no addition of L-CM. In the medium containing the L-CM, macrophages spread very well on the plastic with several dendrites, whereas the cells spread poorly and gradually cytolysed in the medium lacking L-CM. It was found that *E. coli* LPS at 1-10 μg/ml and muramyl dipeptide at 100 μg/ml stimulated the activity 4 to 16 times. Macrophages treated with 1 μM dexamethasone and 10 ng/ml choleragen had a reduced activity (50% of the control). An application of this method to destroying other kinds of microbes, measuring the activity of other phagocytes, and screening of immunomodulators was discussed.

KEYWORDS

Mouse peritoneal macrophages; *in vitro* growth; candidacidal activity; conditioned medium; glucocorticoid; choleragen; lipopolysaccharide; muramyl dipeptide.

INTRODUCTION

The mononuclear phagocytes in blood (monocytes) and tissues (macrophages) play a variety of important roles in host defense responses. A mechanism to control the responses, via mononuclear phagocytic (MP) cells, is by activation of MP cells in the host, as demonstrated by the infection of certain bacteria (Mackaness, 1969). Activated MP cells enhance a variety of cellular functions including killing of intracellular pathogens (Mackaness, 1962; Ruskin, McIntosh and Remington, 1969) and cytotoxicity to tumor cells (Cleveland, Meltzer and Zbar, 1974; Hibbs, Jr., Lambert, Jr. and Remington, 1972; Ruco and Meltzer, 1977). The other mechanism is to control the absolute number of MP cells *in vivo*. The MP cells at a local inflammation site increase in number by the migration of blood monocytes (van Furth and Cohn, 1968; van Furth, Diesselhoff-den Dulk and Mattie, 1973). The migrated cells rapidly proliferate *in vitro* depending on a growth factor produced by lymphocytes (Hadden, Sadlik and Hadden, 1978) or fibroblasts (Defendi, 1976; Lin and Stewart, 1973; Stewart, Lin and Adles, 1975). We examined the effects of certain immunomodulators, glucocorticoid, choleragen and *E. coli* LPS, on the *in vitro* growth of mouse peritoneal macrophages. Furthermore, we devised a simple assay method for candidacidal activity of macrophages. By using the method, the effects of the immunomodulators were investigated.

MATERIALS AND METHODS

Preparation of L-929 conditioned medium. Mouse L-929 cells were cultivated up to confluency in MCDB medium (McKeehan, Hamilton and Ham, 1976), supplemented with 10% heated (56°C, 30 min) fetal calf serum and 100 μg/ml kanamycin sulfate. Cells were removed by treatment with EDTA solution (Nozawa and Guerrant, 1977), cell suspension was divided to one-fourth, and cultivated in a fresh medium for 48 hr. Cultured media were collected, filtered through a Millipore membrane and stored at -20°C until use.

Preparation of normal, TG- and BCG-macrophages. The 4-8 week old ddY male mice were injected intraperitoneally with 1.5 ml TG medium. On the third day, peritoneal exudate cells were collected by washing the cavity with the medium containing 50 unit/ml heparin sulfate. The cells were centrifuged at 150 x g for 2-3 min and washed with the medium. Normal macrophages were prepared from untreated animals. The BCG-macrophages were prepared from animals infected with BCG, as described (Cleveland, Meltzer and Zbar, 1974).

Cultivation of macrophages. The exudate cells were plated in a 16-mm Linbro multidish at 1-2 x 10^4 cells per dish. After 2-3 hr incubation period at 37°C, the media were removed, and the dishes were washed with the medium. Adherent cells to the dish were incubated in 2-ml of the medium containing determined volumes of L-CM in a humidified incubator, with 5% CO_2 and 95% air at 37°C. After an incubation for a set period of time, the media were removed, and the cells were washed with EDTA solution. The cells removed by EDTA solution, after an incubation at 37°C for 30 min, were counted with a Coulter counter.

An assay method for microbicidal activity of normal macrophages. Normal macrophages were cultured overnight with the medium after a removal of nonadherent cells. The macrophages were removed with EDTA, washed and suspended in the medium to 10^5 cells/ml. The 0.1 to 0.2 ml of the cell suspension was plated in a well of Falcon Micro Test II tissue culture plate (96 wells). The medium containing indicated volumes of L-CM added up to 0.25 ml. This medium was incubated for a further 6 hr. *C. parapsilosis*, grown on Sabouraud dextrose agar, was suspended in Puck's saline G, and cell suspension was serially diluted by 2-fold. A 10 to 15 μl of each candida cell suspension was layered on macrophage monolayers. Outgrowth of candida cells in a well was determined after a 48 hr incubation at 37°C, in a CO_2 incubator. An assay was done in duplicate, and outgrowths of candida cells were counted as being in both samples (+), in only one of the two samples (±), or in neither samples (-). The maximum number of the microbes killed (MNMK) in both wells was calculated by separately counting the viable candida cells on Sabouraud agar.

RESULTS

In vitro growth of mouse peritoneal macrophages. The normal, TG- and BCG-macrophages, from mouse peritoneal cavities, were cultivated in the medium with 20% L-CM

(Table 1). Normal macrophages slightly increased in number during a 7-day incubation period. On the other hand, TG- and BCG-macrophages proliferated about 10 times during the same incubation period.

TABLE 1 Growth of Macrophages *in vitro*

Macrophages	Cells per Dish, x 10^{-4}		Increase, fold
	Day 1	Day 8	
Normal	1.89	4.35	2.3
TG	0.93	11.80	12.7
BCG	0.83	8.67	10.5

Peritoneal macrophages were prepared as described and cultured in the medium with 20% L-CM. Experiment was done in triplicate.

Effect of steroid hormones on the growth of macrophages. The TG-macrophages were incubated with various concentrations of steroid hormones, and cell growth as percentage of control was plotted against steroid concentrations (Fig. 1). Glucocorticoids, dexamethasone and hydrocortisone, inhibited growth at physiological concentrations (10-100 nM). Progesterone had 100 times weaker inhibitory effect than hydrocortisone, and diethylstilbesterol and testosterone were 1,000 times weaker. The growth of BCG-macrophages was similarly inhibited by hydrocortisone (61% of control at 1 μM).

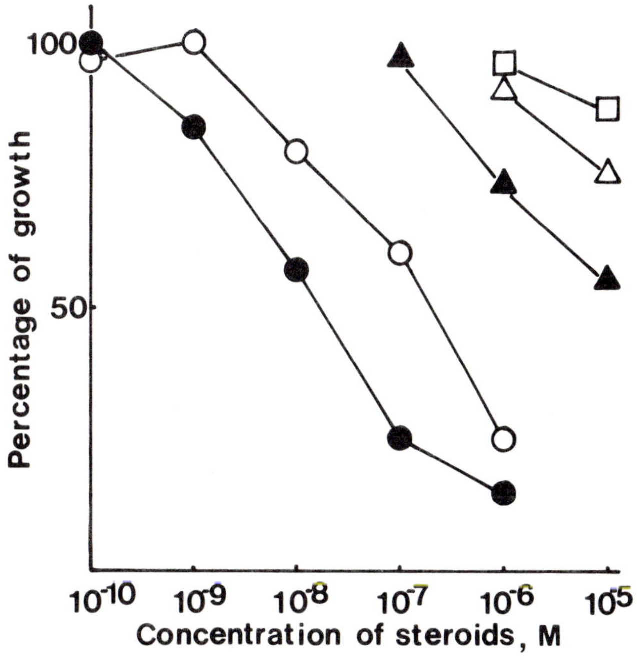

Fig. 1. Dose-response curves of steroids' effects on macrophage growth. The TG-macrophages were cultured with various steroids in the medium containing 25% L-CM for 6 days. —●— , dexamethasone; —○— , hydrocortisone; —▲— , progesterone; —△— ,diethylstilbesterol; —□— , testosterone.

Growth inhibition of macrophages by choleragen. The effect of choleragen on the growth of TG-macrophages was investigated. Very low concentrations of choleragen (10 pg/ml) completely inhibited the growth. A dibutyryl derivative of cyclic AMP also inhibited the growth at a concentration as low as 0.01 mM.

Growth of macrophages in response to E. coli LPS. When *E. coli* LPS was added to TG-macrophages, it induced a marked morphological change on the macrophage. Cells assumed a flat shape with ruffled plasma membrane. Above 10 ng/ml of LPS, however, the growth of the macrophages was inhibited (Fig. 2).

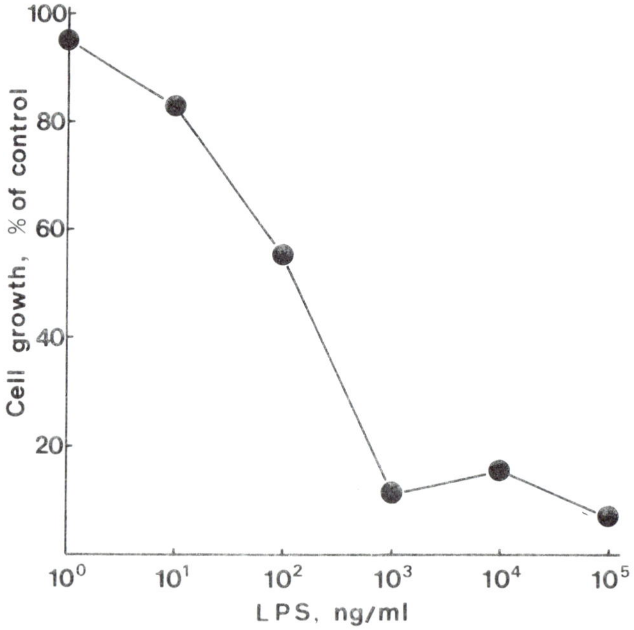

Fig. 2. Dose-response curve of the LPS-effect on macrophage growth. The TG-macrophages were cultured with *E. coli* LPS in the medium containing 20% L-CM for 6 days.

(a)
(b)
(c)
(d)

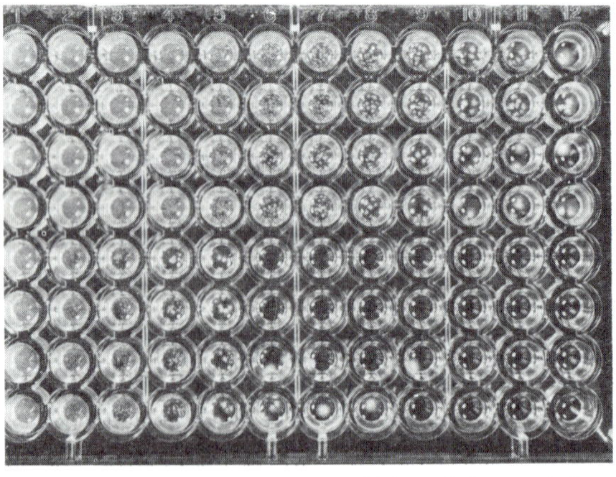

Fig. 3. Effect of L-CM on the candidacidal activity of macrophages. Experimental condition was the same as Table 2. Concentration of L-CM, (a) 0%; (b) 2%; (c) 20%; (d) 10%.

Effect of L-CM on candidacidal activity of normal macrophages. Macrophages were seeded at 10^4 per well, incubated for 6 hr in the medium containing various concentrations of L-CM, and then infected with candida cells (Table 2, Fig. 3). With 0-2%

TABLE 2. Growth of Candida Cells on Normal Macrophage Monolayers

L-CM (%)	Microbial dilution (fold)												
	2^1	2^2	2^3	2^4	2^5	2^6	2^7	2^8	2^9	2^{10}	2^{11}	2^{12}	MNMK
0	+	+	+	+	+	+	+	+	+	+	+	+	$\leqq 5$
2	+	+	+	+	+	+	+	+	+	+	+	+	$\leqq 5$
5	+	+	+	+	+	+	+	+	+	±	+	-	10
10	+	+	+	+	+	+	+	±	±	-	-	-	40
20	+	+	+	+	+	-	-	-	-	-	-	-	640
50	+	+	+	+	+	+	+	±	+	-	-	*	40

Macrophages were seeded at 10^4 per well. Growth of candida cells was expressed as mentioned in the text. *Not determined.

L-CM, the MNMK was less than 5. Above 5% L-CM the MNMK value increased, and with 20% L-CM, macrophage monolayers killed 640 candida cells infected. Thus, L-CM was found to stimulate the candidacidal activity of normal macrophages. With 50% L-CM, however, candidacidal activity of the macrophages decreased drastically, suggesting that a toxic substance to macrophages co-exists in L-CM. Normal macrophages were cultured in the medium with or without L-CM, and cell profiles were photographed (Fig. 4). Without L-CM, the cells spread poorly on plastic and numerous cells remained round. In the presence of L-CM, on the other hand, macrophages spread well with several dendrites, and were highly elongated. By incubating for longer periods of time without L-CM, the cells started to cytolyse and decreased in number (Fig. 5). In the presence of 20% L-CM, the cells slowly proliferated, as also shown in Table 1.

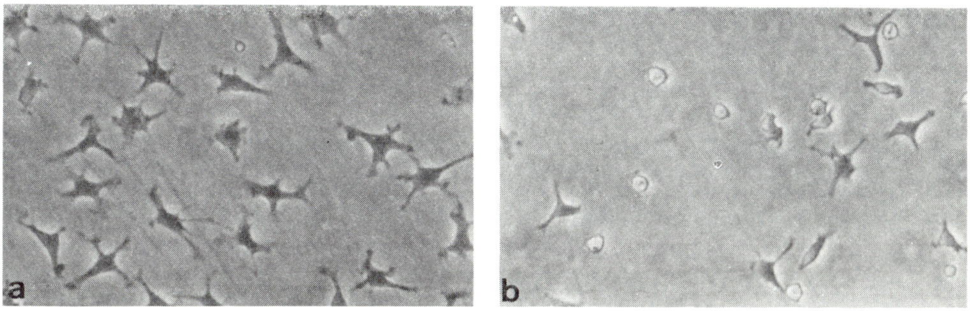

Fig. 4. Cell profiles of macrophages. Macrophages were incubated in a medium either (a) with, or (b) without 10% L-CM for 48 hr. Magnification: x 450.

Stimulation of the candidacidal activity by LPS and muramyl dipeptide. E. coli LPS and muramyl dipeptide (N-acethyl-muramyl-L-alanyl-D-isoglutamine, MDP) were tested in the assay system. Macrophages seeded in the wells were treated with various concentrations of each compound for 6 hr and then infected with candida cells (Table 3). In a condition without L-CM, 100 µg/ml of MDP stimulated by 4 times the macrophage candidacidal activity, expressed by the MNMK value. The MDP at 10 µg/ml had little or no effect. With 5% L-CM, however, the synthetic muramyl peptide,

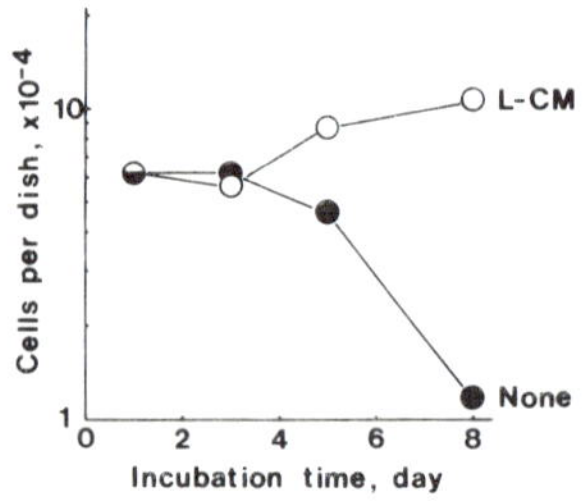

Fig. 5. Effect of L-CM on the maintenance of macrophages *in vitro*. Macrophages were plated in 35-mm Lux plastic tissue culture dishes. On day 1, one half of the dishes were added with L-CM to 20%, -○- , or 0%, -●- , and further incubated. Medium was renewed on day 3. Cells were removed from dish by EDTA treatment and counted by a Coulter counter. Experiment was done in duplicate.

TABLE 2. Effects of Immunomodulators on the Candidacidal Activity of Normal Macrophages

L-CM (%)	Agents added	Activity	
		MNMK	Increase, fold
0		176	
	LPS, 100 μg/ml	88	0.5
	10 μg/ml	352	2
	1 μg/ml	1408	8
	MDP, 100 μg/ml	704	4
	10 μg/ml	176	1
20		2816	16
5		282	
	MDP, 100 μg/ml	282	1
5		≦16	
	LPS, 100 μg/ml	63	≧4
	10 μg/ml	254	≧16
	1 μg/ml	63	≧4
	MDP, 100 μg/ml	≦16	
20		261	
	Choleragen, 10 ng/ml	130	0.5
	Dexamethasone, 1 μM	130	0.5

Macrophages were seeded at 1.5 x 10^4 per well.

even at 100 μg/ml, showed no stimulatory effect. On the other hand, *E. coli* LPS consistently stimulated the macrophage activity much more than MDP. In the absence of L-CM, one μg/ml of LPS stimulated activity by 8 times. The higher concentrations of LPS resulted in less stimulation, and at 100 μg/ml the LPS inhibited the macrophage activity altogether. With 5% L-CM, however, 10 μg/ml of LPS was the most active. Thus, the stimulation of macrophage by MDP and LPS on fungicidal activity was confirmed by our assay. However, the effects of both compounds were found conditional, depending on the concentration of L-CM.

Phagocytic activity of the macrophages treated with L-CM and LPS. Killing of microbes by phagocytes includes two processes: phagocytosis and intracellular killing.

The effect of L-CM on phagocytosis was examined by comparing with that of LPS (Fig. 6). During a 90-min incubation with *C. parapsilosis*, 80% of normal macrophages phagocytosed more than one microbe. Phagocytosis of the macrophage was slightly enhanced by the pretreatment with 20% L-CM for 6 hr, whereby, 90% of the cells phagocytosed more than one microbe. Furthermore, the population of the macrophages phagocytosing more than 6 microbes per cell, was doubling the result without L-CM pretreatment. The phagocytic ability of LPS-treated macrophages increased in a manner similar to the L-CM-treated macrophages.

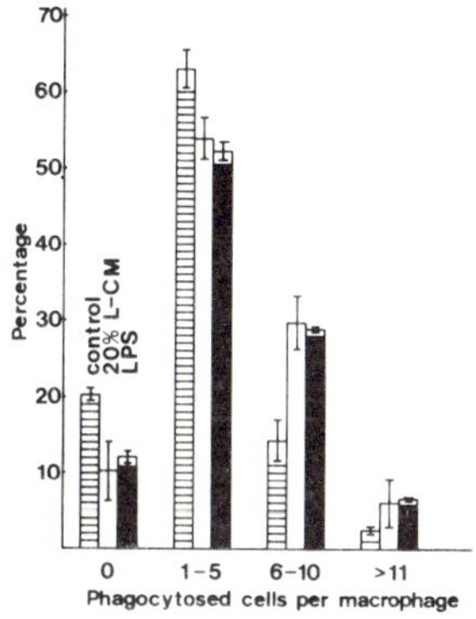

Fig. 6. Phagocytosis of candida cells by macrophage. Macrophages were treated with none, ▤ , 20% L-CM, □ , or 10 μg/ml of LPS, ■ , for 6 hr and then infected with candida cells (Multiplicity of infection: 8). Experiment was done in duplicate. Bar represents standard deviation.

Effects of dexamethasone and choleragen on candidacidal activity. The effect of dexamethasone and choleragen on the candidacidal activity of normal macrophages was examined (Table 3). In the presence of 20% L-CM, the macrophages pretreated with 1 μM dexamethasone and 10 ng/ml choleragen for 6 hr had half of the candidacidal activity of untreated cells.

DISCUSSION

When a local inflammation is induced, macrophages accumulate at the inflammation site within a few days. The increase of the macrophages is caused by the migration of blood monocytes to the site (van Furth and Cohn, 1968; van Furth, Diesselhof-den Dulk, and Mattie, 1973). Glucocorticoid inhibits the macrophages secreting a plasminogen activator, which is essential for the phagocytes to migrate (Vassalli, Hamilton and Reich, 1976). An anti-inflammatory effect of the steroid is partially explained by its inhibitory effect on the migration of macrophage, a mediator cell of inflammation (Davies and Allison, 1976), to the inflammation site. Macrophages accumulated at a local site will also increase by cell division. The mouse macrophages obtained from a peritoneal inflammation site had an enhanced ability to multiply in response to a growth factor produced by mouse fibroblasts, compared with normal peritoneal macrophages (Table 1). We found an inhibitory effect of glucocorticoid on the conditional growth of resident macrophages in hamster (Nozawa and Yokota, 1979), and confirmed the same effect of the steroid on macrophages obtained from an inflammation site (Fig. 1). Therefore, we would like to propose that the steroid exerts its anti-inflammatory effect via macrophage, not only by inhibiting migration, but also by inhibiting cell growth. The combined effects of the steroid, if administered, could reduce drastically the number of MP cells at the inflammation site, as evidenced (Thompson and van Furth, 1970).
A simple, quantitative assay method for activated macrophages was devised using *C. parapsilosis* as target cells. The microbicidal activity of normal macrophages was

greatly stimulated by the L-CM (Table 2). Since the L-CM accentuated the spreading of normal macrophages on plastic (Fig. 4) and was necessary for maintaining macrophages *in vitro* (Fig. 5), these combined effects of L-CM on macrophages should have rendered the cells much more microbicidal than the control cells. Recently, Handman and Burgess (1979) reported that a purified granulocyte-macrophage colony-stimulatin factor stimulates Leishmania killing by macrophages. The colony stimulating factor is identical with macrophage growth factor (Stanley and co-workers, 1976). The latter was found in L-CM (Table 1). Therefore, our result coincides with that of Handman and Burgess. One of the applications of the *in vitro* assay for the activated macrophages is the screening of nonspecific immunostimulants. Well known immunostimulants *in vivo* and *in vitro*, LPS and MDP, were tested (Table 3). The MDP, which activates the cytotoxicity of macrophage to tumor cells (Juy and Chedid, 1975), stimulated the fungicidal activity of the macrophages only at a high concentration, 100 μg/ml, and its stimulatory effect disappeared when L-CM was present. Bacterial LPS, which stimulates the cytotoxicity to tumor cells (Alexander and Evans, 1971), increased the candidacidal activity at a concentration range between 1-100 μg/ml. Since the LPS at the concentrations was toxic to macrophages (Fig. 2), the stimulatory effect by LPS was variable, depending on L-CM. The LPS at 100 μg/ml inhibited the fungicidal activity in the absence of L-CM, but stimulated the activity when L-CM was present, suggesting that L-CM partially neutralizes the toxicity of LPS. The use of bacterial LPS in the treatment of cancer brought inconsistent and unpredictable results (Berendt, North and Kirstein, 1978). One of the reasons for the ambiguous results might be due to LPS's toxicity to macrophages. Thus, an agent which is not cytotoxic to macrophages but stimulates the microbicidal activity of the phagocytes seems to be ideal as an immunostimulant. We are trying to find such stimulant by using this assay method and an assay for macrophage growth *in vitro*.

REFERENCES

Alexander, P., and R. Evans (1971) *Nat. New Biol., 232,* 76-78.

Berendt, M. J., J. R. North, and D. P. Kirstein (1978) *J. Exp. Med., 148,* 1550-1559.

Cleveland, R.P., M.S. Meltzer, and B. Zbar (1974) *J. Nat. Cancer Inst., 52,* 1887-189

Davies, P., and A. C. Allison (1976) In D. S. Nelson (Ed.), *Immunology of the Macrophage.* Academic Press, New York. Chap. 17, pp. 427-461.

Defendi, V. (1976) In D. S. Nelson (Ed.), *Immunology of the Macrophage.* Academic Press, New York. Chap. 11, pp. 275-290.

Hadden, J. W., J. R. Sadlik, and E. M. Hadden (1978) *J. Immunol., 121,* 231-238.

Handman, E., and A. W. Burgess (1979) *J. Immunol., 122,* 1134-1137.

Hibbs, Jr. J. B., L. H. Lambert, Jr., and J. S. Remington (1972) *Nat New Biol., 235,* 48-50.

Juy, D., and L. Chedid (1975) *Proc. Nat Acad. Sci. U. S. A., 72,* 4105-4109.

Lin, H., and C. C. Stewart (1973) *Nat New Biol., 243,* 176-177.

Mackaness, G. B. (1962) *J. Exp. Med., 116,* 381-406.

Mackaness, G. B. (1969) In S. Mudd (Ed.), *Infectious Agents and Host Reaction.* W. B. Saunders, Philadelphia. Chap. 3, pp. 61-75.

McKeehan, W. L., W. G. Hamilton, and R. G. Ham (1976) *Proc. Nat. Acad. Sci. U. S. A. 73,* 2023-2027.

Nozawa, R. T., and R. L. Guerrant (1977) *Exp. Cell Res., 107,* 25-30.

Nozawa, R. T., and T. Yokota (1979) *J. Cell. Physiol.,* Accepted for publication.

Ruco, L. P., and M. S. Meltzer (1977) *Cell. Immunol., 32,* 203-215.

Ruskin, J., J. McIntosh, and J. S. Remington (1969) *J. Immunol., 103,* 252-259.

Stewart, C. C., H-S. Lin, and C. Adles (1975) *J. Exp. Med., 141,* 1114-1132.

Stanley, E.R., M. Cifone, P.M. Heard, and V. Defendi (1976) *J. Exp. Med., 143,* 631-

Thompson, J., and R. van Furth (1970) *J. Exp. Med., 131,* 429-442.

van Furth, R., and Z. A. Cohn (1968) *J. Exp. Med., 128,* 415-435.

van Furth, R., M. M. C. Diesselhof-den Dulk, and H. Mattie (1973) *J. Exp. Med., 138,* 1314-1330.

Vassalli, J-D., J. Hamilton, and E. Reich (1976) *Cell, 8,* 271-281.

THE EFFECT OF ENDOTOXIC SUBSTANCES ON GRANULOPOIESIS

R. Urbaschek and B. Urbaschek

Department of Immunology and Serology, Institute of Hygiene and Medical Microbiology, Klinikum Mannheim, University of Heidelberg, D6, 5, 68 Mannheim, Federal Republic of Germany

ABSTRACT

The stimulatory effect of endotoxins on hematopoiesis is well established. We were interested in the question whether this is a direct effect of endotoxin or whether this is due to histamine or serotonin substances which are released following endotoxin injection. We determined splenic and femoral CFUs and CFUc after injection with histamine in mice. Serum CSF levels were followed after histamine and serotonin injection. The results indicated that histamine had no effect on CFUs and CFUc in vivo similar to that of endotoxin. Both, histamine and serotonin failed to induce elevation in CSF serum levels.

We were interested also in the effect of a methylated preparation extracted according to the method of Nowotny (1963) from S. marcescens endotoxin which has reduced toxicity. We found that this preparation induces within 24 h a nonspecific tolerance against lethal doses of endotoxin and lethal X-irradiation. This substance stimulates hematopoiesis, particularly granulopoiesis, as demonstrated by kinetic studies of blood, splenic and femoral CFUs and CFUc, peripheral differential blood counts and serum CSF levels. These results suggest that this substance increases nonspecific resistance due to its capacity to stimulate granulopoiesis. In the state of nonspecific tolerance CSF levels increased to the same extent as in nontolerant animals. In tolerant mice no inhibitors of CSF activity were found in undiluted serum.

KEYWORDS

Endotoxin; detoxified endotoxin; histamine; serotonin; nonspecific tolerance; radioprotection; granulopoiesis; CFUs; CFUc; CSF;

ABBREVIATIONS: CFUs, colony-forming unit spleen, pluripotent stem cells; CFUc, colony-forming unit culture, granulocytic committed stem cells; CSF, colony-stimulating factor.

INTRODUCTION

The stimulatory effect of bacterial endotoxins is well established. Besides its action on the stem cell compartments (Hanks and Ainsworth, 1965, Monette, Gilio, and Chalifoux, 1974, Quesenberry, 1973, Smith and co-workers, 1966) it induces elevated CSF levels (Chervenick, 1972, Metcalf, 1971, Quesenberry and co-workers, 1972). Many biological activities of endotoxin are mediated through substances such as histamine and serotonin. In this context it was of interest to study the effect of these biogenic amines on hematopoiesis *in vivo*. Byron (1976, 1977) reported that 4-methylhistamine triggered CFUs from the Go state into the S-phase of the cell cycle by *in vitro* treatment of mouse bone marrow cells. We determined splenic and femoral CFUs and CFUc after injection of histamine in mice. We also studied serum CSF levels at different times after histamine and serotonin injection in comparison to CSF levels following *E. coli* endotoxin and an endotoxin extracted by Grehn (1979) from anaerobic bacteria. The histamine and serotonin concentrations used have been reported to be radioprotective in mice (Langendorff and co-workers, 1959, Melching and co-workers 1964, van der Meer and van Bekkum 1959). This fact also could lead to the assumption that these substances do have an effect on hematopoiesis, as shown in the case of the radioprotective effect of endotoxin by Smith (1966) and Hanks and Ainsworth (1967).

Using a methylated endotoxin which has reduced toxicity we found that this substance induces a nonspecific tolerance within 24 hours against lethal doses of endotoxin and lethal X-irradiation (Urbaschek 1967, Urbaschek and Nowotny 1968). This substance induces a marked stimulation of granulopoiesis (Urbaschek and Ringert 1975, Urbaschek, R. and Urbaschek, B., 1977, Urbaschek, R. 1979).

Quesenberry and co-workers (1975, 1978) reported that seven daily injections of endotoxin resulted in subsequent inability to respond to endotoxin with elevated serum CSF levels. In our tolerance model, which is inducable with one pretreatment of detoxified endotoxin 24 hours prior to the challenge injection with endotoxin, CSF levels did increase to the same extent as in nontolerant animals.

HISTAMINE AND SEROTONIN

CFUs, CFUc and serum CSF were determined according the methods of Till and McCulloch (1961), Bradley and Metcalf (1966), and Pluznik and Sachs (1965). Femoral and splenic CFUs were determined by transfering suspensions of bone marrow or spleen cells of mice 6 h, 24 h, and 72 h following i.p. injection of 285 mg/kg histamine into lethally irradiated (650 R) mice. Eight days later the number of colonies formed in the spleen of the irradiated mice were determined. Femoral and splenic CFUc were calculated from the number of colonies that were formed in culture seven days after plating the suspensions of bone marrow or spleen cells.

The results showed that there was no similar effect of histamine on CFUs or CFUc to that observed following endotoxin (Fig. 1). Ten minutes and two hours after i.p. injections of histamine or serotonin serum CSF were measured at different concentrations as shown in Table I. Here the results two hours after injection are presented together with the results obtained two hours after injection of E. coli endotoxin, B. fragilis endotoxin and the methylated endotoxin from S. marcescens. It can be seen that histamine and serotonin did not induce elevated serum CSF levels.

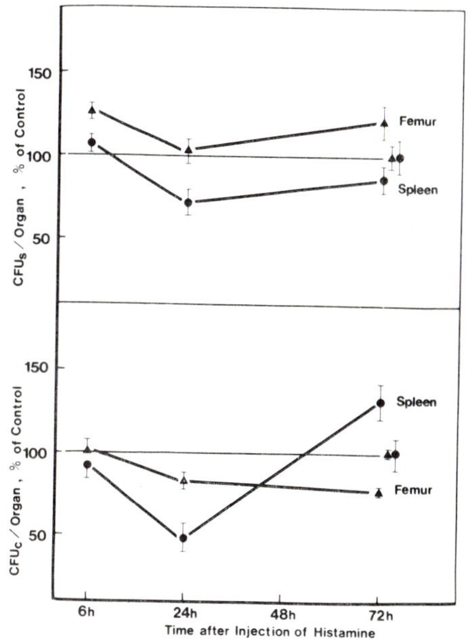

Fig. 1. Femoral and Splenic CFUs and CFUc following Histamine

TABLE 1 Serum CSF in Mice 2 Hours after Intravenous Injection, ±sd

Substance	Colonies/10^5 cells Serum dilution 1:2	Substance	Colonies/10^5 cells Serum dilution 1:2
E. coli endotoxin		Histamine	
5 µg	113.3 ± 2.1	0.3 mg	1.0 ± 0.8
50 µg	118.7 ± 1.5	1.5 mg	1.8 ± 0.9
B. fragilis endotoxin		7.5 mg	1.8 ± 1.3
5 µg	29.7 ± 3.8	Serotonin	
50 µg	84.7 ± 3.1	0.2 mg	10.8 ± 2.8
S. marcescens detoxified endotoxin		0.6 mg	3.5 ± 1.3
		1.8 mg	2.5 ± 1.3
5 µg	77.6 ± 4.2	Saline	
50 µg	147.3 ± 18.5	0.2 ml	1.8 ± 2.1

DETOXIFIED ENDOTOXIN

Boivin-type endotoxin from S. marcescens was treated with potassium methylate according to the method of Nowotny (1963). Femoral, splenic and blood CFUs as well as femoral and splenic CFUc were determined at 6 h, 24 h, 48 h, and 72 h following intravenous injection of 50 µg of detoxified endotoxin, a concentration which induces endotoxin tolerance and X-ray protection. Splenic and blood CFUs were significantely increased 72 hours after injection. The number of blood CFUs were elevated as early as 6 hours after endotoxin. Splenic and femoral CFUc responses are illustrated in Fig. 2 and the CFUs/CFUc ratio in Fig. 3, indicating an increased proliferation of CFUs into CFUc. Differentiation of peripheral blood revealed a marked increase in monocytes 24 hours after injection.

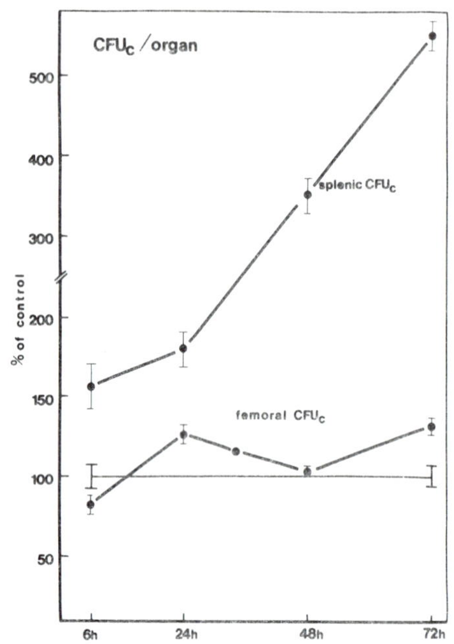

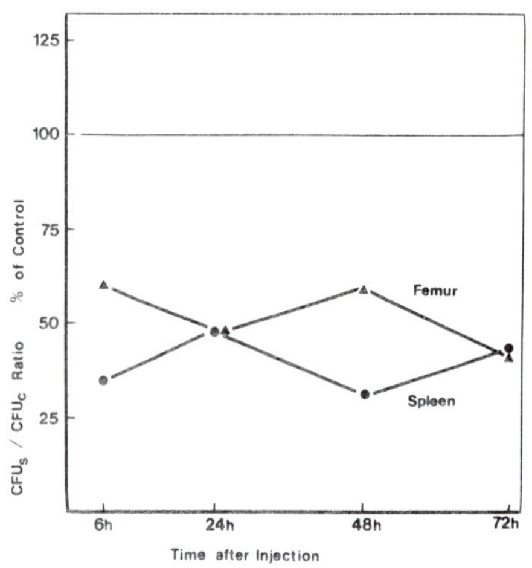

Fig. 2. and Fig. 3. Number of CFUc and CFUs/CFUc ratio at different times after 50 µg detoxified endotoxin

TOLERANCE

Quesenberry and co-workers (1975, 1978) reported the nonresponsiveness in regard to endotoxin-induced elevation of serum CSF of mice which were made tolerant by seven daily injections of endotoxin. We repeated these studies and confirmed that these mice do not respond with elevated serum CSF levels when challenged with 5 µg of endotoxin and noticed that at 50 µg serum CSF levels increase (Fig. 4). In our model, inducing tolerance by one single pretreatment with detoxified endotoxin 24 hours prior to the challenge with endotoxin

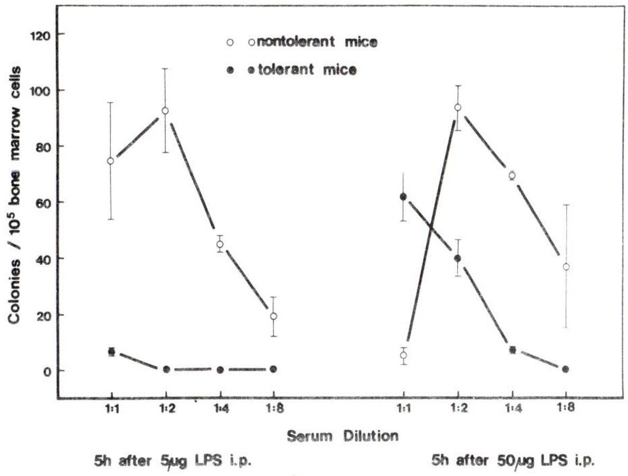

Fig. 4. Serum CSF in Mice made Tolerant by 7 Daily Injections of Endotoxin and in Nontolerant Mice

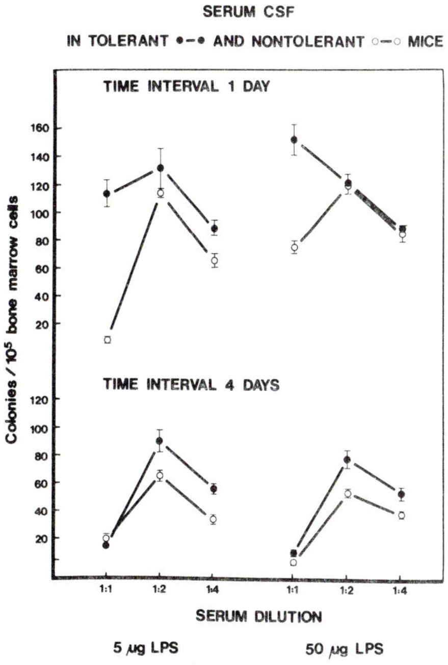

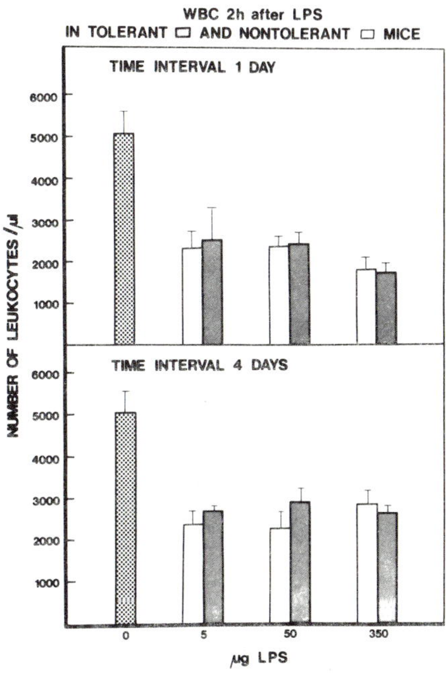

Fig. 5. and Fig. 6. Serum CSF and White Blood Cell Counts (WBC) in Mice made Tolerant with one Injection of Detoxified Endotoxin 24 Hours resp. 4 Days prior to Endotoxin Challenge

serum CSF levels increased by the same amount as in nontolerant animals (Fig. 5). CSF increase also occurred in animals which were challenged 4 days after pretreatment with detoxified endotoxin. In these tolerant mice 100 % survived when challenged with an LD 50 endotoxin concentration at day 1 or at day 4 following injection of detoxified endotoxin. At both time intervals after pretreatment white blood cell counts decreased when endotoxin was injected at 5 μg, 50 μg or 350 μg per mouse. The drop in white blood cell counts does not differ from that in nontolerant animals. Parallel studies using endotoxin as tolerance-inducing substance gave similar results in survival rate, CSF levels and white blood cell counts.

DISCUSSION

The experiments described above do not indicate a major role of histamine or serotonin in mediating the effects of endotoxin on hematopoiesis. Byron (1976 , 1977) had reported the stimulatory effect of 4-methylhistamine on CFUs in vitro and Hirata (1975) demonstrated inhibition of an endotoxin-induced increase in cellularity in bone marrow after injection of antihistaminics. He also produced bone marrow responses by an injection of histamine or serotonin. In our experiments bone marrow cellularity was slightly decreased at all times determined after histamine injection. We also were unable to observe an increase in CSF following histamine or serotonin injections at different concentrations.

Splenic CFUc increase significantly after 50 μg of detoxified endotoxin; this reaction of the granulocytic committed stem cell compartment is similar to that described by Monette (1972) after endotoxin injection. Serum CSF levels increase with a peak two hours after injection, and the CFUs/CFUc ratio determined give evidence for the marked stimulatory effect on granulopoiesis. Detoxified endotoxin might induce nonspecific endotoxin tolerance and radioprotection through its ability to stimulate granulopoiesis.

Mice made tolerant with methylated endotoxin or endotoxin - as indicated by increased postendotoxin survival (100 % versus 50 % in nontolerant animals) occuring at day 1 or at day 4 do react with elevated CSF levels and a decrease in white blood cell counts. We were unable to find nonresponsiveness in these mice as regard to endotoxin-induced CSF elevations as described by Quesenberry (1975, 1978). Injection of 50 μg endotoxin in mice which were rendered tolerant by seven daily injections of 10 μg endotoxin i.p. responsed with an increase in serum CSF while they failed to react with increased CSF when challenged with 5 μg endotoxin (Fig. 4). In regard to the different tolerant status in mice described by Greer and Rietschel (1978) at day 1 and day 4 we could not find different reactivities at this time intervals in the experimental model used. The results in Fig. 4 and Fig. 5 demonstrate that CSF levels in undiluted postendotoxin sera are lower than those in a dilution of 1:2 indicating an inhibition of CSF activity in the bioassay used. In the meantime several inhibitors CSF activity have been discussed. In tolerant mice (Fig. 4 and Fig. 5) with the exception of day 4 interval in Fig. 5 no inhibitors of CSF activity were detectable.

REFERENCES

Bradley, T. R., and D. Metcalf (1966). The growth of mouse bone marrow cells in vitro. J. exp. Biol. med. Sci., 44, 287-300.
Byron, J. W. (1976). Bone-marrow toxicity of metiamide. Lancet II, 1350.
Byron, J. W. (1977). Mechanism for histamine H_2-receptor induced cell-cycle changes in the bone marrow stem cell. Agents and Actions, 7, 209-213.
Chervenick, P. A. (1972). Effect of endotoxin and postendotoxins plasma on in vitro granulopoiesis. J. Lab. clin. Med., 79, 1014-1020.
Greer, G. G., and E. Th. Rietschel (1978). Inverse relationship between the susceptibility of lipopolysaccharide (Lipid A)-pretreated mice to the hypothermic and lethal effect of lipopolysaccharide. Infect. Immun., 20, 366-374.
Grehn, M. Endotoxins of anaerobic gram-negative bacteria. Infection, in press 1979.
Hanks, G. E., and E. J. Ainsworth (1965). The effect of endotoxin on radiosensitivity, proliferation, and migration of colony-forming units in the mouse. Radiat. Res., 25, 195.
Hanks, G. E., and E. J. Ainsworth (1967). Repopulation of colony-forming units in mice. Nature, 215, 20-22.
Hirata, M. (1975). Inhibitory effects of antihistamines and antiserotonins on the bone marrow reactions produced by Escherichia coli endotoxin in mice. J. Infect. Dis., 132, 611-616.
Langendorff, H., H. J. Melching, and H. A. Ladner (1959). 5-Hydroxytryptamine as a radiation protective substance in animals. Internat. J. Radiat. Biol., 1, 24-27.
Melching, H. J., C. Streffer, H. A. Ladner und U. Allert (1964). Zur Frage der Strahlenschutzwirksamkeit von Histamin bei Mäusen. Naturwissenschaften, 51, 266.
Metcalf, D. (1971). Acute antigen-induced elevation of serum colony-stimulating factor (CSF) levels. Immunology, 21, 427-436.
Monette, F. C., B. S. Morse, D. Howard, E. Niskanen, and F. Stohlman, Jr. (1972). Hemopoietic stem cell proliferation and migration following Bordetella pertussis vaccine. Cell Tissue Kinet., 5, 121-129.
Nowotny, A. (1963). Endotoxoid preparations. Nature, 197, 721-722.
Pluznik, D. H., and L. Sachs (1965). The cloning of normal "mast" cells in tissue culture. J. Cell Physiol., 66, 319-324.
Quesenberry, P., A. Morley, F. Stohlman Jr., K. A. Rickard, and D. Howard (1972). Effect of endotoxin on granulopoiesis and colony-stimulating factor. New Engl. J. Med., 286, 227-232.
Quesenberry, P., A. Morley, M. Ryan, D. Howard, and F. Stohlman Jr. (1973). The effect of endotoxin on murine stem cells. J. Cell Physiol., 82, 239-244.
Quesenberry, P., J. Halperin, M. Ryan, and F. Stohlman Jr. (1975). Tolerance to the granulocyte-releasing and colony-stimulating factor elevating effects of endotoxin. Blood, 45, 789-800.
Quesenberry, P., H. Cohen, J. Levin, R. Sullivan, P. Bealmear, and M. Ryan (1978). Effects of bacterial infection and irradiation on serum colony-stimulating factor levels in tolerant and non-tolerant CF_1 mice. Blood, 51, 229-244.
Smith, W. W., G. Brecher, S. Fred, R. A. Budd (1966). Effect of endotoxin on the kinetics of hematopoietic colony-forming cells in irradiated mice. Radiat. Res., 27, 710-717.

Till, J. E., and E. A. McCulloch (1961). A direct measurement of the radiation sensitivity of normal mouse bone marrow cells. Radiat. Res., 14, 213-222.

Urbaschek, B. (1967). Zur Frage des Wirkungsmechanismus bakterieller Endotoxine und seiner Beeinflussung. Habilitationsschrift, Universität Heidelberg.

Urbaschek, B., and A. Nowotny (1968). Endotoxin tolerance induced by detoxified endotoxin (endotoxoid). Proc. Soc. exp. Biol. Med., 127, 650-652.

Urbaschek, B., and R. H. Ringert (1975). The effect of detoxified endotoxin on bone marrow. In Urbaschek, B., R. Urbaschek, and E. Neter (Eds.), Gram-negative bacterial infections and mode of endotoxin actions - Pathophysiological, immunological, and clinical aspects. Springer, Wien/New York. pp. 200-205.

Urbaschek, R., and B. Urbaschek (1977). Zur Wirkung von detoxifiziertem Endotoxin auf die Hämatopoese. Blut, 35, 357.

Urbaschek, R. Effects of bacterial products on granulopoiesis. In Escobar, M. R., and H. Friedman (Eds.), Macrophages and Lymphocytes: Nature, Functions and Interaction. Plenum Publishing Corporation, N.Y. In press, 1979.

van der Meer, C., and D. W. van Bekkum (1959). Mechanism of radiation protection by histamine and other biological amines. Int. J. Radiat. Biol., 1, 5-23.

ACKNOWLEDGEMENT

This investigation was supported by Deutsche Forschungsgemeinschaft SFB 90, Heidelberg. We thank Sylvia Ganninger and Ruth Breunig for their excellent technical assistance.

STUDIES ON LIPID A IMMUNITY IN ANIMALS AND INFECTED CHILDREN

B. Kaijser*, I. Mattsby-Baltzer*, B. Jaup*, U. Jodal** and U. Lindberg****

**Inst. of Med. Microbiology, Univ. of Göteborg, Sweden*
***Dept. of Pediatr., Children's Hospital, Univ. of Göteborg, Sweden*
****Dept. of Gastroenterology, Sahlgren's Hospital, Univ. of Göteborg, Sweden*

ABSTRACT

Enzyme-linked immunosorbent assay (ELISA) was applied for antibody determination against lipid A. It was found to be more sensitive than the generally used indirect hemolysis (IH) or indirect hemagglutination (IHA).

ELISA was also used to study exposure of lipid A on E.coli bacteria as well as in crude antigen preparations. Lipid A was only available in all four crude antigen preparations made from rough E.coli.

Anti-lipid A antibody production was investigated in immunized animals. Animal immunized with lipid A conjugated to bacteria or erythrocytes in general gave an antibody response, in contrast to rabbits immunized with bacteria.

Anti-lipid A antibodies were also analyzed in healthy children and adults, adults with inflammatory bowel disease, IBD (Ulcerative colitis or Mb Crohn), or girls with urinary tract infection (UTI). Antibodies of both IgG and IgM class were found in children and adults. The frequency of IgG antibodies to lipid A was lower in patients with a great extension of their IBD as compared with healthy adults. Children with acute pyelonephritis, cystitis or asymptomatic bacteriuria had higher IgG antibody titres compared to healthy children. Especially high IgG titres were found in patients with progressive kidney damage caused by pyelonephritis. Similar results were observed in infected rats with pyelonephritis. Intraperitoneally injected antiserum to lipid A did not protect rats against experimentally induced pyelonephritis.

In conclusion, lipid A seemed not to be available on the intact bacteria but in the material released from the bacteria. The availability of the antigenic lipid A structure was higher in antigen preparations from rough bacteria defect in the lipopolysaccharide synthesis than in smooth bacteria.

Infection caused by gram-negative bacteria in the urinary tract induced anti-lipid A antibody production although no protection with anti-lipid A serum was afforded against pyelonephritis. Determination of anti-lipid A antibodies might reveal progressive kidney damage in individuals with acute pyelonephritis.

KEYWORDS

Lipid A; Lipopolysaccharide; E.coli; Protection; Diagnosis; Urinary tract infection; Inflammatory bowel disease.

INTRODUCTION

The lipopolysaccharide (LPS), the O antigen, is one of the dominating surface antigens of gram-negative rods. The lipid part, lipid A, of these antigens represents the toxic part of the LPS molecule and is responsible for symptoms like fever in infected individuals (Galanos and co-workers 1971; 1972; Galanos 1975). Earlier investigations have also indicated a tissue damaging effect of lipid A or anti-lipid A by induction of interstitial nephritis in dogs (Westenfelder and Galanos, 1974; Westenfelder, Galanos and Madsen, 1975).

The lipopolysaccharides have been widely used for serological diagnosis of infections caused by gram-negative bacteria (i.a. Jodal, Lindberg and Lincoln, 1975). They have also been suggested for prophylactic immunization against urinary tract infection. A great variety of immunologically different lipopolysaccharides exists, which makes the serological diagnosis or vaccine composition complicated. Therefore the lipid A which is similar in many different gram-negative bacteria, has been suggested to be used as a common antigen for many different strains (Lüderitz, Jann and Wheat, 1968; Lüderitz and co-workers, 1974; Hase and Rietschel 1976; Johns, Bruins and McCabe, 1977). Lipid A has been shown to induce antibody formation when administrered coated onto bacteria or after immunization with some S and R forms of Salmonella (Galanos, Lüderitz and Westphal, 1971).

The aim of the present investigation was to analyse the immunological characteristics of lipid A in animals and infected children, especially in relation to urinary tract infection, caused by E.coli, and in inflammatory bowel disease.

MATERIALS AND METHODS

Patients

Girls treated at the Children's Hospital in Göteborg, for acute urinary tract infection, were included in the study. The diagnosis of acute pyelonephritis, acute cystitis or asymptomatic bacteriuria was defined as earlier described by Jodal, Lindberg and Lincoln (1975). Non-infected children attending the same hospital were included as healthy controls.

Adults treated at the Sahlgren's Hospital in Göteborg for inflammatory bowel disease (Ulcerative colitis or Mb Crohn) were also included.

Animals

Rabbits were used for immunization experiments. Sprague-Dawley rats were used for experimental, ascending pyelonephritis as described by Kaijser, Larsson and Olling (1978).

Immunization

The immunization procedure using isolated lipid A attached to erythrocytes or to hydrolyzed rough Salmonella bacteria was performed as described by Galanos, Lüderitz and Westphal (1971) and immunization with rough E.coli was done as earlier (Mattsby-Baltzer and Kaijser, 1979). Immunization with smooth E.coli was performed as described by Holmgren (1970).

Antigens

Crude O antigen preparations were produced from smooth and rough E.coli and Salmonella minnesota R595 according to Winberg and co-workers (1963). Lipid A was prepared as described recently (Mattsby-Baltzer and Kaijser, 1979) from LPS obtained from E.coli EH100 (Galanos, Lüderitz and Westphal, 1969).

Immunoprecipitation analyses

These were performed according to Wadsworth (1957).

Antibody determinations

The enzyme-linked immunosorbent assay, ELISA, as described by Engvall and Perlmann (1972) was applied for antibody determination against lipid A (Mattsby-Baltzer and Kaijser, 1979). In some experiments the indirect hemolysis, IH, according to Galanos, Lüderitz and Westphal (1971) or indirect hemagglutination, IHA, as originally described by Neter (1956) was used.

Absorption experiments

Inhibition of the lipid A - anti-lipid A reaction as measured with ELISA was performed as shown by Mattsby-Baltzer and Kaijser (1979).

RESULTS

Immunological characteristics of lipid A, antibody assay and immune response in animals

Immunoprecipitation analyses of purified lipid A showed three precipitates indicating a heterogeneity (Mattsby-Baltzer and Kaijser, 1979). Using this purified lipid A for comparison of different antibody assays showed that the ELISA was about 28 times more sensitive than IHA for IgM antibodies and about four thousand times more sensitive than IHA for IgG antibodies (Mattsby-Baltzer and Kaijser, 1979). The ELISA was also more sensitive than indirect hemolysis for IgM antibodies. The indirect hemolysis assay did not reveal IgG antibodies.

Absorption experiments for inhibition of the antibody activity in ELISA to test availability of lipid A on bacteria or in the O antigen in solution showed that lipid A was more exposed in O antigen preparations from rough mutants than in those from smooth strains (Mattsby-Baltzer and Kaijser, 1979) (Table 1). Lipid A seemed not to be available on either smooth or rough bacteria.

Immunization of rabbits with lipid A coated to erythrocytes or to hydrolysed Salmonella minnesota bacteria gave a marked antibody response of both IgG and IgM antibodies (Mattsby-Baltzer and Kaijser, 1979). Immunization of rabbits with whole E.coli bacteria gave an IgM antibody response in 5 out of 36 rabbits. Three of the anti-lipid A antibody producing rabbits where immunized with E.coli rough mutants with possibly more exposed lipid A. Anti-lipid A antibodies was also found in experimentally infected rats that attracted pyelonephritis (Mattsby-Baltzer and co-workers (in manuscript, c)).

TABLE 1 Inhibition, with killed bacteria or crude O antigen preparation, of the lipid A - anti-lipid A reaction as determined with enzyme-linked immunosorbent assay.

Bacteria used for inhibition	% Inhibition with	
	Formalinkilled bacteria	Crude, boiled O antigen preparation
E.coli with O antigen 1, 2, 4, 6, 7, 8, 18 or 75	0	0
E.coli with R1 or R3 antigen	0	90 resp. 55
Salmonella minnesota R595	0	72

Anti-lipid A antibodies in healthy individuals and in girls with acute UTI

80 % of new-borns had detectable anti-lipid A antibodies of the IgG class, but no IgM antibodies (Mattsby-Baltzer and co-workers (in manuscript, a)). Non-infected children aged 4 months to two years had no antibody activity to lipid A. About 50 % of children more than two years of age had IgG as well as IgM antibodies against lipid A.

Girls with acute pyelonephritis, acute cystitis or asymptomatic bacteriuria showed significantly higher levels of IgG antibodies against lipid A compared to healthy children (Mattsby-Baltzer and co-workers (in manuscript, a)). There was no difference concerning anti-lipid A antibody concentrations between patients with acute pyelonephritis, acute cystitis or asymptomatic bacteriuria. However, in females with acute pyelonephritis and with progressive kidney damage the concentration of IgG anti-lipid A antibodies were significantly higher than in others (Mattsby-Baltzer and co-workers (in manuscript, b)).

Anti-lipid A antibodies in inflammatory bowel disease (IBD)

Anti-lipid A antibody activity of IgG class as measured with ELISA was lower in patients with IBD compared to healthy individuals (Mattsby-Baltzer and co-workers (in manuscript, d)). There was no difference between patients with Ulcerative colitis compared to Mb Crohn.

Protection experiments

Passively transferred anti-lipid A antibodies were not protective against experimental, ascending pyelonephritis in rats caused by E.coli O6K13H1 (Mattsby-Baltzer and co-workers (in manuscript, c)).

DISCUSSION

Isolated lipid A in solution does in general not induce antibody formation (Galanos, 1975). The immunogenicity of lipid A can however be increased by conjugation to for example erythrocytes or to hydrolysed, rough Salmonella bacteria. Immunization with such preparations induce antibody production in approximately all immunized rabbits in contrast to immunization of rabbits with whole bacteria, and is therefore preferable for antibody production.

Different techniques have been applied for antibody determination against lipid A. Indirect hemagglutination (Neter, 1956) or indirect hemolysis (Galanos, Lüderitz, Westphal, 1971) have been used earlier. In comparison to enzyme-linked immunosorbent assay, ELISA, these techniques are apparently less sensitive. Furthermore the ELISA-technique is advantagous since it can reveal antibodies of different immunoglobulin classes separately.

Using the ELISA it was also possible to show that lipid A in general is not available for antibodies on bacteria or in O antigen preparations of the bacteria with the smooth type of lipopolysaccharide. In rough bacteria with defect polysaccharide chain of the LPS, lipid A was more available as revealed by better antibody induction in immunized rabbits and by absorption experiments with crude O antigen preparations (Mattsby-Baltzer and Kaijser, 1979). The low availability of lipid A on bacteria might explain why lipid A antibodies seem not to protect against infection as investigated using different animal models (Bruins and co-workers, 1977; Mattsby-Baltzer and co-workers (in manuscript, c)). In contrast antibodies to both E.coli O antigen and K antigen are protective against acute, experimental pyelonephritis (Kaijser and Olling, 1973; Kaijser and Ahlstedt, 1977; Kaijser, Larsson and Olling, 1978).

It is also in accordance with findings that lipid A antibodies might decrease fever reactions and skin necrosis induced by lipopolysaccharide and lipid A as suggested by Rietschel and Galanos (1977).

The possibility to utilize lipid A as a common antigen of Enterobacteriaceae for serological diagnosis of gram-negative infections is because of low immunogenicity and availability as shown in this study limited. However the finding of increased anti-lipid A antibody activity in children with acute pyelonephritis and progressive kidney damage is promising and might be utilized to determine this important group of patients.

In conclusion we have shown the low availability of lipid A on live E.coli bacteria, the advantage of ELISA for antibody determination against lipid A and indicated the usefulness of lipid A antibody determination as a tool to reveal progressive kidney damage in children with acute pyelonephritis.

ACKNOWLEDGEMENT

The skilful technical assistance by Ms Helena Kahu is very much appreciated. The investigation was supported by grants from the Swedish Medical Research Council (project No. 215) and by grants from STU, Sweden (project No. 78-3452).

REFERENCES

Bruins, S.C., R. Stumacher, M.A. Johns, and W.R. McCabe (1977). Immunization with R mutants of Salmonella minnesota. III. Comparison of the protective effect of immunization with lipid A and Re mutant. Infect. Immun., 17, 16-20.

Engvall, E., and P. Perlmann (1972). Enzyme-linked immunosorbent assay, ELISA. III. Quantitation of specific antibodies by enzyme-labelled anti-immunoglobulin in antigen-coated tubes. J. Immunol., 109, 129-135.

Galanos, C. (1975). Physical state and biological activity of lipopolysaccharides.

Toxicity and immunogenicity of the lipid A component. Z. Immunitaetsforsch. Exp. Ther., 149, 214-229.

Galanos, C., O. Lüderitz, and O. Westphal (1969). A new method for the extraction of R lipopolysaccharides. Eur. J. Biochem., 9, 245-249.

Galanos, C., O. Lüderitz, and O. Westphal (1971). Preparation and properties of antisera against the lipid-A component of bacterial lipopolysaccharides. Eur. J. Biochem., 24, 116-122.

Galanos, C., E.T. Rietschel, O. Lüderitz, and O. Westphal (1971). Interaction of lipopolysaccharides and lipid A with complement. Eur. J. Biochem., 19, 143-152.

Galanos, C., E.T. Rietschel, O. Lüderitz, O. Westphal, Y.B. Kim, and W. Watson (1972). Biological activities of lipid A complexed with bovine-serum albumin. Eur. J. Biochem., 31, 230-233.

Hase, S., and E.T. Rietschel (1976). Isolation and analysis of the lipid A backbone. Eur. J. Biochem., 63, 101-107.

Holmgren, J. (1970). Antibody response in rabbits to E.coli K antigen. Int. Arch. Allergy 37, 638-648.

Jodal, U., U. Lindberg, and K. Lincoln (1975). Level diagnosis of symptomatic urinary tract infections in childhood. Acta Paediatr. Scand., 64, 201-208.

Johns, M.A., S.C. Bruins, and W.R. McCabe (1977). Immunization with R mutants of Salmonella minnesota. II. Serological response to lipid A and the lipopolysaccharide of Re mutants. Infect. Immun., 17, 9-15.

Kaijser, B., and S. Ahlstedt (1977). Protective capacity of antibodies against Escherichia coli O and K antigens. Infect. Immun., 17, 286-289.

Kaijser, B., and S. Olling (1973). Experimental hematogenous pyelonephritis due to Escherichia coli in rabbits. The antibody response and its protective capacity. J. Infect. Dis., 128, 41-49.

Kaijser, B., P. Larsson, and S. Olling (1978). Protection against ascending E.coli pyelonephritis in rats and significance of local immunity. Infect. Immun., 20, 78-81.

Lüderitz, O., C. Galanos, V. Lehmann, and E.T. Rietschel (1974). Recent findings on the chemical structure and biological activity of bacterial lipopolysaccharides. J. Hyg. Epidemiol. Microbiol. Immunol., 18, 381-390.

Lüderitz, O., K. Jann, and R. Wheat (1968). Somatic and capsular antigens of gram-negative bacteria. In M. Florkin and E.H. Stolz (ed.), Comprehensive biochemistry., vol. 26 A, Elsevier, New York, pp, 105-228.

Mattsby-Baltzer, I., and B. Kaijser (1979). Lipid A and anti-lipid A. Infect. Immun., 23, 758-763.

Mattsby-Baltzer, I., L.Å. Hanson, U. Jodal, B. Kaijser, U. Lindberg, and H. Peterson. Antibodies to lipid A in urinary tract infections. I. Girls with acute infections and asymptomatic bacteriuria compared with age-matched controls. (In manuscript, a).

Mattsby-Baltzer, I., L.Å. Hanson, U. Jodal, B. Kaijser, U. Lindberg, and H. Peterson. Antibodies to lipid A in urinary tract infections. II. Female patients with renal parenchymal reduction. (In manuscript, b).

Mattsby-Baltzer, I., L.Å. Hanson, B. Kaijser, and S. Olling. Protection against ascending pyelonephritis in rats. Oral immunization with live E.coli O6K13H1 and passively transferred anti-lipid A antibodies. (In manuscript, c).

Mattsby-Baltzer, I., B. Jaup, A. Fasth, B. Kaijser, and L.Å. Nilsson. Anti-lipid A and anti-Tamm-Horsfall antibodies in inflammatory bowel disease (IBD). (In manuscript, d).

Neter, E. (1956). Bacterial hemagglutination and hemolysis. Bacteriol. Rev., 20, 166-188.

Rietschel, E.T., and C. Galanos (1977). Lipid A antiserum-mediated protection against lipopolysaccharide and lipid A-induced fever and skin necrosis. Infect. Immun., 15, 34-49.

Wadsworth, C. (1957). A slide microtechnique for the analysis of immune precipitates in gel. Int. Arch. Allergy, 10, 355-360.

Westenfelder, M., and C. Galanos (1974). Experimental lipid A-induced nephritis in

the dog. Infection, 2, 174-177.
Westenfelder, M., C. Galanos, and P. Madsen (1975). Experimental lipid A-induced nephritis in the dog. Invest. Urology, 12, 337-345.
Winberg, J., H.J. Andersen, L.Å. Hanson, and K. Lincoln (1963). Studies of urinary tract infections in infancy and childhood. I. Antibody response in different types of urinary tract infections caused by coliform bacteria. Br. Med. J., 2, 524-527.

TUMOR REGRESSION CAUSED BY ENDOTOXINS COMBINED WITH TREHALOSE DIMYCOLATE

E. Ribi*, J. L. Cantrell*, A. Nowotny, R. Parker ***, S. M. Schwartzman*, K. B. Von Eschen*, R. W. Wheat**** and C. A. McLaughlin***

**National Institutes of Health, National Institute of Allergy and Infectious Diseases, Rocky Mountain Labs., Hamilton, Montana, USA*
***Univ. of Pennsylvania Center for Oral Health Research, Philadelphia, Pa., USA*
****Hamilton Biochemical Research Lab., Hamilton, Montana, USA*
*****Dept. Microbiology and Immunology, Duke Univ. Medical Center, Durham, North Carolina, USA*

ABSTRACT

The synergistic antitumor activity of two adjuvants, endotoxic glycolipid extracted from Re mutants of gram-negative bacteria and trehalose mycolate isolated from mycobacteria, against guinea pig syngeneic line-10 tumor was abrogated after peptidic substances accompanying the endotoxic extracts had been removed. This activity could be restored by combining peptide-free endotoxin with either cell wall skeleton from Bacillus Calmette-Guérin, a polymeric mycolic acid-arabinogalactan-mucopeptide, or with a combination of two separate components, trehalose dimycolate and synthetic N-acetyl-muramyl-L-alanyl-(L-seryl)-D-isoglutamine (MDP). The tumor regressive activity could also be restored to the refined endotoxin trehalose mycolate mixture by the addition of an essentially nontoxic lipoid side fraction recovered during the isolation of endotoxic glycolipids, which contained a small amount of peptidic substances, or by the addition of nontoxic Braun's lipoprotein known to contain covalently bound MDP moieties. Highly endotoxic lipopolysaccharide (LPS) extracted from wild type Enterobacteriaceae so far tested failed to cause tumor regression. However, acid-hydrolysis of wild type Serratia marcescens LPS led to a residual peptide-containing fraction, designated RESI, which serologically cross-reacted with endotoxins from Re mutant Salmonellae and which, in combination with trehalose dimycolate, provided a cure rate of 90%. This RESI was essentially nonpyrogenic and was about 100 times less toxic than a typical potent endotoxin, suggesting that there was no correlation between the antitumor property and endotoxicity.

KEY WORDS

Endotoxic glycolipid; lipid A;BCG cell wall skeleton; trehalose dimycolate; synthetic muramyl dipeptide; Braun's lipoprotein; porin; antitumor activity.

INTRODUCTION

The transplantable line-10 hepatocellular carcinoma of strain-2 guinea pigs has been used as a model for the study of weakly antigenic malignant tumors (Rapp, 1973). When 6-day-old (10 mm in diameter) dermal tumors were inoculated intralesionally with viable BCG, a significant proportion of such tumors regressed permanently and, as subsequently reported, these results could be equaled by treatment with nonviable mycobacterial cell wall components associated with oil droplets in saline emulsion (Zbar, 1973). A high rate of cures has been obtained with materials unrelated to tubercle bacilli provided they were combined with trehalose dimycolate (P3)[1], a lipoid component removed from the mycobacterial cell walls which is also known as purified cord factor. Particularly effective ingredients were unrefined aqueous phases of phenol-water extracts from polysaccharide-deficient Re mutant strains of Salmonella typhimurium or S. minnesota (Ribi, 1975). Inasmuch as similarly prepared lipopolysaccharide (LPS) extracts from wild type strains of Salmonellae were significantly less active in tumor regression although their endotoxic properties were comparable, it appeared that endotoxicity itself was not the only requirement for tumor regressive potency (Ribi, 1975, 1978).

To determine the structural attributes necessary for tumor regressive potency, we chose as starting materials for fractionation, endotoxic glycolipids extracted with chloroform-methanol (ReGl-CM) from the same Re mutant strains. Because of their solubility in organic solvents, they were expected to be fractionable by preparative microparticulate gel pressure elution chromatography (Ribi, 1974). From a practical point of view our interest centered upon the importance of the toxicity of the extracts.

RESULTS AND DISCUSSION

Antitumor Properties of Endotoxic Extracts from Wild Type vs. Mutant Strains of Enterobacteriaceae.

Table 1 compares tumor regressive properties of endotoxic extracts, alone and in combination with P3. The data show that water-soluble, LPS-containing phenol-water extracts from wild type S. minnesota, S. typhimurium, or Escherichia coli alone failed to cause regression of tumors and only occasional regressions were observed when extracts were tested in combination with P3. These results were similar to those obtained with extracts from wild type S. enteritidis (Ribi, 1975). Water-soluble portions of phenol-water extracts (ReGl-PW) from Re mutant strains of S. minnesota, S. typhimurium or E. coli alone caused only occasional regression of tumors but were highly effective when combined with P3. Most importantly, the tumor regressive activity of the methanol-precipitable portion of chloroform-methanol extracts from Re mutant strains, ReGl-CM, were similar to that of ReGl-PW from the Re mutant bacteria. Re mutant bacteria were also extracted with phenol-

---

[1]Abbreviations: P3 = trehalose dimycolate isolated by microparticulate gel Chromatography (Ribi, 1974); LPS = lipopolysaccharide from wild type gram-negative bacteria (Westphal, 1952); ReGl = endotoxic glycolipids from Re mutant gram-negative bacteria; PW = phenol-water; CM = chloroform-methanol; PCP = phenol-chloroform-petroleum ether; ReGl-PW = ReGl extracted with PW (Westphal, 1952); ReGl-CM = ReGl extracted with CM (Chen, 1973); ReGl-PCP = ReGl extracted with PCP (Galanos, 1969); B4 = chromatographic fraction of ReGl-CM (Ribi, 1979); ACP = acetone-precipitated byproduct of ReGl-CM (Ribi, 1979); lipid A = hydrochloric acid hydrolyzate of LPS or ReGl (Westphal, 1954); RESI = organic solvent-insoluble fraction of lipid A (Chang, 1975); CWS = cell wall skeleton of Bacillus Calmette-Guérin (BCG) (Azuma, 1974); MDP = N-acetyl-muramyl-L-seryl-D-isoglutamine (Schwartzman, in preparation).

chloroform-petroleum ether (ReGl-PCP). Although the lethality and pyrogenicity of ReGl-PCP were similar to those of ReGl-PW and ReGl-CM, it was relatively ineffective in regressing line-10 tumors (Table 1; see also Table 2). This also indicated that endotoxicity *per se* was not sufficient to cure tumors and that at least one additional ingredient which is not readily extracted by the PCP method is needed.

Correlation Between Amino Acid Content of Endotoxic Extracts and Regression of Tumors.

Treatment of ReGl-CM with Triton X-100, which also resulted in abrogation of tumor regressive activity without affecting endotoxicity, was paralleled by a reduction of the amino acid content (Table 2). We have described earlier the removal of peptide-containing fragments of mycobacterial cell wall skeleton (i.e., precursor or autolysis products of the mycolic acid-arabinogalactan-mucopeptide polymer) from trehalose mycolates by pressure elution chromatography through columns of microparticulate silica gel (Azuma, 1974; Ribi, 1974). As shown in Table 2, by processing ReGl with the aid of this technique, the resulting fraction, designated B4, was endotoxic but lacked tumor regressive potency. B4 had a significantly reduced total amino acid content. We noted muramic acid, alanine, and glutamic acid among the principal nitrogenous components present in the untreated ReGl and that the proportion of each of these components was lowered significantly during the preparation of B4 (Table 2). Because they are characteristic components of the peptidoglycan of bacterial cell walls, including those of *Salmonella* species (Adam, 1974), we considered that precursor or autolysis products of the peptidoglycan may have been co-extracted with the endotoxic glycolipids. We reported previously that a combination of ReGl and mycobacterial cell wall skeleton (CWS) possessed tumor regressive potency superior to either component alone (McLaughlin, 1979) and describe here similar results with B4 plus CWS (Table 3). Going one step further, we decided to test N-acetyl-muramyl-L-alanyl-D-isoglutamine, which has been reported to be the minimal structural entity of mycobacterial CWS responsible for adjuvanticity of tubercle bacilli (Ellouz, 1974; Merser, 1975; Kotani, 1975). We chose, however, to use muramyl dipeptide containing L-serine (MDP) rather than the alanine-containing product. It was not surprising that the combination of MDP and a mixture of B4 plus P3 restored the ability of the latter combination to effectively regress tumors. Addition of as little as 0.15 μg of MDP to 150 μg B4 plus 50 μg P3 led to a cure rate of 88% (Table 3).

The activity could also be restored to refined endotoxic B4 by the addition of a nontoxic lipoid side fraction, designated ACP, recovered during the isolation of ReGl which contained a small amount of peptidic substances or by the addition of nontoxic Braun's lipoprotein (Braun, 1970) also a constituent of the outer membrane and known to contain covalently bound MDP moieties (Cantrell and co-workers, submitted to Cancer Immunol. Immunother.). Finally, another outer membrane protein, porin (Nakae, 1976), which was found contaminated with endotoxic glycolipids but was free of peptidoglycolipids, was inactive alone but, as was to be expected, effectively caused tumor regression when combined with Braun's lipoprotein (Table 3). In summary, the data listed in Table 3 show that any of the "nontoxic" fractions (ACP, CWS, Braun's lipoprotein, synthetic MDP), when added to the refined endotoxic fraction (B4) restored antitumor activity. They all contained components characteristic of bacterial cell wall peptidoglycans.

Biological Properties of Crude Lipid A, Acetic Acid-Treated Glycolipid and RESI.

In Re mutants of *Enterobacteriaceae*, the glycolipid is represented only by residues of KDO and the toxic lipid moiety. The term "lipid moiety" was suggested for use instead of "lipid A" by Chang and Nowotny (1975) because the latter term should be reserved for identification of the product obtained by hydrolysis of LPS or ReGl with 1.0 *N* HCl according to the original method of Westphal and

TABLE 1 Antitumor Effect of Endotoxic Extracts from Wild Type and Re Mutant Enterobacteriaceae: No Correlation with Endotoxic Potency

Extract tested	Lethality[a] CELD$_{50}$ (μg)	Tumor regression[b] No. cured/Total Extract alone 300 μg		Extract + P3 300 μg + 150 μg	
Wild type S. minnesota (LPS)	0.005	0/19	0%	3/19	16%
Re mutant S. minnesota (ReGl-PW)	0.035	1/15	7	13/15	87
Re mutant S. minnesota (ReGl-CM)	0.130	7/50	14	81/94	86
Wild type S. typhimurium (LPS)	0.010	0/10	0	3/18	17
Re mutant S. typhimurium (ReGl-PW)	0.042	21/332	6	403/456	89
Re mutant S. typhimurium (ReGl-CM)	0.028	7/50	14	115/126	91
Wild type E. coli (LPS)	0.003	0/10	0	0/10	0
Re mutant E. coli (ReGl-CM)	0.250	0/10	0	8/10	80
Re mutant S. minnesota (ReGl-PCP)	0.013	-	-	3/10	30

[a]CELD$_{50}$: Dose lethal for 50% of 11-day-old chick embryos when inoculated intravenously in aqueous solution (Milner, 1966).

[b]Strain 2 guinea pigs bearing 6- or 7-day-old Line-10 tumors (8-10 mm in diameter) inoculated intralesionally with doses contained in 0.4-ml volumes. Animals were considered cured when tumors had completely disappeared, metastases were not palpable at the first draining lymph node, and rejected challenge to line-10 tumor transplantation 2 months after treatment (Rapp, 1973).

TABLE 2 Correlation Between Amino Acid Content of Endotoxic Extracts from Re Mutants Strains and Regression of Tumors

Fractions tested	Total amino acids (% of original weight)	Lethality[a] CELD$_{50}$ (μg)	Pyrogenicity[b] FI$_{40}$ (μg)	Tumor regression[a] using 150 μg of each fraction combined with 50 μg P3 No. cured/Total	%
ReGl-PW, S. typhimurium	2.47	0.36	0.02	10/10	100
Above after treatment with Triton X-100	0.018	0.110	0.25	1/10	10
ReGl-PCP, S. minnesota	0.265	0.013	0.048	3/10	30
ReGl-CM, S. minnesota[c]	1.28	0.195	0.415	10/10	100
B4 = above ReGl-CM refined by chromatography[c]	0.271	0.167	0.53	1/16	6

[a]See footnotes to Table 1 for further information.

[b]Quantity administered to rabbits giving an area under the fever curve (FI) of 40 cm^2 when plotted by a standard method. Determined in aqueous solution (Haskins, 1961).

[c]Content (%) of	in ReGl-CM, S. minnesota	in B4
Muramic acid	0.253	Not detectable
Alanine	0.136	0.032
Glutamic acid	0.245	0.048

TABLE 3 Antitumor Activity of Toxic and Nontoxic Bacterial Compounds Containing Characteristic Cell Wall Peptidoglycan Components (Muramic Acid, Alanine, Serine, and Glutamic Acid)

Fraction tested	Lethality[a] $CELD_{50}$ (μg)	Tumor regression[a] using 150 μg of each fraction combined with 50 μg P3: No. cured/Total	%
ReGl-CM, untreated	0.195	10/10	100
B4, toxic chromatographic fraction of ReGl-CM	0.167	1/16	6
CWS (mycolic acid-arabinogalactan-peptidoglycan)		1/9	11
B4 + CWS		8/8	100
MDP (synthetic N-acetyl-muramyl-L-seryl-D-isoglutamine)	> 10	6/22	27
B4 + MDP without trehalose dimycolate (P3)		0/7	0
B4 + MDP (150 μg + 0.15 μg)		7/8	88
" (15 μg + 0.15 μg)		4/7	57
" (1.5 μg + 0.15 μg		0/8	0
ACP, nontoxic side fraction of ReGl-CM	> 5	2/17	12
B4 + ACP		27/38	71
Braun's lipoprotein (contains peptidoglycan units)	8.9	0/12	0
B4 + Braun's lipoprotein		8/22	36
Porin (mixture of protein plus endotoxin free of peptidoglycan units)	0.33	0/6	0
Porin + Braun's lipoprotein		11/14	72

[a]See footnotes to Table 1 for further information.

TABLE 4 Comparison of Biological Properties of Lipid A, Acetic Acid-Treated Glycolipid, and RESI

Extract tested	Lethality[a] $CELD_{50}$ (μg)	Pyrogenicity[b] FI_{40} (μg)	Tumor regression[a] using 150 μg extract + 150 μg P3: No. cured/Total
Untreated ReGl-PW (*S. typhimurium*)	0.02	0.62	9/9
Lipid A prepared from ReGl-PW (*S. typhimurium*) by hydrolysis with 0.1 N HCl at 100°C, 30 min.	2.09	~60	2/9
Acetic acid-treated glycolipid prepared from ReGl-PW (*S. typhimurium*) by hydrolysis with acetic acid, 100° C, 2 hr.	0.300	1.6	4/9
RESI from lipid A of LPS from wild type *S. typhimurium* 0901 (total amino acids 23.4%)	Not done	Not done	11/11 (0/10)[c]
RESI from lipid A of LPS from wild type *S. marcescens* 08 (total amino acids 7.25%)	2.30	>100	9/10 (0/10)[c]
Oil droplets in Tween-saline controls	-	-	0/29

[a]See footnotes to Table 1 for further information.
[b]See footnotes to Table 2 for further information.
[c]Results when tested without P3.

Lüderitz (1954). For this study, "entire crude lipid A" was prepared by HCl hydrolysis from ReGl-PW from S. typhimurium. The product was at least 100-fold less toxic and pyrogenic than the starting material (Table 4), which was in agreement with earlier findings in this laboratory (Ribi, 1961; Haskins, 1961). Tumor regressive potency of this product was marginal; only two of nine tumor-bearing animals were cured (Table 4).

The term "lipid A" also has been used to describe preparations obtained by 0.1 N acetic acid hydrolysis of endotoxic glycolipid (Risse, 1967). Because this milder treatment with a more dilute organic acid was considered to bring about different chemical changes than HCl hydrolysis (Ribi, 1961, Haskins, 1961), a sample from the same lot of ReGl-PW hydrolyzed with HCl (Table 4) was hydrolyzed with acetic acid. In accordance with Chang and Nowotny (1975), we designated the water-insoluble sediment "acetic acid-treated glycolipid." In contrast to crude lipid A, its toxicity was only 10-fold rather than 100-fold less ($CELD_{50}$ = 0.3 μg vs. 0.02 μg) and the pyrogenicity only 3-fold less (FI_{40} = 1.6 μg vs. 0.62 μg) than that of the glycolipid prior to hydrolysis. The tumor regressive potency of acetic acid-treated glycolipid was considerably less than that of the untreated starting material (4/9 vs. 9/9). The results obtained with these "free lipids" indicated the lack of correlation between endotoxic potency and antitumor activity.

Chang and Nowotny (1975) recovered the residual activity of the crude lipid A precipitate of wild type LPS in a fraction designated "RESI" and concluded that the activity was due to remnants of incompletely degraded endotoxin, confirming earlier speculation (Ribi, 1961; Haskins, 1961; Nowotny 1963; Milner, 1971). Like Re mutant glycolipids, although about 100 times less toxic and essentially nonpyrogenic, RESI samples were tumor regressive when combined with P3 (Table 4), indicating that the moiety responsible for tumor regression exposed in RESI is not necessarily related to the endotoxic component. RESI samples have been shown to be serologically cross-reactive with ReGl from Enterobacteriaceae (Ng, 1974; 1976). In contrast, the parent wild type LPS of RESI samples which possessed at best only marginal potency to cure line-10 tumors, did not cross-react with ReGl. The ability of RESI to regress tumors may be the result of removal of the polysaccharide moiety of the wild type LPS, which is in agreement with earlier findings that an ReGl may have antitumor activity because of its lack of polysaccharide (Brailovsky, 1973; Nigam, 1975). Hydrolysis of wild type LPS may expose moieties that structurally resemble those similarly exposed in the abnormal tumor cell (Hakamori, 1975). We speculate that endotoxin contaminating fragments of peptidoglycan or synthetic muramyl dipeptide may act as an adjuvant to an antigen which may have cross-reactive determinants associated with the endotoxin itself. Such antigens may be cryptic or sterically hindered from being effective in polysaccharide-rich LPS but are exposed in polysaccharide-deficient ReGl and RESI. It remains to be determined whether this cross-reactive antigen is identical with that shared by BCG, line-10 tumor cells, and malignant melanoma as described by Borsos (1973) and Minden (1976). In addition, Dr. Cantrell of our laboratory, in collaboration with Dr. G.F. Springer, found line-10 tumor cells, ReGl, porin, and B4 to have components that cross-reacted with T antigen, the precursor of human blood group antigen (unpublished communication), whereas no cross-reactivity was observed with ACP or Braun's lipoprotein. Studies are in progress to determine whether cross-reactive antigens shared by the tumor cells and microbial components play a role in tumor regression.

Even though it appears that MDP may replace the putative, essential tumor regressive peptidic ingredient of ReGl, this may not mean that these substances are structurally related, although it is tempting to suggest that this is so. This nontoxic ingredient needed to enable endotoxin to bring about tumor immunity, which we presume to be also present in ACP, RESI, and cell wall skeleton samples, may have structures in common or subantigenic resemblances with the MDP which are cryptic in LPS and exposed in ReGl preparations. We may alternately speculate, therefore, that the hypothetical peptidic component in ACP, ReGl, RESI, or CWS, when associated with P3 on oil droplets, may well function as an antigen, or as a hapten in the case of the low molecular weight synthetic MDP(Audibert, 1978). This alternative speculation proposes that antigenic material of peptidic nature remains associated with endotoxic preparations during extraction with phenol-water or chloroform-methanol. P3, which possesses nonionic surfactant properties may serve to prime the surface of the oil droplets to permit adherence of proteinaceous or peptidic antigenic substances. This binding of antigens to oil droplets by P3 facilitates the development of delayed type hypersensitivity toward the antigens (Granger, 1976). Similarly, in the case of combinations of ReGl and P3 which cause rapid tumor regression, P3 was presumed to facilitate the attachment of the endotoxin carrier-antigen complex to the oil droplets (Ribi, 1975; 1976a; McLaughlin, 1978). Skin testing data had suggested that delayed type hypersensitivity developed against the endotoxin-associated antigens (Ribi, 1976a) as well as against specific tumor antigens (Cantrell, 1978).

Only about one fourth of ReGl was bound to the oil droplets primed with P3 (McLaughlin, 1978). Moreover, exceptionally rapid destruction of tumors also was observed when ReGl was not incorporated into oil droplets but simply added to the aqueous phase into which were suspended oil droplets covered with CWS (McLaughlin, unpublished). The action of endotoxin may not be curative in nature as in the oil droplet-P3 (adjuvant)-antigen system, but rather the result of the well-known endotoxin-mediated hemorrhagic necrosis of tumors. When Re mutant endotoxin is used alone, a line-10 tumor is rarely eliminated and shortly resumes growth (Ribi, 1975; 1976a), but these early antitumor effects may synergistically augment the mechanisms brought into play when, in combination with P3 and oil droplets, certain endotoxic preparations (ReGl, RESI), mycobacterial CWS, or MDP are injected into established tumors.

It also must be emphasized that highly toxic LPS preparations from wild type strains, alone or in combination with P3, failed to cure line-10 tumors although initial strong tumor-damaging effects of hemorrhage and necrosis occurred; the tumors eventually continued their fatal course (Ribi, 1975; 1976b). This is in contrast to the ReGl which induces similar tumor necrosis initially, followed by complete cure of the dermal tumor and immunity against rechallenge. Wild type endotoxin which induced regression of murine tumors with concomitant development of specific systemic tumor immunity, as distinct from hemorrhagic necrosis, is dependent upon the state of T cell-mediated antitumor immunity that is generated only in response to immunogenic tumors (Berendt, 1978). However, the line-10 tumor is weakly immunogenic as classically defined (Rapp, 1973) and thus apparently not immunogenic enough for wild type endotoxin to evoke the generation of T cell-mediated immunity. We believe that it is against weakly immunogenic tumors that clinically useful adjuvant immunotherapy must be developed (Alexander, 1977). Our findings indicate that an immunogen or antigen, in addition to the endotoxin itself, is needed. We conclude that although there is no direct correlation between endotoxic potency and tumor regressive activity, a certain level of toxicity may be required to obtain the highest level of tumoricidal action. From a practical point of view, the findings reported here lend merit to the continued search for products that synergistically enhance the action of CWS or MDP but have low endotoxicity. Finally, we emphasize that the results presented here were exclusively obtained with the aid of the strain 2 syngenic guinea pig-line-10 tumor model and, therefore, the conclusions drawn are limited to this test system and generalizations must be made with caution.

REFERENCES

Adam, A., R. Ciobaru, F. Ellouz, J.F. Petit, and E. Lederer (1974). Adjuvant activity of momomeric bacterial cell wall peptidoglycans. Biochem. Biophys. Res. Commun. 56, 561-567.

Alexander, P. (1977). Back to the drawing board - the need for more realistic model systems for immunotherapy. Cancer 40, 467-470.

Audibert, F., B. Heymer, C. Gros, K.H. Schleifer, P.H. Seidl and L. Chedid (1978).

Absence of binding of MDP, a snythetic immunoadjuvant, to anti-peptidoglycan antibodies. J. Immunol. 121, 1219-1222.

Azuma, I., E.E. Ribi, T.J. Meyer, and B. Zbar (1974). Biologically active components from mycobacterial cell walls. I. Isolation and composition of cell wall skeleton and component P3. J. Natl. Cancer Inst. 52, 95-101.

Berendt, M.J., R. J. North, and D.P. Kirsten (1978). The immunological basis of endotoxin-induced tumor regression. Requirement for T-cell-mediated immunity. J. Exp. Med., 148, 1550-1559.

Borsos, T., and H.J. Rapp. (1973). Antigenic relationship between Mycobacterium bovis (BCG) and a guinea pig hepatoma. J. Natl. Cancer Inst., 51, 1085-1086.

Brailovsky, C., M. Trudel, R. Lallier, and V.N. Nigam (1973). Growth of normal and transformed rat embryo fibroblasts. Effects of glycolipids from Salmonella minnesota R mutants. J. Cell Biol., 57, 124-132.

Braun, V., K. Rehn and H. Wolff (1970). Supramolecular structure of the rigid layer of the cell wall of Salmonella, Serratia, Proteus, and Pseudomonas fluorescens. Number of lipoprotein molecules in a membrane layer. Biochemistry, 9, 5041-5049.

Cantrell, J.L., E. Ribi, and C. McLaughlin (1978). Passive transfer with spleen cells from guinea pigs cured of hepatocarcinoma by nonspecific immunotherapy. Cancer Immunol. Immunother., 4, 21-28.

Chang, C.M., and A. Nowotny (1975). Relation of structure to function in bacterial O-antigens. VII. Endotoxicity of lipid A. Immunochemistry, 12, 19-28.

Chen, C.H., A.G. Johnson, N. Kasai, B.A. Key, J. Levin, and A. Nowotny (1973). Heterogeneity and biological activity of endotoxic glycolipid from Salmonella minnesota R595. J. Infect. Dis., 128, S43-S45.

Ellouz, F., A. Adam, R. Ciorbaru, and E. Lederer (1974). Minimal structural requirements for adjuvant activity of bacterial peptidoglycan derivatives. Biochem. Biophys. Res. Commun., 59, 1317-1325.

Galanos, C., O. Lüderitz, and O. Westphal (1969). A new method for the extraction of R lipopolysaccharides. Eur. J. Biochem., 9, 245-249.

Granger, D.L., K. Yamamoto, and E. Ribi (1976). Delayed hypersensitivity and granulomatous response after immunization with protein antigens associated with a mycobacterial glycolipid and oil droplets. J. Immunol., 116, 482-488.

Hakomori, S.I. (1975). Structures and organization of cell surface glycolipids dependency on cell growth and malignant transformation. Biochem. Biophys Acta, 417, 55-88.

Haskins, W.T., M. Landy, K.C. Milner, and E. Ribi (1961). Biological properties of parent endotoxins and lipoid fractions, with a kinetic study of acid-hydrolyzed endotoxin. J. Exp. Med., 114, 665-684.

Kotani, S., Y. Watanabe, F. Kinoshita, T. Shimono, T. Morisaki, T. Shiba, S. Kusumoto, Y. Tarumi, and K. Ikenaka (1975). Immunoadjuvant activities of synthetic N-acetylmuramyl-peptides or amino acids. Biken J., 18, 105-111.

Lüderitz, O., C. Galanos, V. Lehmann, H. Mayer, E.T. Rietschel, and J. Weekesser (1978). Chemical structure and biological activities of lipid A's from various bacterial families. Naturwissenschaften, 65, 578-585.

McLaughlin, C.A., E.E. Ribi, M.B. Goren, and R. Toubiana (1978). Tumor regression induced by refined microbial components in an oil-in-water emulsion is mediated through their binding to oil droplets. Cancer Immunol. Immunother., 4, 109-113.

McLaughlin, C.A., S. L. Hargrave, W.D. Bickel, and E. Ribi (1979). Synergistic activity of components of mycobacteria and mutant Salmonella in causing regression of line-10 tumors in guinea pigs. Cancer Res., 391, 1766-1771.

Merser, C., P. Sinaÿ, and A. Adam (1975). Total synthesis and adjuvant activity of bacterial peptidoglycan derivatives. Biochem. Biophys. Res. Commun., 66, 1316-1322.

Milner, K.C., and R.A. Finkelstein (1966). Bioassay of endotoxin: Correlation between pyrogenicity for rabbits and lethality for chick embryos. J. Infect. Dis., 116, 529-536.

Minden, P., T.R. Sharpton, and J. K. McClatchy. (1976). Shared antigens between human malignant melanoma cells and Mycobacterium bovis (BCG). J. Immunol., 116, 1407-1414.

Nakae, T. (1976). Identification of the outer membrane proteins of E. coli that produce transmembrane channels in reconstituted vesicle membranes. Biochem. Biophys. Res. Commun., 71, 877-884.

Ng, A.K., C.M. Chang, and A. Nowotny (1974). Comparison of the chemical structure and biological activities of the glycolipids of Salmonella minnesota R595 and Salmonella typhimurium SL1102. Infect. Immun., 10, 938-947.

Ng, A.K., CH. Chen, C.M. Chang, and A. Nowotny (1976). Relationship of structure to function in bacterial endotoxins: Serologically cross-reactive components and their effects on protection of mice against some gram-negative infections. J. Gen. Microbiol., 94, 107-116.

Nigam, V.N. (1975). Effect of core lipopolysaccharides from Salmonella minnesota R mutants on the survival times of mice bearing Ehrlich tumor. Cancer Res. 35, 628-633.

Nowotny, A. (1963). Relation of structure to function in bacterial antigens. II. Fractionation of lipids present in Boivin-type endotoxin of Serratia marcescens. J. Bacteriol., 85, 427-435.

Rapp, H.J. (1973). A guinea pig model for tumor immunotherapy: A summary. Isr. J. Med. Sci., 9, 366-374.

Ribi, E., W.T. Haskins, M. Landy. and K.C. Milner (1961). Preparation and host-reactive properties of endotoxin with low content of nitrogen and lipid. J. Exp. Med., 114, 647-663.

Ribi, E., R. Parker, and K.C. Milner (1974). Microparticulate gel chromatography accelerated by centrifugal force and pressure. In D. Glick (Ed.) Methods of Biochemical Analysis, Vol. 22, John Wiley & Sons, New York. pp. 355-400.

Ribi, E.E., D.L. Granger, K.C. Milner and S.M. Strain (1975). Brief communication: Tumor regression caused by endotoxins and mycobacterial fractions. J. Natl. Cancer Inst., 55, 1253-1257.

Ribi, E., K.C. Milner, D.L. Granger, M.T. Kelly, K. Yamamoto, W. Brehmer, R. Parker, R.F. Smith, and S.M. Strain (1976a). Immunotherapy with nonviable microbial components. Ann. N.Y. Acad. Sci., 277, 228-238.

Ribi, E., K. Milner, M.T. Kelly, D. Granger, K. Yamamoto, C.A. McLaughlin, W. Brehmer, S.M. Strain, R.F. Smith, and R. Parker (1976b). Structural requirements of microbial agents for immunotherapy of the guinea line-10 tumor. In G. Lamoureux, R. Turcotte, and V. Portelance (Eds.), BCG in Cancer Immunotherapy, Grune & Stratton, New York. pp. 51-60.

Ribi, E., C.A. McLaughlin, J.L. Cantrell, W. Brehmer, I. Azuma, Y. Yamamura, S. M. Strain, K.M. Hwang, and R. Toubiana (1978). Immunotherapy for tumors with microbial constituents or their synthetic analogues. A review. In Immunotherapy of Human Cancer, 22nd Annual Clinical Conference on Cancer, The University of Texas System Cancer Center, M.D. Anderson Hospital and Tumor Institute, Houston, Texas, Raven Press, New York. pp. 131-154.

Ribi, E., R. Parker, S. M. Strain, Y. Mizuno, A. Nowotny, K. B. Von Eschen, J. L. Cantrell, C. A. McLaughlin, K. M. Hwang, and M. B. Goren (1979). Peptides as requirement for immunotherapy of the guinea pig line-10 tumor with endotoxins. Cancer Immunol. Immunother., in press.

Risse, H. J., W. Dröge, E. Ruschmann, O. Lüderitz, O. Westphal, and J. Schlosshardt (1967). Serologische und Biochemische Analyse des Heptosekerns von Lipopolysacchariden aus Salmonella minnesota and Salmonella ruirumutantun. Eur. J. Biochem., 1, 216-232.

Westphal, O., and O. Lüderitz (1954). Chemische Erforschung von Lipopolysacchari-der Gramnegativer Bakterien. Angew. Chem., 66, 407-417.

Westphal, O., O. Lüderitz, and F. Bister (1952). Über die Extraktion von Bakterien mit Phenol/Wasser. Z. Naturforsch., 7b, 148-155.

Zbar, B., E. Ribi, and H.J. Rapp (1973). An experimental model for immunotherapy of cancer. In T. Borsos and H. J. Rapp (Eds.), Conference on the use of BCG in therapy of cancer. Natl. Cancer Inst. Monograph No. 39, DHEW Publication No. (NIH) 74-511, pp. 3-9.

BACTERIAL LIPOPOLYSACCHARIDES INDUCE CHANGES IN LIPOPROTEIN AND ACUTE PHASE PROTEINS IN C3H/HeJ 'NON-RESPONDER' MICE[1]

T. C. Bøg-Hansen and U. Back[†]

The Protein Laboratory, University of Copenhagen, and The E. coli Reference Center (WHO), The State Serum Institute, Copenhagen, Denmark

ABSTRACT

The immediate non-immune response to endotoxin (LPS) was studied in mice. We found that circulating LPS is in complex with lipoproteins, (mainly HDL) and that acute phase proteins (haptoglobin, hemopexin, complement C3) increase. This response in independent of expression of the LPS gene, since the response of the 'non-responder' strain C3H/HeJ is similar to that of other strains.

KEYWORDS

Endotoxins; lipoprotein receptor; acute phase proteins; non-responder C3H/HeJ mice; multiple sclerosis.

INTRODUCTION

Bacterial lipopolysaccharides (LPS, endotoxins) cause many physiological changes in mammals (Milner et al. 1971), except in one outstanding mouse strain, C3H/HeJ, that has been shown to be resistant toward LPS. Its unresponsiveness is genetically determined by a single autosomal dominant gene (Watson and Riblet, 1974) and includes the following normal aspects of endotoxicity: polymorphonuclear leucocyte changes (Sultzer, 1969), endotoxic shock (Sultzer, 1972), mitogenicity (Watson and Riblet, 1974), polyclonal B-cell activation (Coutinho et al., 1975), enhancement of nonspecific resistance to infections (Chedid et al., 1976), inhibition of tolerance induction (Skidmore et al., 1976), increase of serum colony-stimulating factor (CSF) (Apte and Pluznik, 1976), increase of serum amyloid protein (SAA) (McAdam and Sipe, 1976), protection against X-irradiation (Urbaschek et al., 1977), adjuvant action (Goodman et al., 1978) and induction of glucocorticoid antagonizing factor (Moore et al., 1978).

The LPS detoxification by serum has been a puzzling question, and deviating evidence of responsible serum factors has accumulated: lipoproteins and non-specific esterase (Skarnes and Chedid, 1964; Skarnes, 1968), complement factors (Johnson and Ward, 1972; May et al., 1972) and a non-lipoprotein LPS inhibitor (Johnson et al., 1977).

---

[1] Presented in part at the International Symposium on Biologically Active Products of Microorganisms, Prague, 1978.

[†] U. Back died on October 2, 1977.

We have been interested in the immediate LPS detoxifying potential of weakened mammals in relation to the pathogenicity of LPS [Back et al., 1976], and we showed that the plasma HDL (high density lipoprotein)-associated arylesterase (E.C. 3.1.1.2) [Brogren and Bøg-Hansen, 1975] binds to LPS in vitro [Back et al., 1976] and that along with acute phase serum proteins arylesterase is induced in SPF (specific pathogen-free) mice in concert with characteristic lipoprotein changes [Bøg-Hansen et al., 1978]. The arylesterase would be a candidate as a LPS-degrading enzyme, and Skarnes [1970] discussed the immediate enzymatic degradation of LPS by the lipoprotein esterase - presumably the same enzyme. On the other hand there is little - if any - direct evidence for degradation of LPS, as reviewed by Olitzki [1972].

On basis of in vivo experiments with C3H/HeJ "non-responder" mice we advanced the idea that HDL might serve directly as an amphiphilic "sink" for lipid toxins like LPS [Bøg-Hansen et al., 1979]. We chose the C3H/HeJ "non-responder" strain for our studies of the immediate reactions towards LPS and in this communication we give evidence that plasma lipoproteins (especially HDL) and albumin serve as receptors for circulating LPS. Characteristic changes in the precipitation pattern in crossed immunoelectrophoresis are described for plasma lipoproteins, arylesterase and albumin in addition to acute phase changes of haptoglobin, hemopexin, complement factor C3 and other plasma glycoproteins.

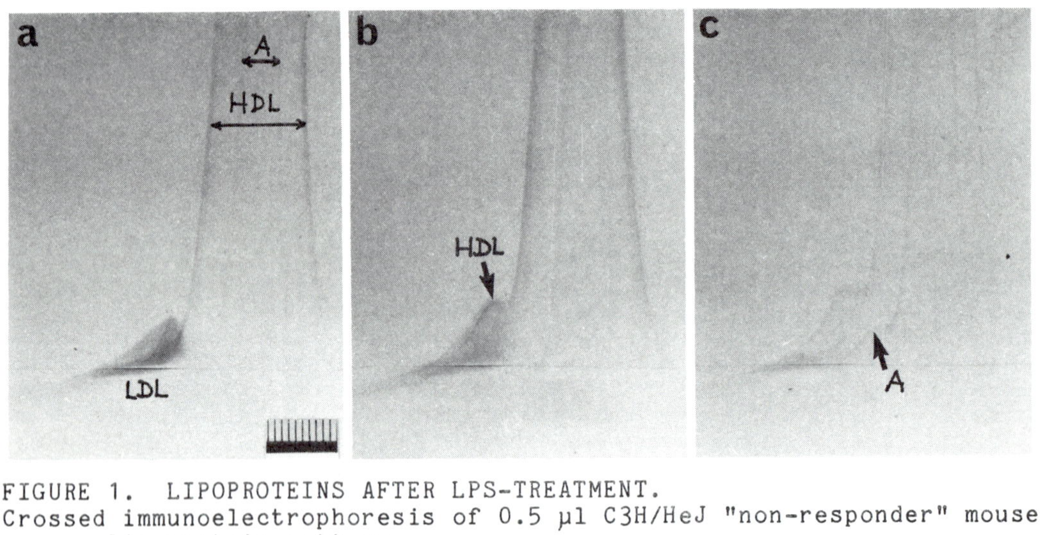

FIGURE 1. LIPOPROTEINS AFTER LPS-TREATMENT.
Crossed immunoelectrophoresis of 0.5 µl C3H/HeJ "non-responder" mouse serum, lipoprotein pattern.
1a. Serum from an untreated mouse.
1b. Serum from a mouse treated intra-venously with 0.6 mg E.coli 055 LPS 10 min before bleeding.
1c. Serum from a mouse treated intra-venously with 0.2 mg E.coli 055 LPS 30 h before bleeding.
LPS: phenolextracted, DIFCO. Abbreviations: A = albumin, HDL = high density lipoprotein, alpha-lipoprotein, LDL = low density lipoprotein, beta-lipoprotein. The bar represents 1 cm. Only the anodal part of the immunoplate is shown (cf. Fig. 5). Stained for lipids with Sudan Black. Antibodies were purified rabbit immunoglobulin fractions of serum from animals immunized with mouse serum. Otherwise as described earlier [Bøg-Hansen et al., 1978].

THE LIPOPROTEIN RECEPTOR

When LPS was given to C3H/HeJ mice by intra-venous and intra-peritoneal injections we noted a characteristic immediate shift in the plasma lipoprotein pattern in crossed immunoelectrophoresis. Fig.1 shows details of the shifts in plasma from mice treated with high doses of LPS from E.coli 055 (corresponding to more than LD-50 in normal mice). Fig.1a is the normal pattern found in untreated mice. HDL (high density lipoprotein) and LDL (low density lipoprotein) are visualized by lipid staining after analysis of serum from different individual mice. Fig.1b shows the pattern 10 min after intra-venous injection of LPS. The lipid staining intensity of the lipoproteins is lower than in untreated animals (especially of LDL) and an electrophoretically deviating component of HDL appears with a staining intensity distinctly greater than for normal HDL (arrow). This component is still present in circulation after more than 2 days (Fig.1c), but the lipid-staining intensity decreases progressively, indicating that the lipid content of the lipoproteins decreases.

Accompanying this shift in lipoproteins, we observe that albumin carries lipid between 24-30 hrs after intra-venous LPS treatment (Fig.1c, arrow).

Similar changes are observed when the LPS is given intra-peritoneally. Fig.2 shows the pattern 16, 24 and 48 hrs after intra-peritoneal injection of LPS. After 4 hrs the extra peak of HDL appears (arrow) and remains for more than two days. In other experiments we could show that this peak also carries arylesterase activity and stain with increasing intensity for this enzyme [Bøg-Hansen et al., 1979].

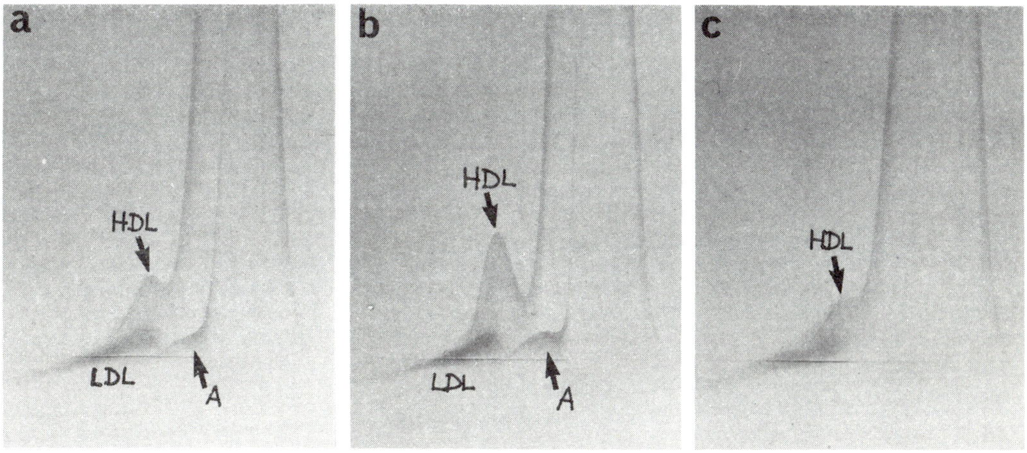

FIGURE 2. LIPOPROTEINS AFTER LPS-TREATMENT.
Crossed immunoelectrophoresis of 0.5 µl C3H/HeJ "nonresponder" mouse serum, stained for lipoproteins.
2a. Serum from a mouse treated intra-peritoneally with 0.6 mg E.coli 055 LPS 16 h before bleeding.
2b. As 2a but treated with LPS 24 h before bleeding.
2c. As 2a but treated with LPS 48 h before bleeding.
A indicates binding of lipid to albumin. Otherwise as for Fig. 1.

With other types of LPS as for instance with Boivin-extracted LPS from E.coli 026 there is a complete shift of the HDL towards the cathode, with the shift more and more pronounced through 1 to 2 days, to reappear in its normal position after about 2 days [Bøg-Hansen et al., 1979]. With a second phenol-extracted LPS (E.coli 0124) we found similar changes in the electrophoretic properties of HDL (the shifts in the first dimension electrophoresis) as shown here in Fig.2 for phenol-extracted E.coli 055 LPS.

The plasma concentration of LDL is somewhat diminished after intra-peritoneal LPS treatment but not as much as after intra-venous injection (compare the staining intensity to that in Fig. 1).

In both cases of injection route, the albumin is capable of staining for lipid up to 24 hrs after treatment (Fig.2, a-arrows). After 30 hrs the albumin does not show lipids associated any more and reappears as the normal albumin without lipid staining.

Several doses of LPS were tested. Figs. 1 and 2 are characteristic of the pattern observed with intra-venous and intra-peritoneal injections (respectively) of LPS in doses that give a lethal response in other strains of mice (e.g. 1-3 times the LD-50 in C3H responder mice and in C57Bl). However, there was a difference in the presence, position and size of the extra peak of HDL. Generally, when the LPS is given by intra-venous injection the time-course of the lipoprotein response is much faster but the same features of the electrophoretic shifts are maintained.

We could quantify lipoprotein by measurement of the area enclosed by the immunoprecipitate and described distinct changes in plasma concentration of HDL with an initial drop succeeded by an increase to the normal level or even to a higher level [Bøg-Hansen et al., 1979].

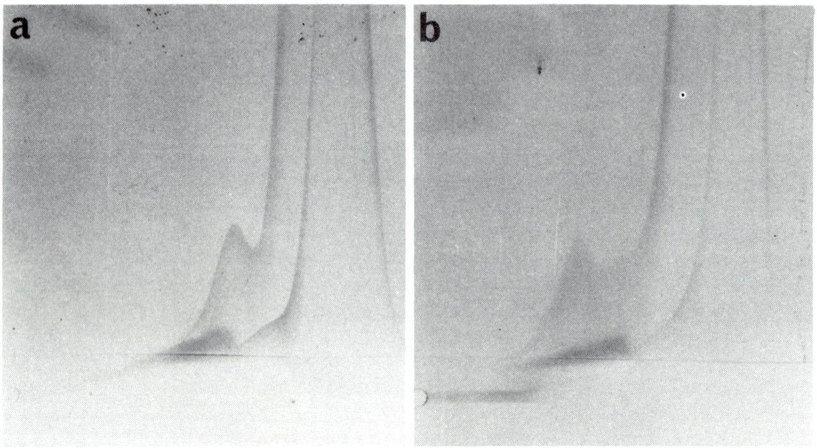

FIGURE 3. LPS-LIPOPROTEIN COMPLEX.
Crossed immunoelectrophoresis of 0.5 μl serum from a C3H/HeJ mouse treated 24 h previously with 0.6 mg E.coli 055 LPS.
3a. Control pattern.
3b. With specific anti 055 LPS in the first dimension gel.
Otherwise as for Fig. 1.

On the basis of Skarnes' early work, cf. [Skarnes, 1970, Moreau and Skarnes, 1973], these studies led us to test the possible complex-formation between serum proteins (especially lipoproteins) and LPS - a complex-formation that might be expected on the basis of the amphiphilic nature of LPS which is well established - including its affinity for cell membrane phospholipids [Rothfield and Horne, 1967 and Springer and Adye, 1975].

We introduced specific, purified anti-LPS antibodies in the first dimension gel according to Platt et al. [1973] and in the intermediate gel according to Svendsen and Axelsen [1973] in crossed immunoelectrophoretic analyses of serum from treated animals. Thus, in Fig.3 is shown the pronounced changes in pattern we observe when anti-LPS is in the first dimension gel: The heavily lipid-stained extra component of HDL and the lipid-stained part of albumin are drawn towards the cathode, and a smear is seen in the first dimension in the antibody-containing gel. This shows that LPS is precipitated in the first dimension gel and that HDL and albumin react with anti-LPS to indicate that these proteins are in molecular complexes with LPS. Anti-LPS in an intermediate gel strengthen this conclusion (Fig. 4). Earlier we showed in an experiment with LPS applied in the first dimension gel in crossed immunoelectrophoresis of human serum proteins that the major proteins reacting with LPS are lipoproteins (HDL with its arylesterase), complement C3 and albumin [Back et al., 1976].

In the experiment shown in Fig. 4 we can discriminate some LPS which is not bound by lipoprotein (Fig. 4b, arrows). This type of experiment does not allow quantification of bound and free LPS. Presumably the amount of free LPS is related to the extremely high

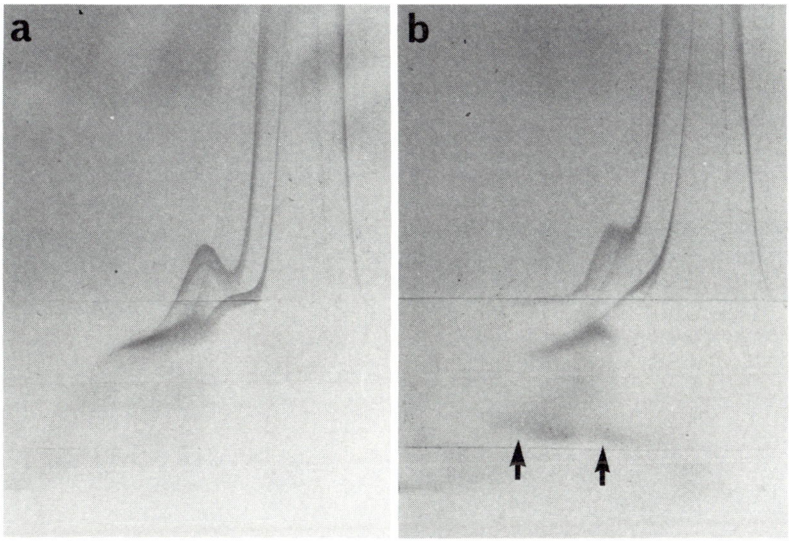

FIGURE 4. LPS-LIPOPROTEIN COMPLEX.
Crossed immunoelectrophoresis of 0.5 µl serum from a C3H/HeJ mouse treated 24 h previouSly with 0.6 mg E.coli O55 LPS.
4a. Control pattern with a blank intermediate gel.
4b. With specific anti O55 LPS in the intermediate gel.
Otherwise as for Fig. 1.

dose the animal was subjected to.

Older reports have implicated lipoprotein as well as other serum factors in the processing and detoxification of endotoxins. Thus Skarnes and coworkers showed a reaction with and changes of lipoproteins after in vivo experiments with LPS [Skarnes, 1966]. Spleen esterase [Rutenberg et al.,1964], lipoprotein esterase [Skarnes and Chedid, 1964] and alpha-globulin LPS inhibitor [Johnsson et al., 1977] have been reported to have an effect on endotoxins, possibly an inactivation. We have not studied the biological effects of lipoprotein complexation with LPS, but our experiments give evidence for the form in which LPS circulates. Moreover, we conclude from our experiments with plasma lipoproteins that they play a role in processing of circulating LPS. Especially HDL seems to serve as a sink and a major receptor for LPS and therefore we regard the plasma lipoproteins as well as albumin as a general amphiphilic sink for toxic lipids.

We presume that the shielding of LPS in the amphiphilic milieu of the lipoproteins is related to expression of the toxicity of the LPS and to the host response. However, our experiments do not give

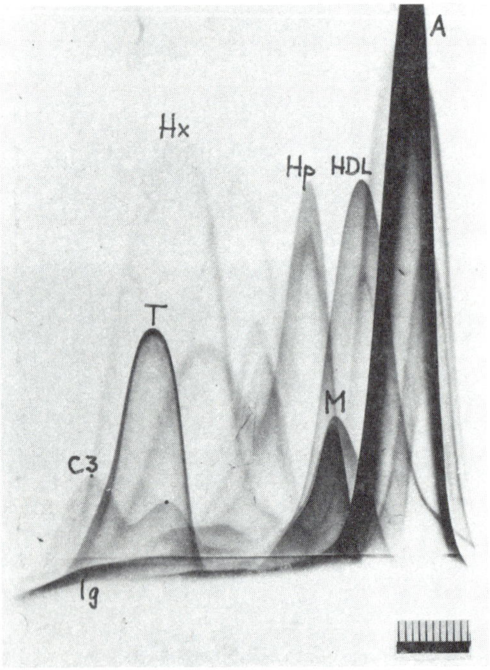

FIGURE 5. MOUSE SERUM PROTEINS. Crossed immunoelectrophoresis of 0.5 µl serum from a C3H/HeJ mouse treated with 0.25 mg E.coli 0124 LPS (phenolextracted) 23 h prior to bleeding. Stained for proteins. Major serum proteins are indicated:
A = albumin,
C3 = complement factor C3,
HDL = high density lipoprotein, alpha lipoprotein,
Hp = haptoglobin,
Hx = hemopexin,
Ig = immunoglobulins,
M = macroglobulins,
T = transferrin.
Otherwise as for Fig. 1. The proteins were identified by reaction in an intermediate gel with specific antibodies against human serum proteins.

any information on the percentual amount of LPS that is bound to proteins or is free in circulation. Probably the lipoprotein shielding is a dominating factor for the effect of serum on the biological activity of LPS, as reported recently by Ulevitch and Johnston [1978]. Increases of serum lipids are observed in animals after LPS-challenge [LeQuire et al., 1959, Hirsch et al., 1964] and in patients with severe infections caused by gram-negative bacilli [Gallin et al., 1969] and further studies are necessary to relate the LPS receptor function of the lipoproteins to the normal lipid metabolism.

LPS, THE LIPOPROTEIN RECEPTOR AND MULTIPLE SCLEROSIS

Endotoxins have been postulated as a pathogenic cause in several diseases including membranoproliferative glomerulonephritis [Back et al., 1976, Fridberg et al., 1978], rheumatic diseases [Larsen, 1976] and in addition to the generally accepted theory of the viral cause of multiple sclerosis, other theories have been advanced to explain the pathology of this disease: Störtebecker [1978] have summarized and speculated upon evidence for possible involvement of toxins of microbial origin and their spreading by the valve-less cranio-vertebral venous system. Thus LPS is a plausible pathogen for the disseminated peri-venous lesions in multiple sclerosis [Störtebecker, 1978]. Our interest in LPS was aroused by this [Back et al., 1976], and in preliminary experiments with multiple sclerosis patients we find changes in lipoproteins and acute phase proteins similar to those described here in mice after LPS treatment. Rieder and Peyer have found that there is a change of the normal balance between beta and alpha lipoproteins (LDL and HDL) with diminished amount of alpha lipoproteins in serum of multiple sclerosis patients [Rieder and Peyer, 1970]. We suggest that by assessment of lipoproteins it will be possible to obtain information on the plasma detoxifying potential and the lipoproteins as factors of significance for progression of multiple sclerosis.

As an approach to the study of the deleterious effects of LPS on the central nervous system we describe in an accompanying paper some experiments with changes in the cerebrospinal fluid of LPS-treated guinea pigs [Boiesen et al., 1980].

ACUTE PHASE PROTEIN INDUCTION

We used the quantitative aspects of crossed immunoelectrophoresis to obtain a quantitative estimation of the concentration increases of the socalled acute phase proteins, serum glycoproteins that increase under various pathologic conditions (see for instance Bacchus [1975]). C3H/HeJ mice were injected with LPS and bled at specified times. The serum was analyzed in parallel to obtain a quantitative expression of changes in protein amounts during the timecourse of the treatment as for lipoprotein above. Some of the acute phase glycoproteins are identified in Fig. 5. The major proteins were measured by planimetry and the changes expressed relatively to the protein content in untreated mice. Thus Figs. 6 and 7 summarize the increases of three characteristic acute phase proteins with <u>E.coli</u> type 055 LPS given intra-peritoneally and intra-venously respectively: Haptoglobin (Fig.6a and 7a), complement C3 (Fig.6b and 7a) and hemopexin (Fig.6c and 7a). Free haptoglobin is absent in serum from untreated control animals, but is present 4-16 hrs after treatment with LPS, except when given in amounts less than 0.2 mg intra-venously. The timecourse of the induction with the different doses appear from the Figure. The higher doses give an earlier increase in the serum. Also intra-peritoneal injections result in a faster acute phase response, most clearly seen for haptoglobin. In other experiments we tested other E.coli LPS types: The induction seen with LPS 0111 starts somewhat earlier than that seen with LPS 0124, but in both cases the maximal amount of haptoglobin is seen after 2 days. Complement increases more than 150% with 0111 and 100% with 0124 after 1 to 2 days after an initial fall (4-6 hrs). Hemopexin increases about 150% with both types of LPS. Other proteins also increase, as for instance macroglobulin with about 100% and immunoglobulin fractions (not shown). At the same time other proteins stay at a constant level as for example transferrin, and other proteins decrease in amount as the earlier mentioned non-specific carboxylic esterase ("B esterase") and albumin [Bøg-Hansen and Back, 1979].

In other experiments the HDL-associated arylesterase was seen to increase in activity (not shown).

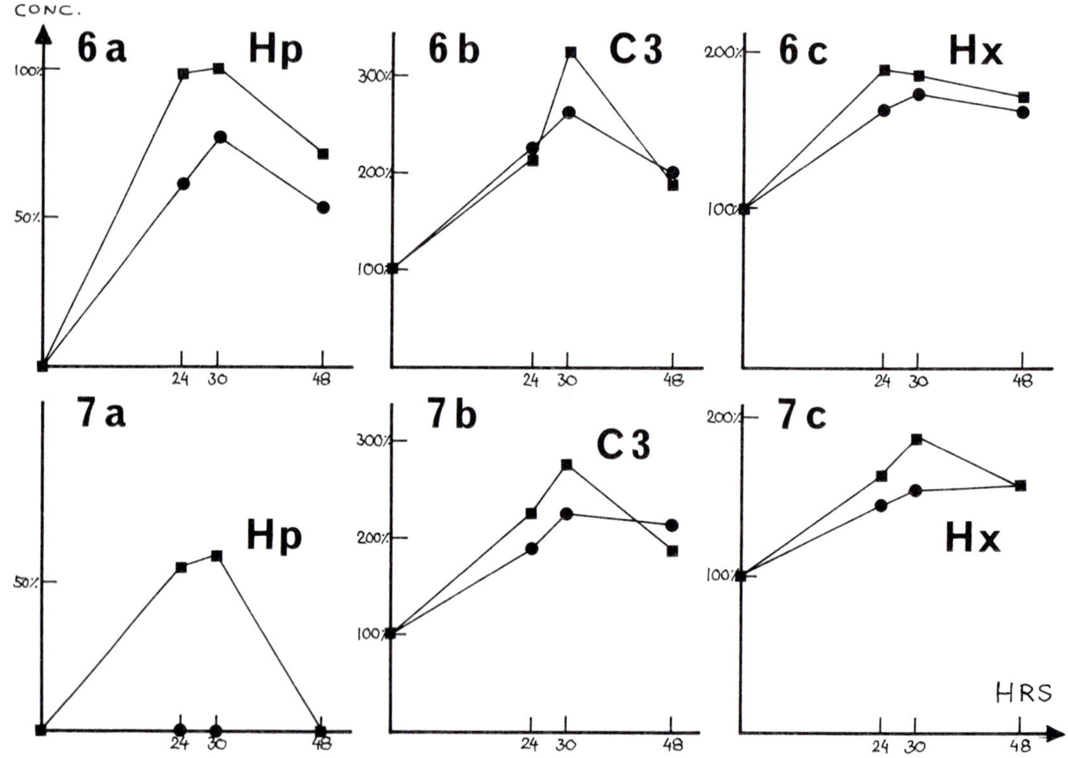

FIGURE 6 AND 7. ACUTE PHASE PROTEINS AFTER LPS-TREATMENT.
Relative concentration of characteristic acute phase proteins: Free haptoglobin (Hp), complement (C3), and hemopexin (Hx).
LPS-treatment:
Fig. 6: E.coli 055 LPS given intra-peritoneally.
Fig. 7: E.coli 055 LPS given intra-venously.
Dosis: 0.2 mg (●——●) and 0.4 mg (■——■). LPS phenolextracted, DIFCO. The relative concentration of specific proteins measured by planimetry of immunoplates as shown in Fig. 5.

On the basis of these experiments we find that C3H/HeJ is capable of a complex response to LPS and that this mouse strain should not be referred to as an over-all non-responder strain.

DISCUSSION

The literature is highly suggestive of reactions between endotoxins and plasma proteins, including detoxifying proteins and lipoproteins [Skarnes, 1970, Moreau and Skarnes, 1973, Johnsson et al., 1978, Bøg-Hansen et al., 1978, Ulevitch and Johnston, 1978] and blood cell receptors [Adye et al., 1973, Springer and Adye, 1975, Thorne et al., 1977] but their relation to the acute phase protein increases studied here is not clear. Earlier we observed characteristic acute phase changes in serum glycoproteins in normal responder mice after LPS treatment [Bøg-Hansen et al., 1978]. The following major changes were noted: Increase of haptoglobin, hemopexin, complement C3 and HDL-associated arylesterase in addition to the increase and shift of high density lipoprotein. On the other hand, as here, we found that other proteins decrease in amounts, as non-specific carboxylesterase (earlier termed "B esterase" [Augustinsson, 1958]) which strengthen the notion of acute phase protein increase.

Earlier Abd-El-Fattah et al. [1976] observed plasma protein changes in rats after challenge with the purified toxic component of LPS, lipid A, and listed increases of acute phase proteins, but they did not analyze for enzyme activities, nor did they describe any electrophortic shift of lipoprotein with lipid A. Similarly with LPS we could show the induction of acute phase proteins in mice (BALB/c) [Bøg-Hansen et al., 1978]. There appears to be differences in the response related to the type, dose and route of injection of the toxin as there appears to be a correlation between macromolecular events taking place between lipoproteins and LPS [Bøg-Hansen et al., 1979, Ulevitch and Johnston, 1978] and the acute phase response [in preparation].

Presumably the environment is of importance for the acute phase resonse since we could distinguish between SPF (specific pathogen-free) and non-SPF mice with respect to the initial level of acute phase proteins: The normal level of acute phase proteins is high in non-SPF animals as compared to a low level or absence in SPF animals. This led us to the conclusion that high levels of acute phase proteins is one of the adaptations to the ever-present endotoxin [Bøg-Hansen et al., 1978]. In this respect the C3H/HeJ strain deviates. At conventional conditions free haptoglobin is not found in the unstimulated state. What concerns the other acute phase proteins, the response is normal. Figs. 5-6 summarize characteristic increases.

We conclude that this strain does not deviate principally in its acute phase protein response from other strains tested.

Recently Haas et al. showed that C3H/HeJ is also capable of an immunological response towards LPS. The suppression of plaque-forming cells (PFC) formation was readily induced with LPS and found to be transferable with spleen cells of LPS-treated C3H/HeJ mice [Haas et al., 1978]. The changes of immunoglobulin fractions as we have seen during our experiments may be part of the normal immunological response still functioning in C3H/HeJ. With the lipoprotein response described recently [Bøg-Hansen et al., 1979] and the acute phase response described here, we argue that the term "non-responder" should be used only with specific reference to certain characteristics, as already advanced in [Bog-Hansen et al., 1979].

Acknowledgments. Drs. K.L.Fennestad, Marina Freudenberg, C.Galanos, Barbara and K.Jann, Ida and F.Ørskov are thanked for their interest and for providing biological material. Ms. Bente Eckert, Ms. Pia Jensen, Ms. Birgit B. Pedersen, Ms. Grethe Rønholt, Mr. W.Pedersen and Mr. W.Rosenbar are thanked for their assistance. The study was supported by the Thorwald Madsen Foundation, the Warwara Larsen Foundation and "Hestehandler Ole Jakobsens Mindelegat"

REFERENCES

Abd-El-Fattah, M., Scherer, R., and Ruhenstroth-Bauer, G. (1976) J.Mol.Med. 1, 211-221.

Adye, J.C., Springer, G.F. and Murthy, J.R. (1973) Z.Immun.Forsch. 144, 491-496.

Apte, R.N. and Pluznik, D.H. (1976) J.Cell.Physiol. 89, 313.

Augustinsson, K.B. (1958) Nature 181, 1786.

Bacchus (1975) Clin.Path. 6, 111-135.

Back, U., Møller, B.B., and Bøg-Hansen, T.C. (1976) Lancet II, 188-191.

Bøg-Hansen, T.C. and Back, U. (1979) Submitted for publication.

Bøg-Hansen, T.C., Krog, H.H. and Back, U. (1978) FEBS Letters 93, 86-90.

Bøg-Hansen, T.C., Hertel-Wulff, B. and Back, U. (1979) FEBS Letters 104, 441-445.

Boiesen, M., Kruger, C. and Bøg-Hansen, T.C. (1980) These proceedings.

Brogren, C.H. and Bøg-Hansen, T.C. (1975) Scand.J.Immunol. 4, Suppl. 2, 37-51.

Chedid, L., Parant, M., Damais, C., Parant, F., Juy, D., and Galleli, A. (1976) Infect.Immun. 13, 722-727.

Coutinho, A., Gronowicz, E. and Sultzer, B.M. (1975) Scand.J.Immunol. 4, 139-143.

Fridberg, M., Larsen, S. and Denneberg, T. (1978) Lancet I, 498-499.

Gallin, J.I., Kaye, D. and O'Leary, W.M. (1969) New Engl.J.Med. 281, 1081-1086.

Goodman, M.G., Parks, D.E. and Weigle, W.O. (1978) J.Exp. Med. 147, 800-813

Haas, G.P., Johnson, A.G. and Nowotny, A. (1978) J.Exp.Med. 148, 1081-1086.

Harboe, N. and Ingild, A. (1973) Scand.J.Immunol. 2, Suppl. 1, 161-164.

Hirsch, R.L., MacKay, D.G. and Travers, R.L. (1964) J.Lipid Res. 5, 563-568.

Johnson, K.J. and Ward, P.A. (1972) J.Immunol. 108, 611-616.

Johnson, K.J., Ward, P.A., Goralnick, S. and Osborn, M.J. (1977) Am.J.Pathol. 88, 559-574.

Larsen, J.H. (1976)

in Dumonde, D.C. (ed.) Infections and Immunology in the Rheumatic Diseases, pp.133-140, Blackwell, London.
LeQuire, V.S., Hutcherson. J.D. and Hamilton. R.L. (1959) J.Exp.Med. 110, 293-309.
May, J.E., Kane, M.A. and Frank, M.M. (1972) J.Immunol. 109, 893-895.
McAdam, K.P.W.J. and Sipe, J.D. (1976) J.Exp.Med. 144, 1121-1127.
Milner, K.C., Rudbach, J.A. and Ribi, E (1971) in General Characteristics in Microbial Toxins. Vol 5. Weinbaum, G., Kadis, S. and Ajl,S.J. (eds.) p1, Academic Press, New York.
Moore, R.N., Goodrum, K.J., Couch, R.E. and Berry, L.J. (1978) Infect.Immun. 19, 79.
Moreau, S.C. and Skarnes, R.C. (1973) J.Infect.Dis. 128, 122-133.
Olitzki, A (1972) Enteric Fevers. Causing Organisms and Host's Reactions. S.Karger, Basel.
Platt, H.S., Sewell, B.M., Feldman, T. and Souhami, R.L. (1973) Clin.Chim.Acta 46, 419.
Rieder, H.P. and Peyer, C (1970) Clin.Chim.Acta, 30, 305-310.
Rothfield and Horne, R.W. (1967) J.Bact. 93, 1705
Rutenburg, S.H., Rutenburg, A.M., Smith, E.E. and Fine, J. (1964) in Bacterial endotoxins (Landy and Braun, eds.) Rutgers University Press, New Brunswick, N.H., pp. 515-521.
Skarnes, R.C. (1966) Ann.N.Y.Acad.Sci. 133, 644-662.
Skarnes, R.C. (1968) J.Bacteriol. 95, 2031-2034.
Skarnes, R.C. (1970) J.Exp.Med. 132, 300-316.
Skarnes, R.C. and Chedid, L. (1964) in Bacterial Endotoxins, M.Landy and W.Brown (eds) Rutgers University Press, New Brunswick, N.J., pp. 575-587.
Skidmore, B.J., Chiller, J.M., Weigle, W.O., Riblet, R. and Watson, J. (1976) J.Exp.Med. 143, 143-150.
Springer, G.F. and Adye, J.C. (1975) Infect.Immun. 12, 978-986.
Störtebecker, T.P. (1978) Cancer - Unnecessary. Microorganisms and Chronic Infections as a Cause of Cancer. Natur och Kultur, Stockholm.
Sultzer, B.M. (1969) J.Immunol. 103, 32-38.
Sultzer, B.M. (1972) Infect.Immun. 5,107-113.
Svendsen, P.J. and Axelsen, N.H. (1972) J.Immunol.Methods 1, 169-176.
Thorne, K.J.I., Oliver, R.C., MacIntyre, D.E., and Gordon, J.L. (1977) J.Cell Sci. 28, 225-236.
Ulevitch, R.J. and Johnston, A.R. (1978) J.Clin.Invest. 62, 1313-1324.
Urbaschek, R., Mergenhagen, S.E. and Urbaschek, B. (1977) Infect.Immun. 18, 860.
Watson, J. and Riblet, R. (1974) J.Exp.Med. 140, 1147-1161.

INTERACTION OF LIPOPOLYSACCHARIDES WITH PLASMA HIGH DENSITY LIPOPROTEIN IN RATS

M. A. Freudenberg*, T. C. Bøg-Hansen, U. Back***, E. Jirillo* and C. Galanos**

**Max-Planck-Institut für Immunbiologie, Freiburg i.Br., Federal Republic of Germany*

***The Protein Laboratory, University of Copenhagen, Copenhagen N, Denmark*

****The Collaboratory Centre of Reference and Research on Escherichia (WHO), The State Serum Institute, Copenhagen, Denmark*

ABSTRACT

Lipopolysaccharides (LPS) and free lipid A after their administration in rats, interact with plasma high density lipoprotein (HLDL) forming a stable complex. They remain in this complex form until they are cleared from the circulation. The LPS-HDL complex was detected by crossed immunoelectrophoresis since it could be precipitated both, by anti LPS- and anti-HDL sera. The electrophoretic mobility of the complex differed from that of free HDL the difference being characteristic for each LPS or lipid A preparation. The results indicate that intact LPS interacts with HDL through its lipid A portion. The interaction with HDL abolishes the known property of LPS and lipid A to sensitize erythrocytes in vitro, since purified rat HDL was found to inhibit attachment of LPS and free lipid A in a dose dependent manner. This may be the reason why in the present study we were not able to detect LPS bound to sheep red cells in vivo. The data suggest that plasma HDL may influence the distribution of LPS in the organism.

KEYWORDS

Lipopolysaccharide, lipid A, high densitiy lipoprotein, complex formation, plasma clearance, erythrocyte binding.

Earlier studies on experimental animals have shown that circulating endotoxin (lipopolysaccharide), is preferentially present in the plasma compartment of the blood (CHEDID and co-workers, 1963). Recently in in vitro experiments the high density lipoprotein was identified as the major LPS binding protein in serum (BØG-HANSEN and co-workers, in preparation). In a study on rats the possible role of HDL as a carrier of circulating LPS in vivo was investigated (FREUDENBERG and co-workers, in preparation).

Protein-free LPS preparations from Salmonella abortus equi S (smooth) form and Salmonella minnesota R595 (Re) in the uniform triethylamine salt form and soluble free lipid A in the triethylamine form obtained from S.minnesota R345 (Rb) were used (GALANOS, LÜDERITZ, 1975; GALANOS and co-workers, 1979). The preparations were injected intravenously in three month old female AS2 rats without detectable antibodies towards the two LPS and lipid A in their serum.

Plasma samples of treated rats were analyzed in crossed immunoelectrophoresis (WEEKE, 1973) with antisera to LPS, rat serum proteins and rat lipoproteins.

Administration of LPS altered the HDL precipitation peak in plasma when analyzed by crossed immunoelectrophoresis. As shown in Fig. 1 changes in HDL immune precipitate induced by LPS appeared as early as 3 minutes after injection and were characteristic for each LPS preparation. With 5 mg of the S form LPS a part of the HDL precipitate was shifted towards the cathode and formed a shoulder on the original HDL peak. With the same amount of the R form LPS all HDL was shifted towards the anode. Apart from the above changes in HDL no alterations in other plasma proteins were observed 3 minutes after LPS injection.

Figure 1.

CHANGES IN RAT PLASMA HDL AFTER LPS (5 MG I.V.) INJECTION

(ANALYSIS WITH ANTI-RAT SERUM ANTIBODIES)

S. ABORTUS EQUI .TEN S. MINNESOTA R595 (RE) .TEN

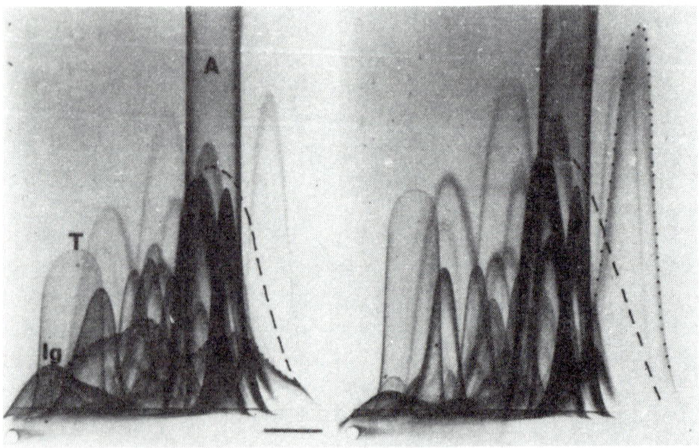

----- ORIGINAL POSITION OF PRECIPITATE

..... POSITION 3 MIN. AFTER LPS

The degree of alteration of HDL was dependent on the dose of LPS injected. With increasing dose of S form LPS (1.25 mg, 5 mg) the amount of altered HDL increased an the amount of original HDL precipitate decreased correspondingly. With very high LPS dose (20 mg) the entire HDL precipitate was shifted towards the cathode and a precipitate at the original HDL position was no longer detectable (Fig. 2).

In contrast to the S form LPS, with the R form preparation all doses used caused a shift of the entire HDL precipitate towards the anode. However, the distance of the new precipitate from the original HDL position increased with increasing amounts of LPS injected (Fig. 2).

With soluble free lipid A changes in the crossed immunoelectrophoretic pattern of HDL were also obtained 3 min. aftr injection. The changes were characterized by a shift of the whole HDL precipitation peak towards the anode which as larger with higher doses of LPS, and were thus comparable to the alterations seen with the R form LPS.

Figure 2.

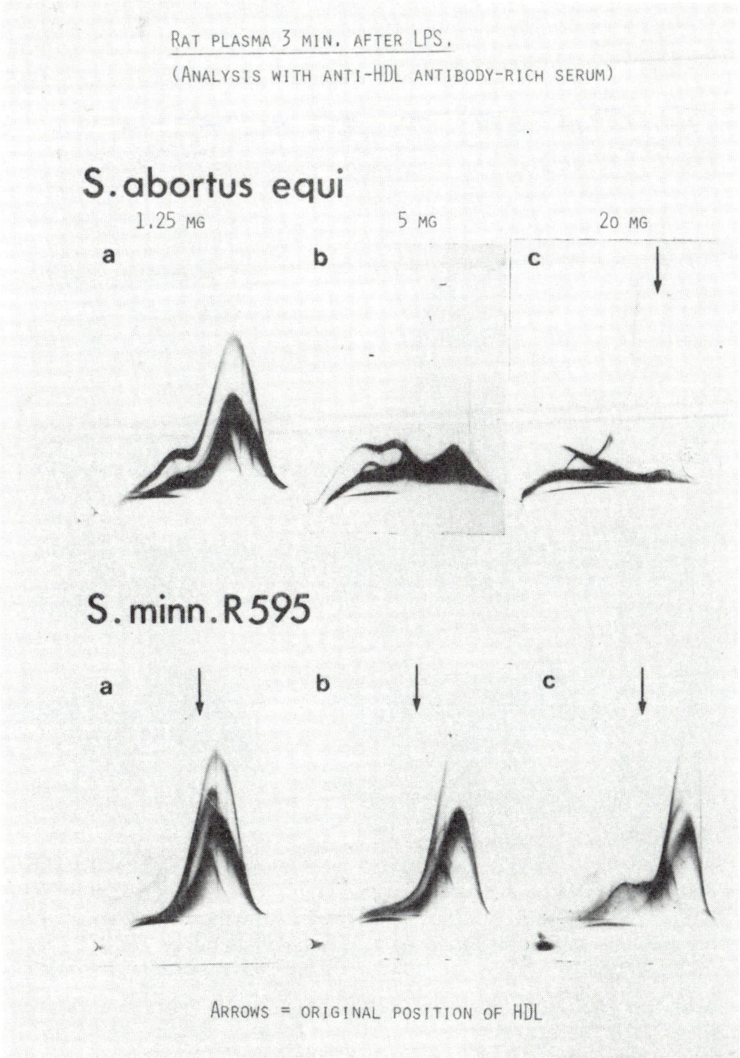

The above changes in HDL were independent of the route of injection of LPS. Thus intraperitoneal injection of S.abortus equi LPS (5 mg) led to a shift of part of the HDL precipitate towards the cathode, forming a shoulder on the original HDL precipitate, as seen with intravenously administered LPS. The changes were seen with plasma collected 6 hours after LPS injeciton, but were not detectable in plasma obtained after 3 min. and 1 hour. The absence of changes in plasma 3 min. and 1 hour after intraperitoneal injection, are explained on account of the delayed appearance of LPS in the blood due to the slow resorption from the peritoneum.

The alterations in HDL precipitation pattern found in plasma of LPS treated rats were identified as being due to complex formation between HDL and LPS. As shown with S form LPS in crossed immunoelectrophoresis with intermediate gel (AXELSEN, 1973), the LPS-

HDL complex was precipitated both by anti-HDL and anti-LPS sera (Fig. 3). Further, from the Fig. 3 it it obvious that after injectin of 5 mg LPS per rat no significant binding of LPS to other serum proteins was detectable.

Figure 3.

CROSSED-IMMUNOELECTROPHORESIS WITH INTERMEDIATE GEL OF RAT PLASMA 1H AFTER LPS

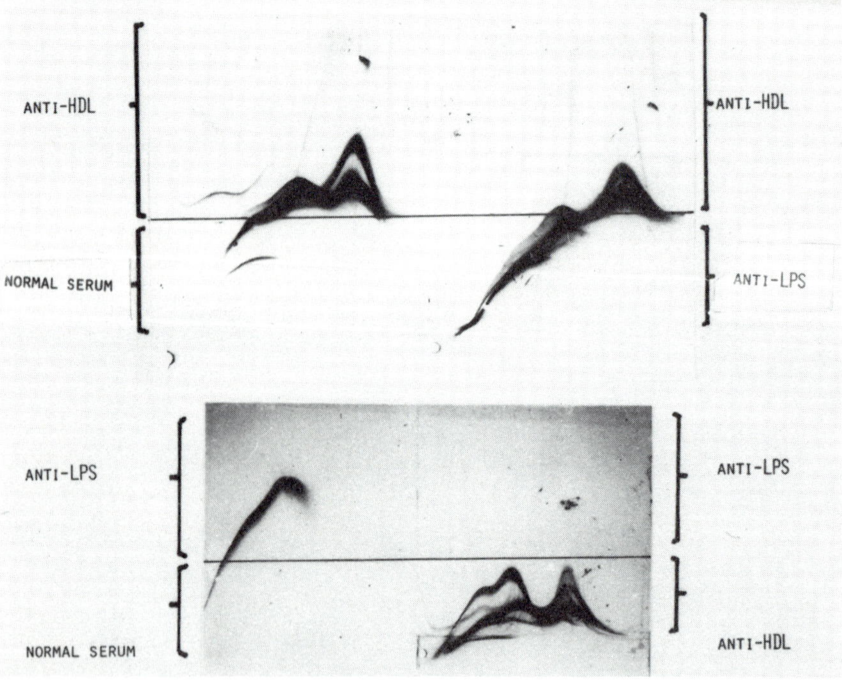

The present results confirm earlier findings of Skarnes (SKARNES AND ROSEN, 1971) that LPS interacts with plasma lipoproteins. As shown in the above experiments the electrophoretic mobility of the LPS-HDL complex differs according to the origin of the LPS used. A reason for this may be the difference in the negative charge of the two LPS, which is responsible for differences in the overall charge of the corresponding complex.

The persistence of the LPS-HDL complex in the circulation was investigated by following the time course of HDL alterations in rats injected with 5 mg LPS. The degree of HDL alterations i.e. the amount of LPS-HDL complex decreased with time, in the case of R form LPS the rate of disappearance was faster (about 6 hours) than with S form LPS (about 2 days).

Plasma clearance studies with ^{14}C-labelled S and R form LPS suggest a correlation between the disappearance of LPS-HDL complex and removal of LPS from circulation.

It should be mentioned that the clearance time for R form LPS (about 6 hours) and also for S form LPS (about 2 days) estimated in our experiments is unusually long compared with those obtained by other outhors (BRAUDE, 1969; CHEDID and co-workers, 1966; HOFMAN and DLABAC, 1974). The high dose of LPS, purity and low molecular weight of the LPS preparations as well as the complete absence of anti-LPS antibodies in the animals employed may all be factors accounting for the slow clearance observed in the present study.

According to the above data HDL represents a carrier protein for circulating LPS and lipid A in plasma. On account of the property of free lipid A to interact with HDL, we assume the intact LPS interacts with HDL via its lipid A portion.

Since lipid A represents the endotoxic principle of all LPS (GALANOS and co-workers, 1977) the question arises of the biological significance of the LPS-HDL interaction. In the present investigation we have not dealt yet with the question of the possible alteration in the biological activity or chemical structure of the LPS following interaction with HDL. Although according to Johnson and co-workers (1978) human lipoproteins are not able to detoxify LPS, earlier studies by Skarnes (SKARNES and ROSEN, 1971) showed that lipoprotein-associated esterases are enzymes involved in the humoral detoxification of LPS. In a recent study in mice it was shown that HDL-associated arylesterase is an acute phase protein inducible by LPS (BØG-HANSEN and co-workers, 1978). Also in our studies we were able to detect arylesterase activity associated with HDL and which persists in the LPS/HDL complex.

In agreement with results of other authors (CHEDID and co-workers, 1963; BRAUDE, 1964), we were not able to detect radioactivity associated with erythrocytes, following i.v. administration of ^{14}C-LPS in rats. For this reason the possible role of HDL in inhibiting the known property of LPS to attach to washed erythrocytes <u>in vitro</u> was investigated by the passive hemolysis test (NETER, 1965) using HDL isolated from fresh rat EDTA-plasma by ultracentrifugation (CAMEJO, 1967).

As shown in Fig. 4 incubation of erythrocytes with <u>S.abortus equi</u> sodium form LPS (PRAINO and co-workers, 1979) in the presence of graded amount of purified HDL inhibited in a dose-dependent manner the attachment of LPS and subsequent lysis by anti LPS serum and complement.

<u>Figure 4.</u>

<u>INHIBITION OF FIXATION OF LPS TO ERYTHROCYTES BY PURIFIED RAT HDL.</u>

(ATTACHMENT OF LPS TO ERYTHROCYTES WAS TESTED BY THE PASSIVE HEMOLYSIS TEST)

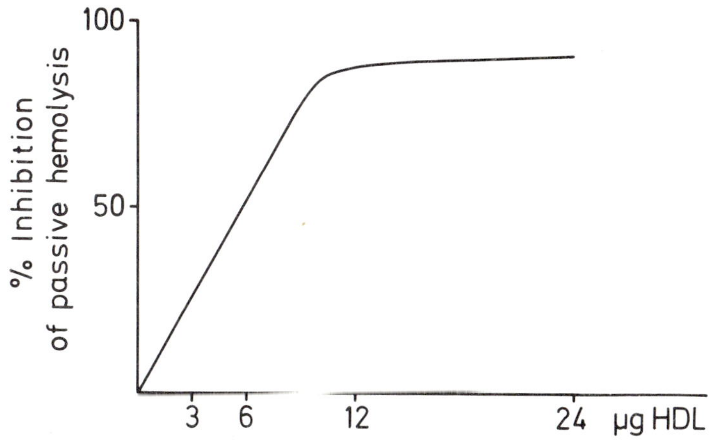

S. ABORTUS EQUI LPS (10 μG) WAS INCUBATED WITH 0.2 ML ERYTHROCYTES IN THE PRESENCE OF DIFFERENT AMOUNTS OF HDL, AND THE CELLS TESTED WITH ANTI-S. ABORTUS EQUI SERUM AND COMPLEMENT.

Under identical experimental conditions HDL also inhibited attachment of free lipid A to erythrocytes, however, to a much higher degree than with the LPS. The present data suggests that plasma HDL due to its binding property may influence the distribution of LPS among humoral and cellular targets in the organism.

ACKNOWLEDGEMENTS

We are grateful to H.Wintersinger, M.Gundelach, C.Serr, C.Bergmann, P.Jensen and W.Pedersen for expert technical assistance.
This study was partly supported by a grant from the VW-Stiftung (C.G.), by The Thorwald Madsen Foundation (U.B.) and The Warwara Larsen Foundation (U.B, T.C.B.-H.).

REFERENCES

Axelsen, N.H. (1973). In N.H.Axelsen, J.Knoll and B.Weeke (eds.), A manual of quantitative immunoelectrophoresis. Methods and Applications. Universitetsforlaget, Oslo-Bergen-Tromso, pp 71-78

Bøg-Hansen-T.C., H.H. Krog, , and U. Back (1978), FEBS letters 93, 86-90.

Braude, A.J. (1964).In M.Landy and W. Braun (eds.), Bacterial Endotoxins, Rutgers University Press, New Brunswick, N.Y., pp. 98-109.

Camejo, G. (1967), Biochemistry 6, 3228-3241.

Chedid, L., R.C. Skarnes and M. Parant (1963), J. Exp. Med. 117, 561-571.

Chedid, L., F. Parant, M. Parant, and F. Boyer (1966). Ann. N.Y. Acad. Sci. 133, 712-726.

Galanos, C., and O. Lüderitz (1975). Eur. J. Biochem. 9, 245-249.

Galanos, C., O. Lüderitz, E.Th. Rietschel., and O. Westphal (1977). In T.W. Goodwin (ed.), Biochemistry of Lipids II. Int. Rev. Biochem., Vol. 14, University Park Press, Baltimore-London-Tokyo, pp. 239-335.

Galanos, C., O. Lüderitz, and O. Westphal (1979) Zbl. Hyg. I Abt. Orig. A 243, 226-244

Hofman, J., and V. Dlabac (1974). J. Hyg. Epidemiol. Microbiol. and Immunol.18, 447-453.

Johnson, K.J., P.A. Ward, S. Goralnick, and M.J. Osborn (1978). Am.J.pathol.88, 559-574.

Neter, E. (1965). Bacteriol. Rev. 20, 166-188.

Praino, M.D., C. Galanos, and E. Neter (1979). Immunol. Comm. 8(1), 85-92.

Skarnes, R.C., and F.S. Rosen (1971). In S. Kadis, G. Weinbaum, and S.J. Ajl (eds). Microbial Toxins, Vol. V, Academic Press, New York and London. Chap. 5, pp. 151-164.

Weeke, L.B. (1973). In N.H. Axelsen, J. Knoll, and B. Weeke (eds.). A manual of quantitative immunoelectrophoresis. Methods and Applications. Universitetsforlaget. Oslo-Bergen-Tromso, pp. 47-56.

EFFECTS OF BACTERIAL ENDOTOXIN ON CEREBROSPINAL PROTEINS IN GUINEA PIGS[1]

(To Uffe Back, in memoriam)

M. Boiesen* **, C. Krüger* and T. C. Bøg-Hansen***

**The Protein Laboratory, University of Copenhagen, Denmark*
***The E. coli Reference Center (WHO), The State Serum Institute, Copenhagen, Denmark*
****Department of Molecular Biology and Biochemistry, The Free University, Berlin*

ABSTRACT

Proteins in the spinal fluid of guinea pigs treated with bacterial lipopolysaccharides for up to 30 days were studied by microgradient gel electrophoresis and quantitative immunoelectrophoresis. We could demonstrate the occurrence of high molecular weight serum proteins in the spinal fluid from 5 to 20 days of challenge. After about 20 days the protein pattern approached normal. The changes in precipitate morphology of antitrypsin indicated release of protease(s) from cells into the cerebrospinal fluid.

KEYWORDS

Endotoxin; blood-brain barrier; alpha-1 antitrypsin; microgradient gel electrophoresis; crossed immunoelectrophoresis; guinea pig.

INTRODUCTION

Endotoxins are the toxic lipopolysaccharide constituents (LPS of the cell wall of Gram-negative bacteria. Of the many biological activities and physiological changes initiated by LPS (Milner et al., 1971; Galanos et al., 1977), their effects on the central nervous system have been studied (Schmahl, 1975). An important question is whether LPS exerts any toxic effect on the blood-brain barrier. Earlier work has shown that parenteral administration of E. coli endotoxin leads to an increased permeability of the blood-brain barrier, permitting the entry of supravital dyes which are normally excluded from the central nervous system (Staab et al., 1965).

We have been interested in the immediate LPS-detoxifying potential of weakened animals in relation to the pathogenicity of LPS (Back et al., 1976), and our earlier studies have dealt with the immediate response expressed in plasma of animals treated with LPS for short time intervals (Bøg-Hansen et al., 1978, 1979; Bøg-Hansen and Back, 1979). In the accompanying paper we have thus shown that high-density lipoprotein (HDL) is the plasma receptor responsible for carrying circulating LPS.

[1]Presented in part at the InternationalSymposium on Biologically Active Products of Microorganisms, Prague, 1978.

This report gives some results on the protein changes observed in cerebrospinal fluid in guinea pigs treated daily for prolonged time (up to 30 days) with E.coli LPS.

EXPERIMENTAL

1. Endotoxin: E.coli type 026:B6 LPS (trichloroacetic acid-extracted) was obtained from Difco. LPS was dissolved in 0.9% saline for injection.

2. Animals: Guinea pigs of an outbread strain kept at conventional conditions at the State Serum Institute were used at the age of 3 months. The animals were given daily intraperitoneal injections of LPS for a period up to 30 days. Each day an animal was killed (24 hours after last injection) and sampled for blood and cerebrospinal fluid. The LPS was given in a dose of 2 mg/kg bodyweight in a volume not exceeding 0.7 ml. Control animals received 0.7 ml of saline. Blood and cerebrospinal fluid were

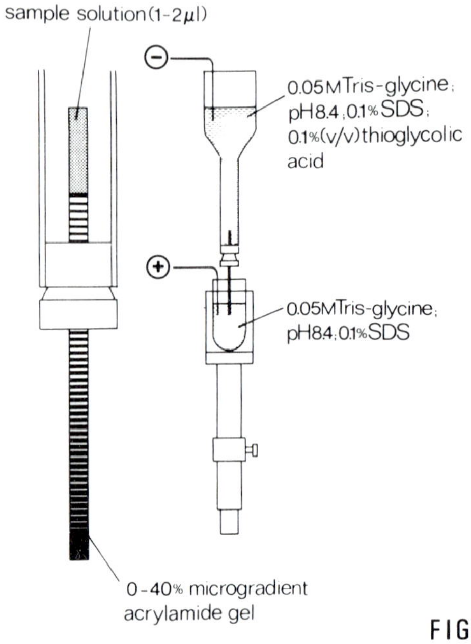

FIG. 1

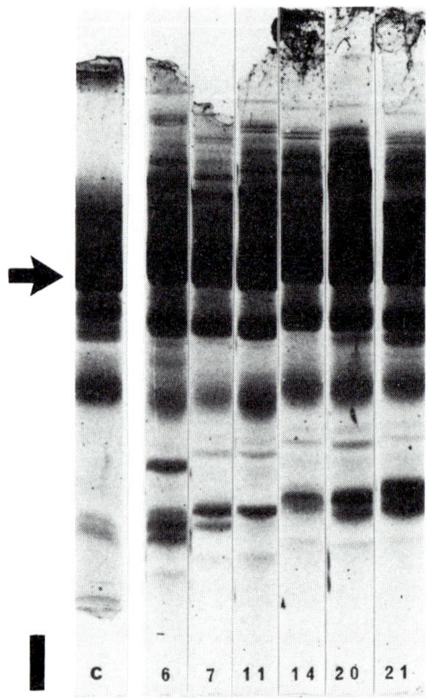

FIG. 2

FIGURE 1. MICROGRADIENT GEL ELECTROPHORESIS, APPARATUS AND SYSTEM. The electrophoreses were run at 40 V for 5 min, then at 80 V until the marker (bromo-phenol blue) was out of the gel, then for 30 min at 100 V. Capillary tubes were from Blaubrand (cat no. 709109, 10 ul, 32 mm).The gels were processed and stained according to [Rüchel et al., 1973].

FIGURE 2. MICROGRADIENT GELS. The protein pattern of guinea pig cerebrospinal fluid in microgradient electrophoresis. Patterns of control animal (C) and of animals treated with LPS each day until sampling (6-21 days). The arrow indicates albumin. The bar signifies 1 mm.

obtained after killing the animal with ether. The blood was allowed to clot at 4 C and the serum was separated after centrifugation. The cerebrospinal fluid was obtained by laying-free the atlantooccipital membrane and pierzing it with a pointed capillary tube [Moreland, 1965, Federspil, 1972]. The serum and cerebrospinal fluid were frozen at -20 C. until analyzed.

3. Microgradient gel electrophoresis: Acrylamide and bisacrylamide were recrystallized from analytical grade reagents. The power supply was obtained from E.Schütt (Göttingen, Germany) and the electrophoresis stand for the microcapillaries was home built (see Fig. 1).

4. Crossed immunoelectrophoresis was performed as described earlier for mouse (Bøg-Hansen et al.,1978). Antibodies were obtained from DAKO Immunoglobulins (Copenhagen, Denmark).

RESULTS

Microgradient Gel Electrophoresis

We used two types of sensitive electrophoresis systems to monitor protein changes: microgradient gel electrophoresis and quantitative immunoelectrophoresis. In Fig. 1 we show a schematical representation of the microgradient gel electrophoresis apparatous and electrophoresis system [Rüchel et al., 1973]. With normal spinal fluid we observed a small number of protein bands, but when animals were given daily intraperitoneal injections of LPS the number of protein bands increased (Fig. 2). Moreover we observed lasting changes in the banding pattern.

The most remarkable change in the microgradient gels was the appearance of high and low molecular weight components after about three days. The high molecular weight components were present in the cerebrospinal fluid until about the 20th day of LPS-treatment and disappeared afterwards. The low molecular weight proteins stayed in the cerebrospinal fluid during at least 30 days of LPS treatment.

The nature of the protein bands is not clear, but we expect the high molecular weight bands represent immunoglobulin fractions or macroglobulins.

Crossed Immunoelectrophoresis

In order to obtain more information on the proteins, we employed crossed immunoelectrophoresis of normal cerebrospinal fluid and of corresponding serum (Fig. 3). Some proteins were identified by cross-reaction with specific antibodies against human serum proteins, and the main components in cerebrospinal fluid are: Albumin (A), antitrypsin (AT) and transferrin (T). Both in serum [Kobayashi et al., 1974] and in spinal fluid, antitrypsin appears as a characteristic double peak (arrows).

Corresponding to changes observed in the microgradient gel pattern, we find additional protein precipitates between day 3 and day 20. Also we noticed a considerable individual variation in the number of additional precipitates, their size and intensity, but albumin and transferrin remained at an increased level.

Most characteristic were the changes in the antitrypsin peak. In contrast to the normal antitrypsin (Fig. 3) the antitrypsin precipitate from cerebrospinal fluid of treated animals became much more irregular and diffuse, often showing additional peaks with total or partial identity to the original antitrypsin (Fig. 4, arrows). Such precipitates for antitrypsin has been described by Hochstrasser et al. [1972] after complexation with leukocyte proteases.

We interpret the change of pattern seen here as a similar indication of complex formation with protease(s).

DISCUSSION

The experiments with cerebrospinal fluid of guinea pigs treated with LPS are our approach to the study of the deleterious effects of toxic bacterial components on the central nervous system, a line of research which we persue because endotoxins (LPS) have been postulated as a pathogenic cause in several diseases including diseases of the central nervous system, cf. discussion in [Bøg-Hansen and Back, 1980]. Thus, Störtebecker [1978] recently summarized and discussed the evidence for involvement of toxins of bacterial origin in the demyelination proces.

The most remarkable change we observed in the microgradient gels of cerebrospinal fluids was the appearance of high and low molecular weight compounds after about 3 days of treatment with endotoxin. We interpret the presence of these components as a result of a damage to the blood-brain barrier. However, when we measured the protein ratio between cerebrospinal fluid and serum for specific proteins, we could not demonstrate this ultimately, probably due to the large variation in both the treated and untreated group of animals (data not shown).

The nature and origin of these bands represent an interesting question. The high molecular weight bands may be immunoglobulins or macroglobulins, either originating from plasma or from local production.

To approach this question, we performed crossed immunoelectrophoresis, a method which is very useful for characterization of proteins. In addition to antiserum against brain proteins, we used antiserum against guinea pig serum proteins, as these proteins constitute the main part of the total protein content of the cerebrospinal fluid [Glasner, 1975]. The crossed immunoelectrophoresis from both treated and untreated animals shows several precipitates. Three distinct precipitates have been identified as albumin, antitrypsin and transferrin. Of special interest is the antitrypsin, as this protein changes drastically in its immunoelectrophoretic properties after only a few doses of endotoxin (Fig. 4). Similar changes are not observed in the corresponding serum, a fact which indicate special pathophysiological processes in the cerebrospinal fluid behind the blood-brain barrier after intraperitoneal endotoxin treatment. Based upon the character of antitrypsin as a proteinase inhibitor, we interpret the observations as consequences of proteinase release into the cerebrospinal fluid giving rise to complex formation between antitrypsin and proteinase(s), changing the electrophoretic properties of antitrypsin.

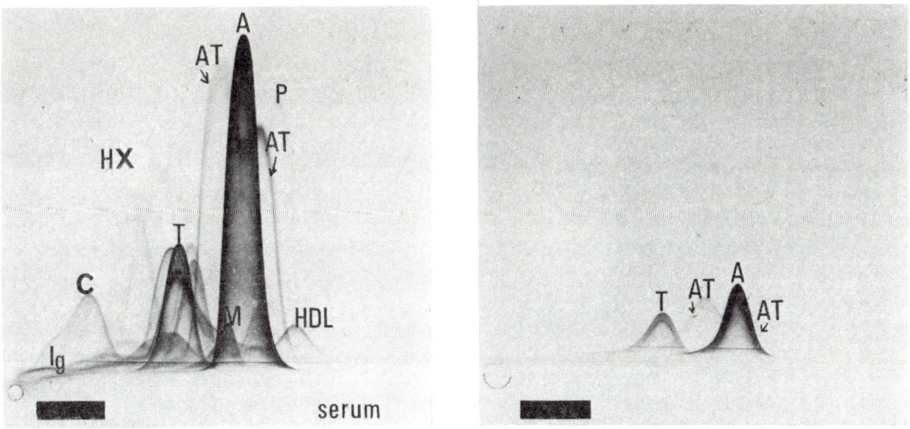

FIGURE 3. CROSSED IMMUNOELECTROPHORESIS OF NORMAL GUINEA PIG SERUM AND CEREBROSPINAL FLUID. The major proteins are indicated. Abbreviations:
A = albumin,
AT = alpha-1 antitrypsin,
C = complement C3,
HDL = alpha lipoprotein,
Hx = hemopexin,
Ig = immunoglobulins,
M = alpha-2 macroglobulin,
P = prealbumin,
T = transferrin.
Amounts analyzed: 0.5 ul serum and 15 ul CSF; antibody concentration: 6 ul/cm^2 (for serum) and 3 ul/cm^2 (for CSF). The bar represents 1 cm.

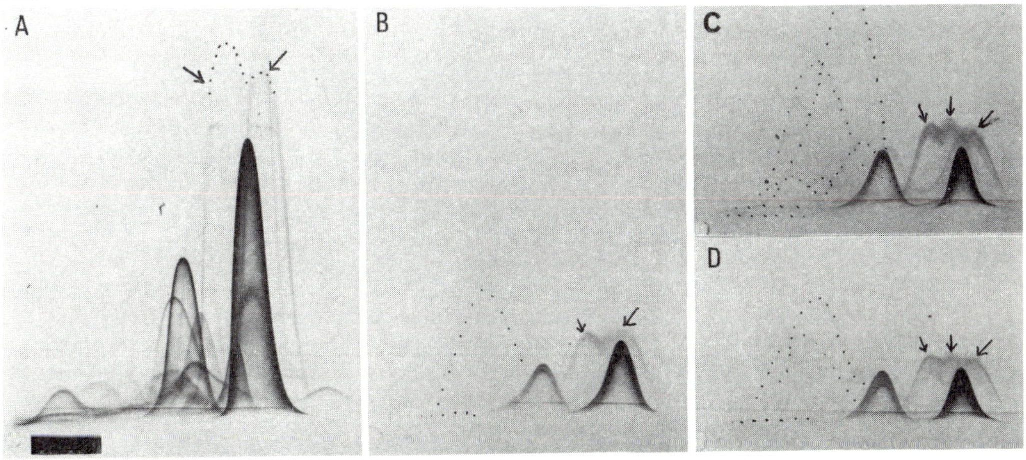

FIGURE 4. CROSSED IMMUNOELECTROPHORESIS OF CEREBROSPINAL FLUID FROM GUINEA PIGS TREATED WITH ENDOTOXIN (LPS).
A and B: serum and cerebrospinal fluid from a guinea pig treated with LPS each day for 21 days (daily dosis 2 mg/kg), compare Fig. 3.
C and D cerebrospinal fluids from two guinea pigs treated for 7 days (dayly dosis 1 mg/kg).
The arrows indicate alpha-1 antitrypsin. Weak additional precipitates indicated by dots. Otherwise as for Fig. 3.

We find it likely that the enzyme release is a result of tissue damage related to the endotoxin treatment.

In this connection it appears to be noteworthy that Adams et al. [1971] have found that proteolytic enzymes may play a role at an early stage in the pathogenesis of the multiple sclerosis plaque. By histochemical techniques it was shown that basic protein is degraded at the margin of the acute plaque, preceeding disintegration of myelin lipids [Adams et al., 1971]. Even more recently, Cammer et al. [1978] have found that proteinases from activated macrophages will selectively digest the basic protein moiety of myelin.

Acknowledgements.
Drs. K.L.Fennestad, Lis Specht Hansen, Ida and F.Ørskov are thanked for their interest. Ms. Pia Jensen and the staff at the guinea pig house at the State Serum Institute are thanked for their assistance. The study was supported by "Hestehandler Ole Jakobsens Mindelegat" and the Warwara Larsen Foundation.

REFERENCES

Adams, C.W.M., Hallpike, J.F. and Bayliss, O.B. (1971) J.Neurochem. 18, 1479-1483.

Back, U., Møller, B.B., and Bøg-Hansen, T.C. (1976) Lancet II, 188-191.

Bøg-Hansen, T.C. and Back, U. (1979) Submitted for publication.

Bøg-Hansen, T.C., Krog, H.H. and Back, U. (1978) FEBS Letters 93, 86-90.

Bøg-Hansen, T.C., Hertel-Wulff, B. and Back, U. (1979) FEBS Letters 104, 441-445.

Cammer, W., Bloom, B.R. and Norton, W.T. (1978) Proc.Natl.Acad.Sci. U.S.A. 75, 1554-1558.

Federspil, Von P. (1972) Z.Versuchstierk. 14, 341-346.

Galanos, C., Lüderitz, O., Rietschel, E.T. and Westphal, O. (1977) Intl.Rew.Biochem. 14, 239-235.

Glasner, H. (1975) Eur.Neurol. 13, 304-314.

Hochstrasser, K., Schuster, R., Reichert, R., Heimburger, N. (1972) Hoppe-Seyler's Z.Physiol.Chem. 353, 1120-1124.

Kobayashi, S. and Nagasawa, N. (1974) Biochim.Biophys.Acta 342, 372-381.

Milner, K.C., Rudbach, J.A. and Ribi, E. (1971) in General Characteristics in Microbial Toxins. Vol 5. Weinbaum, G., Kadis, S. and Ajl, S.J. (eds.) pl, Academic Press, N.Y.

Moreland, A.F. (1965) Methods of Animal Experimentation. Vol 1. Gay, W.I. (ed.) pp. 21-23.

Rüchel, R., Mesecke, S., Wolfrum, D.I. and Neuhoff, V. (1973) Hoppe-Seylers Z.Physiol.Chem. 354, 1351-1368.

Schmahl, F.W. (1975) in Gram-negative Bacterial Infections and Mode of Endotoxin Actions. Urbaschek, B., Urbaschek, R. and Neter, E. (eds.) Springer Verlag, Wien, pp. 338-345.

Staab, E.V., Good, R.A. and Condie, R.M. (1965) Proc.Soc.Exp.Biol.Med. 119, 1o30-1034.

Störtebecker, T.P. (1978) Cancer-Unnecessary. Microorganisms and Chronic Infections as a Cause of Cancer. Natur och Kultur, Stockholm.

STRUCTURE AND TOXICITY OF LIPID A FROM *VIBRIO CHOLERAE*

S. Raziuddin

Department of Immunopathology, Scripps Clinic and Research Foundation, La Jolla, California 92037, USA

ABSTRACT

Lipid A moiety of the lipopolysaccharide (LPS) represent the endotoxic principle of the Gram-negative bacteria. The significance of lipid A for the functional and structural integrity of the bacterial cell membrane and the central role it plays in the endotoxicity of endotoxins prompted studies on structure, biological and immunological activities from various antigenically different strains of Vibrio Cholerae. Structural studies revealed that lipid A from V. cholerae 569 B (Inaba) contains a glucoasamine backbone, and the fatty acids are bound to the hydroxyl and amino groups of glucoasamine residues. Approximately, equal amounts of palmitic, oleic and 3-hydroxy lauric acids were involved in ester linkages, and 3-hydroxymyristic acid was the only amide-linked fatty acid in this lipid A molecule. The LPS of V. cholerae do not contain 2-keto-3-deoxyoctonate (KDO), the typical linking sugar of lipid A and polysaccharide moiety of LPS from enterobacteriaceae. The de-O-acylated lipid A (water soluble product of lipid A) obtained as a result of mild alkaline methanolysis was proved to be a mixture of phosphorylated oligosaccharides. De-o-acylated lipid A on fractionation using Sephadex G-25 gave three major fractions, F1, F2 and F3. These fractions of lipid A, the intact purified LPS and lipid A/BSA have been studied for various biological activities. It was noted that LPS, lipid/BSA and F1 fractions exhibited local Shwartzman reaction in rabbits, gelated the limulus lysate, were lethal to chick embryos and were pyrogenic in rabbits. The results of these tests showed that LPS from these bacteria were toxic but high doses were required to exhibit these toxic effects. The structural part responsible for various biological activities of LPS was its lipid A moiety. The alkaline digestion (0.3 N NaOH, 105 C, 30 min) of lipid A which cleaves the ester linked fatty acids from it resulted in complete loss in toxicity of the lipid A from V. cholerae. These results reveal that ester-linked fatty acids in lipid A plays a central role in toxicity of LPS and lipid A's. Antiserum prepared against the lipid A of V. cholerae prevented the local Shwartzman reaction in rabbits. In all rabbits treated with lipid A antiserum, lipid A/BSA did not provoke a positive reaction.

KEYWORDS

Vibrio cholerae; lipopolysaccharides; lipid A; lipid-A antiserum; structure, toxicity.

INTRODUCTION

The lipopolysaccharide component of the cell wall of gram-negative bacteria is the endotoxic principle and has received considerable attention during the past several decades due to its ubiquitous capacity to perturb or activate a wide spectrum of eukaryotic cells. Generally lipopolysaccharides consist of three regions with different chemical and biological activities. The O-specific side chain polysaccharide (region I) carries the main serological specificity of bacteria. It is linked to a core polysaccharide (region II) that is common to groups of bacteria. This polysaccharide core is linked through a 2-keto-3-deoxyoctonate (KDO) trisaccharide to the lipid component, termed lipid A. The lipopolysaccharides are synthesized in the inner cytoplasmic membrane of the bacterial cell and, immediately after completion, are exported to the outer membrane, where with proteins they form the external face of the bilayer. Lipopolysaccharides, being anchored on the surface of the bacterial cell through the lipid A component and thus occupying an exposed position, certainly play a significant role in the interaction of bacteria with the host during infection because of their unique biological properties.

The structure of lipid A moiety of lipopolysaccharide from a large number of gram-negative bacteria has been elucidated, and studies on structure-function relationship has already yielded significant results. Lipid A is covalenty bound within the lipopolysaccharides, from which it can be released by gentle acid hydrolysis, which simultaneously liberates polysaccharides. Chemical investigations on lipid A's from Salmonella R-mutants, have revealed that lipid A consists chemically of B-1, 6-linked D-glucoasamine disaccharide units, which are interlinked by pyro phosphate bridges between position 1 and 4 of neighboring disaccharides. Studies carried out in several laboratories have shown that B1, 6-linked glucoasamine residues also form the backbone of lipid A in a number of lipopolysaccharides. In the last two decades numerous studies attempted to correlate biological activity with the various physical and/or chemical properties of endotoxin preparations with results implicating both the polysaccharide and the lipid regions of the lipopolysaccharide as having the predominant biological activity. Kasai (1966) suggested that neither fraction alone could elicit full biological activity but rather that the macromolecular complex formed by the chemical bonds linking the lipid A with the polysaccharide was required for the manifestation of full biologic activity. The separation and isolation of the lipid A fractions, their chemical identification, and their biological assays for endotoxic activities were commenced several years ago mainly by Nowotny and others (1966) and Lüderitz and others (1973). But it was not until the isolation and characterization of a heptose deficient mutant strain of a gram-negative organism (the R595 mutant of Salmonella minnesota) that the biological activity of lipid A preparations was firmly established. The demonstration by a number of investigators that lipopolysaccharide prepared from these polysaccharide-deficient (rough) mutants still manifest virtually all of the endotoxic properties of polysaccharide-containing endotoxins firmly established that lipid A plays a dominant role in endotoxicity (Galanos and others, 1977). Thus most of the physiopathological reactions expressed by lipopolysaccharides or endotoxins during infection reside in the lipid A moiety, which is an ubiquitous structure in bacteria. Many activities including lethal toxicity, pyrogenicity, complement inactivation, adjuvanticity, and tumor necrosis, bone marrow reaction, limulus lysate gelation, interferon release, induced abortion in mice, B-lymphocyte mitogenicity and activation of Hageman factor, were demonstrated with free isolated lipid A (Morrison and Ulevitch, 1978). Lipid A exhibits a high affinity to cell membranes, proteins and lipids, and this property is assumed to initiate biological reactions. Galanos and others (1971) have shown that lipid A, when exposed on the surface of bacterial cells, acts as an immunogen, giving rise to the production of specific antilipid A antibodies. They are stimulated under defined conditions in rabbits, dogs, goats, mice and other animals. Furthermore, natural antibodies with lipid A specificity have been detected in the sera of various species including man. Since these natural antibodies react with free lipid A from Salmonella, this is taken as an additional evidence that the immunological specificity of free lipid A is not an artifact. According to the structural similarities of lipid A among Enterobacteriaceae, antilipid A antibodies cross-react with lipid A obtained from otherwise serologically unrelated lipopolysaccharides. These findings prompted investigations into the biological significance of lipid A antisera of different bacterial species.

The main features of the structure of Escherichia Coli and Salmonella lipid A have been evaluated. These toxic lipid A preparations contain both hydroxy and non hydroxy fatty acids as essential main constituents. It has also been found that the lipid A precursors prepared from Salmonella (Osborn and others, 1974), whose structure lacks non-hydroxylated fatty acids, is highly toxic for mice and moderately pyrogenic in rabbits. These and other findings have stimulated investigations in various laboratories to identify the minimal structural conditions for endotoxicity. Various approaches can be used. Selective stepwise degradation of endotoxin or lipid A may lead to the identification of the smallest fragments still exhibiting biological activities. Inactive fragments of lipid A can be used for restoration of activity by partial chemical re-synthesis. In spite of these various approaches, it still remains obscure why and by which mechanisms these lipid A preparations exhibit their extraordinary diversity of biological activities and which are the minimal structural requirements for these properties. Investigations on lipid A from species other than Escherichia Coli and Salmonella may represent a further route for exploring biologically essential structures. Therefore as a part of our continuing program in determining the toxic principles of gram-negative bacterial endotoxins, the lipid A moiety of the lipopolysaccharides from antigenically different strains of Vibrio cholerae, V. cholerae 569 B (Inaba) and V. cholerae el-tor (Inaba) have been studied in relation to structure and toxicity. Lipopolysaccharides were extracted from the cell walls of these bacterial species (Raziuddin and Kawasaki, 1976) by phenol-water extraction procedures of Westphal and Jann (1965). The lipid A, being hydrophobic, is insoluble in aqueous solvents and thus may be easily separated from the partially degraded, although antigenically intact, polysaccharide either by centrifugation or extraction into organic solvents. In this study lipid A was released by mild acid hydrolysis of lipopolysaccharides using 1% acetic acid at 105°C for 2.5 hrs (Raziuddin, 1977). Each hydrolysate was separated into chloroform-soluble, water soluble and interfacial materials by thorough mixing with an equal volume of chloroform, followed by low speed centrifugation at 18000 g for 20 min. The chloroform layer was isolated, washed twice with water and dried to give lipid A, and purified as described (Raziuddin and Ambegaokar, 1976; Raziuddin and Kawasaki, 1976). Fatty acid residues (ester- and amide-linked) were removed from lipid A by hydrazinolysis with anhydrous hydrazine at 100°C for 10 h, and lipid A was de-o-acylated by mild alkaline methanolysis. The water soluble products from lipid A were fractionated by column chromatography using Sephadex G-25. Elution was carried out with 20% (v/v) methanol and fractions were analysed for phosphorus and were then pooled according to the respective peaks and analyzed. Fatty acids were liberated from lipid A with 2.0 M HCl or 10% (w/v) KOH in 50% (v/v) methanol, and methylesters of the free fatty acids prepared by reaction with diazomethane were trimethysilylated and analyzed by gas-liquid chromatography (Raziuddin, 1976, 1977). The relative proportions of O- and N-substitution with fatty acids were also determined. Lipid A and their fractions were also analyzed for various sugars and aminosugars. Lipid A was made soluble by complexing with bovine serum albumin (BSA) and various toxic activities such as local Shwartzman reaction in Rabbits, chick embryo lethality, limulus lysate gelation and pyrogenicity were studied from lipid A/BSA complex and their fractions. Effects of alkaline digestion, and ethylenediamino-tetraacetic acid (EDTA) treatments on lipid A's were also investigated (Raziuddin, 1978). Lipid A antiserum prepared was tested for certain anti endotoxic activities.

RESULTS

Structure of Lipid A: The lipid A moiety of the lipopolysaccharides obtained from V. cholerae 569 B (Inaba) and V. el-tor (!naba) showed the presence of glucosamine, the only aminosugar it contained. After hydrolysis of lipid A in 1M HCl at 105°C for 4 h traces of glucose, fructose and heptose were detected. Apart from glucose, fructose and heptose, other sugars tested were completely absent from these lipid A preparations. Thin-layer chromatography of lipid A preparations on silica gel G using chloroform-methanol-water (65:25:4, by vol) showed a considerable heterogeneity, which could partly be due to the existence of extended structures in which acylated disaccharide units are linked together by phosphodiester or pyrophosphate bridges.

The structural studies of the backbone of lipid A can be simplified by the prior removal of fatty acid residues. Hydrazinolysis was therefore used to remove the fatty acids, both ester- and amide-linked, from the lipid-A preparations. The de-O-acylated lipid A (water-soluble products of lipid A), obtained as a result of mild alkaline methanolysis, was proved to be a mixture of phosphorylated oligosaccharides. De-O-acylated lipid A was further fractionated by column chromatography on Sephadex G-25, giving the results shown in Fig. 1. Three major fractions designated F1, F2 and F3 were resolved by fractionating of the de-O-acylated lipid A of these bacteria.

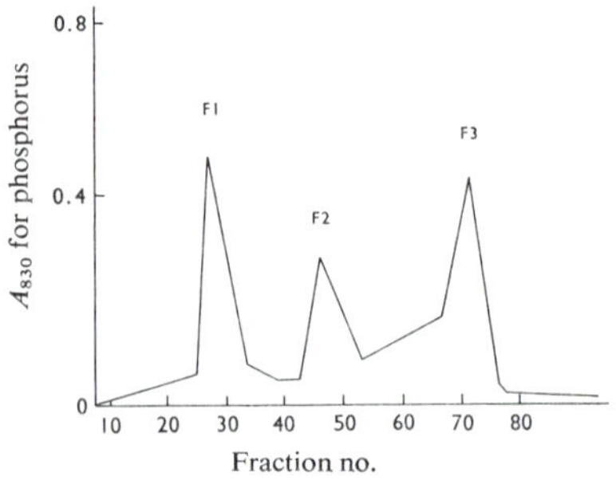

Fig. 1: FRACTIONATION OF DE-O-ACYLATED LIPID A FROM V. CHOLERAE

The water-soluble products (de-O-acylated lipid) from lipid A (15 mg) were fractionated on a column of Sephadex G-25 (1.5 cm x 70 cm). Elution was carried out with 20% (v/v) methanol at a flow rate of 10 ml/h. Fractions (2 ml) were collected and screened for phosphorus content and were then pooled and analysed as described in Table I. Similar results were obtained for V. cholerae 569 B (Inaba) and V. el-tor (Inaba).

The distribution of components between the fractions of de-O-acylated lipid A, F1, F2 and F3 are given in Table I. Glucoasmine and phosphorus were present at different concentrations in F1, F2 and F3 fractions.

Table I: Analysis of Fractions of de-O-acylated Lipid A From V. Cholerae and V. El-Tor

	V. cholerae		*V. el-tor*	
Fractions	Glucosamine (μg)	Total phosphorus (μg)	Glucosamine (μg)	Total phosphorus (μg)
F1	250	12.5	280	28
F2	190	20.0	65	18
F3	405	60.0	510	48

The results of the g.l.c. analysis of the fatty acids liberated by acidic (2.0M-HCl, 2.5h 105°C) and alkaline (10% KOH in 50% methanol; 2.5h refluxing) hydrolysis of lipid A from V. cholerae and V. el-tor are given in Table 2. Both of the hydrolytic procedures used gave an identical quantitative fatty acid pattern, with $C_{14:0}$, $C_{16:0}$, $C_{16:1}$ and $C_{18:1}$ fatty acids, 3-hydroxy-$C_{12:0}$ and 3-hydroxy-$C_{14:0}$ as the major fatty acids, and differing only in $C_{16:1}$ fatty acid content. The alkaline hydrolysis of lipid A yielded a smaller amount of $C_{16:1}$ fatty acid. 3-Hydroxy-$C_{12:0}$ was the main fatty acid component of lipid A from V. cholerae and V. el-tor. Moreover, hydroxy fatty acids were absent from free lipids and phospholipids of these bacteria (Raziuddin, 1976; Raziuddin and Kawasaki, 1976).

Table 2: Fatty Acid Composition Determined by Acid and Alkaline Hydrolysis of Lipid A from V. Cholerae and V. El-Tor

	V. cholerae		*V. el-tor*	
Fatty acids	Acid hydrolysis (%, w/w)	Alkaline hydrolysis (%, w/w)	Acid hydrolysis (%, w/w)	Alkaline hydrolysis (%, w/w)
$C_{14:0}$	12.8	10.2	13.4	10.8
$C_{15:0}$	1.0	0.6	1.6	0.8
$C_{16:0}$	9.2	11.4	13.6	12.2
$C_{16:1}$	10.8	4.2	12.8	3.8
$C_{18:0}$	2.8	Trace	3.0	Trace
$C_{18:1}$	12.8	11.6	11.8	10.6
3-OH-$C_{10:0}$	2.5	1.6	1.8	0.6
3-OH-$C_{12:0}$	28.6	26.4	22.4	25.4
3-OH-$C_{14:0}$	14.2	13.4	15.6	14.2

Mild alkaline methanolysis was used to distinguish between the ester- and amide-linked fatty acids from lipid A. Methanolysis transesterifies O-acyl residues into methyl esters, but in contrast, amide-linked fatty acids are not liberated by this treatment and are still present in the de-O-acylated lipid A, obtained after the centrifugation of the methanolysates as a sediment. Strong alkaline hydrolysis (4M-NaOH, 6h, 105°C) was therefore used to release amide-linked fatty acids from these products. In the de-esterfied sediments of lipid A from V. cholerae and V. el-tor, 3-hydroxymyristic acid was the only fatty acid component identified by g.l.c. Therefore these results indicate that 3-hydroxymyristic acid is an amide-linked fatty acid in lipid A of V. cholerae and V. el-tor. On the other hand, ester-linked fatty acids were identified in the supernatants, obtained after the centrifugation of the methanolysates, in the form of methyl esters. The ester-bound major fatty acids from lipid A of V. cholerae and V. el-tor were $C_{16:0}$, $C_{16:1}$ and $C_{18:1}$ fatty acids and 3-hydroxylauric acid. Of these ester-bound fatty acids, 3-hydroxylauric acid was the main component and 3-hydroxymyristic acid was not detected (Table 3). Thus these results clearly indicate that 3-hydroxymyristic acid is an amide-linked fatty acid, and $C_{16:0}$, $C_{16:1}$, $C_{18:1}$ fatty acids and 3-hydroxylauric acid are ester-linked fatty acids in lipid A of V. cholerae and V. el-tor.

The relative proportion of O- and N-substitutions in fatty acids of lipid A from V. cholerae and V. el-tor are given in Table 3. Hydroxylaminolysis of lipid A showed that $C_{14:0}$, $C_{18:0}$ and 3-hydroxy-$C_{10:0}$ fatty acids were O-linked in V. cholerae, whereas the $C_{18:1}$ fatty acids was O-linked in V. el-tor. Similarly, N-linked fatty acids were $C_{16:1}$ from V. cholerae and $C_{16:1}$ and 3-hydroxy-$C_{10:0}$ from V. el-tor. Approximately equal amounts of O-linked $C_{16:0}$ and $C_{18:1}$ fatty acids and 3-hydroxylauric acid were found to be involved in ester linkages. Except for these above-mentioned differences, all other fatty acids were present as both the O-acyl and N-acyl esters.

Table 3: Quantification of Fatty Acids in Methanolysates of Lipid A and Relative Proportions of O- and N-Linked Esters of Fatty Acids from V. Cholerae and V. El-Tor

Fatty acids	*V. cholerae* Total (%)	*V. cholerae* *O*-Acyl (%)	*V. cholerae* *N*-Acyl (%)	*V. el-tor* Total (%)	*V. el-tor* *O*-Acyl (%)	*V. el-tor* *N*-Acyl (%)
$C_{14:0}$	6.8	6.8	—	5.4	3.2	0.5
$C_{15:0}$	Trace	3.0	6.8	1.2	7.1	4.2
$C_{16:0}$	18.6	16.4	12.5	16.0	14.4	10.2
$C_{16:1}$	11.8	—	14.8	10.2	—	18.2
$C_{18:0}$	8.0	11.4	—	8.8	10.2	2.4
$C_{18:1}$	22.2	12.8	14.5	20.8	10.8	—
3-OH-$C_{10:0}$	1.4	1.2	—	3.2	—	9.8
3-OH-$C_{12:0}$	32.2	32.6	26.8	34.0	30.4	34.0
3-OH-$C_{14:0}$	—	18.0	24.4	—	24.0	16.2

The fractionation of lipid A released by mild acid hydrolysis of lipopolysaccharides disclosed a variety of compounds such as free fatty acids and glucosamine on the one hand and unaltered phosphorylated aclpolyglucosamine of different chain lengths on the other hand. Thus, it is difficult to visualize lipid A as a simple linear structure consisting of a phosphorylated polyglucosamine chain with ester- and amide-linked fatty acids. More likely, lipid A possesses a branched structure consisting of several polyglucosamine chains of different lengths linked together through phosphodiester linkages, as demonstrated by fractionation of the de-O-acylated lipid A (Fig. 1) from V. cholerae and V. el-tor. The lipid A moiety of these bacteria have the same overall architecture as those present in enterobacteriaceae; but they differ from enterobacterial and various other gram-negative bacterial lipopolysaccharides in lacking 2-keto-3-deoxyoctonate (KDO), which typically links lipid A and polysaccharide moieties.

Toxicity of lipid A: The toxicity, local Shwartzman reaction in rabbits, chick embryo lethality, limulus lysate gelation and pyrogenicity of lipid A/BSA, intact purified lipopolysaccharides and the fractions of lipid A (F_1, F_2 and F_3 fractions as shown in Fig. 1) of V. cholerae are summarized in Table 4.

Table 4: Toxicity of Lipopolysaccharide and Lipid A of V. Cholerae

Strains	Preparations	Local Shwartzman Reaction (100 ug)	Chick Embryo-lethality (LD_{50} ug)	Pyro-genicity MPD-3 [1] (ug/kg)	Limulus lysate gelation (ug/ml)
V. cholerae	LPS [2]	13x13mm	0.030	0.10	10^{-13}
	Lipid A/BSA	12x12mm	0.021	0.08	10^{-11}
	F_1	NR [3]	0.31	0.22	NR
	F_2	NR	NR	NR	NR
	F_3	NR	NR	NR	NR
V. el-tor	LPS	17x17mm	0.025	0.08	10^{-10}
	Lipid A/BSA	15x15mm	0.018	0.07	10^{-8}
	F_1	NR	0.25	0.15	NR
	F_2	NR	NR	NR	NR
	F_3	ND [4]	ND	NR	NR

[1] MPD-3 = Minimum pyrogenic dose tested in 3 rabbits to cause 0.5°C rise in temperature after intravenous injection of the samples.

[2] LPS = Lipopolysaccharides

[3] NR = No reaction

[4] ND = Not done

These toxicity studies showed that lipopolysaccharide and lipid A/BSA complex are toxic from these bacterial species, but high doses are needed to exhibit these toxic effects. Among the different lipid A fractions F_1, F_2 and F_3 tested for these biological activities, some residual activity (chick embryo lethality and pyrogenicity) was present in the major fraction F_1. Other lipid A fractions F_2 and F_3 were inert in these activities. The treatments of lipid A/BSA with alkali (0.3 N NaoH at 56°C for 1.5 hr) cleaves the ester-linked fatty acids from it and such preparations tested for lethal toxicity in mice were found to be non-toxic in comparison with untreated samples (Raziuddin, 1979). These results clearly show that ester-linked fatty acids in lipid A moiety plays an essential role in toxicity. However the treatments of lipid A/BSA either with ethylenediaminotetraacetic acid or sodium dodecyl sulphate did not affect their toxic activities.

The antiserum prepared against the lipid A of V. cholerae prevented the local Shwartzman reaction in rabbits. In all rabbits (5 Nos.) treated with lipid A antiserum, lipid A/BSA did not provoke a positive reaction (Table 5).

Table 5: Prevention of the local Shwartzman reaction in rabbits by lipid A/BSA and lipo polysaccharide antiserum from V. cholerae

Intravenous injection Preparation	Dose (ug)	Positive Shwartzman reaction Normal rabbit serum	Lipid A antiserum	Lipopoly-saccharide antiserum
Lipopolysaccharide	100	4/5[1]	1/5	0/5
Lipid A/BSA	100	5/5	0/5	4/5

Normal rabbit serum (5 ml) or lipid A antiserum (5 ml) or lipopolysaccharide antiserum (5 ml) were given 3 hr before the challenge dose of lipopolysaccharide or lipid A.
[1] Number of rabbits with positive reaction/number of rabbits tested.

It has been noted in V. cholerae that lipid A antiserum is more effective in immunizing the rabbits against some of the endotoxic activities than did lipopoly saccharide antiserum. The lipid A antiserum was precipitated with ammonium sulphate, and on chromatography using Sephadex G 200 column gave two serologically active protein fractions corresponding to IgM and IgG immunoglobulin. These IgM and IgG immunoglobulin fractions showed antilipid A activity in the passive hemolysis test (Raziuddin, 1979). This is in agreement with the previous findings by Galanos and others (1971) in Salmonella minnesota R595 that antibodies against lipid A are detected in the IgM and IgG immunoglobulin fractions.

Lipid A has been shown as a potent activator of both the classical and the alternative (properdin) pathways of complement, and the role of the complement system in the pathophysiological effects produced by endotoxins has long been under discussion. Lipid A's from V. cholerae showed high anticomplementary activity. But the anticomplementary activity of these bacterial lipid A's was not correlable with endotoxin lethality. The chemical, immunological and toxic investigations carried out on V. cholerae lipid A and similar such studies from other gram negative bacteria have led to the supposition that the lipid A component of the bacterial lipopolysaccharides are structurally very much related.

CONCLUSIONS

The results of these studies provide strong support that as in other gram negative bacterial lipopolysaccharides, lipid A moiety is the main toxic principle in *V. cholerae*. The investigations on the structure of lipid A showed that it is made up of a central backbone of B 1, 6-linked D-glucosamine disaccharide substituted at position '4 and '1 by pyrophosphate bridges. Long chain hydroxylated as well as non hydroxylated fatty acids represent major components which are bound to the hydroxyl and amino groups of glucosamine backbone through ester and amide linkages. They are responsible for the hydrophobic properties of lipid A and seem to play a role in its endotoxic activity, because their removal by alkaline digestion leads to preparations of reduced endotoxic activities. Thus lipid A is an amphoteric molecule, carrying both acidic and basic functional groups. Its unique chemical architecture endows lipid A with affinities and specificities which make it a vital constituent of the bacterial membrane and also one of the most potent biologically active non protein molecules, expressing a great variety of distinct endotoxic and immunological activities.

ACKNOWLEDGEMENTS

I am very grateful to Dr. David C. Morrison for his guidance and encouragement, and to Mrs. Monica Bartlett for preparation of the manuscript. My current address is the Department of Microbiology, Emory University, Atlanta, GA.

REFERENCES

Galanos, C., O. Lüderitz, and O. Westphal (1971). Eur. J. Biochem., 24, 116-122.
Galanos, C., O. Lüderitz, E. T. Rietschal, and O. Westphal (1977). In: Biochemistry of Lipids II, Vol. 14, T. W. Goodwin (ed.), University Park Press, Baltimore, pp. 239-335.
Kasai, N. (1966). Ann. N. Y. Acad. Sci., 133, 486-507.
Lüderitz, O., C. Galanos, V. Lehmann, M Nurminen, E. T. Rietschel, G. Rosenfelder, M. Simon, and O. Westphal (1973). J. Infect. Dis., 128, 17-29.
Morrison, D. C., and R. J. Ulevitch (1978). Am. J. Pathol., 93, 527-618.
Nowotny, A., K. Cundy, N. Neale, A. M. Nowotny, R. Radvany, S. Thomas, and D. Tripodi (1966). Ann. N. Y. Acad. Sci., 133, 586-603.
Osborn, M. J., P. D. Rick, V. Lehman, E. Rupprecht, and M. Singh (1974). Ann. N. Y. Acad. Sci., 235, 52-65.
Raziuddin, S. (1976). J. Gen. Microbiol., 94, 367-372.
Raziuddin, S., and S. D. Ambegaokar (1976). Indian J. Biochem. Biophys., 13, 57-61.
Raziuddin, S., and T Kawasaki (1976). Biochim. Biophys. Acta, 431, 116-126.
Raziuddin, S. (1977). Biochem. J., 167, 147-154.
Raziuddin, S. (1978). Immunochemistry, 15, 611-614.
Raziuddin, S. (1979). J. Infect. Dis., in press.
Westphal, O., and K. Jann (1965). Methods Carbohydr. Chem., 5, 83-89.

This is publication #1892 from the Research Institute of Scripps Clinic.

ESCHERICHIA COLI ENDOTOXIN AND ENTEROTOXIN IMPLICATION ON PHARMACOKINETICS OF DRUGS

H. Rašková*, R. Lapka, M. Langmeicrová**, Z. Urbanová***, J. Černy***, J. Vaněček**, A. Kubiček***, and L. Polák******

**Inst. Pharmacol. Czechosl. Acad. Sci., Prague, Czechoslovakia*
***Charles University, Prague, Czechoslovakia*
****Veterinary Postgrad. Institute, Dukovany, Czechoslovakia*
*****State Veterinary Service, Prague, Czechoslovakia*

ABSTRACT

Calves are extremely sensitive to *E. coli* endotoxin (LD_{100}= 0.4 μg/kg intravenously). Sulphadimidine, acetylsalicylic acid, sulphadiazine and trimethoprim have higher plasma levels in calves with diarrhoea. Filtrates from isolated *E. coli* strains produced fluid accumulation in ligated rabbit small intestine loops. In rabbits, *E. coli* filtrates from diarrhoeic calves led to an increase of sulphadimidine levels. Intravenous injection of *E. coli* endotoxin(Difco) had the opposite effect on sulphadimidine, sulphadiazine and trimethoprim plasma levels. The adsorption rate in diarrhoeic animals is increased. In endotoxin-treated animals the plasma levels of all investigated drugs were significantly lower. The importance of differences in pharmacokinetics after the administration of various toxins is discussed.

KEYWORDS

E. coli endotoxin; sensitivity in calves; pharmacokinetics; enterotoxin; endotoxin; sulphadimidine; sulphadiazine; aceytlsalicylic acid; trimethoprim.

INTRODUCTION

We are interested in changes produced by bacterial toxins in the pharmacokinetics and eventual metabolism of drugs. Of special interest are toxins in natural model diseases. Calves are especially interesting in this respect. They suffer from *E. coli* enterotoxin-induced diarrhoea. In the early postnatal period lethal Gram-negative bacteraemia and septicaemia are common in calves insufficiently protected by colostrum (Smith and Halls, 1967; Fey, 1971; Rašková and Raška, 1977). Therefore, the sensitivity of calves to endotoxin was tested. Changes of pharmacokinetics of sulphadimidine, acetylsalicylic acid and trimethoprim-sulfadiazine were investigated in calves with diarrhoea. Because of the high sensitivity of calves to endotoxin, the endotoxin-drug experiments had to be performed in rabbits.

EXPERIMENTAL

Experimental Animals and Drugs

Cross-bred (Friesians Czech red) calves 1-60 days old were taken into the experiments. Adult chinchilla rabbits weighing 2.5-3 kg were used. Endotoxin was from Difco, Detroit, sulphadimidine and acetylsalicylic acid were from Messrs SPOFA. Trimethoprim-sulphadiazine was a gift from Messrs Wellcome.

Procedures. Endotoxin was injected into calves 3 hours after feeding (9 a.m.) in doses of 0.01, 0.02 and 0.04 μg/kg. Rectal temperature was taken and blood was withdrawn from the jugular vein at intervals indicated in the relevant figures. Blood element counts were performed. The changing activity of lymphocyte nucleoli was determined in smears of the peripheral blood stained with toluidine blue for RNA (Smetana, Lejnar and Potměšil, 1969; Busch and Smetana, 1970), which facilitated the classification on nucleoli according to their biosynthetic activity and distribution of RNA-containing components (Smetana, 1971). The percentage of lymphocytes with compact nucleoli or nucleoli with nucleolonemas (active nucleoli synthesizing RNA), ring-chaped nucleoli (resting nucleoli with decreased RNA synthesis) and micronucleoli (inactive nucleoli without RNA synthesis) was determined in 50-100 lymphocytes for each investigated sample.

Sulfadimidine, acetylsalicylic acid (50 mg/kg), trimethoprim (5 mg/kg) and sulphadiazine (25 mg/kg) were administered orally to healthy and diarrhoeic calves. *E. coli* filtrates from diarrhoeic calves were checked on ligated small intestine segments of rabbits (Moon and Whipp, 1971). In some experiments, sulphadimidine was injected simultaneously. Drugs were administered to rabbits one hour after the intravenous injection of 2, 20 or 200 μg of endotoxin per kg. The method of Bratton and Marshall (1939) was used for sulphonamide determination. Schwartz, Koechlin and Weinfeld's (1969) method was used for determination of trimethoprim.

Pharmacokinetic analysis. All values obtained were processed by an ADT-4136 computer using a one-compartment model. Curves were fitted by the iterative method of residues.

RESULTS

Endotoxin Activities in Calves

Pyrogenicity was found from 0.01 μg/kg and upward. Figure 1 presents the course of the pyrogenic response after the administration of 0.02 μg endotoxin per kg body weight. The febrile peak is achieved between the first and second hour after administration. There is some seasonal variation. The experiments were performed directly in the field. It takes 12-13 hours before the initial values are obtained. When the ambient temperature in winter is very low the pyrogenicity increases. Even after 0.01 μg/kg a febrile response of almost 2° C was observed. In these cases general symptoms were also observed. Typical changes of the leucocyte count seen. Forty-five minutes after the endotoxin injection leukopenia was present. This is still detectable after three hours. Lymphocyte activation (after 0.02 μg /kg) appeared within one hour and was still present after eight days of daily checking (Fig. 2). The dependence of clinical signs on dosage is presented in Fig. 3. (tremor, tachycardia, tachypnoea, diarrhoea and circulatory failure). A dose of 0.4 μg/kg was attempted for pharmacokinetic experiments and was 100% lethal. All of the animals (5 calves) died in shock within a short period.

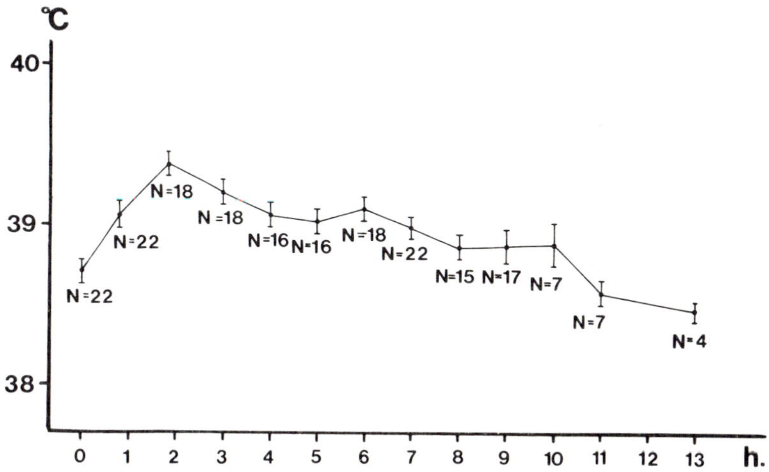

Fig. 1. Pyrogenic response in calves.
Abscissa = time in hours,
N = number of animals

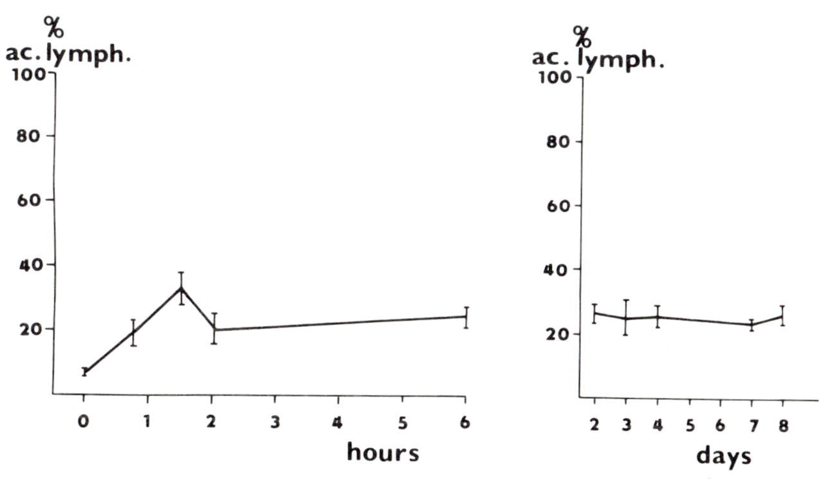

Fig. 2. Endotoxin-induced activation of lymphocytes in calves.

Escherichia coli Enterotoxin and Pharmacokinetics of Drugs

Sulphadimidine (SDM). Table 1 indicates the differences in the half-time of absorption and the half-time of elimination of healthy and diarrhoeic calves. As may be seen, there is a highly significant increase in absorption and elimination rates. The differences in the pharmacokinetics of sulphadimidine are even more apparent in Fig. 4, which presents one healthy (No 605) and one diarrhoeic (No 680) animal. The earlier and higher peak is evident, as is also the more rapid elimination. The same trend is seen in rabbits when sulphadimidine was injected together with *E. coli* enterotoxic filtrate into the ligated segment of the small intestine (Fig. 5).

TABLE 1 Pharmacokinetic Parameters of Sulphadimidine*

Parameter Units	Healthy	Diarrhoeic	Significance
Distribution volume	0.82±0.03	0.79±0.03	n.s.
Half-time of absorption (hours)	7.3±0.3	2.52±0.04	p<0.0005
Half-time of elimination (hours)	26±1	17.7±0.5	p<0.005

* 50 mg/kg was administered to 6 diarrhoeic and 18 normal calves. Values are mean ± SDM.

Acetylsalicylic acid. The higher plasma levels of total salicylates after the administration of acetylsalicylic acid (50 mg/kg) perorally to diarrhoeic calves in comparison with healthy animals is presented in Fig. 6. In this case the time of observation was only six hours, so no data on elimination were obtained.

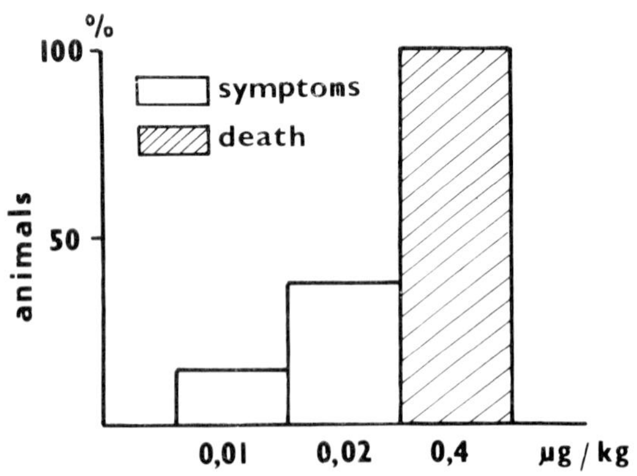

n = 10 n = 20 n = 5

Fig. 3. General symptoms after endotoxin administration to calves. The main symptoms, more frequent with increased dosage, were: tachypnoea, tachycardia, diarrhoea, apathy, laying on side. The lag period after administration of endotoxin was about 1 hour. After 0.4 µg/kg the animals died with irreversible shock symptoms within 1 - 3 hours.

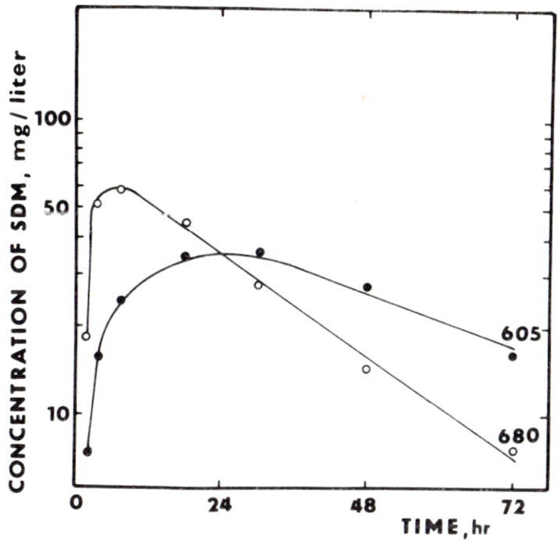

Fig. 4. Pharmacokinetics of sulphadimidine in calves. 605 = normal, 680 = diarrhoeic. (Figure reproduced from Drug Metabolism and Disposition 6, 639, (1977) by permission of the editor.)

Trimethoprim-sulphadiazine. The difference in trimethoprim plasma levels between normal and diarrhoeic calves is highly significant, the levels being much higher in the diarrhoeic animals (Fig. 7). Table 2 shows some pharmacokinetic parameters. The distribution volume is lower and the plasma clearance is significantly depressed. The levels of sulphadiazine are also elevated in diarrhoeic animals, but the changes are not as pronounced as with trimethoprim or sulphadimidine. The youngest calves show the greatest changes.

TABLE 2 Pharmacokinetic Parameters of Trimethoprim*

Parameter Units	Healthy	Diarrhoeic	Significance
Distribution volume (l/kg)	11.6 ± 1.5	5.3 ± 1.4	p<0.02
Half-time of adsorption (hours)	1.17 ± 0.19	1.00 ± 0.23	n.s.
Half-time of elimination (hours)	3.76 ± 0.67	4.18 ± 0.87	n.s.
Plasma clearance (ml/min/kg)	42.3 ± 10.0	16.8 ± 3.8	p<0.05

*5 mg/kg was administered to 6 diarrhoeic and 6 healthy calves. Values are mean ± SEM.

E. coli Endotoxin and Pharmacokinetics of Drugs

Sulphadimidine administered per os one hour after the intravenous injection of 2, 20 or 200 μg of endotoxin per kilo had dose-dependent plasma levels lower than in the controls. Figure 8 presents data obtained after the administration of 200 μg of endotoxin per kg body weight. During the comparatively short (6 hours)

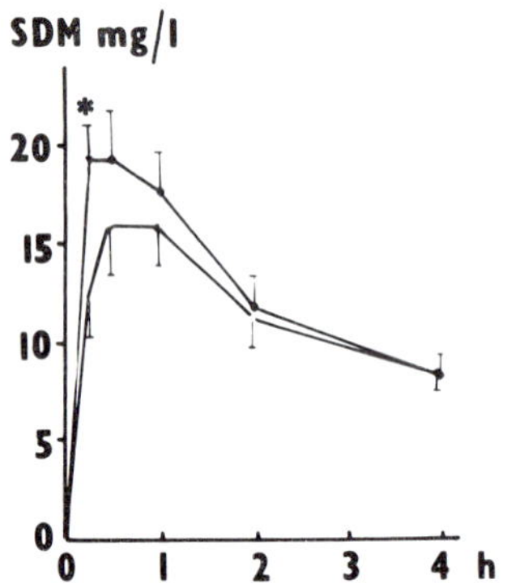

Fig. 5. Sulphadimidine phamacokinetics in rabbits (intestinal loop). Upper curve, enterotoxin. n = 5

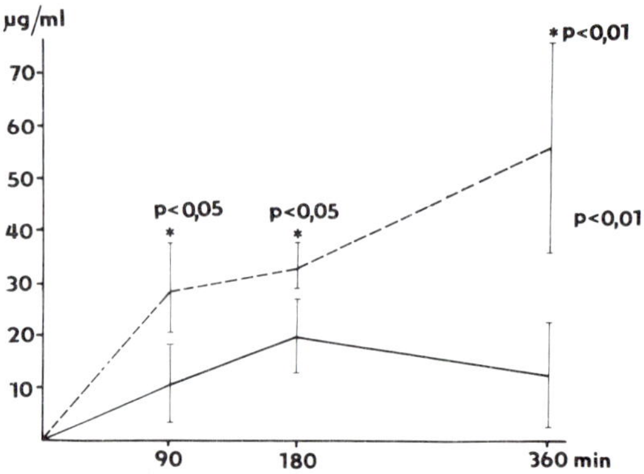

Fig. 6. Pharmacokinetics of salicylates in calves. Full line, normal; dotted line, diarrhoeic. n = 60. (Reproduced from Arzneimittelforschung, 29, 806, (1979) by permission of the editor.)

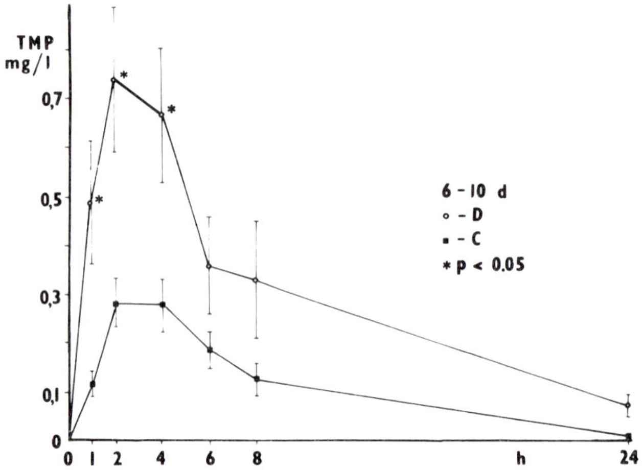

Fig. 7. Trimethoprim pharmacokinetics in calves. C = normal, D = diarrhoeic, d = age in days. n = 12 (6 D and 6 C).

experimental period rabbits in general did not die.

Trimethoprim. Under otherwise the same conditions trimethoprim (10 mg/kg) had maximal plasma levels of 0.06 mg per liter. The animals served as their own controls one week later. After the administration of 200 µg of endotoxin per kilo almost no TMP could be detected in the plasma. For this set of rabbits the endotoxin dosage was too high: 50 percent of the animals died within 7 hours following the injection.

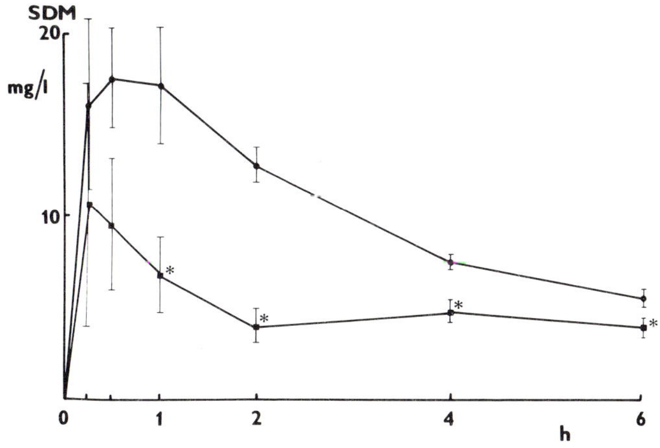

Fig. 8. Pharmacokinetics of sulphadiminine in rabbits after 200 µg/kg of endotoxin. Upper curve, controls (n = 6). Lower curve, endotoxin pre-treated (n = 6).

DISCUSSION

From our data one can conclude that calves are extremely sensitive to endotoxin. Injection of 0.5 µg endotoxin into a 50 kg calf produces a pyrogenic and eventually even a general effect. The fever is dose dependent and the changes are typical for endotoxin. The second fever peak typical for endotoxin-induced fever in rabbits is less pronounced in calves. Early leukopenia precedes the onset of the febrile response. The activation of lymphocytes was previously demonstrated after endotoxin administration into rabbits in vivo (Líkovský and Koníčková, 1977). A long-lasting lymphocyte nucleoli activation is now demonstrated in calves, and a longer time is required for the animals to return to their normal temperature.

The 100 percent lethal dose was only 0.4 µg/kg. It was not feasible to determine the LD_{50}, as the work was done directly in the field with farm animals. The extreme sensitivity of the calf to endotoxin explains the high mortality of calves with Gram-negative bacteraemia.

Four different drugs, sulphadimidine, acetylsalicylic acid, trimethoprim and sulphadiazine have practically the same pharmacokinetics upon oral administration to diarrhoeic calves. Plasma level peaks are earlier and higher than in healthy animals. Apparently, the absorption rate is increased. Whether the decrease in distribution volume and the changed clearance also play a role depends on the severity of the dehydration. The fact that drugs of different chemical types behave in essentially the same way indicates the necessity to keep in mind the altered pharmacokinetics of drugs in diarrhoeic animals.

Our observation of the lower plasma levels of sulphadimidine after intravenous injection of endotoxin into rabbits is in agreement with earlier experiments in which sulphadimidine-Na was also administered intravenously. The literature on fever and drug pharmacokinetics is more extensive than that on diarrhoea. Sulphonamides, salicylates and trimethoprim were tested in this respect. In mice, lower plasma levels of salicylate were observed (Hurwitz, Furtado and Low, 1975). Whether higher or lower levels compared to the controls are observed apparently depends on the endotoxin dose. At low endotoxin doses the plasma sulphonamide levels are higher than in the controls, whereas significantly lower levels have been observed after shock-producing doses (Van Miert, Van Gogh and Witt, 1976). Lower plasma levels and an increase of the peripheral compartment were found for trimethoprim in febrile rabbits (Ladefoged, 1977). The changes in pharmacokinetics thus depend on the dose of endotoxin. As both *E. coli* enterotoxins and endotoxin change the pharmacokinetics of drugs, attention must be paid to appropriate dosage. Animal models should be chosen to maximize the possibility of feedback to pathological conditions in animals and man.

REFERENCES

Bratten, A. C., and E. K. Marshall (1939). J. Biol. Chem., 128, 537-538.

Busch, H., and K. Smetana (1970). The Nucleolus, Academic Press, New York.

Fey, H. (1971). Ann. N. Y. Acad. Sci., 176, 49-63.

Hurwitz, A., D. Furtado, and R. R. Low (1975). J. Pharmacol. Exp. Therap., 192, 236-241.

Ladefoged, O. (1977). Acta Pharmacol. Toxicol., 41, 507-514.

Lapka, R., Z. Urbanová, B. Kobylka, H. Rašková, J. Vaněček, and L. Polák (1978). Drug. Metab. Dispos., 6, 637-639.

Líkovský, Z., and Z. Koníčková (1977). Life Sci., 21, 1425-1428.

Moon, H. W., and S. C. Whipp (1971). Ann. N. Y. Acad. Sci., 176, 197-211.

Rašková, H., and K. Raška (1977). Biochem. Pharmacol., 26, 1103-1108.

Schwartz, D. B., B. A. Koechlin, and R. E. Weinfeld (1969). Chemotherapy, 14, 22-29.

Smetana, K. (1971). Nucleoli of human non-leukemic blood lymphocytes. In: J. Libánský and L Donner (Eds.), Present Problems in Hematology, Excerpta Medica, Avicenum, Amsterdam, Prague, pp. 185-192.

Smetana, K., J. Lejnar and M. Potměšil (1969). Folia Haematol., 91, 381-394.

Smith, H. W., and S. Halls (1967). J. Path. Bact., 93, 499-531.

Van Miert, A. S. P. A. M., H. van Gogh, and J. G. Witt (1976). Vet. Rec., 99, 480-481.

Edema and Purpura-Producing Toxins

STUDIES ON TOXICITY AND IMMUNOGENICITY OF STAPHYLOCOCCAL EXFOLIATINS A AND B

I. Kondo and S. Sakurai

Department of Microbiology, The Jikei University School of Medicine, Tokyo, Japan

ABSTRACT

The following results were newly obtained from our recent studies on the staphylococcal exfoliatin A and B. 1) The A type exfoliatin is a kind of metallotoxin containing one atom of copper per molecule. 2) Exfoliatin toxoids were successfully prepared by azo-coupling to or nitration of the toxin. 3) Conventional mice are generally unable to produce an antibody against the native toxin of exfoliatin. However the azo- or nitro-toxoids can elicit an antibody production not only to the toxoids but also to the native toxins in these mice. 4) The H-2 locus of mice seems to contain the so-called Ir gene responsible for producing a specific antibody to the native toxins of both types. Haprotype d was found to be a high responder but haprotype b a non-responder and haprotypes a and k were low responders to these toxins. 5) SDS fraction extracted from the skin tissue of neonatal mice makes a specific complex with the purified toxin and inactivates the latter. A receptor substance with ganglioside moiety could be extracted from this SDS fraction.

KEYWORDS

Staphylococcal toxin; staphylococcal scalded skin syndrome (SSSS); staphylococcal exfoliatin; metallotoxin; toxoid; Ir-gene; receptor for toxin; ganglioside as receptor.

INTRODUCTION

Staphylococcal exfoliatin has recently been regarded as the causative toxin for the so-called staphylococcal scalded skin syndrome (hereafter abbreviated as SSSS) which includes Ritter's disease, bullous impetigo, and staphylococcal scarlatiniform rash. This toxin also attracts much interest by its very strict organ- and host-specificity. Except for man, the mouse is the only animal susceptible to this toxin. Even in mice, only newborn mice less than 5 days old are susceptible. The susceptibility rapidly decreases after this critical age and it is lost in adult mice. A similar situation is also observed in SSSS in man. Ritter's disease is encountered exclusively in infants even within a half year of age, whereas impetigo is a children's disease, and adults do not suffer from either disease at all. On the other hand, the lesions in SSSS and those caused by this toxin are exclusively to epidermis. Generalized exfoliation of epidermis is caused by subcutaneous injection of neonatal mice with this toxin. The so-called Nikolski sign, one of the conspicuous symptoms in Ritter's disease, i.e., a peeling off of the epidermis caused by a slight rubbing of the skin with fingertips can also be seen. A splitting of the corneal epidermis accompanying the granular layer in the skin of the suffed mice as well as that of the patients of Ritter's disease, but no hemorrhage or accumlation of leukocytes occurs. These findings show a good resemblance to those in the patients of Ritter's disease. We have previously reported that there are at least two kinds of exfoliatin, A and B, which are distinctly different from each other in their serological features and some other physicochemical properties (Kondo et al, 1973, 1974, 1975). Exfoliatin A, abbreviated hereafter as Ex-A, corresponds to the toxins reported by Melish (1970), Kapral (1971), Wiley (1974) and their coworkers, whereas exfoliatin B, abbreviated as Ex-B, was newly isolated by Kondo et al (1974) from the staphylococcal isolates from the patients of Ritter's disease or staphylococcal impetigo, not belonging to the phage group II. Thermosusceptibility is another conspicuous difference between them. Ex-A is thermostable, resisting 100 C for 20 min, whereas Ex-B thermolabile and easily inactivated at 60 C for 30 min. In this paper the following five subjects will be described.

1) Characterization of the exfoliatin A as a kind of metallotoxin.
2) Preparation of Ex-toxoids by chemical modification.
3) Immunogenicity of exfoliatins to mice.
4) A possible receptor substance for exfoliatin isolated from mice.
5) Model receptor experiment using bovine brain ganglioside.

MATERIAL AND METHOD

Bacterial strain. S. aureus ZM and SU were exclusively used as the standard strains respectively producing Exfoliatin A and B.

Toxin. Exfoliatin samples used in this experiment are all those highly purified by the method described in the previous paper (Kondo et al, 1973). Exfoliatin A is finally purified into four toxic proteins, a, b, c, and d, in polyacrylamide disc electrophoresis whereas Exfoliatin B into a single fraction corresponding to the b fraction of the former. The Ex-A sample used in this experiment is a mixture of the toxic proteins b, c and d unless especially noticed.

Test animals. Neonatal mice of the ICR strains within four days of age were used for the examination of the exfoliative toxicity. Congenic strains of the B 10 series which were introduced the H-2 loci of various haplotypes were used for the examination of the immunological response to exfoliatin. They were kindly provided by Dr. Moriwaki from the National Institute of Genetics in Japan.

Radio activation analysis. The detection and determination of the essential metal contained in the exfoliatins were performed by radio activation analysis. Purified toxin samples (820 μg of E -A/c and 95 μg of Ex-A/b) were each sealed in polyethylene containers and subjected to integrated neutron exposure at a dose rate of 4×10^{13} neutron/cm^2/sec for 20 min in a reactor, JRR-4. The gamma ray energy of the essential element was measured by a gamma ray spectrometer (a multichannel analyser). The concentration of the element contained in the toxin was determined by comparing of the height of the photopeak of the essential element of an Ex-A sample on the gamma ray spectrum with that of the authentic element (metal) of a known concentration which was radioactivated in the same container.

RESULTS AND DISSCUSSIONS

CHARACTERIZATION OF EXFOLIATIN A AS A METALLOTOXIN

In our previous study (Kondo and Sakurai, 1976), Ex-A was found to lose its toxicity when treated with ethylene-diamin-tetra-acetate (EDTA) and the detoxified sample restored the toxicity when added with some salts of di-valent metals, Mg, Zn, Co and

Cu. Ex-B was not affected at all by EDTA treatment. From these findings Ex-A was suggested to be a kind of metallotoxin and the contained metal is concerned with its extreme thermostability. This conception has recently been supported by neutron activation analysis (Sakurai and Kondo, 1978). Samples of purified exfoliatin A and B as well as some metal elements sealed in polyethylene containers were subjected to integrated neutron exposure, at a dose rate of 4 x 10^{13} neutron/ cm^2/sec for 20 min in a reactor, JRR-4. As shown in Table 1, after radioactivation 95 μg of Ex-A pure sample and 20 μg of copper metal gave net counts of gamma-ray energy 158 and 11,365 respectively at 255 channel, but no count was detected with 95 μg of Ex-B sample. According to the values obtained from the calculations indicated in the table, the copper content of Ex-A was estimated to be approximately one g atom per molecule, on an assumption that the molecular weight of Ex-A is 24,000.

TABLE 1 Copper Contents of S. aureus Exfoliatin A

Materials ($4x10^{13}n/cm^2/sec$ 5 min with JRR-4)	Net counts at 255 channel	mg Cu/g	g Cu/mole	Copper to toxin ratio
Cu (20.3 μg)	2,000			
Ex-A (ZM-c) (820 μg)	165	2.44	58.54	0.9 g atom/mole
Ex-B (SU) (740 μg)	0			

PREPARATION OF EX-TOXOIDS BY CHEMICAL MODIFICATIONS

Rabbits can produce specific antibodies to exfoliatin, and the two serotypes A and B were classified by rabbit antisera to these toxins. However rabbits are not susceptible to these toxins even when new born rabbits are used for the test.

On the contrary, neonatal mice are the only susceptible animals other than men, but the mice are generally unable to produce any antibody to these toxins even when massively immunized by the native toxins mixed with Freund's adjuvant. Attempts to elevate this poor immunogenicity of exfoliatin to mice through chemical modifications resulted in somewhat unexpected findings. Azo-coupling or nitration with tetranitromethan-ethanol were performed respectively according to the method of Tabachnik et Sobotka (1960) and that of Cuatrecasas et al (1968). After these treatments the azo- or nitro- toxins of both exfoliatins were observed to have lost their toxicities for neonatal mice, but retained the immunogenicities as well as the specific response to the homologous rabbit antiserum. In other words they have been altered into toxoid. The aminoacid residues which are most reactive to these chemical modifications are tyrosine, histidine and lysine for diazonium arsenylic acid and tyrosine and cystein for tetranitromethane. Cystein is known not contained in both toxins from the results of aminoacid analysis. So, tyrosine, the common aminoacid is presumed to be the one which received the modification resulting the detoxification in both toxins. As a matter of fact, Table 2 indicates the results of aminoacid analysis of Ex-A and Ex-B as well as their nitrated samples. Three of five residues of tyrosine are observed to be lost during the process of 60 min nitration.

On the other hand, Fig. 1 shows a part of the elution profile of the hydrolysed nitrotoxoid of Ex-A. Mononitrotyrosine is observed to be eluted after the peak of phenylalanine. The same result was also obtained with nitrotoxoid of Ex-B. These evidences support the afore-mentioned concept that the chemical modification of tyrosine residue or residues results in the detoxification in both of types of exfoliatins, suggesting that the aminoacid tyrosine is necessary for toxicity of both exfoliatins.

TABLE 2 RESULTS OF AMINOACID ANALYSIS OF NATIVE TOXINS AND NITROTOXOIDS OF EXFOLIATIN A (ZM-B) AND EXFOLIATIN B (SU)

Amino acid	Native ZM-b	Nitro ZM-b	Native SU	Nitro SU
Lys	16.1	16.3	16.4	16.1
His	5.1	5.1	4.8	4.6
Arg	6.5	6.8	6.7	6.6
Asp	24.6	25.4	24.7	25.1
Thr	8.5	8.5	8.8	8.9
Ser	11.6	12.2	11.6	11.9
Glu	18.7	19.0	19.3	18.9
Pro	7.7	8.2	8.3	8.4
Gly	21.3	20.1	19.5	19.8
Ala	11.2	10.5	10.6	11.0
Cys	0	0	0	0
Val	9.3	8.6	8.8	8.5
Met	0	0	0	0
ILeu	11.6	11.5	11.6	12.3
Leu	12.7	13.2	12.7	13.4
Tyr	4.5	2.0	5.3	2.2
Phe	6.5	6.8	7.3	6.6
Try	-*	-*	-*	-*

Nitration was perfored for 60 min at 37 C.
Results were expressed as moles of the aminoacid per mole of the toxin.
-* : not determined.

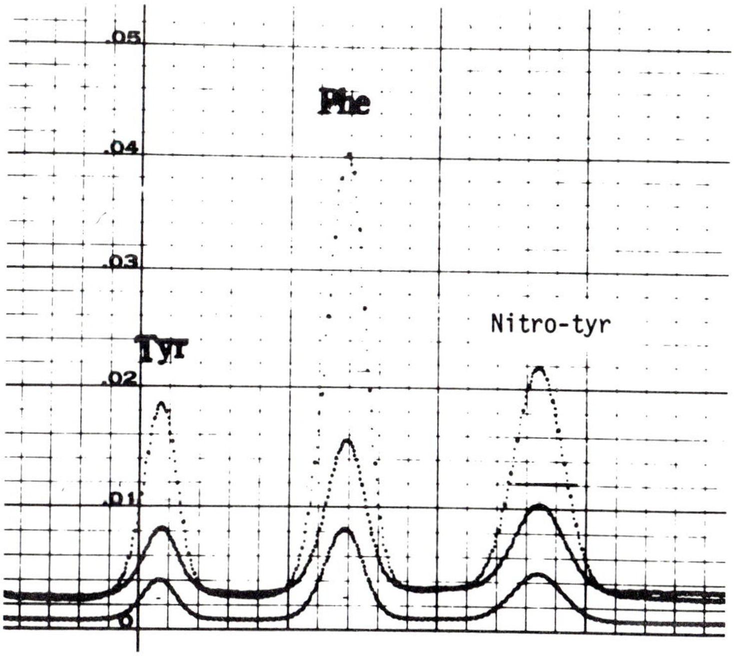

Fig. 1. Elution Patern of Nitrototyrosine in Aminoacid Analysis of Nitrotoxoid of Exfoliatin B (SU).

IMMUNOGENICITY OF EXFOLIATIN TO MICE

Another striking evidence is that these azo- and nitrotoxoids were found to have acquired immunogenicities to mice which are unable to produce any antibody to the native toxin (Kondo and Sakurai, 1976). It was found that the mouse antiserum obtained by immunizing the homozygous hairless mouse with nitro-toxoid of Ex-A produces an identical, fused precipitation line towards the native, nitro- and azo- toxins of Ex-A series, but not to nitro-Ex-B. These toxoids can also be utilized for vaccination of the mother mouse in order to protect her new-born litters against exfoliatin. The new-borns from the immunized mother manifested a resistance approximately four times greater than the control mice. The mice to which were referred up to now are confined to conventional mice, ICR or hairless strains etc. We have recently examined inbred mice of B10 series which were introduced the H-2 loci of various haplotypes and found that only the haplotype d was the so-called high responder to the native toxins of both types, whereas the haplotypes a and k were low responders and the b type a non-responder. Furthermore the F_1 between $H\text{-}2^d$ and $H\text{-}2^b$ was also found to be a high responder (Kondo and Sakurai, 1979). Although further analyses should be completed, these evidences suggest that the so-called Ir gene responsible for producing a specific antibody to exfoliatins exists in the H-2 locus of mice.

A POSSIBLE RECEPTOR SUBSTANCE FOR EXFOLIATIN ISOLATED FROM MICE

Since the target organ is strictly confined to the epidermis in SSSS patients and the mice injected with this toxin, some specific receptor is assumed to locate in the skin layer of men and mice. Our recent experimental results support this inference. SDS extract from newborn mouse skin was found to be able to form a specific complex with exfoliatin causing an inativation of the latter. The heads, limbs and viscera of neonatal and adult mice and newborn rats and hamsters were removed, and skin tissue emulsions were prepared from the remaining trunks. Water soluble (WS), sodium deoxycholate (DOC) and sodium dodecyl sufate (SDS) fractions were respectively extracted from all these emulsions. When 50 mg of these extracts were respectively incubated with 60 µg of Ex-A sample at 37 C for 3 hours, only the SDS fraction from neonatal mice was found to strongly inactivate the toxin. The same fraction from adult mice also showed but a weak inactivation. But neither WS and DOC fractions of mice nor all kinds of fractions from rats and hamsters were able to inactivate the toxin. On the other hand, 300 µg of these extracts were respectively mixed with 50 µg of Ex-A and incubated at 37 C for 30 hours, and then subjected to polyacrylamide gel electrophoresis. When the toxin was incubated with the SDS fraction of neonatal mice, the toxin did not migrate remaining at the top together with this water insoluble fraction. Whereas the original electrophoretic pattern of Ex-A (the b, c and d toxin bands) manifested unchanged when the toxin was incubated with the other fractions. All thses evidences may be ascribed to the presence of a receptor substance of this toxin in this SDS fraction from newborn or adult mice. Such a specific substance may be masked or changed into an inefficient form as the mouse grows old. Chemical nature of this receptor substance was further examined. At first its ability to neutralize or combine with the exfoliatin was not lost by trypsin or pronase digestion as well as by heating at 100 C for 30 min, suggesting that the receptor is not of protein nature at least. Whereas water soluble and active substance could further be isolated from this SDS fraction by means of long term digestion of the fraction with pronase E. About 4.8 g of the lyophilized sample was dissolved in Tris-HCl buffer and digested at 37 C by pronase E for 70 hours, and then heated at 100 C for 30 min. After centrifuged the supernatant was subjected to ultrafiltration by PM-10 and then by UM-2 membrane. The final filtrate through UM-2 was shown to have the receptor activity, indicating the molecules of the active substance to be of molecular weight less than one thousand at most. Subsequently this final filtrate was subjected to two dimensional silica gel thin layer chromatography on TLC or PLC plates with the following two kinds of solvents.

1st solvent : n-butanol:acetone:acetic acid:water
35 35 7 23
2nd solvent:n-butanol:isopropanol:0.5% boric acid
35 50 20

The migration pattern of sugar containing components was examined by color reaction to naphtalenediol-H_2SO_4-ethanol reagent. Four spots were stained dark green. Aminoacid or peptide containing spots were revealed on the second plate by color reaction to ninhydrin. Purple red spots were stained. The upper two spots in this plate correspond to those of sugar components demonstrated on the previous plate. Among all these spots located either on the first plate or the second one, the uppermost spot which reacted to color with both reagents possesses the receptor activity. In the other words, the receptor substance contained in the SDS fraction is essentially a small molecule of aminosugar with a M.W. less than 1000 at most.

MODEL RECEPTOR EXPERIMENT USING BOVINE BRAIN GANGLIOSIDE

Recently various types of gangliosides have been marked as the receptor substances for some bacterial toxins such as cholera toxin (Heyningen, 1974), tetanus toxin (Heyningen, 1974) or alpha toxin of S. aureus (Kato & Naiki, 1976). Table 3 shows the result of examination of the bovine brain ganglioside, hereafter abbreviated as BBG, purchased from Sigma Co. Ltd. About 0.38 µg of ExA- b was mixed with different volumes of the BBG samples in Tris-HCl buffer. After incubation at 37 C for 2 hours with gentle shaking, the mixtures were subcutaneously injected to neonatal mice. As shown in the table the so-called Nikolski sign, afore explained, could be blocked with 900 µg BBG sample at least during 5 hours after the injection of BBG-toxin mixture.

TABLE 3 INACTIVATING CAPACITY OF NEURAMINIDASE-TREATED GANGLIOSIDES ON THE TOXICITY OF STAPHYLOCOCCAL EXFOLIATIN

After subcutaneously injection	ExA-b (μg) 0.38	bovine brain gangliosides (μg) Control 900	Neuraminidase-treated 400
3 hr	++	-	-
5 hr	+++	-	-
7 hr	+++	+	-
10 hr	++++	+++	-

Since the sample of BBG used in this experiment is not a pure sample of a single ganglioside but a mixture of various types of gangliosides, the next question is what type ganglioside contained in this sample is really responsible for the receptor activity. Analysis is still under way, but the following results are highly suggestive in this respect. A one mg portion of BBG sample was treated with 0.5 U of neuraminidase overnight at 30 C in 0.2 M citrate buffer, pH 5.0. After inactivating the neuraminidase contained in the reaction mixture at 90 C for 3 min, the solution was filtrated through collodion bag to remove the sialic acid residues released during the digestion, and the concentrate in the bag was used as the digested BBG sample. Under a similar condition as afore mentioned, the toxin of 0.38 μg was mix-incubated with various volumes of this digested BBG sample and then the mixtures were injected into neonatal ICR mice. The receptor activity was much enhanced in these digested samples in comparison to that in the original sample. As also shown in the Table 3 above mentioned, the digested sample was found to block the Nikolski sign with only 400 μg until 10 hours or more after the injection.

TABLE 4 VARIOUS TYPES OF BRAIN GANGLIOSIDE

NANA-NANA-Gal-Glu-Ceramide $GalNH_2$ Gal-NANA <u>SGGnSSLC</u> (GT_1)	NANA-NANA-Gal-Glu-Ceramide $GalNH_2$ Gal <u>GGnSSLC</u> (GD_{1B})
NANA-Gal-Glu-Ceramide $GalNH_2$ Gal-NANA <u>SGGnSLC</u> (GD_{1A})	NANA-Gal-Glu-Ceramide $GalNH_2$ Gal <u>GGnSLC</u> (GM_1)
NANA-Gal-Glu-Ceramide $GalNH_2$ <u>GnSLC</u> (GM_2)	NANA-Gal-Glu-Ceramide <u>SLC</u> (GM_3)

NANA : N-acetylneuraminic-acid : sialic acid : <u>S</u>

<u>G</u> : Galactose <u>Gn</u> : $GalNH_2$: N-acetyl galactosamine

<u>L</u> : Lactose : Gal-Glu <u>C</u> : Ceramide

Table 4 shows simplified structures of the six best known ganglioside types together with their McCluer's abbreviated nomenclatures underlined and Svennerholm's in the parentheses. As to the symbols in the parentheses, G means ganglioside, T, D and M the number of the sialic acid residues contained, namely tri, di and mono-gangliosides, and the numerals after the symbols the migration grade of the compounds, the larger the number the longer the distance of migration. Circled NANA presents the sialidase labile N-acetylneuraminic acid, and the arrows the direction of sialidase digestion. All these ganglioside types are considered to be contained in the original BBG sample in a definite proportion but this proportion may naturally change in the digested sample and this change is probably responsible for the enhanced receptor activity in the digested sample.

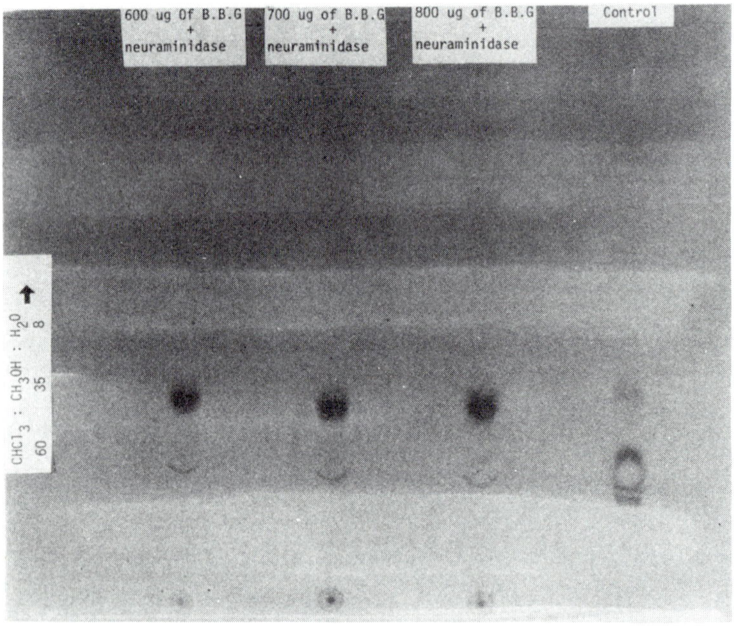

Fig. 2. Thin Layer Chromatography of the original and Sialidase-digested Samples of Bovine Brain Ganglioside (B.B.G.)

Figure 2 demonstrates the result of the thin layer chromatography with the original and the digested samples. As shown in the figure, the original sample developed at least six discernible bands and the three lower bands, especially the 1st and the 2nd bands from the bottom, are much more dense than the other upper ones. The maps of the three digested samples are the same as that of the non digested control sample except for the three lower bands. The color of the 1st and 2nd became faint and instead the 3rd one increased in thickness and darkness. It is difficult to determine exactly the type of these bands. However, because of their slow migration and the increase in density of the 3rd band instead of the decrease of that in the 1st and 2nd bands after sialidase treatment, the 1st band probably corresponds to GT_1, and the 2nd to GD_1A or B and the 3rd one is considered to be the GM_1 which resulted from GT_1 and GD_1A or B removed of their sialidase labile N-acetyl neuraminic acid residues. From these results obtained up to now through this receptor model experiment, GM_1 type ganglioside is most likely to be an essential receptor for this toxin.

ACKNOWEGEMENT

The authors would like to express their gratitude to Dr. K. Moriwaki, National institute of Genetics, Japan, for his kind distribution of the congenic strains of B-10 mice and also to Dr. M. Shibuya, National Institute of Agrecultural Science, Japan, for his kind help to the radio activation analysis experiment.

REFERENCE

Cuatrecasas, p., S. Fuchs, and C. B. Anfinsen (1968). J. Biol. Chem., 243, 4787-4798.
Heyningen, W. E. (1974). Nature, 249, 415-417.
Kapral, F. A. and M. M. Miller (1971). Infect. Immun., 4, 541-545.
Kato, I. and M. Naiki (1976). Infect. Immun., 13, 289-291.
Kondo, I., S. Sakurai, and Y. Sarai (1973). Infect. Immun., 8, 156-164.
Kondo, I., S. Sakurai, and Y. Sarai (1974). Infect. Immun., 10, 851-861.
Kondo, I., S. Sakurai, Y. Sarai, and S. Futaki (1975). J. Clin. Microbiol., 1, 397-400.
Kondo, I., and S. Sakurai (1976). Zbl. Bakt. Hyg. I. Abt. Suppl. 5, 489-498.
Kondo, I., and S. Sakurai (1979). Studies on staphylococcal exfoliatin A and B. Proceeding 79th ASM Meeting, Honolulu, Hawaii.
Melish, M.E., and L. A. Glasgow (1970). N. Engl. Med. J., 282, 1114-1119.
Sakurai, S., and I. Kondo (1978). Japan. J. Med. Sci. Bio., 31, 208-211.
Tabachnick, M., and H. Sobotka (1960). J. Biol. Chem., 235, 1051-1054.
Wiley, B. B., S. Allman, M. Rogolsky, C. W. Norden and L. A. Glasgow (1974). Infect. Immun., 9, 636-642.

THERMAL ANALYSIS AND NUCLEAR MAGNETIC RESONANCE AS PROBES FOR THE STUDY OF EDEMA INDUCED IN RAT SKIN BY SOME BACTERIAL TOXINS

A. Ohsaka*, K. Yoshikawa, M. Momota*** and S. Iwasa******

**The 2nd Dept. of Bacteriology, National Institute of Health, Tokyo 141, Japan*
***College of General Education, University of Tokushima, Tokushima 770, Japan*
****Rigaku Corporation, Tokyo 196, Japan*
*****Dept. of General Biologics Control, National Institute of Health, Tokyo 141, Japan*

ABSTRACT

1) Simultaneous TG-DTA and nuclear magnetic resonance were applied to the study of edema induced in skin tissue by bacterial toxins and by hypersensitivity reactions. The methods have been proved to be useful for studying edema, and the water in biological systems in general.
2) For the understanding of the mechanism of edema formation, changes in the physical state and the amount of water and other substances in the tissue concerned should be determined during the course of edema formation.
3) Edema is divided into at least two types, in respect to change in the amount of 'bound' water. With edema resulting from skin hypersensitivity reactions, a large portion of the 'free' water which had increased in the early phase of the reactions was lost through transformation into 'bound' water. The amount of 'bound' water did not decrease in any phases of the edema formation. In contrast, with edema induced by bacterial toxin the amount of 'bound' water decreased dramatically to a level lower than the normal one as the edema progressed, although a temporary increase of the amount of 'bound' water was seen in the early phase of the reaction. It appears therefore that the physiological role of 'bound' water in normal tissue is as a regulator for the amount of 'free' water.

KEYWORDS

Thermal analysis; simultaneous TG-DTA; nuclear magnetic resonance; biological water; mass spectrometry; edema; bacterial toxin; Clostridium; immediate hypersensitivity; delayed hypersensitivity.

INTRODUCTION

Edema results from the abnormal accumulation of body fluid in the cells and/or in the intercellular tissue spaces. In spite of its clinical importance in a number of diseases, including bacterial infections, edema is still very incompletely understood. This has largely been due to the lack of a suitable method for characterizing and quantitating water in biological systems. Another problem with the subject of biological water has been the imprecise use of such terms as 'free', 'bound', 'ordered', 'structured' and 'icelike' water, and 'water of hydration' (James, 1975). Since it is not really possible at present to define these terms exactly, we will use them as follows: 'free' water is defined as that water in its natural unbound state in tissues which is readily available for transfer, while 'bound' water is defined as that water in tissues which is not readily available for transfer.
We have recently applied thermal analysis (simultaneous TG-DTA) and nuclear

magnetic resonance (NMR) to the study of water of edema induced in rat skin by the toxin of Clostridium oedematiens (Ohsaka and co-workers, 1979a, 1979b, 1979c and also by the α-toxin of Clostridium perfringens (Yoshikawa, Ohsaka, Yamakawa, 1979) administered intracutaneously. For comparison, a study was also made of the edema resulting from the immediate (IH) and delayed (DH) skin hypersensitivity reactions induced in mouse paw (Iwasa, Ohsaka, Momota, 1979; Ohsaka, Momota, 1979b; Yoshikawa, Ohsaka, Iwasa, 1979).

The purpose of this presentation is to review these data obtained in our laboratory and to discuss the usefulness of thermal analysis and nuclear magnetic resonance as probes for the study of edema in general.

METHODS

Thermal analysis: The method used for thermal analysis was simultaneous thermogravimetry (TG)-differential thermal analysis (DTA) (Momota, Ohsaka, 1979; Ohsaka, Momota, 1979b).

The simultaneous TG-DTA apparatus used in this study was model "Thermoflex TG-DTA" manufactured by Rigaku Corporation, Tokyo, Japan. The apparatus consists of (a) two sample holders surrounded by a furnace, (b) an electric balance, (c) DTA, TG and DTG control units, (d) a temperature control unit and (e) a recorder. One sample holder is used to contain the test smaple and the other serves to hold the reference material. The test sample and the reference (α-Al_2O_3) are put in two aluminium pans without sealing and each pan is put in contact with the thermocouple junction of its respective holder; the two holders are tied together and suspended on the beam of a balance. The holders are heated at a rate controlled by a programmer. The sample weight is continuously monitored by the balance and recorded as a function of the sample temperature. When the sample undergoes a chemical or physical reaction, the sample thermocouple will reflect the endothermal or exothermal difference between the sample temperature and the reference temperature, and an electromotive force or ΔT will be generated proportional to this temperature difference. The magnitude of the ΔT is proportional to the heat of the total reaction.

In the present study, all samples (25-26 mg) were heated at 2.5°C per minute in a continuously flowing air environment (flow rate: 65 ml/min) at temperature ranging from room temperature to 150°C. All energy changes observed were endothermic.

Mass spectrometry: A mass spectrometer (model "TE-600", ANELVA Corporation) was coupled to the simultaneous TG-DTA apparatus (model "Thermoflex TG-DTA", Rigaku Corporation). This allowed continuous mass spectrometric analysis of the volatile components evolved from the biological systems (Ohsaka, Momota, 1979b).

Nuclear magnetic resonance: Any nucleus with a nonzero magnetic moment will interact with electromagnetic radiation in the presence of an external magnetic field and absorb energy. It is possible to study selected nuclei independent of others (e.g. ^{1}H, ^{2}H, ^{13}C, ^{15}N, ^{31}P). NMR, being a non-destructive method of analysis, will give information about the environment and molecular freedom of most of the atoms present in the biological systems. In the present study ^{1}H(100MHz)-and ^{13}C(25 MHz)-NMR spectra of the skin samples were taken in a 5-mm sample tube and a 10-mm sample tube, respectively, with an FT-NMR spectrometer, model Jeol JNM-FX100. T_1 measurements of $^{1}H_2O$ were carried out by Fourier transforms using 180°C-τ-90°C pulse sequence.

RESULTS AND DISCUSSION

For ease of presentation, our studies of water in biological systems will be divided into two parts. The first is concerned with edema induced in rat skin by the toxin of Clostridium oedematiens. The second considers edema resulting from the immediate and delayed types of hypersensitivity produced in mouse paw.

Edema induced in rat skin by the toxin of Clostridium oedematiens

The abdomens of white female rats of Wistar strain were shaved with an electric shaver and then depilated with a saturated solution of barium sulfide (Ohsaka, Momota, 1979b). This was done under intraperitoneal Nembutal anesthesia 48 hrs prior to the intracutaneous injection of toxin or a 0.85% NaCl solution in a dose of 0.1 ml into the central part of the abdomen. Ether anesthesia was used at the time of the injection. The skin samples from the site of injection were taken at 3, 4.5, 6, 9, 12, 18, 24, 48, 72 and 120 hrs from animals injected with toxin; the control skin samples were taken at 3 and 24 hrs from animals injected with a 0.85% NaCl solution and also from non-injected animals. A group of two to three animals was used for each time point. The complete experiment as described above was repeated four times. Each of the skin samples taken was put in a polyethylene bag and kept in an ice jar until testing. After fluid had been removed from the surface of the skin samples with a piece of filter paper, the samples were cut into pieces and these were analyzed immediately by means of thermal analysis or nuclear magnetic resonance. Great care was taken to minimize the evaporation of water from the samples during the handling (Ohsaka, Momota, 1979b).

As a first step, pure water was submitted to thermal analysis. It was found that, when heated in a continuously flowing air environment (flow rate: 65 ml/min), pure water evaporated with the endothermal peak of the DTA curve between 40° and 50°C. The control rat's skin was then submitted to thermal analysis. On the basis of the above results with pure water, the peak of the DTA curve seen between 40° and 50°C in the resulting thermogram (Fig. 1) is interpreted as being due to the evaporation of 'free' water in the tissue. The endothermal peaks seen at higher temperatures are interpreted as being due to the evaporation of 'bound' water. From the TG and DTG curves, the amounts of 'free' and 'bound' water in the tissue were calculated. Thus, the average amount of 'free' water per gram of dry weight of the skin from 6 male and 6 female rats weighing 150-170 g (11-weeks old) was estimated to be 0.46 ± 0.03 g (n=12), while that of 'bound' water was estimated to be 0.96 ± 0.04 g (n=12) (Ohsaka, Momota, 1979b).
In the interpretation of the thermogram (Fig. 1), we have assumed that the observed endothermal peaks of the DTA curve as well as the recorded weight loss of the skin sample (TG curve) are due solely to the evaporation of water. To demonstrate this experimentally, all of the evolved volatiles from the rat skin had to be identified by mass spectrometric analysis. This was performed by using a mass spectrometer connected with the simultaneous TG-DTA apparatus. The results obtained demonstrated that the recorded weight loss of the control rat's skin was due solely to the evaporation of water without detectable amounts of any other gases being evolved (Ohsaka, Momota, 1979b).
In Fig.2 is shown typical thermogram of rat's skin taken at 3 hrs after intracutaneous injection of C. oedematiens toxin. From this and other thermograms, the amounts of 'free' and 'bound' water in the affected tissues at the indicated time were determined (Ohsaka, Momota, 1979b). During the course of edema formation induced in rat skin by the toxin, the amount of 'free' water increased in 3 hrs, decreased temporarily in 4.5 hrs and again increased in steps at the 9th-12th hrs and the 24th hr (Fig. 3); the 'free' water content then tended to decrease up to the 5th day to a normal level with a temporary increase at the 3rd day. On the other hand, the amount of 'bound' water temporarily increased 3 hrs after the toxin injection and then decreased, reaching a level lower than the normal one in 12 hrs and this was maintained up to the 5th day (Fig. 4). It was demonstrated that the increase in the content of 'free', 'bound' and total water of the skin of rats 3 hrs after toxin injection was proportional to the dose of the toxin injected (Ohsaka, Momota, 1979b).
The mechanism involved in the changes in the amounts of 'free' and 'bound' water occurring during the course of development of edema is not well understood. The toxin increases vascular permeability (Izumi, Kondo, 1978). The fluid (water) which has leaked from the microcirculation, most probably from the arteriole side of the capillaries may be absorbed partly by the venule side of the capillaries and partly by the lymphatic system (lymphatic capillaries). The observed accumulation of 'free' and 'bound' water in the affected tissue in 3 hrs may be

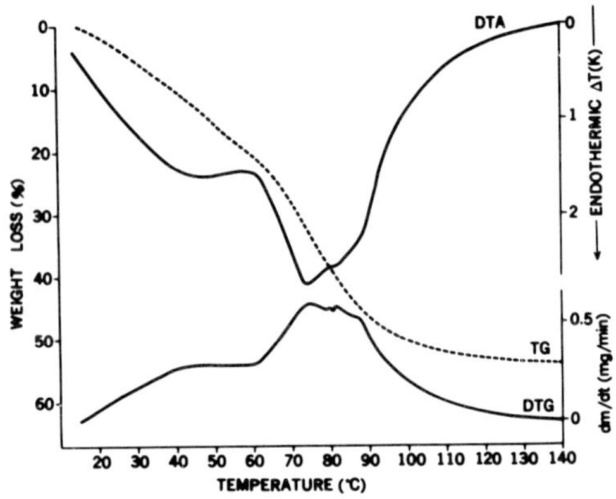

Fig. 1. Thermogram of control rat's skin.

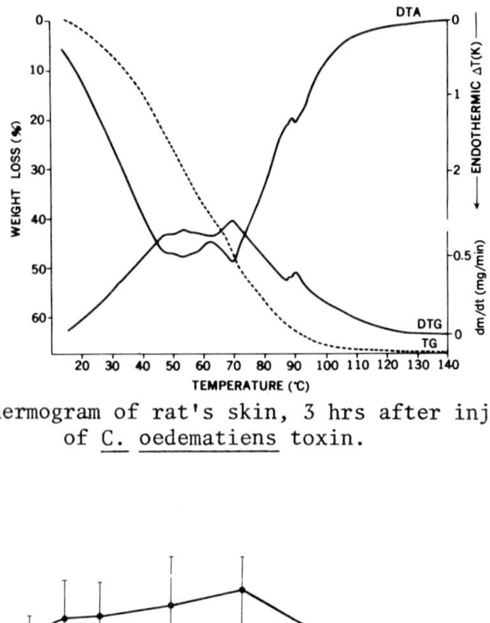

Fig. 2. Thermogram of rat's skin, 3 hrs after injection of C. oedematiens toxin.

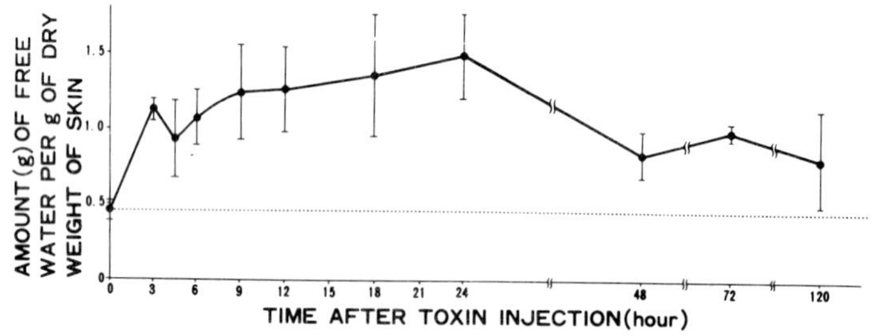

Fig. 3. Change in the amount of 'free' water during the course of edema formation induced in rat skin by C. oedematiens toxin. Each point represents the mean from 5 rats, except for the control value (dotted line) and the value for 120 hrs, the former being the mean from 12 rats and the latter the mean from 2 rats. Each vertical bar represents the 95% confidence interval of the mean.

interpreted as indicating that the amount of the fluid leaked is greater than that absorbed. This interpretation, however, is not sufficient to explain all of the observed changes, during the course of edema formation, in the amount of 'free' and 'bound' water, especially those in the latter. We must assume that the 'free water-holding capacity' and the 'water-binding capacity' of the tissue change as the action of toxin on the tissue progresses. The decrease in the 'water-binding capacity' observed with the affected tissue at the later stage, may be indicative of the occurrence of some damage to the tissue (Ohsaka, Momota, 1979b).

In addition to thermal analysis, we studied the edema induced in rat skin by the same toxin by means of nuclear magnetic resonance (NMR) (Ohsaka, Yoshikawa, 1979c). We demonstrated that the rat skin contained a considerable amount of triglyceride(s) 'observable' by ^{1}H- and ^{13}C-NMR (Yoshikawa, Ohsaka, 1979) and that the ratio of the amount of 'free' water to that of the triglyceride(s) varied during the course of edema formation (Ohsaka, Yoshikawa, 1979c). Figure 5 shows the change in the value of the longitudinal relaxation time (T_1) of the water proton in the skin tissue during the course of edema formation (Ohsaka, Yoshikawa, 1979 c); the value for T_1 increased in the 3 hrs following the toxin injection, decreased temporarily in 4.5 hrs and again increased in the 6th-24th hrs. T_1 then tended to decrease up to the 5th day to a normal level with a temporary increase at the 3rd day. Apparently, the change of T_1 with time resembled closely that of the amount of 'free' water as determined by thermal analysis (Fig. 3), indicating that T_1 of the water proton, being a measure of the mobility of water, is a useful parameter to follow up the development of edema in the tissue.
NMR study revealed also an interesting fact that the physical state of triglyceride changed with time in the affected tissue (Ohsaka, Yoshikawa, 1979c). Figure 6 shows the temperature dependence of the intensity of the proton signal of triglyceride in the skin affected by C. oedematiens toxin; the triglyceride in the control tissue began to 'freeze' at -30°C, whereas it began to 'freeze' at much higher temperatures in the affected tissues. Apparently, the change in the physical state of the tissue lipid is concerned with the course of edema formation.

All these results from thermal analysis as well as NMR provide a clue for elucidating the mechanism of edema formation.

Edema resulting from the immediate and delayed types of hypersensitivity produced in mouse paw

Hypersensitivity reaction is regarded as a particular kind of self-protecting reaction. The physical state of water in hypersensitized tissues may be different from that of water in tissues of pathophysiological state as induced by bacterial toxins.
With these points in mind, we have recently applied thermal analysis and nuclear magnetic resonance to the study of the water of edema resulting from the immediate (IH) and delayed (DH) skin hypersensitivity reactions produced in experimental animals (Iwasa, Ohsaka, Momota, 1979; Ohsaka, Momota, 1979b; Yoshikawa, Ohsaka, Iwasa, 1979).

Human serum albumin (HSA) and methylated human serum albumin (MHSA) were used as antigens. An appropriate amount of antigen was dissolved in a 0.85% NaCl solution and sterilized by filtration through a Millipore filter. Aluminium hydroxide gel-adsorbed HSA (Al-HSA) was prepared by mixing equal volumes of solutions of HSA and aluminium hydroxide gel (8 mg of $Al(OH)_3$/ml). An aliquot of the sterilized antigen solution was emulsified with an equal volume of complete (CFA) or incomplete Freund adjuvants (IFA). Mice were injected subcutaneously into the belly skin, with 20 μg of MHSA in CFA for induction of delayed skin hypersensitivity and with 100 μg of HSA in IFA for induction of immediate

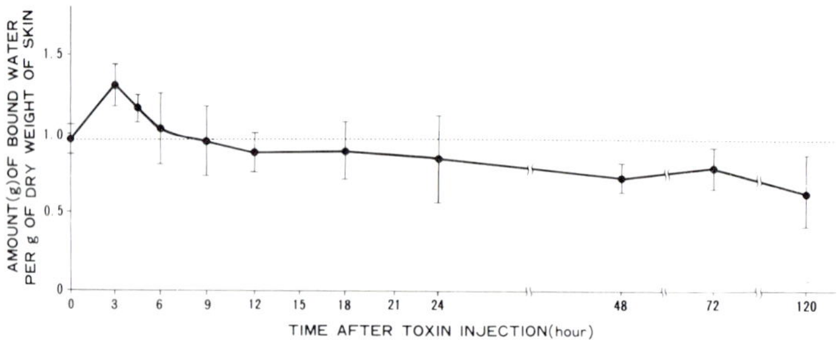

Fig. 4. Change in the amount of 'bound' water during the course of edema formation induced in rat skin by C. oedematiens toxin. Each point represents the mean from 5-8 rats, except for the control value (dotted line) which is the mean from 12 rats. Each vertical bar represents the 95% confidence interval of the mean.

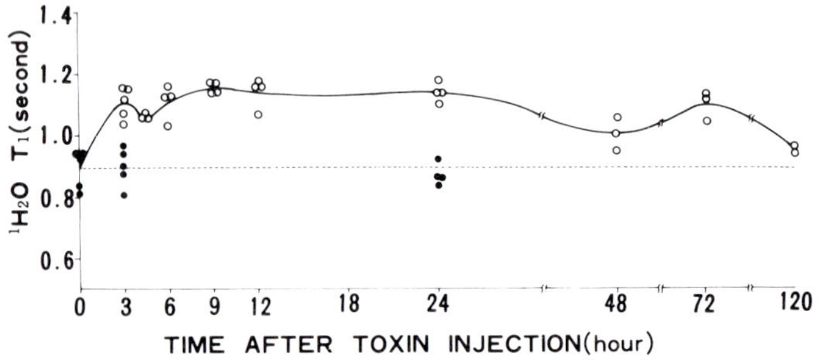

Fig. 5. Change in T_1 value of water proton during the course of edema formation induced in rat skin by C. oedematiens toxin. ●, Control rat; ○, rat injected with toxin.

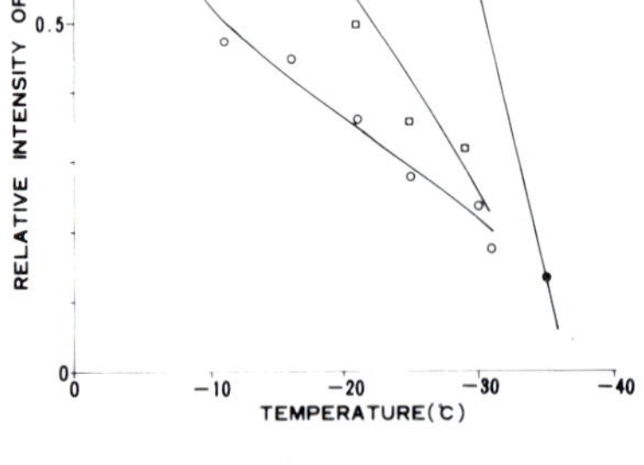

Fig. 6. Temperature dependence of the intensity of lipid proton signal in the skin of rat injected with C. oedematiens toxin. Intensity at room temperature was taken as unity. ●, Control; □, 3 hrs after toxin injection; ○, 24 hrs after toxin injection.

skin hypersensitivity. On the 10th day after the sensitization, the elicitation was made by injection with 50 μg of antigen into the right hind paws at the ventral side; MHSA was used for the former mice and Al-HSA for the latter mice (Ohsaka, Momota, 1979b). Saline or aluminium hydroxide gel without antigen was injected into the left hind paws at the ventral side of the same mice to serve as a control.
Mice sensitized with MHSA in CFA, when elicited with MHSA, developed DH reaction without any signs of IH reaction, confirming the finding of Crowle and co-workers (1968) that MHSA as a sensitizing protein antigen leads mice to develop DH to the antigen preferentially. The specific swelling in the hind paw reached up to 60×10^{-2} mm in 24 to 48 hrs. In contrast, animals sensitized with HSA in IFA produced IH reactions which reached a peak (specific swelling, 50×10^{-2} mm) in 2 to 3 hrs after the elicitation, followed by the appearance of DH reactions when the former reaction had subsided.

Figure 7 shows a typical thermogram of the skin taken from the left hind paws of DH-sensitized mice, 24 hrs after challenge with a 0.85% NaCl solution*. The skin taken 48 hrs after challenge with a 0.85% NaCl solution gave a similar thermogram. The endothermal peak observed at around 50°C is due to the evaporation of 'free' water, while those observed at higher temperatures is due to the evaporation of 'bound' water. The skin samples of the right hind paws of mice hypersensitized with MHSA were taken separately at 24 and 48 hrs after elicitation with the antigen and were subjected to thermal analysis; typical thermograms are depicted in Figs. 8 and 9. These thermograms are apparently different from that shown in Fig. 7.
From repeated such experiments the average contents of 'free' and 'bound' water in skin samples were calculated (Ohsaka, Momota, 1979b). The results are summarized in Fig. 10. It was concluded that the 'free' water content of the skin from the right hind paws of mice having a delayed hypersensitivity reaction, significantly increased in the 24 hrs following elicitation. This increased portion of the 'free' water was lost in the subsequent 24 hrs when the reaction reached its peak, with a concomitant increase in 'bound' water content. It may be justifiable to interpret these results as indicating that a large portion of the 'free' water which had increased in the early phase of the reaction was lost through transformation into 'bound' water.

The skin showing IH reaction was next investigated. Typical thermograms of the skin sample from the left hind paws taken at 2 hrs and those from right hind paws taken at 2 and 4 hrs are shown in Figs. 11, 12 and 13, respectively.
From such experiments repeated several times the average contents of 'free' and 'bound' water in skin samples were calculated. The results are summarized in Fig. 14. It was demonstrated that only the 'free' water content of the skin from the right hind paws of mice having an immediate hypersensitivity reaction, significantly increased in the 2 hrs following elicitation. This increased portion of the 'free' water was lost in the subsequent 2 hrs when the reaction subsided, with a concomitant increase in 'bound' water content. This increase is probably due to the conversion into the 'bound' water form of the 'free' water portion which had increased with the development of edema.

In Table I are shown T_1 values of water protons in the skin tissues from the hind paws of normal mice and those of mice having delayed and immediate hypersensitivity reactions. It is apparent that the T_1 value of the water proton is larger in the skin tissue of mice having either type of hypersensitivity than in the skin tissue of normal mice, indicating an increased mobility of water in hypersensitized tissues. Increased mobilities of ^{13}C atoms in hypersensitized tissue were also suggested from the sharpening of ^{13}C signals in NMR spectra. NMR study also demonstrated an increase in the amount of fermentation products

* An almost identical thermogram was obtained with the skin from the right hind paws of unsensitized mice, 24 hrs after challenge with MHSA.

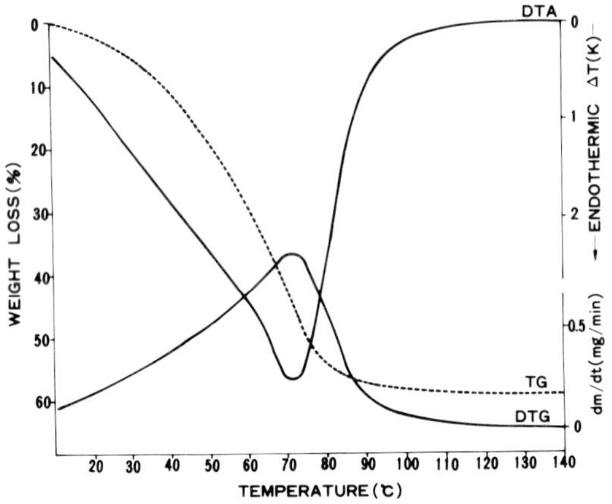

Fig. 7. Thermogram of the skin taken from the left hind paws of DH-sensitized mice, 24 hrs after challenge with a 0.85% NaCl solution.

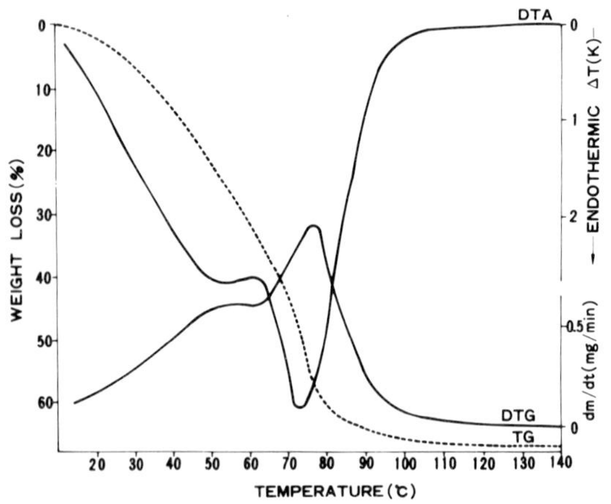

Fig. 8. Thermogram of the skin taken from the right hind paws of DH-sensitized mice, 24 hrs after elicitation with MHSA.

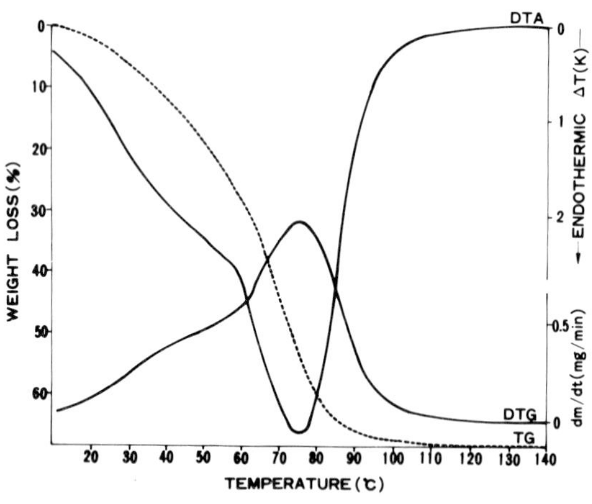

Fig. 9. Thermogram of the skin taken from the right hind paws of DH-sensitized mice, 48 hrs after elicitation with MHSA.

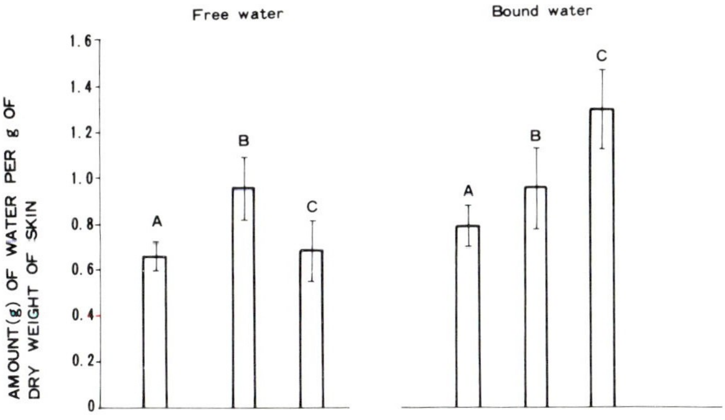

Fig. 10. The contents of 'free' and 'bound' water in the skin from the hind paws of DH-sensitized mice. The skin samples from the left hind paws were taken separately at 24 hrs and 48 hrs after challenge with a 0.85% NaCl solution. Since no difference in water contents was found between the two samples, both were combined to serve as a control for 24 hrs and 48 hrs (Column A). The skin samples from the right hind paws were taken at 24 hrs (Column B) and 48 hrs (Column C) after elicitation with MHSA. Each column represents the mean and each vertical bar the 95% confidence interval of the mean.

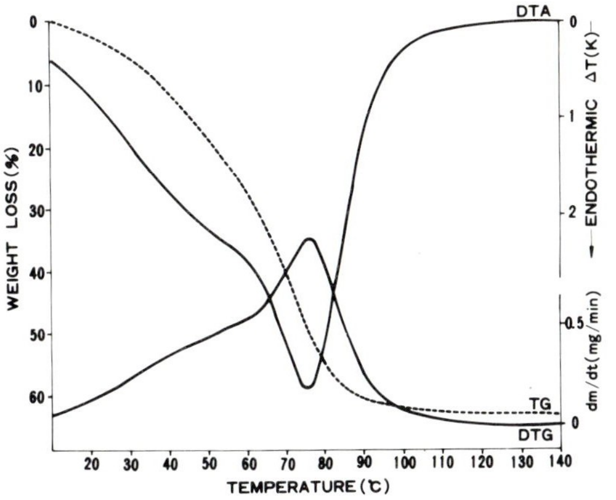

Fig. 11. Thermogram of the skin taken from the left hind paws of IH-sensitized mice, 2 hrs after challenge with aluminium hydroxide gel.

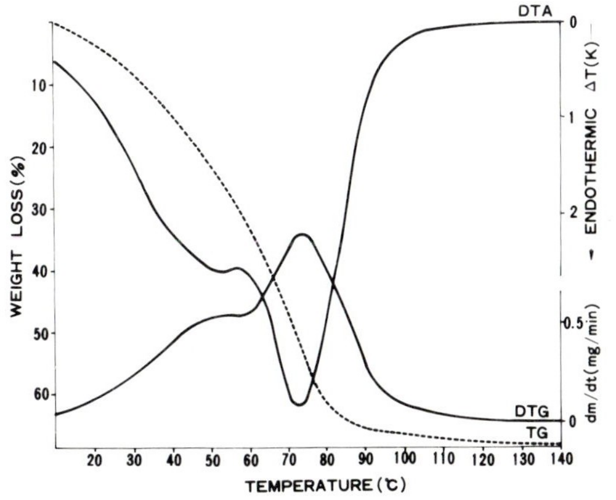

Fig. 12. Thermogram of the skin taken from the right hind paws of IH-sensitized mice, 2 hrs after elicitation with Al-HSA.

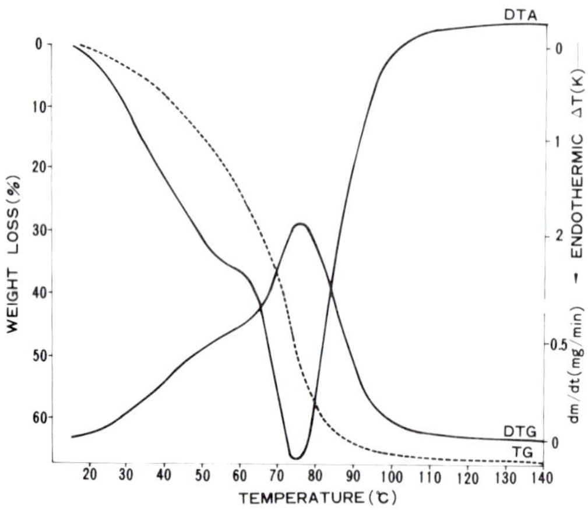

Fig. 13. Thermogram of the skin taken from the right hind paws of IH-sensitized mice, 4 hrs after elicitation with Al-HSA.

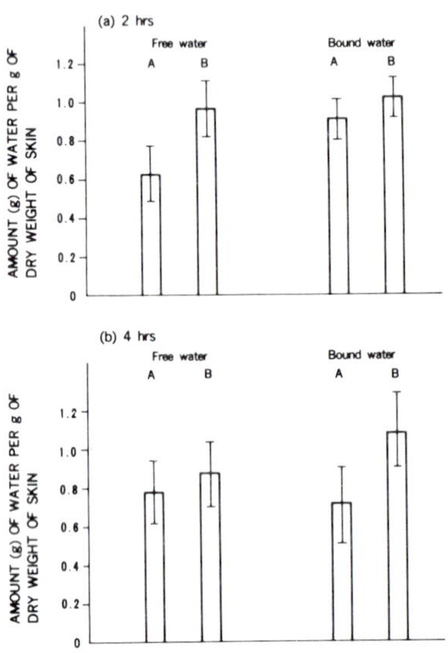

Fig. 14. The contents of 'free' and 'bound' water in the skin from the hind paws of IH-sensitized mice. The skin samples were taken from the left hind paws (Column A) at 2 hrs (a) and 4 hrs (b) after challenge with aluminium hydroxide gel and also from the right hind paws (Column B) at 2 hrs (a) and 4 hrs (b) after elicitation with Al-HSA. Each column represents the mean and each vertical bar the 95% confidence interval of the mean.

TABLE 1. T_1 Values of Water Proton in the Skin Tissues from the Hind Paws of Normal Mice and Those of Mice having Delayed and Immediate Hypersensitivity Reactions

Skin tissue	T_1 (sec)
Control	0.76 ± 0.02
Delayed hypersensitivity, 48 hrs (Classical type)	1.04 ± 0.02
Control	0.79 ± 0.04
Immediate hypersensitivity, 2 hrs	1.04 ± 0.04

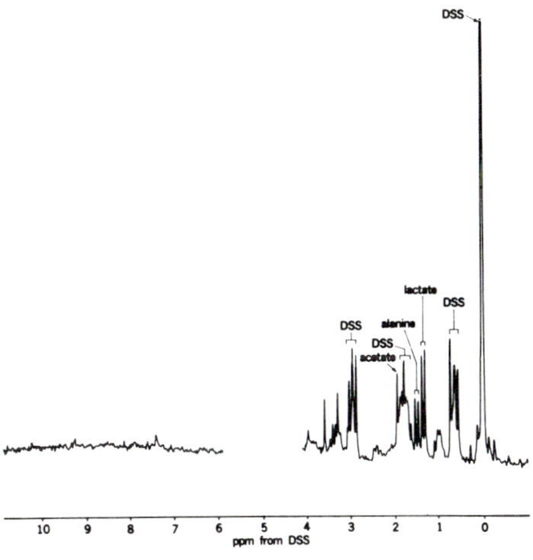

Fig. 15. 100 MHz ^{1}H-NMR spectrum of the extract with a 0.85% NaCl solution in D_2O of the skin tissue taken from DH-sensitized mice, 24 hrs after challenge with a 0.85% NaCl solution. Chemical shift is shown in ppm from internal DSS.

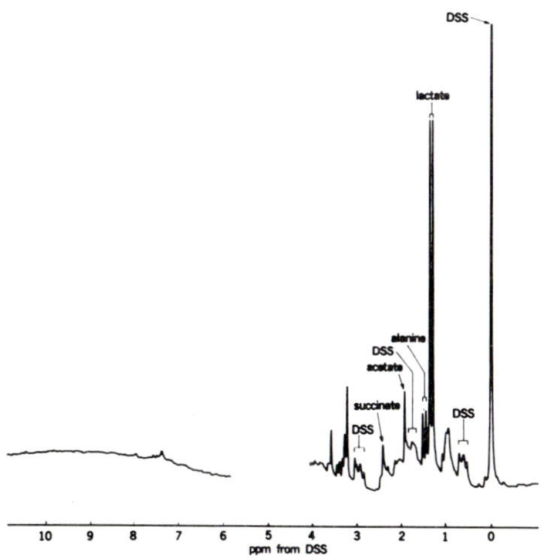

Fig. 16. 100 MHz ^{1}H-NMR spectrum of the extract with a 0.85% NaCl solution in D_2O of the skin tissue taken from DH-sensitized mice, 24 hrs after elicitation with MHSA. Chemical shift is shown in ppm from internal DSS.

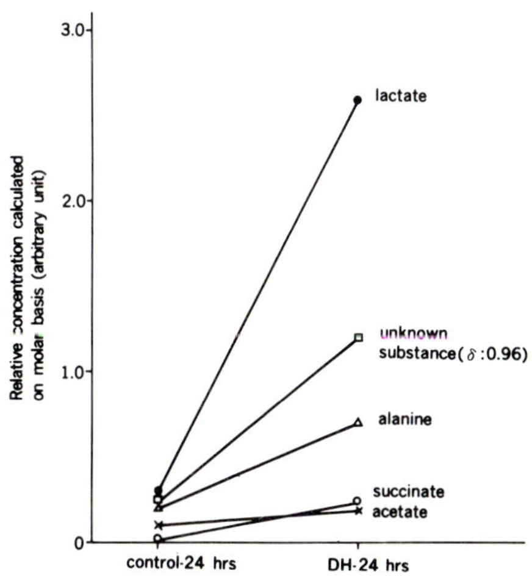

Fig. 17. Increase in the amount of fermentation products in the skin tissue of DH-sensitized mice, taken at 24 hrs after elicitation with MHSA. The relative concentration of the products were calculated from ^{1}H-NMR spectra of the extract of the skin tissue with a 0.85% NaCl solution in D_2O.

in hypersensitized tissue. The skin tissues from normal mice and mice having delayed hypersensitivity reaction were extracted with 0.85% NaCl in D_2O and ^1H-NMR spectra of these extracts were compared (Figs. 15 and 16). The results summarized in Fig. 17 demonstrated increases in the amount of such fermentation products as lactate, alanine, succinate, acetate and an unidentified substance (δ: 0.96). It is apparent that fermentation is accelerated in the hypersensitized tissue.

All these results from thermal analysis as well as NMR provide a clue for elucidating the mechanisms involved in hypersensitivity reactions.

ACKNOWLEDGEMENTS

We thank the Institute for Molecular Science, Okazaki, Japan for making FT NMR spectrometer available to us. Work was performed under a grant to A. O. (1977-1978) from the Ohyama Health Foundation, Inc., Tokyo, for which we wish to thank.

REFERENCES

Crowle, A. J., C. C. Hu and A. Patrucoo. (1968). Preferential development by mouse of delayed hypersensitivity to purified basic protein. J. Allergy, 42, 140-156.

Iwasa, S., A. Ohsaka and M. Momota. (1979). Characterization of immediate and delayed types of hypersensitivity produced in mouse paw by simultaneous thermogravimetry - differential thermal analysis. In preparation.

Izumi, N. and H. Kondo. (1978). Studies on Clostridium oedematiens toxin with special reference to differentiation of the lethal, oedematous, hemolytic and lecithinase activities. Japan. J. Med. Sci. Biol., 31, 219.

James, T. L. (1975). 'Nuclear Magnetic Resonance in Biochemistry. Principles and Applications', pp.298-388. Academic Press, New York.

Momota, M. and A. Ohsaka. (1979). Simultaneous thermogravimetry (TG)-differential thermal analysis (DTA) for the study of water in foodstuffs: Instrumentation and technology. In L. B. Rockland and G. F. Stewart, (eds.), Influences of Water and Water Activity on the Quality and Stability of Foods, Academic Press, New York, in Press.

Ohsaka, A., M. Momota, N. Izumi and H. Kondo. (1979a). The use of differential thermal analysis and thermogravimetry to study the free and bound water of edema induced in rat skin by the toxin of Clostridium oedematiens. Japan. J. Med. Sci. Biol., 32, 124-125.

Ohsaka, A. and M. Momota. (1979b). The use of differential thermal analysis and thermogravimetry to study free and bound water in foodstuffs and animal tissues. In L. B. Rockland and G. F. Stewart (eds.), Influences of Water and Water Activity on the Quality and Stability of Foods, Academic Press, New York, in press.

Ohsaka, A. and K. Yoshikawa. (1979c). Nuclear magnetic resonance as a probe for the study of edema induced in rat skin by the toxin of Clostridium oedematiens. In preparation.

Yoshikawa, K., A. Ohsaka and Y. Yamakawa. (1979). Nuclear magnetic resonance study of edema induced in rat skin by α-toxin of Clostridium perfringens. In preparation.

Yoshikawa, K., A. Ohsaka and S. Iwasa. (1979). NMR as a probe for the study of skin hypersensitivity produced in mouse paw. In preparation.

Yoshikawa, K. and A. Ohsaka. (1979). Nuclear magnetic resonance of rat skin. Physiol. Chem. Physics, 11, 185-188.

Novel Bacterial Toxins

CLOSTRIDIUM DIFFICILE AND PSEUDOMEMBRANOUS COLITIS IN HUMANS

J. G. Bartlett, N. Taylor, S. Willey and T.-W. Chang

Veterans Administration Hospital and Tufts University School of Medicine, Boston, Massachusetts, USA

ABSTRACT

The studies summarized here provide compelling evidence that C. *difficile* is the putative agent of all, or nearly all, cases of antibiotic-associated pseudomembranous colitis (PMC). The organism is regularly recovered from stool of afflicted patients, but is infrequently encountered in the fecal flora of healthy persons. The vast majority of patients also have a cytotoxin in stools which may be neutralized by C. *sordelli* antitoxin. C. *difficile* has been found to produce a similar or identical cytotoxin in vitro. This organism or its partially purified cytotoxin produce a similar disease with intracecal injection into experimental animals. Thus, Koch's postulates have been satisfied for the role of C. *difficile* as an enteric toxigenic pathogen. These observations have evolved rapidly during the past three years, and they have eventuated in the most encouraging finding, which is successful treatment using oral vancomycin directed against the responsible agent. Nevertheless, the final chapter in PMC has obviously not been written. Particularly enigmatic at this juncture is the association of C. *difficile*, its toxin and its clinical expression , almost exclusively in the presence of antibiotic exposure. There is little precedent for this type of relationship in other infectious diseases caused by bacterial toxins. Also perplexing is the source of the organism, since it is uncertain if patients who develop PMC are a subset of those who were previously colonized by the organism, or if C. *difficile* was acquired from an environmental source. Finally, the mechanism of action of C. *difficile* toxin on the intestinal mucosa is unclear. Studies in tissue cultured cells show changes in ultrastructure, but other biologic effects of the toxin are ill-defined. A final comment is that toxin purification studies have focused on the cytotoxin, but there is no absolute assurance that this is the only toxin produced by C. *difficile*.

KEYWORDS

Clostridium difficile; *Clostridium sordellii* antitoxin; antibiotic-associated diarrhea; clindamycin; cytotoxin; pseudomembranous colitis; tissue culture; typhilitis.

INTRODUCTION

Diarrhea is a relatively common complication of antibiotic usage. Anatomical studies of the colon in these patients show a variety of pathologic changes. However, the most serious and most characteristic lesion is pseudomembranous colitis (PMC) characterized by intralumenal exudative plaques attached to an inflamed colonic mucosa. Work during the past three years implicates *Clostridium difficile* as the major cause of antibiotic-associated PMC. Evidence to support this conclusion is based on two separate, but mutually complementary lines of investigation. The first is tissue culture assays of stools showing a cytopathic toxin which appears to be identical to the cytotoxin produced by C. *difficile* in vitro. The second line of investigation concerns experimental animal studies which implicate C. *difficile* as the cause of a similar disease induced by antibiotic administration in hamsters. The purpose of the present report is to review the data implicating C. *difficile* as the cause of this disease, and to characterize the cytotoxin.

EXPERIMENTAL ANIMAL STUDIES

It has long been known that most antibiotics are lethal to hamsters and guinea pigs. The only consistent pathologic finding at necropsy in these animals is an intensely congested cecum which is distended with bloody, liquid contents. Our initial work concerned the cause of this lesion in hamsters given clindamycin. It was noted that 96% of animals given clindamycin expired within three to five days due to the hemorhaggic typhilitis. The LD_{50} for clindamycin was approximately 50 μg, both the oral and parenteral routes of administration caused the disease and a variety of other antimicrobials were also lethal with similar lesions noted at necropsy. Attempts were made to identify a transmissible agent using intracecal innoculations of cecal contents into healthy recipients. This work showed that the disease could be transferred with five serial passes. The substance responsible for transferrable pathogenicity could be passed through a 0.02 μm filter and was completely neutralized by preincubation with gas gangrene antitoxin. This suggested a clostridial toxin and attempts were then made to recover a clostridial species which would reproduce the disease using intracecal injections of broth cultures. One organism, C. *difficile,* satisfied this criterion (Bartlett and others, 1977). Cultures were then performed on stools from hamsters with a focus of attention on this clostridia. C. *difficile* was not detected in specimens from any of 15 healthy animals, and it was found in concentrations of $10^{6.8}$ to $10^{10.1}$ per g wet weight in each of 35 animals which were moribund following antibiotic exposure. Extensive environmental cultures have failed to reveal a source of C. *difficile* and it is possible that healthy animals harbor the organism in the colonic flora in concentrations which are too low to detect with our culture techniques. Thus, the source of the organism is not clear, but its association with the disease process is firmly established.

TISSUE CULTURES

During the course of the previously noted experiments with animals, an attempt was made to recover a virus as well as bacterial agents (Chang and others, 1978a). This work failed to reveal a virus, but it did uncover a tissue culture assay which has become a favored diagnostic test in antibiotic-associated colitis. It was noted that stools from hamsters with antibiotic-induced colitis contained a cytotoxin which is neutralized by C. *sordellii* antitoxin. This toxin is not present in the stools of healthy animals, but it was found in specimens from each of 546 hamsters which expired after antibiotic exposure (Bartlett and others, 1978b). Low concentrations of the toxin were initially detected at 12-36 hours after clindamycin administration, and concentrations gradually increased to levels of 10^{-5} to 10^{-7} dilutions at time of death. A direct correlation was noted between toxin titres, concentrations of C. *difficile* and severity of the disease. The cytotoxin was also noted in the blood in moribund animals, suggesting mucosal absorption in the terminal stages.

CLINICAL STUDIES

The relevance of the animal work to clinical practice became apparent when both the cytotoxin and *C. difficile* were found in patients with antibiotic-associated PMC. The first patient studied in our laboratory had lethal antibiotic-associated PMC due to cephalothin in June 1977. Stool obtained on the day prior to death showed a cytotoxin in a concentration of 10^{-7} dilutions, and *C. difficile* was recovered in a concentration of $10^{6.8}$/g wet weight. Intracecal injection of cell-free supernatant from the stool and cell-free supernatant of broth cultures of the organism into hamsters reproduced the pathologic lesion found with antibiotic administration to these animals; both preparations were completely neutralized by the addition of *C. sordellii* antitoxin (Bartlett and others, 1977). Subsequent work in this laboratory and several others has verified these initial observations (Bartlett, 1979; George, R.H. and others, 1978; Keighley and others, 1978; Larson and Price, 1977).

Our experience with the tissue culture assay in patients with diarrheal complications of antibiotics is summarized in Table 1.

TABLE 1 Tissue Culture Assays of Stools

	No. Tested	No. Positive*
Patients with antibiotic-associated diarrhea PMC	102	98 (96%)
Diarrhea without confirmed PMC	255	50 (20%)
Gastrointestinal diseases without antibiotic exposure	170	4 (2%)
Antibiotic recipients without diarrheal complications	40	0
Healthy adults	70	0
Healthy neonates	82	2 (2%)

*Criterion for positive assay is a cytopathic toxin which is neutralized by *C. sordellii* antitoxin.

These tests have been performed using stool supernatant applied to WI-38 cells or primary human amnion cells. The criterion for a positive response is the demonstration of cytopathic changes which are neutralized by *C. sordellii* antitoxin. It is noted that this toxin was found in 96% of patients with antibiotic-associated PMC. The cytotoxin was also found in approximately 20% of specimens from patients with antibiotic-associated diarrhea in which endoscopy failed to reveal pseudomembranes or else was not performed. The toxin was present in four patients of 170 patients with gastrointestinal diseases which were unrelated to antibiotic exposure; three of these four patients had PMC, but denied exposure to antimicrobials during the three months prior to symptoms. The toxin has not been found in healthy adults, but stools from asymptomatic neonates occasionally yield the toxin. Toxin titres have been performed using serial 10-fold dilutions of stool supernatant. This shows a median titre of 10^{-3} dilutions in patients with PMC, and 10^{-2} dilutions in patients with antibiotic-associated diarrhea without demonstrable pseudomembranes. There appears to be a crude correlation between the severity of the clinical disease and the titre, but marked exceptions to this trend have been noted.

Bacterial cultures of stool are complicated by the complexity of the fecal flora. This factor is the presumed explanation for the consistent failure to identify the cause of antibiotic-associated colitis in both patients and animals, despite extensive studies using conventional culture techniques spanning three decades. The indirect methods previously described in the hamster model led to a focus of attention on clostridia, and subsequently on *C. difficile*. Recent work with a search for this organism has now verified the association of *C. difficile* and PMC in several laboratories (Bartlett, 1979; George, W. L. and others, 1979; Keighley and others, 1978; Larson and others, 1978). In our experience, this organism has been detected in stools from 52 of 53 patients with antibiotic-associated PMC. The median concentration of *C. difficile* in these patients was $10^{5.8}$ per g wet weight. However, as with toxin titres, there has been only a crude correlation between concentrations of *C. difficile* and the severity of the disease process. Also important is the observation that this organism accounts for a relatively small portion of the total bacterial counts, indicating that it would be difficult to detect with direct Gram stain. The carrier rate of *C. difficile* in healthy adults is not well established, but is believed to be only about 3% (George, W. L. and others, 1978). Carrier rates in neonates appear to be substantially higher (Hall and O'Toole, 1935; Larson and others, 1978).

Clostridium difficile

There is considerable precedent for the role of various clostridia as enteric pathogens. Well established causes of diarrheal diseases in clinical and veterinary medicine include *Clostridium perfringens* (types A, B, C and D), *C. sordellii*, *C. septicum* and *C. colinum*. *C. difficile* represents a new addition to this group. Enteritis necroticans, which is caused by *C. perfringens*, type C, is somewhat similar to pseudomembranous colitis in that both are enteric clostridial diseases characterized by inflammation of the intestinal mucosa in patients. One major difference between the two is that *C. perfringens*, type C, invades the mucosa, whereas penetration of epithelial cells has not been observed with *C. difficile*.

C. difficile has rarely been implicated in diseases other than antibiotic-associated diarrhea or colitis. The organism was originally described by Hall and O'Toole (1935) as a component of the normal fecal flora in neonates. The original name, *Bacillus difficilis*, reflects the difficulty encountered by these investigators in isolating and maintaining the organism. Subsequent work by Hafiz and Oakley, 1976) showed that *C. difficile* could be isolated from stools of numerous animal species and was widely distributed in the environment. Clinical studies have shown that *C. difficile* has been infrequently recovered from extraintestinal infections (Gorbach and Thadepalli, 1975). Thus, this organism has been regarded as a rare and relatively unimportant pathogen until the recent work implicating its role in antibiotic-associated diarrhea. A unique feature is the intimate association between antibiotic exposure and *C. difficile* colonization, toxin production and colonic inflammation. *C. difficile* has recently been implicated as a cause of neonatal diarrhea in hares (Dabard and others, 1979). However, with this exception, *C. difficile* has been implicated as a cause of enteric disease almost exclusively in patients and experimental animals exposed to antibiotics. A logical conclusion is that this represents a superinfection in which a resistant pathogen fluorishes when the competing flora are suppressed. Against this thesis is the observation that a major portion of *C. difficile* isolates have proven susceptible to the agents responsible for PMC. Ampicillin, for example, is implicated in a major portion of cases, and virtually all strains of *C. difficile* are highly susceptible to this agent (George, W. L. and others, 1978).

Clostridium difficile TOXIN

It was noted in the original description of C. *difficile* that subcutaneous injection of cell-free filtrates of broth cultures are lethal to guinea pigs and rabbits (Hall and O'Toole, 1935). Subsequent work showed that cats, dogs, rats and pigeons are also susceptible to parenteral administration of C. *difficile* broth supernatant (Snyder, 1937). More recent work has shown that the cell-free supernatant is cytopathic to all cell lines tested to date. These preparations also cause lethality upon intraperitoneal injection into mice, increased capillary permeability upon intradermal injection in guinea pigs, lethal cecitis upon intracecal injection into hamsters and fluid accumulation in the rabbit ileal loop assay (Aswell and others, 1979; Bartlett and others, 1977; Humphrey and others, 1979; Rifkin and others, 1977). In each instance, the different biologic effects are neutralized by C. *sordellii* antitoxin.

The original observation that C. *sordellii* antitoxin neutralized the cytotoxin in stool from patients with PMC posed a dilemma concerning which clostridial species was actually responsible for PMC. C. *sordellii* is known to cause enterotoxemia in cattle, so the precedent for this as an enteric pathogen was well established (Smith, 1975). Nevertheless, stool cultures consistently failed to yield C. *sordellii*, and broth cultures of numerous C. *sordellii* failed to produce the actinomorphic changes in tissue-cultured cells which were seen with stool analyses. This issue has subsequently been resolved by showing that cell-free supernatant of C. *difficile* broth cultures produce typical cytopathic changes which can be neutralized by C. *sordellii* antitoxin (Bartlett and others, 1978c). The rate of neutralization in this reaction is almost instantaneous, and a zone of equivalence is readily demonstrated. However, the union between the toxin and anti-toxin can be readily disassociated by simple dilution, by ammonium sulfate precipitation followed by dilution or by continued incubation of the toxin-antitoxin mixture. The potency of C. *sordellii* antitoxin from different sources also shows a poor correlation with values reported for mouse protection tests against C. *sordellii* toxin. All of these observations are consistent with antigenic cross-reactivity in which there is relatively little serologic specificity or affinity (Chang and others, 1978b).

Studies have been conducted in our laboratory to determine if all strains of C. *difficile* produce the cytopathic toxin. This was of great interest in view of the observation that occasional adults and many infants harbor the organism in the colonic flora without detectable toxin in stools and without apparent clinical consequences. Initial tests were performed to determine the optimal method to detect in vitro toxin production (Bartlett and others, 1978c). This work showed that the highest titres (10^{-3} - 10^{-5} dilutions) were noted with glucose-containing media using sonicates obtained after incubation for 24-48 hours, and broth supernatants obtained after 72-96 hours. The high toxin levels noted with broth supernatants occurred at the termination of log phase growth. Studies using continuous culture indicate that, unlike some toxigenic clostridia, the cytotoxin of C. *difficile* is not associated with sporulation (Onderdonk and others, 1979). Subinhibitory concentrations of clindamycin, an antibiotic which is commonly implicated in PMC, failed to enhance toxin concentrations. Thus, induction of the toxin by antibiotics is an unlikely explanation for the association of C *difficile* cytotoxin and antimicrobial exposure.

On the basis of these observations, 200 strains of C. *difficile* from a variety of sources were examined for cytotoxin production using supernatants of chopped-meat glucose broth cultures after incubation for five days. All supernatants caused actinomorphic changes in tissue cultures, including stool isolates from some patients who had no cytotoxin in the original specimen. Similar testing with 146 clostridial species representing 23 species other than C. *difficile* failed to reveal any which produced typical changes in tissue-cultured cells. It would appear that all strains of C. *difficile* are toxigenic, and that no other clostridial species is known to produce a toxin similar to the cytotoxin found in stools of patients with PMC. These results, coupled with the high isolation rate of C. *difficile* in stools, provide compelling evidence that this organism is responsible for the cytotoxin found in nearly all patients with antibiotic-associated PMC.

As previously noted, the cytotoxin produced by C. *difficile* appears to be cytopathic to all tissue-cultured cells. These include primary human amnion, human fibroblast, baby hamster kidney, mouse fibroblast, human chroion, human brain, human embryonic tonsil, Chinese hamster ovary and Y-1 adrenal cells. With monkey kidney, human amnion and fibroblast cells there is retraction of the cell membrane with stringing of cytoplasmic processes, giving characteristic actinomorphic changes. Scanning electron microscopy with primary human amnion monolayer cells shows changes in the ultrastructure of cell membranes which are detected within one hour of exposure. The patterns of surface changes are specific for two different types of cells in this monolayer. Cells with demarkated borders show rearrangement of microvilli into globular chains or ridges which align with the branching membrane. Cells without demarkated borders exhibit stud-like microvilli arranged into ridges or globular chains. These pathogenic changes are similar to those seen with other toxins which bind cell membranes and lead to cell destruction(Bernheimer, 1974). The rapidity of the changes indicates that this in unlikely to reflect an effect on cell mitosis, since cell proliferation activity in primary amnion cultures is extremely low.

Partial purification of C. *difficile* cytotoxin was previously reported by Taylor and Bartlett (1979), using ultrafiltration, ammonium sulfate precipitation, Sephadex G-200 chromatography and DEAE-Sepharose CL6B chromatography. This resulted in a 1500-fold purification of the cytotoxin from the starting material (Table 2). Polyacrylamide gel electrophoresis of the partially purified cytotoxin shows one

TABLE 2 Purification of Cytotoxin from *Clostridium difficile* Supernatant

	Total Protein (mg)	Total Cytotoxic Units*	Cytotoxic Units/mg Protein	Fold Purification	Recovery
Starting material	5320	2500	0.47	1	100%
Ultrafiltration	496	2000	4.0	6	80%
70% $(NH_4)_2SO_4$	78	725	9.3	10	30%
Sephadex G-200	13.5	750	55.6	90	30%
DEAE-Sepharose CL6B	0.7	500	714.3	1500	20%

*Cytotoxic units = amount of toxin necessary to give actinomorphic changes in WI-38 cell cultures at 10^{-3} dilutions.

major band and 3 or 4 very faint bands. Preparations containing 60 picograms/ml elicited typical cytophathic changes in tissue-cultured cells. This cytotoxin is inactivated by heat (56°C, 1 hour), by alkali (pH 10.4, 1 hour at 37°C). The partially purified cytotoxin is negative for hemolysisn, lecithinase, lipase and proteolytic activity. Molecular weight estimates performed using Sephadex G-200 with protein standards indicate a molecular weight of approximately 240,000. Aswell and others (1979), using a somewhat different purification method, has reported a molecular weight of 550,000-600,000.

REFERENCES

Aswell, J. E., M. Erlich, R. L. Van Tassell, C. C. Tsai, L. V. Holdeman and T. D. Wilkins (1979). Characterization and comparison of *Clostridium difficile* and other clostridial toxins. In: Microbiology 1979, D. Schlessinger (Ed.), Amer. Soc. Microbiol. Washington, pp 272-275.

Bartlett, J. G. (1979). Antibiotic-associated pseudomembranous colitis. Rev. Infect. Dis., 1, 530-539.

Bartlett, J. G., T. W. Chang, M. Gurwith, S. L. Gorbach, and A. B. Onderdonk (1978a) Antibiotic-associated pseudomembranous colitis due to toxin producing clostridia. New Engl. J. Med., 290, 531-534.

Bartlett, J. G., T. W. Chang, N. Moon, and A. B. Onderdonk (1978b). Antibiotic-induced lethal enterocolitis in hamsters: Studies with eleven agents and evidence to support the pathogenic role of toxin-producing clostridia. Amer. J. Veterin. Res., 39, 1525-1530.

Bartlett, J. G., N. Moon, T. W. Chang, N. Taylor, and A. B. Onderdonk (1978c). The role of *Clostridium difficile* in antibiotic associated pseudomembranous colitis. Gastroenterology, 75, 778-782.

Bartlett, J. G., A. B. Onderdonk, R. L. Cisneros, and D. L. Kasper (1977). Clindamycin-associated colitis due to a toxin-producing species of *Clostridium* in hamsters. J. Infect. Dis., 136, 701-705.

Bernheimer, A. W. (1974). Interactions between membranes amd cytolytic bacterial toxins. Biochim. Biophys. Acta, 344, 27-50.

Chang, T. W., J. G. Bartlett, S. L. Gorbach, and A. B. Onderdonk (1978a). Clindamycin-induced enterocolitis in hamsters as a model of pseudomembranous colitis in patients. Infect. Immun., 20, 526-529.

Chang, T. W., S. L. Gorbach, and J. G. Bartlett (1978b). Neutralization of *Clostridium difficile* toxin by *Clostridium sordellii* antitoxin. Infect. Immun., 22, 418-422.

Dabard, J., F. Dubos, L. Martinet, and R. Ducluzean (1979). Experimental reproduction of neonatal diarrhea in young gnotobiotic hares simultaneously associated with *Clostridium difficile* and other *Clostridium* strains. Infect. Immun. 24, 7-11.

George, R. H., J. M. Symonds, F. Dimock, J. D. Brown, Y. Arabi, N. Shinagawa, M. R. B. Keighley, J. Alexander-Williams, and D. W. Burdon (1978). Identification of *Clostridium difficile* as a cause of pseudomembranous colitis. Brit. Med. J., 1, 695.

George, W. L., V. L. Sutter, D. Citron, and S. M. Finegold (1979). Selective and differential medium for isolation of *Clostridium difficile*. J. Clin. Microbiol. 9, 214-219.

George, W. L., V. L. Sutter, and S. M. Finegold (1978). Toxicity and antimicrobial susceptibility of *Clostridium difficile*, a cause of antimicrobial agent-associated colitis. Curr. Microbiol., 1, 55-58.

Gorbach, S. L., and H. Thadepalli (1975). Isolation of *Clostridium* in human infections. J. Infect. Dis., 131, 581-585.

Hafiz, S. L., and C. L. Oakley (1976). *Clostridium difficile*: isolation and characteristics. J. Med. Microbiol., 9, 129-137.

Hall, I. C., and E. O'Toole (1935). Intestinal flora in new-born infants with a description of a new pathogenic anaerobe, *Bacillis difficilis*. Amer. J. Dis. Child., 49, 390-402.

Humphrey, C. D., C. W. Condon, J. R. Cantey, and F. E. P. Honan (1979). Partial pirification of a tosin found in hamsters with antibiotic-associated colitis. Gastroenterology, 76, 468-476.

Keighley, M. R. B., C. W. Burdon, Y. Arabi, J. Alexander-Williams, H. Thompson, D. Youngs, M. Johnson, S. Bentley, R. H. George, and G. A. G. Mogg (1978). Randomized controlled trial of vancomycin for pseudomembranous colitis and postoperative diarrhea. Brit. Med. J., 2, 1667-1669.

Larson, H. E., and A. B. Price (1977). Pseudomembranous colitis: presence of clostridial toxin. Lancet, 2, 1312-1314.

Larson, H. E., A. B. Price, P. Honour, and S. P. Borriello (1978). *Clostridium difficile* and the aetiology of pseudomembranous colitis. Lancet, 1, 1063-1066.

Onderdonk, A. B., B. R. Lowe, and J. G. Bartlett (1979). Effect of environmental stress on *Clostridium difficile* toxin levels during continuous culture. Appl. Environ. Microbiol., in press.

Rifkin, G. D., F. R. Fekety, J. Silva, Jr., and R. Fekety (1977). Antibiotic-induced colitis: implication of a toxin neutralized by *Clostridium sordellii* antitoxin. Lancet, 2, 1103-1106.

Smith, L. D. S. (1975). *Clostridium sordellii*. In: The Pathogenic Anaerobic Bacteria, Charles C. Thomas, Springfield, Ill., pp 291-298.

Snyder, M. D. (1937). Further studies on *Bacillis difficilis*. J. Infect. Dis., 60, 223-229

Taylor, N. S., and J. G. Bartlett (1979). Partial purification and characterization of a cytotoxin from *Clostridium difficile*. Rev. Infect. Dis., 1, 379-385.

STUDIES ON THE CLOSTRIDIAL TOXIN ASSOCIATED WITH ANTIBIOTIC-INDUCED PSEUDOMEMBRANOUS COLITIS

T. Wilkins*, M. Ehrich*, R. Van Tassell* and E. Balish**

**VPI and SU Anaerobe Laboratory, Blacksburg, Va., USA*
***Dept. of Surgery, Univ. of Wisconsin Med. Center, Madison, Wisc., USA*

ABSTRACT

The toxin of Clostridium difficile is considered responsible fcr pseudomembranous colitis which may follow antibiotic chemotherapy, This toxin can be produced in broth culture. After purification by gel filtration, ammonium sulfate precipitation, and ion-exchange chromatography, 12.5 picograms protein was cytotoxic to Chinese hamster ovary cells. Gnotobiotic rats were associated with a strain of C. difficile which produced large amounts of toxin. A spontaneous mutant was isolated from the ceca of these mice that produced 10,000-fold less toxin. This toxin had the same molecular weight as that produced by the parent and was neutralized by antitoxin to C. difficile. We have produced antitoxin to C. difficile that will neutralize the mouse LD_{100} (ip, 16 h) of the toxin at a dilution of 1:8000.

KEYWORDS

Clostridium difficile toxin, antitoxin, mutant, pseudomembranous colitis.

INTRODUCTION

Pseudomembranous colitis may follow therapy with antibiotics, including cephalosporins, tetracycline, ampicillin, and clindamycin (Hutcheon, 1978; Lusk, 1977; Medline, 1976). This rare side effect has a mortality rate between 27 - 44% (Anonymous, 1978). The antibiotic most closely associated with pseudomembranous colitis is clindamycin, a drug that is often used for infections caused by anaerobic bacteria. Fecal filtrates from patients who have received clindamycin and developed pseudomembranous colitis are cytotoxic (Bartlett, 1978, 1979; Chang, 1978a; Larson, 1977; Rifkin, 1977, 1978). This cytotoxicity is preventable by pretreatment of the fecal filtrate with antitoxin to C. sordellii (Chang, 1978b; Rifkin, 1977, 1978), but C. sordellii has not been isolated from these stool samples. C. difficile has been isolated from such stools and its toxin is neutralized by the C. sordellii antitoxin from the U.S. Bureau of Biologics (Chang, 1978a; R. George, 1978; W. George, 1978). We previously reported that the antitoxin to C. sordellii from the U.S. Bureau of Biologics is unusual in its ability to neutralize C. difficile toxin (Aswell, 1979). C. sordellii antitoxins produced in our laboratory and that obtained from Lederle Laboratories did not neutralize C. difficile toxin. In this paper we report our continued work on the production and reactivity of antisera prepared against the toxins of C. difficile and C. sordellii as well as purification of the toxin to C. difficile.

METHODS

To produce C. difficile or C. sordellii toxin 75-100 ml of saline was placed in dialysis tubing suspended in 3 L of brain heart infusion (BHI) broth. The saline was inoculated with 0.2 ml of an overnight BHI culture and incubated for 48-72 hours. Cells were harvested from within the dialysis tubing by centrifugation at 8000 x *g* for 20 min. The supernatant was filter sterilized and stored at 4° C.

Toxicity Determinations

Toxicity was determined in mice and in tissue culture. Eight mice were used per dilution of toxin. The toxin was injected intraperitoneally and the percent mortality was calculated at 16 hours from integrated data (Reed and Muench, 1938). The 50% and 100% lethal doses (LD_{50} and LD_{100}) were determined graphically from these results. Toxicity was determined in tissue culture by observing rounding of Chinese hamster ovary cells (CHO-K1) cultured in F-12 medium with 2% fetal calf serum. Titers were the lowest dilution of toxin yielding 40-60% cell rounding and were expressed as the reciprocal of this dilution.

C. difficile Antitoxin

Antitoxin to C. difficile was produced in rabbits, goats, and chickens following administration of toxoid and Freund's adjuvant. The toxoid was prepared by incubating toxin with 0.3 - 0.5% formaldehyde for 30-36 h at 37 C. The rabbits and chickens were given 6 weekly intramuscular injections before bleeding, 3 injections of 1:1 formaldehyde-inactivated toxin with Freund's complete adjuvant and 3 injections of toxoid with Freund's incomplete adjuvant. Goats were administered the toxoid/adjuvant suspensions by subcutaneous injection on the same schedule as the rabbits.

To determine the activity of antiserum in mice, serial dilutions of the antiserum were mixed with the LD_{100} of C. difficile toxin. After one hour at room temperature, the mixture was injected intraperitoneally to mice. The titer of the antitoxin was that dilution at which all mice survived.

C. sordellii Antitoxin

Antitoxin to C. sordellii was produced in rabbits after 6 weekly intramuscular injections of toxoid and Freund's adjuvants on the same schedule as described above for production of antitoxin to C. difficile. Cross-reactivity between the toxins and antitoxins of C. sordellii and C. difficile was determined in mice by mixing serial dilutions of the antitoxins and the LD_{100}'s of the toxins (culture filtrates).

Molecular Weight Determinations

Toxins were applied to an agarose 6B column (1.5 x 90 cm) and molecular weights were determined by comparison to standard proteins. Polyacrylamide gel electrophoresis was done on 2.5-27% gradient gels with Tris(hydroxymethyl)aminomethane borate buffer at 125 volts for 16 hours for molecular weight determinations.

Purification of Toxins

The toxin of C. difficile (VPI 10463) produced in BHI culture was purified as follows. The filter sterilized supernatant from the dialysis tubing was concentrated

10-20 times with an Amicon XM-100 filter (Amicon, Lexington, Mass.). This concentrate was applied to an AcA34 column (LKB, Bromma, Sweden) (5 x 30 cm). Toxicity was tested at each step using Chinese hamster ovary cells. The toxin, which was in the void volume of the AcA34 column, was precipitated with ammonium sulfate at 45% saturation. The pellet was resuspended in 0.025 M Tris HCl, pH 7.0, dialyzed against the same buffer, and then applied to a DEAE-Biogel A column (1 x 5 cm), (Bio-Rad, Richmond, Calif.). A step-wise sodium chloride gradient from 0.0 to 0.5 M with 0.05 M increments of 20 ml each was used to elute the column. The toxin eluted at 0.15 to 0.20 M. Proteins were estimated using the Bio-Rad Protein Determination (Bio-Rad, Richmond, Calif.).

Gnotobiotic Rats

Twelve Spague Dawley rats, males and females, 90-120 days old, were housed in plastic isolators maintained at the Gnotobiotic Laboratory at the University of Wisconsin. They were given food (Ralston Purina 5010-C) and water *ad libitum*. Animals which survived the initial oral introduction of *C. difficile* were sacrificed at 29 days for autopsy.

RESULTS

Antitoxin

Using the procedure described above, we obtained good production of antitoxin to *C. difficile* in rabbits, goats, and even in chickens. Antitoxin prepared to partially purified *C. difficile* toxin had a titer of 1/8000 (a 1:8000 dilution neutralized the LD_{100} in mice). This antitoxin, as well as antitoxin made to concentrated culture filtrates, had very little cross reactivity with *C. sordellii* toxin.

TABLE 1

Toxin	Neutralization Titer *C. difficile* Antitoxin
C. difficile (VPI 10463)	1/8000
C. sordellii (VPI 8827)	1/128

We also produced *C. sordellii* antitoxin. The *C. sordellii* antitoxin from the U.S. Bureau of Biologics neutralized *C. difficile* toxin almost as well as *C. sordellii* toxin. Our antiserum, however, did not neutralize *C. difficile* toxin.

TABLE 2

Toxin	Neutralization Titer *C. sordellii* Antitoxin	
	VPI 8827	Bureau of Biologics
C. sordellii	1/128	1/512
C. difficile	0	1/256

Purification of Toxin

The toxin of *C. difficile* was purified to a single band as detected by gradient polyacrylamide gels (Table 3).

TABLE 3 Purification of Toxin from C. difficile

STAGE OF PURIFICATION	TCD_{50}*	FOLD PURIFICATION
CULTURE SUPERNATANT (DIALYZED)	600	--
ULTRAFILTRATION, XM100	350	1.7
GEL EXCLUSION (AcA34)	80	7.5
$(NH_4)_2SO_4$ PRECIPITATION (45% SATURATION)	40	15
ION EXCHANGE (DEAE) (0.2M NaCl)	12.5	48

*) Tissue culture dose, picograms protein, for 50% rounding.

When this band was eluted from the gels it was toxic to CHO cells. The specific activity of this preparation was very high - 12.5 picograms resulted in rounding of 50% of the CHO cells. The toxin had an undenatured molecular weight of 550,000 as determined both on gradient polyacrylamide gels and agarose 6B column chromatography.

Association with Germfree Rats

We considered that the large molecular weight of the toxin could be an artifact of the cultural conditions. Therefore, we associated 12 germfree rats with *C. difficile*. Three of the rats died within 24 hrs. In the survivors there was little physiological evidence of toxin activity. The ceca were reduced in size at 29 days from 6 percent to 3.3 percent of body weight, and there was some sloughing of the epithelium and hypercellularity of the lamina propria. However, the massive destruction which occurs in hamsters (Lusk, 1978) did not occur. Toxin was present in the cecal contents in relatively high amounts (dilutions of 10^{-4} to 10^{-6} rounded CHO cells). The toxin in these cecal contents had the same molecular weight as the toxin found in BHI cultures.

During growth in the gnotobiotic rats the *C. difficile* culture produced a less-toxic spontaneous mutant (or loss of plasmid, phage, etc) which was present in very low numbers. One colony of 100 picked was of this phenotype. The mutant (tox R) produced only one ten-thousandth as much toxin, but toxin could be demonstrated and was of the same high molecular weight (Table 4). The tox R *C. difficile* was introduced into gnotobiotic rats in the same manner as the wildtype strain. All rats survived the administration of this mutant. Cecal weights were 4.5 percent of body weight when these rats were sacrificed.

TABLE 4 Relative Toxicities of C. difficile Toxin Produced in Broth Culture and that Obtained from the Cecal Filtrates of Gnotobiotic Rats Monoassociated with C. difficile

SOURCE OF TOXIN	ASSAY	TITER	PROTEIN CONCENTRATION*
PURE CULTURE SUPERNATANTS (DIALYZED)			
WILDTYPE	CHO	$5.0 - 1.5 \times 10^6$	0.2 - 1.0 NANOGRAMS
	MICE	$2.5 - 1.2 \times 10^3$	200 - 500 NANOGRAMS
TOXR	CHO	$10^3 - 10^4$	5 - 9 MICROGRAMS
	MICE	NOT DETECTED	
CECAL FILTRATES Gnotobiotic Rats			
WILDTYPE	CHO	$10^4 - 10^6$	5 - 500 NANOGRAMS
TOXR	CHO	10^1	250 - 400 MICROGRAMS

*) The amount of protein that will cause 40 - 60% rounding of CHO cells or 50% mouse mortality.

DISCUSSION

As well as we have been able to determine, we have the only antitoxin that has been prepared against the toxin of C. difficile. For production of antitoxin, we used normal immunization procedures with formalinized toxoid and Freund's complete adjuvant. Our success may be due to the strain of C. difficile that we have used. The toxin from this strain is a good antigen in that very small amounts of toxoid elicited antibody production. Antitoxin was even formed to crude culture filtrates of the less toxic mutant. We currently are injecting rabbits with our most purified preparation to prepare completely monospecific antitoxin. Our present antitoxins were produced to partially purified preparations of toxin but still are much better than the C. sordellii antitoxin currently used. This goat antisera is available from us. In the near future, enzyme-linked immunoassay may be possible through the use of the antisera or antitoxin raised to purified preparations.

Purification procedures of C. difficile toxin were first described by Taylor and Bartlett (1979) at a symposium held in Boston in July 1978. At that time we briefly mentioned our preliminary data on purification as well as the appropriate molecular weight of 600,000 (Wilkins, 1979). Additional data on purification has been presented at the ICAAC meeting by ourselves (Wilkins, 1978), by Bartlett's research group (Taylor, 1978), and by Harvie (1978). The results were at variance in regard to the molecular weight of the toxin. We always have obtained a molecular weight of about 550,000 but the other investigators reported somewhat lower values. More recently Rolfe and Finegold (1979) reported apparent purification of the toxin by following essentially the same procedures first reported by Taylor and Bartlett (1979). Rolfe and Finegold agree with our data concerning an undenatured molecular weight of 550,000 to 600,000. They were successful in breaking the toxin into apparent subunits of 50,000 with SDS which we were not able to do. The large molecular weight does not appear to be aggregated medium components or an artifact of growth conditions since we obtained the same molecular weight for toxin produced in gnotobiotic rats.

It is possible however that, as far as molecular weight determinations are concerned, the data may still require clarification. Many hydrophobic molecules aggregate with membrane components to form large molecular weight complexes that can be "purified." C. botulinum toxin also was originally "purified" attached to hemagglutinating protein (DasGupta and Boroff, 1967). We therefore intend to use hydrophobic chromatography in a search for an active toxin of low molecular weight.

ACKNOWLEDGEMENTS

This work was supported by Public Health Service grant 1 R01 AI15749-01 from the National Institute of Health.

REFERENCES

Anonymous (1978). Antibiotic-associated colitis: A progress report. Br. Med. J., 1, 699-671.

Aswell, J. E., M. Ehrich, R. L. Van Tassell, C-C Tsai, L. V. Holdeman and T. D. Wilkins (1979). Characterization and comparison of Clostridium difficile and other clostridial toxins. Microbiology-1979, 272-275.

Bartlett, J. G., T. W. Chang, M. Gurwith, S. L. Gorbach, A. B. Onderdonk (1978). Antibiotic-associated pseudomembranous colitis due to toxin-producing clostridia. N. E. J. Med., 298, 531-534.

Bartlett, J. G., T. W. Chang, N. S. Taylor and A. B. Onderdonk (1979). Colitis induced by Clostridium difficile. Rev. Infect. Dis., 1, 370-378.

Chang, T. W., J. G. Bartlett, S. L. Gorbach and A. B. Onderdonk (1978a). Clindamycin-induced enterocolitis in hamsters as a model of pseudomembranous colitis in patients. Infect. Immun., 20, 526-529.

Chang, T. W., S. L. Gorbach and J. G. Bartlett (1978b). Neutralization of Clostridium difficile toxin by Clostridium sordellii antitoxin. Infect. Immun., 22, 418-422.

DasGupta, B. R. and D. A. Boroff (1967). Chromatographic isolation of hemagglutinin-free neurotoxin from crystalline toxin of Clostridium botulinum type A. Biochim. Biophys. Acta., 147, 603-605.

George, R. H., J. M. Symonds, F. Dimock, J. D. Brown, Y. Arabi, N. Shinagawa, M. R. B. Keighley, J. Alexander-Williams and D. W. Burdon (1978). Identification of Clostridium difficile as a cause of pseudomembranous colitis. Brit. Med. J., 2, 695.

George, W. L., V. L. Sutter, E. J. C. Goldstein, S. L. Ludwig, S. M. Finegold (1978). Aetiology of antimicrobial-agent-associated colitis. Lancet, i, 802-803.

Harvie, N., S. Ellis, D. Mason, N. Allo, G. Rifkin, J. Silva and R. Fekety (1978). Isolation and purification of a Clostridium difficile toxin that causes colitis in the Syrian hamster. 18th International Science Conference, Antimicrob. Agents Chemotherap., Atlanta, Oct., Abstract # 130.

Hutcheon, D. F., F. D. Milligan, J. H. Yardley and T. R. Hendrix (1978). Cephalosporin-associated pseudomembranous colitis. Am. J. Digest. Dis., 23, 321-326.

Lusk, R. H., F. R. Fekety, Jr., J. Silva, T. Bodendorfer, B. J. Devine, H. Kawanishi, L. Korff, D. Nakauchi, S. Rogers and S. B. Siskin (1977). Gastrointestinal side effects of clindamycin and ampicillin therapy. J. Infect. Dis., 135, S111-S119.

Lusk, R. H., R. Fekety, Jr., J. Silva, R. A. Brown, D. H. Ringler and G. D. Abrams (1978). Clindamycin-induced enterocolitis in hamsters. J. Infect. Dis., 137, 464-475.

Medline, A., D. H. Shin and N. M. Medline (1976). Pseudomembranous colitis associated with antibiotics. Human Pathol., 7, 693-703.

Reed, L. J., and H. Muench (1938). A simple method of estimating fifty percent endpoints. Amer. J. Hyg., 493-497.

Rifkin, G. D., F. R. Fekety, Jr., J. Silva and R. B. Sack (1977). Antibiotic-induced colitis implication of a toxin neutralized by Clostridium sordellii antitioxin. Lancet, ii, 1103-1106.

Rolfe, R. D. and S. M. Finegold (1979). Purification and characterization of Clostridium difficile toxin. Infect. Immun., 25, 191-201.

Taylor, N. S., A. B. Onderdonk and J. G. Bartlett (1978). Partial purification and characterization of Clostridium difficile colitis toxin. 18th International Science Conference, Antimicrob. Agents Chemotherap., Atlanta, Oct., Abstract # 127.

Taylor, N. S. and J. G. Bartlett (1979). Partial purification and characterization of a cytotoxin from Clostridium difficile. Rev. Infect. Dis., 1, 379-385.

Wilkins, T. D., C-C Tsai, J. E. Aswell, M. Ehrich, R. L. Van Tassell and L. V. Holdeman (1978). Toxins of Clostridium difficile and C. sordellii. 18th International Science Conference, Antimicrob. Agents Chemotherap., Atlanta, Oct. 1-4, Abstract # 437.

Wilkins, T. D. (1979). Discussion at symposium entitled "Virulence Factors of Anaerobic Bacteria," Boston, July 17-18, 1978. Rev. Infect. Dis., 1, 397.

INTERACTION OF *CLOSTRIDIUM DIFFICILE* TOXIN WITH HUMAN LUNG FIBROBLASTS *IN VITRO*

M. Thelestam and M. Brönnegård

Dept. Bact., Karolinska Institutet, S-104 01 Stockholm 60, Sweden

ABSTRACT

Partially purified toxin from Clostridium difficile induced a characteristic morphological change in fibroblasts from human embryonic lung and intestine. The toxin bound to as yet unidentified receptors at the surface of these cells. The toxin-induced actinomorphic changes closely resembled the effects induced by the fungal metabolite cytochalasin B. Indirect immunofluorescence with anti-actin antiserum on lung fibroblasts demonstrated that the C.difficile toxin (as well as cytochalasin B) disrupted the straight actin filament bundles seen in normal fibroblasts. The cytopathogenic effect became apparent in 3-5 h after exposure to the toxin but irreversible intoxication occurred already within 20 min of exposure. The experimental evidence so far is consistent with two possible different modes of action of the toxin, leading to microfilament disruption: 1. Transmembrane signal by surface-bound toxin via microfilament-linked integral membrane protein(s) and 2. Penetration of surface-bound whole toxin or an active fragment, followed by its intracellular action.

KEYWORDS

Clostridium difficile toxin, pseudomembranous colitis, human lung fibroblasts, microfilaments, cytotoxicity, mode of action, cytochalasin B.

INTRODUCTION

Recent research has indicated that a cytotoxic factor produced by strains of Clostridium difficile is responsible for antibiotic associated enterocolitis in both hamsters and man (Chang, 1978). This factor has recently been highly purified and shown to be a high-molecular weight glycoprotein (Rolfe and Finegold, 1979). The toxin causes a characteristic morphological change in cultured human amnion cells and in lung fibroblasts after contact with the cells for 24 h (Larson and Price, 1977; Chang, 1978). Chang and colleagues (1979) reported cytopathogenic effects to human amnion cells after 3-5 h and changes in the ultrastructure of the surface of toxin-treated amnion cells after 1 h. It was suggested that the toxin from C.difficile is a cytolysin.

Our preliminary experiments indicated that the C.difficile toxin possessed no hemolytic activity, nor any membrane damaging activity against human lung fibroblasts as tested with a sensitive assay (Thelestam and Möllby, 1975). Thus further experiments were undertaken with the aim of clarifying the cytotoxic mode of action of the C.difficile toxin.

PREPARATION OF TOXIN

C.difficile (ATCC 9689) was cultivated in pre-reduced chopped meat medium for 72 h. Extracellular toxin was obtained by centrifugation (8 000 x g, 4°C) and filtration of the supernatant. The filtrate was partially purified by fractionation on a Sepharose 6B column, eluted with tris-buffered saline (TBS), i.e. 0.15 M NaCl in 0.02 M tris-HCl at pH 7.0. The cytotoxic fractions, which eluted in a single peak, were pooled, concentrated and stored at -70°C. The cytotoxic activity was abolished by treatment of the toxin with trypsin and pronase (100 µg/ml) for 30 min at 37°C, by warming to 56°C for 30 min and by goat antiserum against C.difficile toxin (kindly supplied by T. Wilkins, VPI (see separate chapter this volume). The toxin was devoid of proteolytic or phospholipase C activities.

MORPHOLOGICAL EFFECTS OF TOXIN AND CYTOCHALASIN B ON FIBROBLASTS

The C.difficile toxin induced a characteristic actinomorphic change in human embryonic intestinal fibroblasts (Flow 11000) as well as in human embryonic lung fibroblasts (MRC-5). In the toxin treated cells the cytoplasm became contracted, leaving long processes radiating in a star-like pattern from the rounded cell-body (Thelestam and Brönnegård, 1979). Cytochalasin B, which is known to disrupt cellular actin microfilaments (Weber, 1976), in both lung and intestinal fibroblasts induced a similar actinomorphic effect to that observed with C.difficile toxin.

The morphological change caused by CB occurred already in 30 min after addition of CB to the cells. By contrast there was a latency period of 3-5 h before the toxin-induced effect appeared, and the effect occurred with the same latency even if the toxin was removed after only a brief incubation with the cells. Thus the toxin seemed to bind rapidly to the cell surface.

Pre-treatment for 30 min of lung fibroblasts with 2,4-dinitrophenol (DNP) (10 mM) inhibited subsequent development of cytopathogenic effect with either the C.difficile toxin or cytochalasin B. Thus uncoupling of oxidative phosphorylation from mitochondrial respiration prevented the activities of both toxin and CB.

EFFECT OF TOXIN AND CYTOCHALASIN B ON CELLULAR MICROFILAMENTS

Indirect immunofluorescence with anti-actin antiserum on toxin treated lung fibroblasts demonstrated that the actinomorphic change was parallelled with disruption of the straight actin microfilament bundles seen in control cells. Similar changes occurred in cells treated with cytochalasin B (Fig. 1).

The microfilament breakdown caused by CB was completely reversible within 30 min after removal of CB from the medium, as reported by others (Miranda, 1974). By contrast the toxin-induced effect was irreversible. This was shown by trypsinization and reseeding of the cells at various time intervals after addition of the toxin (Fig. 2).

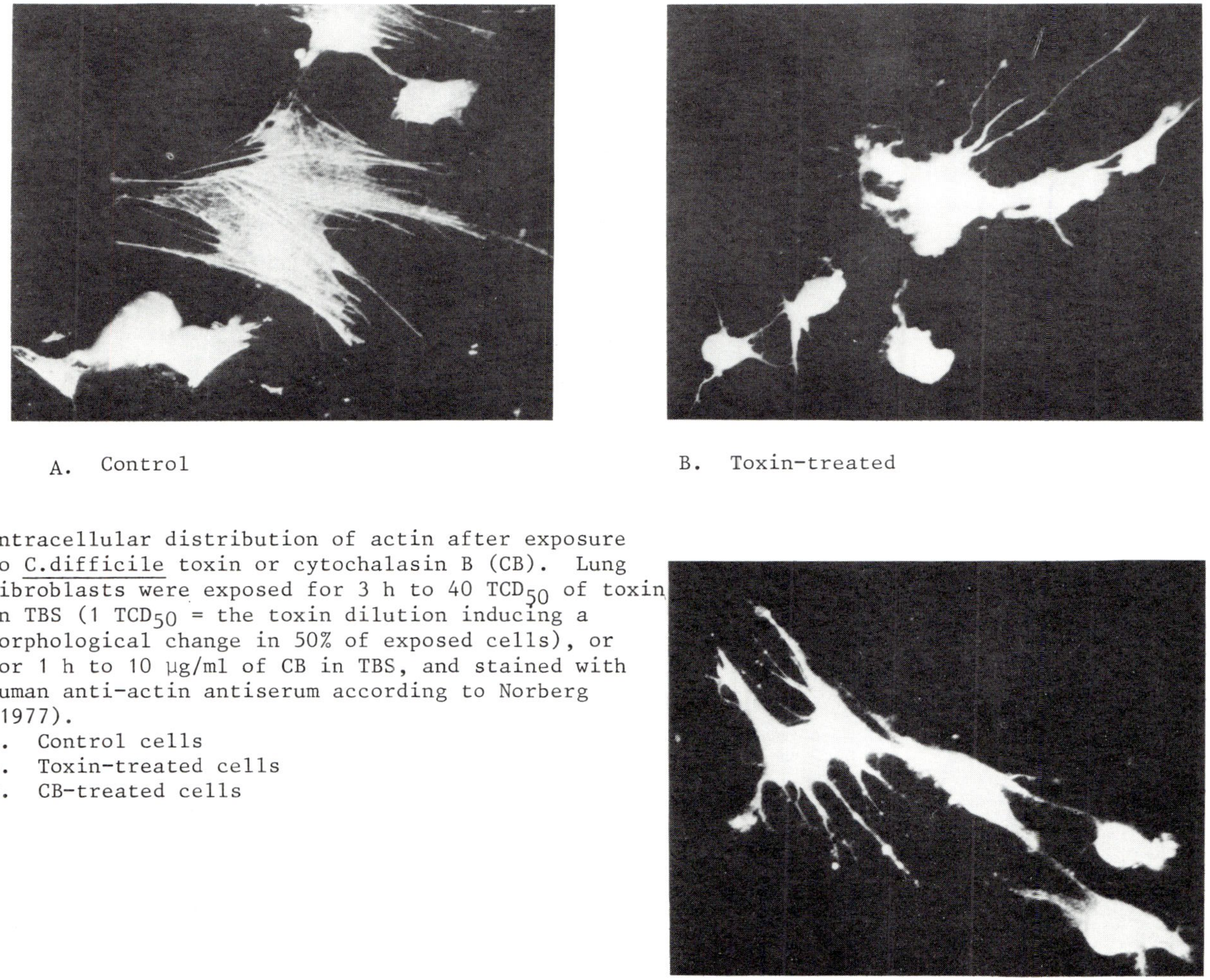

A. Control

B. Toxin-treated

C. Cytochalasin B treated

Fig. 1. Intracellular distribution of actin after exposure to C.difficile toxin or cytochalasin B (CB). Lung fibroblasts were exposed for 3 h to 40 TCD_{50} of toxin in TBS (1 TCD_{50} = the toxin dilution inducing a morphological change in 50% of exposed cells), or for 1 h to 10 µg/ml of CB in TBS, and stained with human anti-actin antiserum according to Norberg (1977).
A. Control cells
B. Toxin-treated cells
C. CB-treated cells

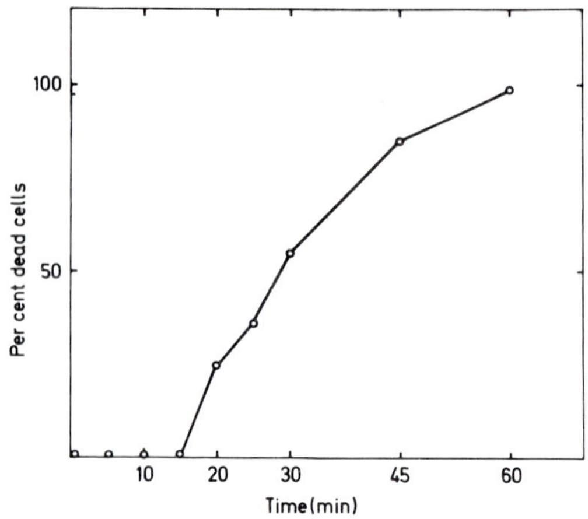

Fig. 2. Time course for induction of irreversible cytopathogenic effects in lung fibroblasts.
Cells were exposed to toxin (40 TCD_{50} in TBS) and trypsinized after the time intervals indicated. Trypsinized cells were suspended in fresh growth medium and seeded in new flasks immediately. Per cent dead cells was scored 20 h later by counting 10 randomly selected fields of view per flask. Cells unable to attach and regain the typical fibroblastic morphology were classified as dead.

As seen from the figure some cells were irreversibly intoxicated already in 20 min after first contact with the toxin. The same time course was found when the toxin was only allowed to bind to the cells for 1 min at 37°C and the cells were then incubated in medium until the trypsinizations. The intoxicated cells still excluded trypan blue and were thus not "dead" according to the dye exclusion criterion. However, they could not attach to the solid substratum and regenerate their typical shape during up to 10 days after toxin-treatment. Eventually these cells degenerated.

THE NATURE OF CELL SURFACE RECEPTORS FOR C.DIFFICILE TOXIN

Since the toxin was rapidly adsorbed by cells in monolayers, attempts were made to identify the nature of the cell surface receptor for the toxin. Lung fibroblasts or toxin were pre-treated for 15 min at 37°C with the various enzymes and other substances listed in Table I.

TABLE I

Pre-treatment of cells		Pre-treatment of toxin	
Trypsin	1.25 mg/ml	Cholesterol	1 µg/ml
Pronase	100 µg/ml	Ganglioside-mixture	200 µg/ml
Beta-galactosidase	5 U/ml	Lecithin	50 µg/ml
Phospholipase C	0.5 U/ml		
Streptolysin O	10 HU/ml*		
EDTA	0.02 %		

*Haemolytic units

None of the treatments of the cells would alter their characteristic morphological response to subsequent toxin treatment. Neither did pre-treatment of the toxin with cholesterol, gangliosides or lecithin abolish its subsequent cytotoxic activity. Thus the toxin receptor appeared neither to be a peripheral membrane protein, sensitive to enzymatic cleavage, nor phospholipid, cholesterol or ganglioside in nature.

COMPARATIVE BINDING PROPERTIES OF C.DIFFICILE TOXIN AND CYTOCHALASIN B

Since the toxin induced a similar effect as CB it was of interest to investigate if these substances would compete in their actions. It was found that the toxin bound to cells already morphologically affected by 10 or 5 µg/ml of CB. Toxin and CB did not seem to compete when a mixture was applied to cells. They probably have different receptors at the cell surface and/or cause the same symptom, microfilament breakdown, by different intermediate steps. (For further details see Thelestam and Brönnegård, 1979.)

CONCLUSIONS

The most obvious symptom of cellular intoxication with C.difficile toxin is a depolymerization of microfilament bundles. Preliminary results indicate that the toxin also inhibits phagocytosis and chemotaxis (Jan Palmblad, Nikos Venizelos and M.T., unpublished) giving further support to the analogy with cytochalasin B. The latter is known to inhibit cytokinesis, single cell movement and phagocytosis, activities which are dependent on functioning microfilaments (Wessells, 1971; Stossel, 1977). An important difference, however, between the actions of cytochalasin B and the C.difficile toxin is that the former is completely reversible whereas the toxin-induced effects are irreversible. Thus the processes controlling the polymerization of microfilaments or the relaxation of hypercontracted microfilaments (Miranda, 1974) might be affected by the toxin. How this effect is brought about is not yet clear.

The experimental evidence so far is consistent with either of two possible modes of action of the toxin:
1. Transmembrane signal by surface-bound toxin via microfilament linked integral membrane protein(s) and
2. Penetration of surface-bound whole toxin or active fragment, followed by its intracellular action.

To distinguish between these possibilities further investigation is needed concerning early intracellular changes as well as phenomena occurring at the cell surface after exposure to toxin.

Besides being of clinical interest the toxin from C.difficile may become important in the study of processes governing cytoskeletal breakdown and repolymerization.

ACKNOWLEDGEMENTS

Carl-Erik Nord is gratefully acknowledged for focusing our attention at Clostridium difficile and for providing the strain of the bacterium. Astrid Fagraeus generously supplied anti-actin antiserum. Greger Blomquist, Eva Brännkärr, Lena Norenius and Gunnel Sigstam provided excellent technical assistance. This investigation was supported by grants from Nordiska Samfundets Stiftelse and Karolinska institutets fonder.

REFERENCES

Chang, T.W., J.G. Bartlett, S.L. Gorbach, and A.B. Onderdonk (1978). Clindamycin-induced enterocolitis in hamsters as a model of pseudomembranous colitis in patients. Infect. Immunity, 20, 526-529.

Chang, T.W., P.S. Lin, S.L. Gorbach, and J.G. Bartlett (1979). Ultrastructural changes of cultured human amnion cells by Clostridium difficile toxin. Infect. Immunity, 23, 795-798.

Larson, H.E., and A.B. Price (1977). Pseudomembranous colitis: presence of clostridial toxin. Lancet, ii, 1312-1314.

Miranda, A.F., G.C. Godman, and S.W. Tanenbaum (1974). Action of cytochalasin D on cells of established lines. II. Cortex and microfilaments. J. Cell Biol., 62, 406-423.

Norberg, R., G. Biberfeld, A. Fagraeus, K. Lidman, R. Thorstensson, and G. Utter (1977). The reaction of cells with anti-actin sera in relation to the amount of cellular actin. Clin. exp. Immunol., 28, 512-516.

Rolfe, R.D., and S.M. Finegold (1979). Purification and characterization of Clostridium difficile toxin. Infect. Immunity, 25, 191-201.

Stossel, T.P. (1977). Endocytosis. In, P. Cuatrecasas and M.F. Greaves (Eds.), Receptors and recognition, Series A, Volume 4, Chapman and Hall, London, pp. 103-141.

Thelestam, M. and M. Brönnegård (1979). Interaction of cytopathogenic toxin from Clostridium difficile with cells in tissue culture. Scand. J. Inf. Dis. (in press).

Thelestam, M. and R. Möllby (1975). Determination of toxin-induced leakage of different size nucleotides through the plasma membrane of human diploid fibroblasts. Infect. Immunity, 11, 640-648.

Weber, K. (1976). Biochemical anatomy of microfilaments in cells in tissue culture using immunofluorescence microscopy. In, S.V. Perry et al. (Eds.), Contractile systems in non-muscle tissues,. Elsevier/North-Holland Biomedical Press, pp. 51-66.

Wessels, N.K., B.S. Spooner, J.F. Ash, M.O. Bradley, M.A. Luduena, E.L. Taylor, J.T. Wrenn, and K.M. Yamada (1971). Microfilaments in cellular and developmental processes. Science, 171, 135-143.

THE EFFECT OF *PSEUDOMONAS AERUGINOSA* EXOTOXIN A ON ANTIBODY FORMING MOUSE SPLEEN CELLS

O. R. Pavlovskis*, B. Wretlind* and M. L. Hale**

**Department of Microbiology, Naval Medical Research Institute, Bethesda, Maryland, 20014, USA*
***Department of Preventive Medicine, Uniformed Services University of the Health Sciences, Bethesda, Maryland, 20014, USA*

ABSTRACT

Pseudomonas aeruginosa exotoxin A inhibits protein synthesis in vitro and in vivo, and this effect may involve antibody production. We have studied the response of antibody forming spleen cells (AFC) to exotoxin A in mice immunized with sheep red blood cells (RBC) and in vitro using the Marbrook technique. The effect on IgM and IgG AFC was examined on the 4th and 13th days, respectively, following immunization with RBC.

In vivo a linear decrease from 75 - 30% in IgM AFC was observed in mice receiving exotoxin between 2 days prior and 3 days post immunization. The decrease of IgG AFC was about 30-35% in mice injected with exotoxin at the day of and up to 10 days post immunization. The exotoxin has no significant effect on IgG production when injected on the 11th or 12th day. It appears that at least 2 days are required for the exotoxin to significantly affect antibody production.

KEY WORDS

Pseudomonas aeruginosa, exotoxin, antibody forming cells, hemolytic plaque assay.

INTRODUCTION

Pseudomonas aeruginosa is an opportunistic pathogen which causes serious infections in patients with impaired host defenses such as in the case of extensive burns, hematologic malignancies, and solid tumors. In recent years the P. aeruginosa exotoxin A (Liu 1966; Liu and others, 1973a, Callahan 1974,1976; Leppla, 1976), which is produced by most clinical strains (Bjorn and others, 1977; Pollack and others, 1977) has been established as one of the major virulence factors of the organisms (Atik and others, 1968; Pavlovskis and Shackelford, 1974b; Pavlovskis and others, 1974a, 1975, 1976, 1977, 1978; Liu and Hsieh, 1973b; Iglewski and others, 1977; Saelinger and others, 1977; Stieritz and Holder, 1978). Biochemical studies have shown that the exotoxin inhibits protein synthesis (Pavlovskis and Gordon, 1972; Pavlovskis and others, 1974a; Pavlovskis and Shackelford, 1974b; Pavlovskis and others, 1975) in a manner similar to diphtheria toxin (Iglewski and Kabat, 1975; Iglewski and others, 1976, 1977). The exotoxin catalyses the transfer of the adenosine diphosphate ribose (ADP-ribose) moiety of nicotinamide adenine dinucleotide to elongation factor 2 (EF2) in mammalian ribosomes. The resultant ADP-ribose-EF2 complex is inactive in protein synthesis, and, as functional EF-2 is depleated, there is a corresponding reduction in protein synthesis.

Since antibody production requires protein synthesis, and since exotoxin is produced during experimental infections (Pavlovskis and others, 1977, 1978; Saelinger and others, 1977; Stieritz and Holder, 1978) and in patients (Pollack and others 1976; Pollack and Young, 1979), we can expect a marked reduction in antibody production during pseudomonas infection. We have examined the effect of exotoxin on the formation of hemolytic plaque-forming spleen cells in mice inoculated with sheep red blood cells (RBC). The results presented indicate that exotoxin reduces antibody production.

IN VIVO STUDIES

Method

At various time intervals from 2 days prior (-2) to 12 days post (+12) immunization (day 0) with RBC (0.1 ml of 50% suspension) mice were injected i.v. with an exotoxin dose producing 75% mortality in about 48-72 hrs. Mice were killed by cervical dislocation either on day +4 or day +13, spleens excised, cells separated, and plated in various concentrations according to a modified Jerne hemolytic plaque assay technique (Hanna and Hale, 1975). The plates were incubated for 3 hrs at 37°C, and for the detection of IgM forming cells they were covered with guinea pig complement. To detect IgG antibodies the plates were incubated with rabbit anti-mouse IgG serum (1:40 dil.) before complement was added.

The Effect on IgM Antibody Production

The effect of exotoxin on IgM antibody production was examined on day +4(Fig. 1). A significant decrease in IgM antibody forming cells (AFC) was observed in mice treated

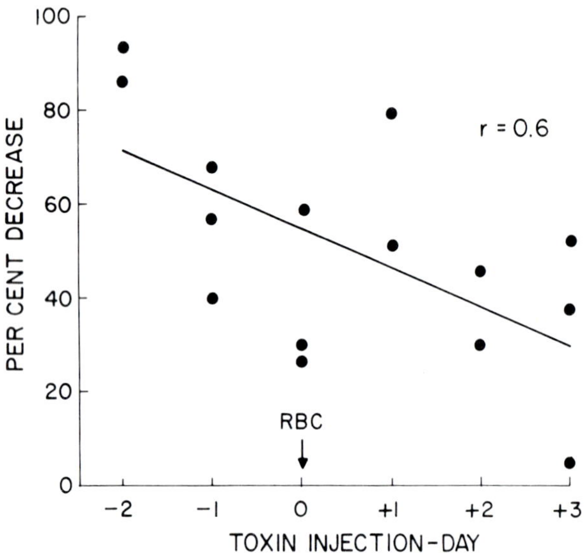

Fig. 1 Temporal relationship between the percent decrease of IgM AFC and the time of exotoxin administration.

with exotoxin between days -2 and +3. Analysis of 15 experiments by linear regression (Fig. 1) demonstrated a linear relationship between the time of exotoxin administration and the inhibition of antibody production ($r = -0.6$, $0.02>P>0.01$). The percent decrease varied from 75% on day -2 to about 30% on day +3.

The Effect on IgG Antibody Production

The number of IgG AFC was determined on day +13, because, in our experiments IgG AFC were at maximum and IgM AFC at minimal level. No significant decrease in AFC was observed in mice treated with exotoxin on days -2 and -1 (Fig. 2).

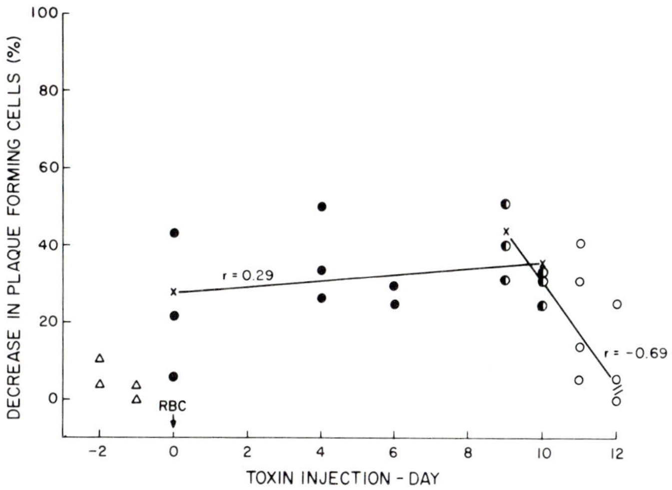

Fig. 2 Temporal relationship between the percent decrease of IgG AFC and the time of toxin administration.

Analysis of 21 experiments by linear regression (Fig. 2) showed that at day 0 IgG AFC was reduced by 30-35% and remained constant to day +9. Mice injected with exotoxin few days prior AFC determination i.e. between +9 and +12 showed a reduction of the effect of exotoxin similar to that seen with IgM AFC (Fig. 1). The results suggest that at least 2 days are required for exotoxin to significantly affect the number of AFC.

IN VITRO STUDIES

Method

Mouse spleen cells (30×10^6) were cultured with RBC (1×10^6) in Marbrook vessels in the presence and absence of exotoxin (Hanna and Hale, 1975). After either 4 or 12 days cultures were assayed for the presence of anti-RBC AFC by hemolytic plaque assay as indicated above.

In Vitro Effect of Exotoxin

Five nanograms of exotoxin completely abolished in vitro antibody response (Table 1) whereas at lower concentrations (0.5 ng or less) exotoxin exerted a pronounced stimulatory effect on the IgG response of the spleen cells (+12). No significant change was seen on day +4.

TABLE 1 The In Vitro Effect of Exotoxin on Antibody Forming Response

Exotoxin (ng)	Number of AFC	
	4 Day response	12 Day response
0	1560	21
5	0	0
0.5	1645	240
0.005	1670	560

To determine which cell population was predominantly affected by exotoxin, mouse spleen cells (30 x 10^6) were separated into macrophages (adherent spleen cells), bone-marrow-derived cells (B-cells), and thymus-derived cells (T-cells) (Hale and Hanna, 1976). Individual cell populations were treated with 0.005 ng exotoxin (1 hr), following which the exotoxin treated cell population was reconstituted with the other two untreated cell populations and cultured in the presence of RBC. On day 4 and 12 cultures were assayed for AFC. No significant changes occurred with any of the treated cell populations on day 4. On day 12, however, a 600 fold increase in AFC was observed with the exotoxin treated T-cell population, while the exotoxin treated macrophage and B-cell populations remained unchanged. The results indicated that exotoxin at low levels affected primarily the T-cell population.

COMMENTS

The data presented in this preliminary communication indicates that purified exotoxin inhibits antibody production both in vitro and in vivo. The in vivo stimulating effect of low doses of exotoxin on thymus derived cells requires further study. In light of this evidence immunization during pseudomonas infection might be of limited value. It suggests that in cases where the underlying trauma predisposes the patient to pseudomonas infection, immunization should be started early while the patient can still respond immunologically.

ACKNOWLEDGEMENTS

We thank Dr. E. Weiss for his suggestions and comments throughout this study and Dr. R. DeBell for providing purified exotoxin A. We are also grateful to D. Anderson, G. Hare, and L. Lewis for their expert technical assistance.

This study was supported by the U.S. Naval Research and Development Command, Research Work Unit No. M0095PN002.5059. The opinions and assertions contained herein are the private ones of the authors and are not to be construed as official or reflecting the views of the Navy Department or the Naval Service at large.

The experiments reported were conducted according to the principles set forth in the "Guide for the Care and Use of Laboratory Animals," Institutes of Laboratory Resources, National Research Council, DHEW, Pub. No. (NIH) 78-23.

REFERENCES

Atik, M., P.V. Liu, B.A. Hanson, S. Amini, and C.F. Rosenberg (1968). J.A.M.A., 205, 134-140.

Bjorn, M.J., M.L. Vasil, J.C. Sadoff, and B.H. Iglewski (1977). Infect. Immun., 16, 362-366.

Callahan, L.T.,III (1974). Infect. Immun.,9, 113-118.

Callahan, L.T.,III (1976). Infect. Immun.,14,55-61.

Hale, M.L., and E.E. Hanna (1976). J.Cellular Immunol.,26, 168-177.

Hanna, E.E., and M. Hale (1975). Infect. Immun.,11, 265-272.

Iglewski, B.H., and D. Kabat (1975). Proc. Natl. Acad. Sci. U.S.A.,72,2284-2288.

Iglewski, B.H., L.P. Elwell, P.V. Liu, and D. Kabat (1976). In S. Shaltiel (Ed.), Proc. Internatl. Symposium on the Metabolic Interconversion of Enzymes, Springer Verlag, New York. Comparative Toxicities of Diphtherial Toxin and Pseudomonas aeruginosa Exotoxin A: Evidence for different cell receptors, pp.333-337.

Iglewski, B.H., P.V. Liu, and D. Kabat (1977). Infect. Immun., 15, 138-144.

Leppla, S.H. (1976). Infect. Immun., 14,1077-1086.

Liu, P.V. (1966) J. Infect. Dis., 116, 481-489.

Liu, P.V., S. Yoshii, and H. Hsieh (1973a). J. Infect. Dis., 128, 514-519.

Liu, P.V., and H. Hsieh (1973b). J. Infect. Dis., 128, 520-526.

Pavlovskis, O.R. and B.F. Gordon (1972). J.Infect. Dis., 125,631-636.

Pavlovskis, O.R., L.T. Callahan III, and R.D. Meyer (1974a). J.Infect.Dis. 130, Suppl., S100-S102.

Pavlovskis, O.R. and A.H. Shackelford (1974b). Infect. Immun. 9,540-546.

Pavlovskis, O.R., L.T. Callahan III, and M. Pollack (1975). In D. Schlessinger (Ed.) Microbiology 1975, American Society for Microbiology, Washington, D.C. Pseudomonas aeruginosa exotoxin, pp. 252-256.

Pavlovskis, O.R., F.A. Voelker, and A. H. Shackelford (1976). J. Infect. Dis., 133, 253-259.

Pavlovskis, O.R., M. Pollack, L.T. Callahan, III, and B.H. Iglewski (1977). Infect. Immun., 18, 596-602.

Pavlovskis, O.R., B.H. Iglewski, and M. Pollack (1978). Infect. Immun.,19, 29-33.

Pollack, M., N.S. Taylor, and L.T. Callahan III (1977). Infect.Immun.,15, 776-780.

Pollack, M. and L.S. Young (1979). J. Clin. Invest.,63,276-286.

Saelinger, C.B., K. Snell, and I.A. Holder (1977). J.Infect.Dis.,136,555-561.

Stieritz, D.D. and I.A. Holder (1978). J. Med. Microbiol.,11,101-109.

Toxins With Intracellular Targets

INVESTIGATIONS INTO THE RELATIONSHIPS BETWEEN STRUCTURE AND FUNCTION OF DIPHTHERIA TOXIN FRAGMENT B

P. Falmagne*, P. Lambotte*, C. Capiau*, J.-M. Ruysschaert and J. Dirkx***

**Lab. de Chimie biologique et de Biophysique, Univ. de l'Etat à Mons, Mons, Belgium*
***Lab. de Chimie physique des Macromolécules aux Interfaces, Univ. Libre de Bruxelles, Bruxelles, Belgium*

ABSTRACT

On the basis of N-terminal automated Edman degradation, circular dichroism measurements and liposomes studies of its CNBr peptides, fragment B of diphtheria toxin has been shown to contain at least two different lipid-associating domains: the first one, of the surface type, is located at its N-terminus; the second one, of the transverse type, is located in its middle region.

KEYWORDS

Diphtheria toxin; fragment B structure; protein sequencing; cell penetration; protein lipid interaction.

INTRODUCTION

Diphtheria toxin is a 62 000 daltons proenzyme activated by proteolytic nicking into two fragments, A (21 150 daltons) and B (40700 daltons), which remain connected together by a disulfide bridge. The biological activity of fragment B is to bind to specific membrane receptors of sensitive eukaryotic cells and to mediate the entry of the enzymically active fragment A into the cytoplasm where the latter catalyzes the ADP-ribosylation of elongation factor 2 (EF 2) and inhibits in this way the protein biosynthesis. The 17 000 daltons C-terminal region of fragment B participates in the binding to the cell receptors while its 23 000 daltons N-terminal moiety contains a hydrophobic domain (Boquet and co-workers, 1976) that could be inserted into the phospholipid bilayer of the cell membrane.

In a previous work, we isolated and characterized the CNBr peptides of fragment B whose proposed alignment is shown in Fig. 2 (Falmagne, Lambotte and Dirkx, 1978).

Using automated Edman degradation (Brauer, Margolies and Haber, 1975; Klapper, Wilde and Capra, 1978), we have determined the almost completę amino acid sequences of CB4 and CB5, and the N-terminal sequences of CB1, CB2 and CB3. They are shown in Fig. 1; the sequences of residues in brakets remain to be confirmed.

```
        1     5         10         15         20         25         30
CB4     S V G S S L K C I S L D W D V I R D K M K T K I E S L K E H G
             35        40
        P I K N(N G K T Q)M

        1     5         10         15         20         25         30
CB2     S E S P N K T V S E E K A K Q Y L E E F T Q T A L E S P E I E
             35
        N I K A V - - -

        1     5         10         15         20         25
CB5     G I A D G A V H H N T E E I V A Q S I A L(S)S L M

        1     5         10         15         20         25         30
CB1     V A Q A I P L V G E L V D I G F A A Y N F V E S I I N L F Q V
             35
        V H N N Y N - - -

        1     5         10         15         20
CB3     R C R A I D G D V T F C R P K S P V Y V G D - - -
```

Fig. 1. Amino acid sequences of CNBr peptides CB4 and CB5 and N-terminal sequences of CNBr peptides CB1, CB2 and CB3.

Conformation prediction analysis (Chou and Fasman, 1974) on these peptide sequences as well as circular dichroism measurements and liposomes studies of the corresponding peptides have led to a refinement in the molecular topography of the region of fragment B containing the hydrophobic domain and to a better understanding of the mechanism of interaction of this fragment with the phospholipid bilayer.

PEPTIDES CB4 AND CB2

The amino acid sequence of CB4 and the N-terminal sequence of CB2 provide the covalent structure of the N-terminal part of fragment B. This segment of 77 residues is highly hydrophilic; its polarity index, calculated according to Capaldi and Vanderkooi (1972), is 0.61. The predicted secondary structure contains 66% α-helix (26% in CB4 and 40% in CB2); molecular models of these helices show an amphipatic topography, i.e., one apolar and one polar faces. The very large polar faces contain pairs of negatively and positively charged residues that should complement the charged head groups of the phospholipid molecules;

Both CB4 and CB2 form stable complexes with dimyristoyl phosphatidyl cholin (DMPC) multilamellar liposomes. Circular dichroism spectra of CB4 and CB2 in aqueous solvents show little or no helicity, which coul mean that the interaction of the charged residues with water renders the predicted helical structures rather unstable, whilst they are stabilized by the hydrocarbon environment of the cell membrane phospholipid bilayer.

In other words, this 77 residues N-terminal hydrophilic sequence of fragment B exhibits the general properties of the surface lipid-associating domains of the plasma apolipoproteins, as described by Segrest and Jackson (1977). Comparison of this amino acid sequence with the sequence of human apolipoprotein A1 (Apo A1) shows interesting homologies; in the following comparison, residue 155 of human Apo A1 is aligned on residue 1 of fragment B (F_B):

```
         155       160       165       170       175       180
Apo A1   H V D A L R T H L A P Y S D E L R Q R L A A R L E A L K E
         +   -     +   +           - -   +   +     +   -     + -
F_B      S V G S S L K C I S L D W D V I R D K M K T K I E S L K E
                       +         -   -     + - +   +   +   -   + -
         1       5         10        15        20        25

          185       190       195       200       205       210
Apo A1   N G G A R L A E Y H A K A T E H - L S T L S E K A K P A L
                 +     -   +   +     - +               - +   +
F_B      H G P I K N(N G K T Q)M S E S P N K T V S E E K A K Q Y L
         +       +       +         -         +       - - +   +
         30        35        40        45        50        55

             215       220       225       230
Apo A1   E D L R Q G L L P V L E S F K V S F L S A
         - -   +               -     +
F_B      E E F T Q T A L E S P E I E N I K A V
         - -             -     -   -     +
           60        65        70        75
```

Therefore, this N-terminal region of fragment B could have surface phospholipid-binding properties similar to those of apolipoproteins. These surface interactions are known to be reversible.

PEPTIDES CB5 AND CB1

The amino acid sequence of CB5 and the N-terminal sequence of CB1 provide the covalent structure of the middle part of the fragment B molecule. This region is highly hydrophobic. The polarity indexes of the CB5 sequence is 0.44, and 0.32 for the N-terminal sequence of CB1. The latter value is similar to the polarity indexes of the hydrophobic segments of membrane protein like cytochrome b5 (0.30), cytochrome b5 reductase (0.35) and Semliki Forest Virus glycoprotein (0.28). Like these proteins, CB1 forms stable complexes with multilamellar liposomes of dimyristoyl phosphatidyl cholin.

The predicted secondary structures of these sequences contain 73% α-helix for CB5 and 86% for CB1. The predicted helical region of CB1 represents about 30% of the whole peptide and may well account for its 30% helical content measured by circular dichroism in aqueous solutions. The helix of CB1 is also amphipatic but, in contrast to the helices of CB4 and CB2, the apolar face is the largest and the polar face contains very few charged amino acid residues.

These properties confer to the hydrophobic helical amphipatic region located in the middle of the fragment B molecule a strong resemblance with the hydrophobic transverse lipid-associating domains of intrinsic membrane proteins wich span the phospholipid bilayer (Segrest and Jackson, 1977). These transverse interactions have been shown to be quite irreversible.

Fragment B might thus interact with the phospholipid bilayer in at least two ways (Fig. 2). The first one should involve the hydrophilic N-terminal part of fragment B, the amphipatic helices of CB4 and CB2 being half-buried at the interface between the hydrocarbon chains and the polar heads of the phospholipid molecules, in an orientation parallel to the membrane surface, i.e., perpendicular to the fatty acyl chains. The second one should involve the hydrophobic middle region of fragment B, the amphipatic helix of CB1 being inserted into the phospholipid bilayer, in an orientation parallel to the hydrocarbon chains of the fatty acids, i.e., perpendicular to the cell surface; this type of association would anchor fragment B in the membrane by formation of a more stable complex.

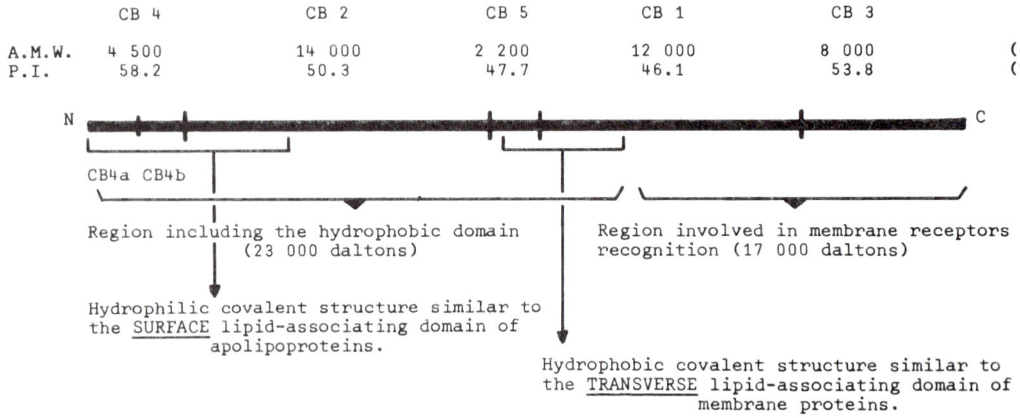

Fig. 2. Proposed alignment of the CNBr peptides of diphtheria toxin fragment B

PEPTIDE CB3

From conformational prediction analysis, the N-terminal amino acid sequence of CB3 contains mostly β-sheet structure. Two cysteinyl residues are located at positions 2 and 12 of CB3 and would participate to its disulfide bridge. The closure of that bridge, situated at about 8 000 daltons from the C-terminal end of fragment B, would induce the clustering of four basic amino acid residues, three arginines and one lysine, that would render the corresponding region of fragment B highly sensitive to the action of cellular proteases.

REFERENCES

Boquet, P., M. S. Silverman, A. M. Pappenheimer, Jr., and W. B. Vernon (1976). Proc. Natl. Acad. Sci. USA, 73, 4449-4453.

Brauer, A. W., M. N. Margolies, and E. Haber (1975). Biochemistry, 14, 3029-3035.

Capaldi, R. A., and G. Vanderkooi (1972). Proc. Natl. Acad. Sci. USA, 69, 930-932.

Chou, P. Y., and G. D. Fasman (1974). Biochemistry, 13, 211-222 and 222-245.

Falmagne, P., P. Lambotte, and J. Dirkx (1978). Biochim. Biophys. Acta 535, 54-65.

Klapper, D. G., C. E. Wilde, III, and J. D. Capra (1978). Anal. Biochem., 85, 126-131.
Segrest, J. P., and R. L. Jackson (1977). In R. A. Capaldi (Ed.), Membrane Proteins and their Interactions with Lipids, M. Dekker, Inc., New York and Basel, pp. 21-45.

RICIN INHIBITION OF FUNGI MITOCHONDRIAL AND CHLOROPLASTIC PROTEIN SYNTHESIS

L. J. G. Kohn*, A. A. J. Lugnier*, E.-E. Creppy*, H. Küntzel, O. Tiboni***, O. Ciferri*** and G. Dirheimer***

**Lab. Toxicol. Biol. Mol., Fac. Pharmacie, Université Louis Pasteur, and I.B.M.C. du C.N.R.S., 15 rue René Descartes, 67084 Strasbourg, France*
***Max-Planck-Institut für Experimentelle Medizin, Abt. Chemie, Göttingen, Federal Republic of Germany*
****Istituto Microbiologia Fisiologia Vegetale, Università Pavia, 27100 Pavia, Italy*

ABSTRACT

Ricin, a glycoprotein from *Ricinus communis* L. seeds, strongly inhibits eukaryotic, but not procaryotic, protein synthesis. It is therefore interesting to examine the action of ricin on organellar protein synthesis since both mitochondrial and chloroplastic protein synthesis systems have been classified, on the basis of both structural and functional criteria, as prokaryotic-like systems. We report here that, in contrast to what one would expect, ricin inhibits protein synthesis in the mitochondria of baker's yeast and *Neurospora crassa* and the chloroplasts of spinach. The inhibitory action of ricin occurs in intact organelles as well as on sub-organellar polypeptide synthesizing systems.

KEYWORDS

Ricin ; *Ricinus communis* L. seeds ; plant toxin ; mitochondria ; baker's yeast ; *Neurospora crassa* ; chloroplasts ; *Spinacia oleracea* L. ; protein synthesis.

INTRODUCTION

Ricin (molecular weight : 66,600 daltons, Lugnier and co-workers, 1976b) inhibits protein synthesis in eukaryote (Dirheimer and co-workers, 1967, 1968 ; Olsnes and Pihl, 1972 ; Lugnier, 1974, 1975 ; Lugnier and co-workers, 1974, 1977b), but not in prokaryote (Olsnes and co-workers, 1973). In this study action of ricin on organelle (mitochondria and chloroplasts) protein synthesis was investigated.

MATERIALS AND METHODS

Ricin was purified as previously described (Lugnier and Dirheimer, 1971). Baker's yeast mitochondria were prepared according to the method of Lugnier and co-workers (1976a) and the translation mixture was that of Lamb and co-workers (1968). *Neurospora crassa* mitochondria were isolated as described earlier (Küntzel and Blossey, 1974). The sub-mitochondrial polypeptide-synthesizing system (S-30 fraction) was prepared and incubated with tritiated-phenylalanine at 37°C in the absence of exogenous messenger RNA as described (Lugnier and co-workers, 1976a). Spinach chloroplasts and the corresponding sub-chloroplastic polypeptide-synthesizing system were obtained according to Tiboni and co-workers (1976). Various concentrations of ricin were added in the system (final volume : 250 µl) containing 80 µg of poly (U) per ml and 40 pmol of $[^{14}C]$ phenylalanyl-tRNA. After incubation for 30 min at 37°C, the reaction was stopped by adding 0.2 ml of 10% trichloroacetic acid and heated to 90°C for 15 min. The cooled precipitate was recovered by filtering through Oxoid Nuflow membrane filters (pore size : 0.45 µm). The radioactivity incorporated in the precipitate was then determined in a liquid scintillation spectrometer after different washes in ethanol and ether (Kohn and co-workers, 1978). *Escherichia coli* cell-free protein synthesis was prepared as described (Lugnier and co-workers, 1976a).

RESULTS

Phenylalanine Incorporation into Proteins of Intact Yeast Mitochondria

Incorporation of radioactive phenylalanine into yeast mitochondria was measured in presence of 20 µg ricin/50 mg mitochondrial proteins/ml and was equivalent to the control amino acid incorporation in presence of both cycloheximide (that inhibits residual cytoplasmic protein synthesis) and chloramphenicol (which inhibits mitochondrial protein synthesis) as shown in Table 1.

TABLE 1 Percent of Radioactivity Incorporated into Intact Yeast Mitochondria Proteins in the Presence of Antibiotics and Ricin

Addition to the mitochondria*	Percent of the total radioactivity**
None	100
Cycloheximide	60
Cycloheximide plus chloramphenicol	1
Ricin (20 µg/ml)	1

*The system contains 50 mg baker's yeast mitochondrial protein per ml.
**The radioactivity is measured after 30 min at 32°C.

Protein Synthesis in a *Neurospora crassa* S-30 System

When ricin (12 µg/ml) was added to this sub-mitochondrial protein synthesizing system, incorporation of tritiated-phenylalanine into proteins was 80% inhibited (Fig. 1). Contamination of cytoplasmic 77-S ribosomes in the mitochondrial preparation was negligible since the cycloheximide-control was identical to the control without antibiotic. With 24 µg ricin/ml, a 90% inhibition of protein synthesis is obtained.

Protein Synthesis in Spinach's Chloroplasts

On a sub-chloroplastic protein-synthesizing system, protein synthesis is inhibited to about 80% in presence of 40 µg ricin/ml. Figure 2 shows the percentages of protein synthesis inhibition obtained according different concentrations of ricin. The same inhibition level is obtained with isolated chloroplasts-ribosomes and chloroplasts-translation factors.

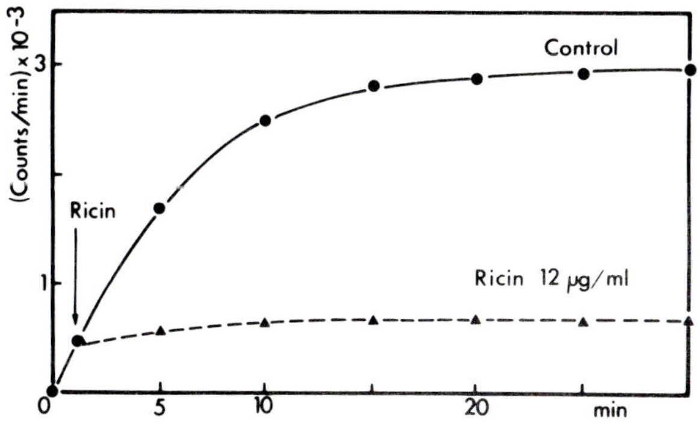

Fig. 1. Kinetic of a *Neurospora crassa* sub-mitochondrial protein synthesis in presence of ricin or not (control). The control plus cycloheximide was only 0.5% lower than the control.

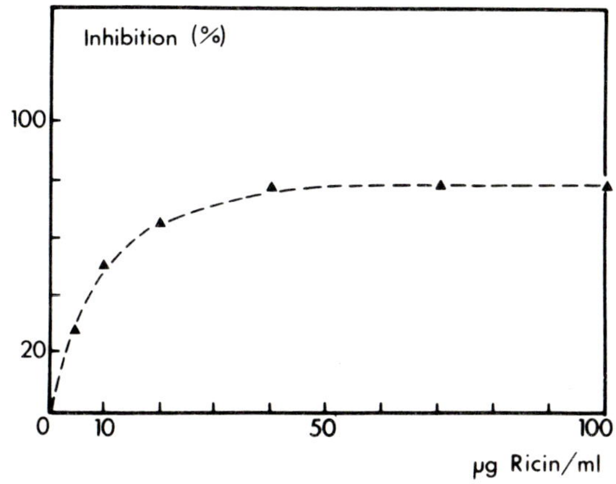

Fig. 2. Percentages of protein synthesis inhibition in a sub-chloroplastic protein synthesizing system according to different concentrations of ricin.

Escherichia coli Cell-Free Protein Synthesis

No inhibition of protein synthesis in an *in vitro Escherichia coli* system is obtained even with the use of very high doses of ricin (Table 2).

DISCUSSION AND CONCLUSION

Ricin inhibits fungi mitochondrial and chloroplastic protein synthesis though these organelles are regarded as prokaryotic-like whereas this toxin is inactive in a prokaryotic (*Escherichia coli*) cell-free protein synthesizing system. However, it must be emphasized that these mitochondrial and chloroplastic protein synthesis inhibitions are obtained with higher doses (respectively about 60 and 200 times more) than those required to obtain the same inhibition level (80%) in an eukaryotic cell-free (rabbit reticulocyte lysate) protein synthesizing system (Lugnier, 1974 ; Lugnier and co-workers, 1976a, 1977a, 1977b).

TABLE 2 Action of Ricin on *Escherichia coli* Cell-Free Protein Synthesis

Reaction mixture	Percent of incorporated radioactivity*
Complete	100
Ricin (20 μg/ml)	100
Ricin (500 μg/ml)	98

*The radioactivity is measured after 30 min at 37°C.

To our knowledge, ricin represents the first substance that inhibits both the cytoplasmic and organellar (mitochondria and chloroplasts) protein synthesis in eukaryotes, at least in fungi and in plants, but not the prokaryotic protein synthesis. However, there might be differences in the sensitivity of mitochondrial protein synthesizing systems to ricin since Greco and co-workers (1974) did not obtain an inhibition of protein synthesis by ricin in a rat liver mitochondrial system.

ACKNOWLEDGEMENTS

This work was supported by grants from the Institut National de la Santé et de la Recherche Médicale (CRL INSERM 79.1.154.3), from the Fondation pour la Recherche Médicale Française and from the Deutsche Forschungsgemeinschaft. The authors are grateful to the Société Française du Ricin (Marseille, France) for its generous gifts of *Ricinus communis* L. seeds. The authors also would like to thank Professor Y. Boulanger for the correction of the English of the manuscript.

REFERENCES

Dirheimer, G. , F. Haas, and P. Métais (1967). Hépatonéphrite Expérimentale Provoquée par la Ricine. *VIIIème Réunion Nationale des Centres de Lutte contre les Poisons*, Grenoble (France), 28-29 April. Communication n° 6.

Dirheimer, G., F. Haas, and P. Métais (1968). In L. Roche (Ed.), *Hépatonéphrites Toxiques*, Masson et Cie, Paris. Toxicol. Méd. Série B, pp. 45-50.

Greco, M., L. Montanaro, F. Novello, C. Saccone, S. Sperti, and F. Stirpe (1974). Inhibition of Protein Synthesis by Ricin : Experiments with Rat Liver Mitochondria and Nuclei and with Ribosomes from *Escherichia coli*. *Biochem. J.*, *142*, 695-697.

Kohn, L., A.A.J. Lugnier, O. Tiboni, and O. Ciferri (1978). Inhibition of Spinach's Chloroplasts Protein Synthesis by Ricin, the Toxin of *Ricinus communis* L. Seeds. *XIIth FEBS Meeting*, Dresden (G.D.R.), July 2-8. Abstract n° 1816-F16.

Küntzel, H., and H.-C. Blossey (1974). Translation Products *in vitro* of Mitochondrial Messenger RNA from *Neurospora crassa*. *Eur. J. Biochem.*, *47*, 165-171.

Lamb, A.J., G.D. Clark-Walker, and A.W. Linnane (1968). The Biogenesis of Mitochondria. 4. The Differenciation of Mitochondrial and Cytoplasmic Protein Synthesizing System *in vitro* by Antibiotics. *Biochim. Biophys. Acta*, *161*, 415-427.

Lugnier, A.A.J. (1974). Isolation and Study of Physical, Chemical, Biochemical and Biological Properties of Ricin, a Toxic Protein from the Castor-Oil Plant (*Ricinus communis* L.). *Thèse de Doctorat d'Etat ès-Sciences*, Université Louis Pasteur, Strasbourg (France), October 18, pp. 701 ; ref. 1337 ; fig. 111 ; tabl. 42.

Lugnier, A.A.J. (1975). Kinetics of Eukaryotic Protein Synthesis Inhibition by Ricin, the Toxalbumin of *Ricinus communis* L. Seeds. *Xth FEBS Meeting*, Paris (France), July 20-25. Abstract n° 488.

Lugnier, A.A.J., E.-E. Creppy, and G. Dirheimer (1977a). Inhibition of Cytoplasmic and Organelle Protein Synthesis by Ricin, the Phytotoxin of *Ricinus Communis* L. Seeds. *Hoppe-Seyler's Z. Physiol. Chem.*, *358*, 1242-1243.

Lugnier, A.A.J., E.-E. Creppy, M.-A. Le Meur, P. Gerlinger, and G. Dirheimer (1977b) Reciprocal Interactions of Ricin from *Ricinus communis* L. Seeds with Eukaryote Ribosomes. *FEBS Lett.*, *76*, 166-172.

Lugnier, A.A.J., and G. Dirheimer (1971). Extraction, Purification et Détermination du Poids Moléculaire de la Ricine, Toxalbumine de *Ricinus communis* L. *C.R. Acad. Sci. Paris*, *273D*, 704-707.

Lugnier, A.A.J., H. Küntzel, and G. Dirheimer (1976a). Inhibition of *Neurospora crassa* and Yeast Mitochondrial Protein Synthesis by Ricin, a Toxic Protein Inactive on *E.coli* Protein Synthesis. *FEBS Lett.*, *66*, 202-205.

Lugnier, A.A.J., M.A. Le Meur, P. Gerlinger, and G. Dirheimer (1974). Inhibition of *in vitro* Protein Synthesis in a Rabbit Reticulocyte Cell-Free System by Toxic Tryptic Peptides from Ricin. *Biochimie (Paris)*, *56*, 1287-1289.

Lugnier, A.A.J., M.-A. Le Meur, P. Gerlinger, and G. Dirheimer (1976b). Isolation and Biochemical Properties of Toxic Tryptic Peptides of Ricinotoxin from *Ricinus communis* L. Seeds. *Eur. J. Toxicol.*, *6*, 323-333.

Olsnes, S., R. Heiberg, and A. Pihl (1973). Inactivation of Eucaryotic Ribosomes by the Toxic Plant Proteins Abrin and Ricin. *Mol. Biol. Reports*, *1*, 15-20.

Olsnes, S., and A. Pihl (1972). Ricin - A Protent Inhibitor of Protein Synthesis. *FEBS Lett.*, *20*, 327-329.

Tiboni, O., G. Di Pasquale, and O. Ciferri (1976). Ribosomes and Translation Factors from Isolated Spinach Chloroplasts. *Plant Sci. Lett.*, *6*, 419-429.

INHIBITION OF HEPATOMA TISSUE CULTURE CELL GROWTH AND OF CELLULAR PROTEIN, DNA AND RNA SYNTHESIS BY RICIN AND TWO OF ITS TRYPTIC PEPTIDES

E.-E. Creppy* **, A. A. J. Lugnier* **, G. Beck* and G. Dirheimer**

**Laboratoire de Toxicologie et de Biologie Moléculaires, Faculté de Pharmacie, Université Louis Pasteur, Strasbourg, France*
***Institut de Biologie Moléculaire et Cellulaire du C.N.R.S., 15 rue René Descartes, 67084 Strasbourg, France*

ABSTRACT

The effect of ricin, the phytotoxin from castor beans, as well as two of its isolated tryptic peptides, was studied on hepatoma tissue cell suspension cultures (HTC). The toxin at a 0.3 μg/ml concentration, for $3 \cdot 10^5$ cells/ml, has a cytostatic effect . Protein synthesis measured by the incorporation of tritiated-leucine in the cell begins to be inhibited after 30 min of incubation with ricin, 45 min and 60 min with respectively the peptides II_{1c} and II_{2a}, although protein synthesis is completely blocked after 2 h for a toxin concentration of 0.3 μg/ml. DNA synthesis is inhibited from 1 h on. Finally the level of the DNA slows down from 3 h on, whereas the level of RNA abruptly falls between 4 and 5 h.

KEYWORDS

Ricin ; hepatoma tissue culture ; tryptic peptides ; protein synthesis ; DNA synthesis ; RNA synthesis.

INTRODUCTION

Ricin, the glycoproteic toxin from castor beans (*Ricinus communis* L.) is extremely toxic to animals producing hepatonephritic symptoms (Dirheimer and co-workers, 1966, 1967, 1968). It has been purified (Ishiguro and co-workers, 1964 ; Lugnier and Dirheimer, 1971) and has a molecular weight of 66,600 daltons (Lugnier and Dirheimer, 1971 ; Lugnier and co-workers, 1976). It was first shown (Dirheimer and co-workers, 1967, 1968) that ricin inhibits protein synthesis at the ribosomal level and later it was established that it inhibits protein synthesis both in intact cells (Lin and co-workers, 1971 ; Refsnes and co-workers, 1974) and in cell-free protein-synthesizing systems (Olsnes and Pihl, 1972a). This toxin is formed by two polypeptide chains A and B joined by a disulfide bond (Funatsu and Funatsu, 1968 ; Olsnes and Pihl, 1972b), but only the intact (or reassociated molecule) has a toxic effect on animals and cultured cells whereas in cell-free systems all the toxic activity is due to the A-chain alone (Olsnes and co-workers, 1974).

In this paper we study the action of ricin as compared to that of its tryptic peptides on hepatoma tissue culture (HTC) cells grown in suspension and on the cellular synthesis of proteins, DNA and RNA. It was previously shown that the tryptic hydrolysate of ricin contains several peptides which are highly toxic on animals (Lugnier and co-workers, 1976) and that these toxic peptides have an inhibitory effect on protein synthesis in a rabbit reticulocyte cell-free system (Lugnier and co-workers, 1974). Here we report the isolation of two of these peptides in a pure state and their action on hepatoma tissue culture cells as compared to that of ricin.

MATERIALS AND METHODS

Ricin was prepared as described before (Lugnier and Dirheimer, 1971). It was homogeneous in polyacrylamide disc gel electrophoresis and had no hemagglutinating effect.

Trypsin Hydrolysis and Isolation of Tryptic Peptides

As native ricin is resistant to trypsin action it was first denatured as previously described and hydrolyzed with chymotrypsin-free trypsin (Lugnier, 1974 ; Lugnier and co-workers, 1976). The tryptic digest was chromatographed on Sephadex G200 and yielded a toxic peak II. This toxic mixture of polypeptides gave two peaks II_1 and II_2 by chromatography on CM-cellulose. From II_1 we obtained on DEAE-cellulose a toxic peptide II_{1c} which was homogeneous on polyacrylamide disc gel electrophoresis (Creppy and co-workers, 1978).

When peak II_2 was charged on DEAE-cellulose perfused by a 10 mM pH 6.8 buffer it was retained. A homogeneous polypeptide called II_{2a} could be eluted by a 10 mM potassium phosphate buffer pH 6.8 supplemented with $1 \cdot 10^{-6}$ M Fe^{3+} which is known to elute ricin from DEAE-cellulose according to Funatsu and Funatsu (1968).

The molecular weight of polypeptides II_{1c} and II_{2a} are respectively of 22,000 and 18,000 daltons. By β-mercaptoethanol reduction followed by disc gel electrophoresis they were shown to be composed by parts of the A- and B-chains of ricin. They were six times less toxic than pure ricin, on animals. LD_{50} (24 h) in rat are respectively of 20 μg/kg and 18 μg/kg for II_{1c} and II_{2a} (Creppy, 1978).

Cell Protein, DNA and RNA Synthesis

For HTC cell protein synthesis determination the cells were isolated, washed and resuspended as previously described (Creppy and co-workers, 1979). Ricin at 0.3 μg/ml was added and the cells were incubated in a shaking waterbath at 37°C. Simultaneously, with ricin or 2 h after ricin action, tritiated-leucine (specific activity : 53 Ci/mmol ; C.E.A., Saclay, France) at a concentration of 5 μCi per 30 ml was added. Samples were removed, and the radioactivity incorporated into proteins was determined as previously described (Creppy and co-workers, 1979).

DNA and RNA synthesis were measured as described (Creppy and co-workers, 1979).

RESULTS

Figure 1A shows the results of cell growth experiments in the presence of different concentrations of ricin. From $5 \cdot 10^{-3}$ pmol/ml to 5 pmol/ml ricin displays a cytostatic action towards HTC cells. With 10 pmol/ml this action becomes cytotoxic and an important cytolysis is observed after 72 h. As shown in Fig. 1B the tryptic peptides are about 3 to 4 times less toxic on HTC cells as compared to ricin. The same results were obtained when their action on protein synthesis, followed by the incorporation of tritiated-leucine into cell proteins, were tested. At a concentration of 5 pmol ricin per ml this inhibition begins after 30 min of incubation (Fig. 2). It is complete after 2 h. Tryptic peptides inhibit protein synthesis too but after a longer lag time (45 to 60 min) and to a lesser extent although their concentrations are about 3 times higher than that of ricin (Fig. 2). To ensure that protein synthesis was completely inhibited after 2 h, cells were incubated for this time with the toxins and tritiated-leucine only added thereafter. No more incorporation of radioactivity into cell proteins occurred.

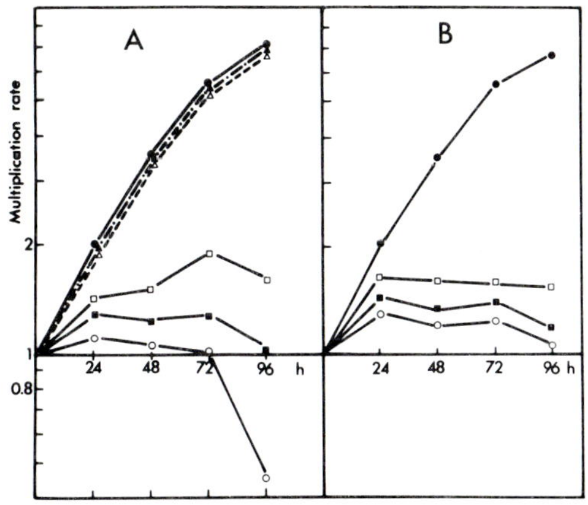

Fig. 1. HTC cells multiplication rate in presence of :
A : ricin - (△---△) ricin $5 \cdot 10^{-3}$ pmol/ml ;
(▲-•-▲) ricin 0.5 pmol/ml ;
(□——□) ricin 2.5 pmol/ml ;
(■——■) ricin 5 pmol/ml ;
(○——○) ricin 10 pmol/ml ;
(●——●) control (without ricin).
B : tryptic peptides -
(■——■) II_{1c} 15 pmol/ml ;
(□——□) II_{2a} 18 pmol/ml ;
(○——○) ricin 5 pmol/ml ;
(●——●) control (without toxin).

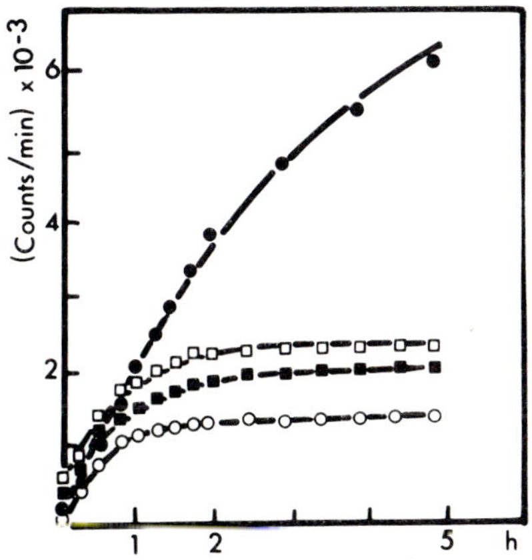

Fig. 2. HTC cells protein synthesis in presence of :
(○——○) ricin 5 pmol/ml ;
(■——■) II_{1c} 15 pmol/ml ;
(□——□) II_{2a} 18 pmol/ml ;
(●——●) control (without toxin).

Under the same experimental conditions, DNA synthesis is inhibited about 15% by ricin after 1 h of culture ; afterwards the incorporation of tritiated-thymidine into DNA diminishes dramatically. After 3 h one even sees a decrease in the level of DNA reaching 50% of the control at 5 h. The results were similar for the two polypeptides II_{1c} and II_{2a}, but the residual level of DNA were slightly higher than with ricin (Fig. 3).

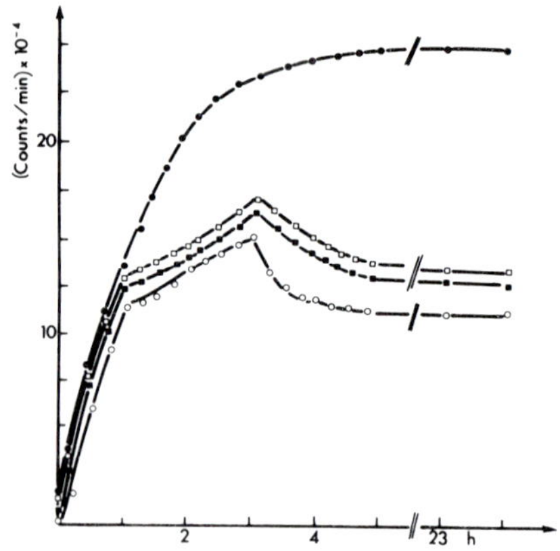

Fig. 3. HTC cells DNA synthesis in presence of :
(○—○) ricin 5 pmol/ml ;
(■—■) II_{1c} 15 pmol/ml ;
(□—□) II_{2a} 18 pmol/ml ;
(●—●) control (without toxin).

Practically no change in cellular RNA synthesis was seen during the first 4 h of culture (Fig. 4).

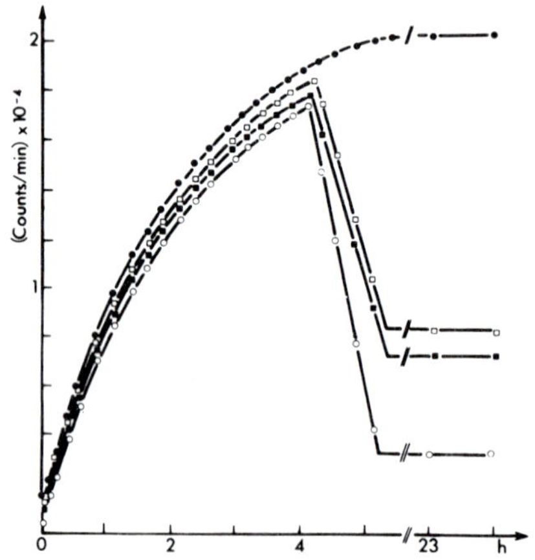

Fig. 4. HTC cells RNA synthesis in presence of :
(○—○) ricin 5 pmol/ml ;
(■—■) II_{1c} 15 pmol/ml ;
(□—□) II_{2a} 18 pmol/ml ;
(●—●) control (without toxin).

However, between the 4th and 5th h of culture, the level of RNA fell abruptly reaching about 10% of the original level in presence of ricin and respectively 25% and 30% in presence of the peptides II_{1c} and II_{2a}. These levels were maintained for a culture period of 24 h (Fig. 4).

DISCUSSION

Lin and co-workers (1971) had described a DNA synthesis inhibition in ricin treated Ehrlich ascite tumor cells, but they followed it for only 3 h. They also looked for $[^{14}C]$-uridine incorporation into RNA but did not see a significant effect. This is probably due to the fact that they only followed this biosynthesis for 3 h whereas we have seen that the RNA degradation starts after 4 h. But the inhibitory effect on DNA synthesis always starts later than protein synthesis inhibition and is very likely a consequence of it. The degradation of DNA however may be a direct effect of ricin on DNA because with ochratoxin, which inhibits protein synthesis too in HTC cells, no inhibition of DNA synthesis nor decrease of the level of DNA occurs (Creppy and co-workers, 1979). It is important to noticed that in these tests, HTC cells were in a culture medium where they normally continue to grow for at least 4 days.

Tryptic peptides are less toxic than ricin on HTC cells. This can be explained by the binding to cell membrane. It was established that only the B-chain of ricin binds to cell membrane and let the A-chain into cell (Olsnes and co-workers, 1974). We have shown that the two peptides have only a part of the B-chain so they might bind less strongly to cell membrane receptors. This hypothesis was corroborated by the fact that α-lactose at a 0.1 M concentration can prevent the toxicity of the peptides even if it is added to the cells 30 min after them although it no more prevents the toxicity of ricin. The lower toxicity of the peptides can also be explained by the presence of only a part of the toxic A-chain. The toxic effects of ricin and peptides are not reversible when they penetrated into cell. Only sugar compounds like β-galactose, α-lactose under determined conditions can avoid the fixation on cell membrane and as a consequence the entry in cell and the toxic effects of both ricin and tryptic peptides.

ACKNOWLEDGEMENTS

The present study was supported by grants from the Institut National de la Santé et de la Recherche Médicale (CRL INSERM n° 76.10613). We are grateful to the Société Française du Ricin (Marseille) for its generous gifts of *Ricinus communis* L. seeds. We wish to thank Professor Yves Boulanger for reviewing the English of the manuscript.

REFERENCES

Creppy, E.-E. (1978). Action of Ricin, of Two of its Isolated Tryptic Peptides and of Ochratoxin A on Cells in Cultures and on *in vitro* Protein Synthesizing Systems. *Thèse de Doctorat d'Etat ès Sciences-Pharmaceutiques*, UER Sciences Pharmaceutiques, Université Louis Pasteur, Strasbourg (France), December 18. pp. 196 ; ref. 101 ; fig. 68 ; tabl. 7.

Creppy, E.-E., A.A.J. Lugnier, G. Beck, and G. Dirheimer (1978). Isolement et Etude des Peptides Toxiques obtenus par Hydrolyse Trypsique de la Ricine. *Ann. Méd. Nancy (France)*, *17*, 323-327.

Creppy, E.-E., A.A.J. Lugnier, G. Beck, R. Röschenthaler, and G. Dirheimer (1979). Action of Ochratoxin A on Cultured Hepatoma Cells. - Reversion of Inhibition by Phenylalanine. *FEBS Lett.*, *104*, 287-290.

Dirheimer, G., F. Haas, and P. Métais (1966). Modifications Biochimiques du Sang au Cours de l'Intoxication du Rat par la Ricine. *C.R. Soc. Biol. (Paris)*, *160*, 2458-2461.

Dirheimer, G., F. Haas, and P. Métais (1967). Hépatonéphrite Experimentale Provoquée par la Ricine. *VIIIème Réunion Nationale des Centres de Lutte Contre les Poisons*, Grenoble (France), 28-29 April. Communication n° 6.

Dirheimer, G., F. Haas, and P. Métais (1968). In L. Roche (Ed.), *Hépatonéphrites Toxiques*. Masson et Cie, Paris. Toxicol. Méd. Série B, pp. 45-50.

Funatsu, M., and G. Funatsu (1968). Toxicity and Chemical Structure of a Toxin from the Common Castor Beans (in japanese). *Tampakushitsu Kakusan Kôso (Protein, Nucleic Acid, Enzyme)*, *13*, 905-912.

Funatsu, M., G. Funatsu, M. Ishiguro, and S. Nanno (1968). Chemical Structure and Toxicity of Ricin D. *15th Symposium on Toxins*, Suita-shi,Osaka (Japan), July 20-21. Abstract n° 40.

Funatsu, M., G. Funatsu, M. Ishiguro, and S. Nanno (1970). Chemical Structure and Toxicity of Ricin D. *Japan. J. Med. Sci. Biol.*, *23*, 264-267.

Ishiguro, M., T. Takahashi, G. Funatsu, K. Hayashi, and M. Funatsu (1964). Purification of Ricin. *J. Biochem. Tokyo*, *55*, 587-592.

Ishiguro, M., T. Takahashi, K. Hayashi, and M. Funatsu (1964). Molecular Weight and some Physicochemical Properties of Cristalline Ricin D. *J. Biochem. Tokyo*, *56*, 325-327.

Lin, J.-Y., K. Liu, C.-C. Chen, and T.-C. Tung (1971). Effect of Crystalline Ricin on the Biosynthesis of Protein, RNA, and DNA in Experimental Tumor Cells. *Cancer Res.*, *31*, 921-924.

Lugnier, A.A.J. (1974). Isolation and Study of Physical, Chemical, Biochemical and Biological Properties of Ricin, a Toxic Protein from the Castor-Oil Plant (*Ricinus communis* L.). *Thèse de Doctorat d'Etat ès-Sciences*, Université Louis Pasteur, Strasbourg (France), October 18. pp. 701 ; ref. 1337 ; fig. 111 ; tabl. 42.

Lugnier, A.A.J., E.-E. Creppy, M.-A. Le Meur, P. Gerlinger, and G. Dirheimer (1977). Reciprocal Interactions of Ricin from *Ricinus communis* L. Seeds with Eukaryote Ribosomes. *FEBS Lett.*, *76*, 166-172.

Lugnier, A.A.J., and G. Dirheimer (1971). Extraction, Purification et Détermination du Poids Moléculaire de la Ricine, Toxalbumine de *Ricinus communis* L. *C.R. Acad. Sci. Paris*, *273D*, 704-707.

Lugnier, A.A.J., H. Küntzel, and G. Dirheimer (1976). Inhibition of *Neurospora crassa* and Yeast Mitochondrial Protein Synthesis by Ricin, a Toxic Protein inactive on *E.coli* Protein Synthesis. *FEBS Lett.*, *66*, 202-205.

Lugnier, A.A.J., M.-A. Le Meur, P. Gerlinger, and G. Dirheimer (1974). Inhibition of *in vitro* Protein Synthesis in a Rabbit Reticulocyte Cell-Free System by Toxic Tryptic Peptides from Ricin. *Biochimie (Paris)*, *56*, 1287-1289.

Lugnier, A.A.J., M.-A. Le Meur, P. Gerlinger, and G. Dirheimer (1976). Isolation and Biochemical Properties of Toxic Tryptic Peptides of Ricinotoxin from *Ricinus communis* L. Seeds. *Eur. J. Toxicol.*, *9*, 323-333.

Lowry, O.H., N.J. Rosebrough, A.L. Farr, and R.J. Randall (1951). Protein Measurement with the Folin-Phenol Reagent. *J. Biol. Chem.*, *193*, 265-275.

Olsnes, S., and A. Pihl (1972a). Ricin - A Potent Inhibitor of Protein Synthesis. *FEBS Lett.*, *20*, 327-329.

Olsnes, S., and A. Pihl (1972b). Treatment of Abrin and Ricin with β-Mercaptoethanol Opposite Effects on their Toxicity in Mice and their Ability to Inhibit Protein Synthesis in a Cell-Free System. *FEBS Lett.*, *28*, 48-50.

Olsnes, S., K. Refsnes, and A. Pihl (1974). Mechanism of Action of the Toxic Lectins Abrin and Ricin. *Nature (London)*, *249*, 627-631.

Olsnes, S., E. Saltvedt, and A. Pihl (1974). Isolation and Comparison of Galactose-Binding Lectins from *Abrus precatorius* and *Ricinus communis*. *J. Biol. Chem.*, *249*, 803-810.

Refsnes, K., S. Olsnes, and A. Pihl (1974). On the Toxic Proteins Abrin and Ricin. Studies of their Binding To and Entry into Ehrlich Ascites Cells. *J. Biol. Chem.*, *249*, 3557-3562.

ACTION OF RICIN ON STEROID MEDIATED INDUCTION OF TYROSINE AMINOTRANSFERASE IN HEPATOMA TISSUE CULTURE CELLS

E.-E. Creppy* **, A. A. J. Lugnier* **, G. Beck* and G. Dirheimer* **

**Laboratoire de Toxicologie et de Biologie Moléculaires, Faculté de Pharmacie, Université Louis Pasteur, Strasbourg, France*
***Institut de Biologie Moléculaire et Cellulaire du C.N.R.S., 15 rue René Descartes, 67084 Strasbourg, France*

ABSTRACT

Ricin, at a concentration of 5 pmol/ml, inhibits completely protein synthesis measured by incorporation of radioactive-leucine into HTC cell proteins, but a slight induction of tyrosine aminotransferase (TAT) by dexamethasone still takes place. Only higher doses of ricin (25 pmol/ml) impair completely this induction. This could be due either to a high affinity of the messenger RNA of TAT for the ribosomes or to the presence of several still active ribosomes liberated from ricin-blocked ribosomes.

KEYWORDS

Ricin ; protein synthesis ; tyrosine aminotransferase ; enzymatic induction ; hepatoma tissue culture ; ribosomes ; polysomes ; dexamethasone.

INTRODUCTION

In a previous paper (Creppy and co-workers, 1979), we described the action of ricin, the glycoproteic toxin from castor beans, as well as of its two polypeptide A- and B-chains, on hepatoma tissue cell suspension cultures (HTC cells). Ricin at a 5 pmol/ml concentration for $3 \cdot 10^5$ cells/ml, has a cytostatic effect, whereas the isolated A-and B-chains had no action. In the presence of ricin, the protein content of the cells decreases and protein synthesis measured by the incorporation of a labelled-amino acid into proteins starts to be inhibited 30 min after the treatment and is completely blocked 2 h later. DNA synthesis is inhibited from 1 h on, and the level of DNA slows down from 3 h. Finally the level of RNA abruptly falls between 4 and 5 h. It was therefore interesting to study the action of ricin on the induction of a specific protein, tyrosine aminotransferase (TAT).

MATERIALS AND METHODS

HTC cells (initial concentration : $3 \cdot 10^5$ cells/ml) were grown in Swim's S-77 medium supplemented with 10% calf serum at 37°C in shaker suspension cultures (30 or 45 ml). Their generation time was approximately 28 h, and growth continued for 3 to 4 days before reaching the stationary phase. Their multiplication was followed as previously described (Creppy and co-workers, 1979). For TAT induction, the steroid, dexamethasone (in ethanol solution), was added to a final concentration of 1 μM.

Ricin was prepared as previously described (Lugnier and Dirheimer, 1971).

For the TAT determination 2 ml of cell culture were centrifuged at 600 x *g* for 3 min at 4°C. The cells were washed twice with NaCl 0.9% and recentrifuged. They were then disrupted in 1 ml potassium phosphate buffer 50 mM, pH 7.6, α-ketoglutarate 5 mM, EDTA sodium salt 5 mM, pyridoxal phosphate 0.2 mM, by sonication for 2 x 20 s at 70 V in a Sonicator type 250TS 20K (Ultrasons, Annemasse, France). The TAT activity was assayed by the enzymatic method of Diamondstone (1966) and expressed as specific activity. Proteins were estimated by the technic of Lowry and co-workers (1951).

For the analysis of the cellular ribosomes and polysomes of ricin treated cells, 900 ml of cell culture ($3 \cdot 10^5$ cells/ml) were preincubated with ricin (0.3 μg/ml or 1.5 μg/ml) and centrifuged for 7 min at 1500 x *g* at 4°C. The pellets were first washed with cold 0.9% NaCl, then with buffer A (Tris-HCl 25 mM, pH 7.2, KCl 25 mM, $MgCl_2$ 5 mM). They were then taken up by "x" ml (one volume) of buffer A to which 100 μg/ml of heparine were added to inhibit RNAases. After 10 min chilling and swelling in ice the cells were disrupted in a Potter by 2 times 10 strokes, allowing to stand 2 min between each set of strokes. After microscopic control to ensure that cells were broken but the nuclei intact, 0.125 volume of 2 M sucrose was added (final concentration : 0.25 M). After 10 min centrifugation at 2600 x *g*, the supernatant was centrifuged for 25 min at 112500 x *g*. The concentration of the polysomes and ribosomes was determined by measuring their optical density at 280 and 260 nm. The analysis of the polysomes was done on a 10-40% sucrose gradient in buffer A with heparine (total volume of the gradient : 13 ml). An amount of polysomes corresponding to 2-20 O.D. units at 260 nm were put on the gradient and centrifuged for 2 h at 23000 x *g* at 4°C (Beckman ultracentrifuge L5-75, rotor SW41, without brake setting). The O.D. profile was monitored in an Isco densitometer.

RESULTS

Inhibition of Induced TAT Synthesis by Ricin

Inhibition of protein synthesis in HTC cells is complete after 2 h when a concentration of 5 pmol/ml (0.3 μg) of ricin is added to the cell culture medium (Creppy and co-workers, 1979). We tested in these conditions what happens with a specific steroid induced protein, the tyrosine aminotransferase (TAT). Kinetics of TAT induction mediated by dexamethasone (1 μM) in absence or presence of ricin (5 pmol per ml) were followed. Figure 1 shows a high stimulation of TAT induction in the control, but in the presence of ricin a slight formation of TAT is observed between the second and the third hour. This slight, but measurable, induction of TAT can be completely suppressed if higher concentrations of ricin were used (25 pmol/ml) as shown in Fig. 1.

When the cells are pretreated with ricin (5 pmol/ml) for 2 h before addition of dexamethasone no TAT induction takes place (Fig. 2).

To see if ricin interacts with dexamethasone, experiments with a 10 times more glucocorticoid hormone were carried out. The results obtained were comparable to those obtained in Fig. 1 with only 1 μM dexamethasone. Dexamethasone and ricin therefore do not interact.

Irreversibility of the Inhibition of TAT Synthesis by Ricin

HTC cells were pretreated for different times with ricin. Cells were then extensively washed to remove ricin and resuspended in culture medium. Dexamethasone (1 μM) was then added to induce TAT synthesis. Every 2 h TAT was estimated. No TAT induction took place even after only 2 h of pretreatment. This shows that ricin has an irreversible effect on TAT synthesis.

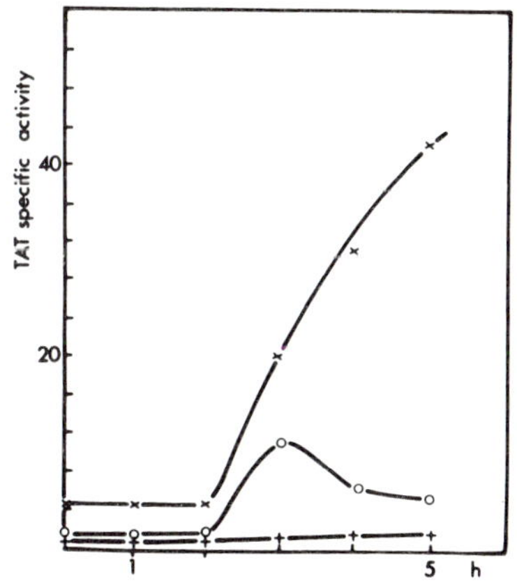

Fig. 1. Dexamethasone induced synthesis of tyrosine amino-transferase in presence of ricin.
(x——x) control ; (o——o) ricin 5 pmol/ml ;
(+——+) ricin 25 pmol/ml.

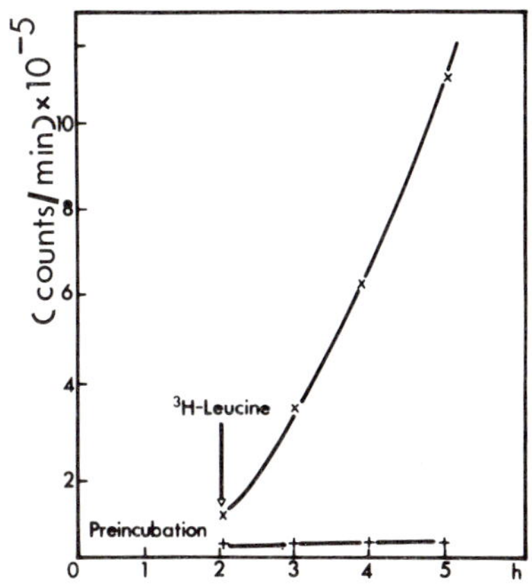

Fig. 2. TAT induction in HTC cells pretreated for 2 hours with ricin.
(x——x) induced control ; (+——+) ricin 5 pmol/ml.

Analysis of the Ribosomes and Polysomes

The analysis of the ribosome of ricin treated cells (5 pmol/ml) shows (Fig. 3) the presence of free forms and of polysomes. As compared to the control, the light polysomes (fraction A) have practically disappeared ; fraction B polysomes are present to a greater extent in ricin treated cells, whereas the heavy polysomes (fraction C) have practically disappeared.

When the cells were treated with a 5 fold higher concentration of ricin (25 pmol/ml), a lower amount of free ribosomes but a higher amount of fraction B polysomes were observed (Fig. 4) and only a few heavy polysomes corresponding to fraction C were left (Fig. 4).

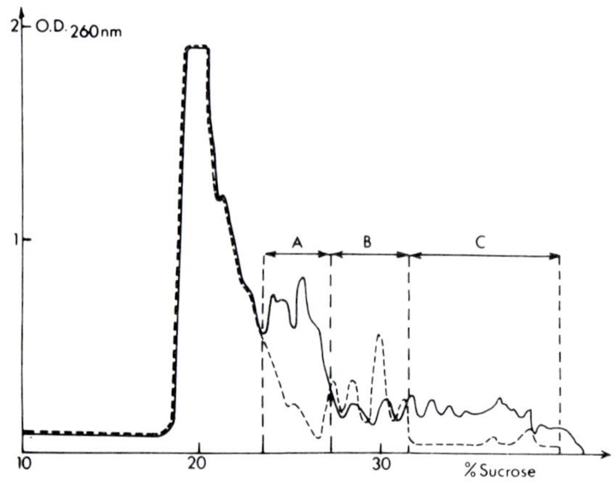

Fig. 3. HTC polysomes and ribosome profile.
(———) control ; (-----) HTC cells treated by ricin (5 pmol/ml) for 2 hours.

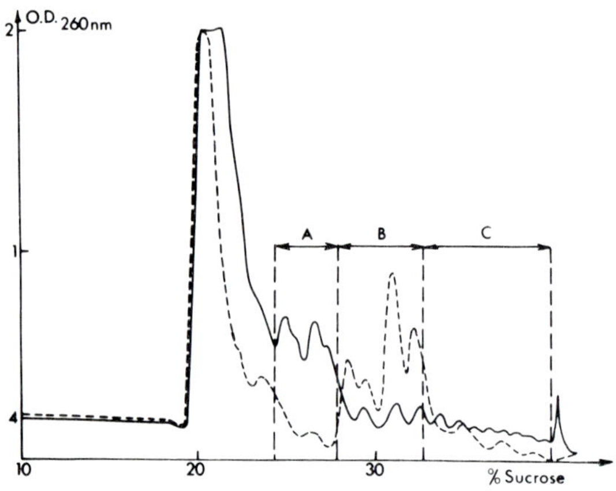

Fig. 4. HTC polysomes and ribosome profile.
(———) control ; (-----) HTC cells treated by ricin (25 pmol/ml) for 2 hours.

DISCUSSION

Dexamethasone induces after 2 h lag period the synthesis of tyrosine aminotransferase in a HTC cell culture (Thompson and co-workers, 1966). The presence of a 5 pmol/ml ricin inhibits almost completely this phenomenon. The presence of ricin in the culture medium is not necessary for this action because cells which have been treated with ricin for 2 h, washed and resuspended in ricin-free medium, cannot be induced anymore. This inhibition is due to the action of ricin on cell protein synthesis which seems to be completely blocked after 2 h (Creppy and co-workers, 1979). The slight induction of TAT shown in Fig. 1 then remains to be explained. It does not appear anymore when the ricin concentration is higher, for example 25 pmol/ml. It seems therefore that more ricin is needed to inhibit induced protein synthesis than to inhibit general protein synthesis. More experimentation is necessary to explain this result but the following hypotheses might be suggested.

When the TAT mRNA reaches the polysomes blocked by ricin (Lugnier and co-workers, 1977) it desplaces the ribosomes, some of them being still active as was shown by Fodstad and Olsnes (1977). These are able to give active polysomes with the TAT mRNA and to synthesize a small number of TAT molecules before being also inactivated by ricin. This supposes that the induced TAT mRNA has a higher affinity for the ribosomes than the other mRNAs. Similar hypotheses concerning different affinities or different messengers have been proposed by Sonenshein and Brawerman (1976) for immunoglobulins and by Lodish (1974) for haemoglobin.

Another hypothesis was suggested by the results obtained in the study of ribosomes and polysomes of ricin treated cells. During the synthesis of common proteins, the cytoplasm contains either free ribosomal subunits or polysomes engaged in protein synthesis. Only these are blocked by ricin (Lugnier and co-workers, 1977). The inactivation of a single ribosome of a polysome blocks those which follow it on the mRNA, but not the preceding ones which can continue the protein biosynthesis and are liberated in an active state if they are not themselves inactivated by ricin on the polysome. Such liberated free ribosomes or ribosomal subunits exist in large amounts in ricin treated cells (Fig. 3). Furthermore the polysomes are proportionally shorter than the polysomes of the non-treated cells. This could explain the accumulation of fraction B and the diminution of fraction C (Fig. 3).

At high concentrations, ricin may not only inhibit the elongation step but also block the initiation as has been suggested for abrin by Skorve and co-workers (1977). According to another hypothesis practically all free ribosomes are blocked, the number of ricin molecules being sufficient to inactivate simultaneously several ribosomes on the polysomes. This would diminish the number of free ribosomes or ribosomal subunits as seen in Fig. 4. Thus the increase in the ricin concentration would block more rapidly a larger number of ribosomes and even hinder the translation of induced messengers.

ACKNOWLEDGEMENTS

This work was supported by grants from the Institut National de la Santé et de la Recherche Médicale (CRL INSERM n° 79.1.154.3). We wish especially to thank Dr. Jean-Paul Beck for reviewing the manuscript and Marie-Thérèse Hotz for her technical assistance.

REFERENCES

Creppy, E.-E., A.A.J. Lugnier, G. Beck, and G. Dirheimer (1979). Action of Ricin and its Polypeptide Chains on Cultured Hepatoma Cells. *Arch. Toxicol.* Accepted for publication.

Diamondstone, T.I. (1966). Assay of Tyrosine Transaminase Activity by Conversion of *p*-hydroxyphenylpyruvate to *p*-hydroxybenzaldehyde. *Anal. Biochem.*, *16*, 395-401.

Fodstad, Ø., and S. Olsnes (1977). Studies on the Accessability of Ribosomes to Inactivation by the Toxic Lectins Abrin and Ricin. *Eur. J. Biochem.*, *74*, 209-215.

Lodish, H.F. (1974). Model for the Regulation of mRNA Translation Applied to Haemoglobin Synthesis. *Nature (London)*, *251*, 385-388.

Lowry, O.H., N.J. Rosebrough, A.L. Farr, and R.J. Randall (1951). Protein Measurement with the Folin-phenol Reagent. *J. Biol. Chem.*, *193*, 265-275.

Lugnier, A.A.J., E.-E. Creppy, M.-A. Le Meur, P. Gerlinger, and G. Dirheimer (1977). Reciprocal Interactions of Ricin from *Ricinus communis* L. Seeds with Eukaryote Ribosomes. *FEBS Lett.*, *76*, 166-172.

Lugnier, A.A.J., and G. Dirheimer (1971). Extraction, Purification et Détermination du Poids Moléculaire de la Ricine, Toxalbumine de *Ricinus communis* L. *C.R. Acad.*

Sci. Paris, *273D*, 704-707.
Skorve, J., A.K. Abraham, S. Olsnes, and A. Pihl (1977). Effect of Abrin on Peptide Chain Initiation. *Eur. J. Biochem.*, *79*, 559-564.
Sonenshein, G.E., and G. Brawerman (1976). Regulation of Immunoglobuline Synthesis in Mouse Myeloma Cells. *Biochemistry*, *15*, 5497-5501.
Thompson, E.B., G.M. Tomkins, and J.F. Curran (1966). Induction of Tyrosine α-ketoglutarate Transaminase by Steroid Hormones in a Newly Established Tissue Culture Cell Line. *Proc. Natl. Acad. Sci. USA*, *56*, 296-303.

EFFECT OF CHOLERA TOXIN ON RICIN ACTIVITY

M. Tomasi, C. Delfini, M. Sargiacomo, M. Cardelli, G. Oberholtzer and G. D'Agnolo

Laboratorio di Biologia Cellulare e Immunologia, Istituto Superiore di Sanità, Roma, Italy

ABSTRACT

The effect of cholera toxin on ricin activity, binding and distribution have been studied in HeLa cells. Cells pre-treated with cholera toxin are more resistant than untreated cells to ricin intoxication and retain appreciable levels of protein synthesis. The protection of protein synthesis afforded by cholera toxin is both time and concentration dependent. Cholera toxin does not affect either ricin binding to the cell or the distribution of ricin on cell membranes. At the same time ricin does not affect the stimulation of adenylate cyclase produced by cholera toxin. The simple occupation by cholera toxin of its receptor sites does not lead to any effect on ricin binding, but it does inhibit the efficiency of the mechanism of ricin uptake into the cell.

KEYWORDS

Cholera toxin, ricin, toxins competition, toxin uptake, penetration mechanism, receptor distribution.

INTRODUCTION

Many efforts have recently been devoted to the understanding of the mechanism by which protein of diverse physiological and pathological activities do enter the cells. Receptor-mediated transport processes, followed by internalization of the protein via pynocitosis, have been described for several hormones (Goldstein and co-workers, 1979). The transport mechanism and the interaction between the receptor and transport process in the case of other well studied proteins, such as ricin, diphteria and cholera toxin remain still unknown.

Cholera toxin, the agent responsible for fluid accumulation in clinical cholera through the stimulation of membrane bound adenylate cyclase, is a protein of 84 000 M.W., composed of three polypeptide chains α, β and γ and has a molecular formula $\alpha\gamma\beta_5$ (Finkelstein, 1973; Gill, 1976; Sigler and co-workers, 1977). Treatment of the toxin with dithiothreitol gives selective reduction of a disulfide bridge, linking two distinct functional regions (Tomasi and co-workers, 1978, 1979), which are consistent with a two step model for the entry of cholera toxin into the cells. The first step involves the binding of the toxin through the $\gamma\beta_5$ region to the oligosaccharide moiety of ganglioside GM1, containing a terminal galactose residue, while the second step the α region penetrates into the membrane and reaches its site of

action. A similar two step mode of entry into the cells has been suggested for other toxins like ricin. Ricin a potent inhibitor of protein synthesis in mammalian cells, is a protein of 66 000 M.W. composed of two polypeptide chains A and B, linked through a disulfide bond (Olsnes and Phil, 1976). The B chain binds the toxin to the cell membrane recognizing receptor sites containing galactose residues and facilitates the penetration of the B chain into the sensitive cells, where it inactivates protein synthesis (Sperti and co-workers, 1973). Thus, cholera toxin and ricin have a similar structure consisting of two functional regions connected to each other by a disulfide bond.
The present paper describes the competition for cell surface receptors of the two toxins, which have a remarkable structural similarity but a different mechanism of action.

MATERIALS AND METHODS

L-4,5-[^{3}H]-Leucine, [^{3}H]-acetic anhydride and the cyclic AMP assay kit were purchased from the Radiochemical Centre (Amersham, England). The tritiated ganglioside GM1, prepared according to Ghidoni, Tettamanti and Zambotti (1976), was the generous gift of prof. G. Tettamanti (Istituto di Chimica Biologica, Università di Milano). Beef brain gangliosides were purchased from Supelco (Bellefonte, Pa., USA). Ricin was prepared according to Nicholson and Blaustein (1972). FITC-Ricin was obtained from Miles Italiana (Milano, Italy). Cholera toxin was purified as previously described (Tomasi and co-workers, 1979). [^{3}H]-acetyl derivatives of both toxins were prepared according to the method of Riordan and Vallee (1972).
HeLa cells were maintained in monolayer in Eagle medium (MEM) containing 10% fetal calf serum as described by Benedetto and co-workers (1972). Serum-free MEM containing 2 µg of cholera toxin per ml was added to the confluent monolayers in 24-well tissue culture Limbro plates. After 30 min, at 37°C, each well was washed three times with the serum free MEM and was additioned with ricin at the concentrations indicated in the single experiments. After 3 h at 37°C the cells, washed three times with the serum free medium, were exposed to 1.5 ml per well of [^{3}H]-leucine (0.05 µCi/ml), and further incubated for 1 h. After the incubation, monolayers were washed five times with 0.9% (w/v) NaCl and extracted with 0.2 ml of 2% (w/v) sodium dodecyl sulfate. This extract was precipitated with 10% (vol/vol) trichloroacetic acid, collected on Millipore filters, and counted for radioactivity after addition of 10 ml of Aquasol 2 (New England Nuclear, Dreieichenhain, FRG) in a Packard Tri Carb liquid scintillation spectrometer. The amount of radioactivity incorporated indicated the HeLa cells (total) protein synthesis. In additional determinations the amounts of cholera toxin employed and the time intervals of incubation were as indicated in the single experiments. Functional incorporation of gangliosides into cell membranes was achieved by exposing the monolayers to serum-free MEM supplemented with various concentrations of ganglioside (0-10 µg/ml), for 1 h at 37°C (Callies and co-workers, 1977). For cyclic AMP determinations, HeLa monolayers containing approximately 2 x 10^6 cells in 25 cm^2 Falcon bottles, were scraped from the bottles with a rubber policeman in the presence of ethanol and the resulting suspension was dried under vacuum. Cyclic AMP levels were determined on the residue, dissolved in 1 ml of water, using the cyclic AMP assay kit.

RESULTS AND DISCUSSION

The earliest demonstrable effect of ricin, acting directly on the 60 S ribosomal subunits, on HeLa cells in culture is the inhibition of protein synthesis (Sperti and co-workers, 1973; Olsnes and Phil, 1976). The monitoring of tritiated leucine incorporation into cellular proteins after addition of cholera toxin to the cell culture medium showed that protein synthesis had become less sensitive to the presence of ricin (Fig. 1).

The protective effect of cholera toxin on ricin-induced inhibition of protein synthesis was maximal at a concentration of 1-2 μg/ml. At higher concentrations cholera toxin itself had an inhibitory effect on protein synthesis (Fig. 2).

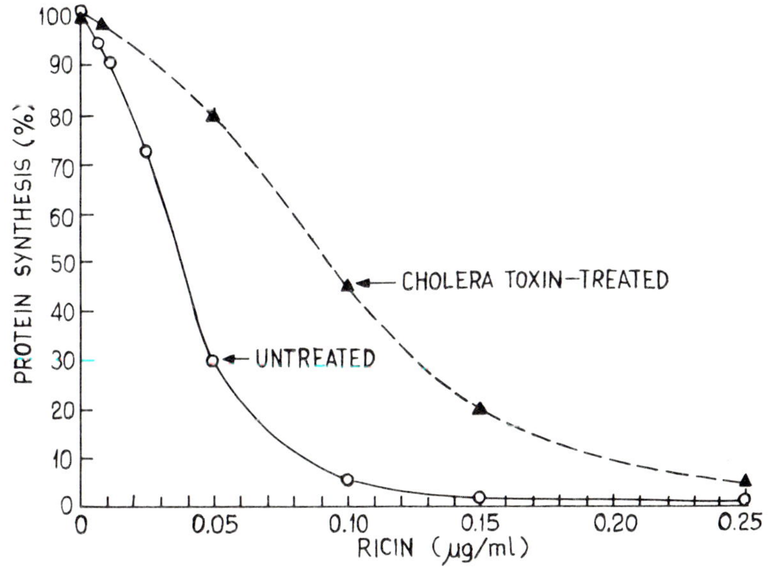

Fig. 1. Protection effect of cholera toxin on ricin-induced inhibition of protein synthesis.

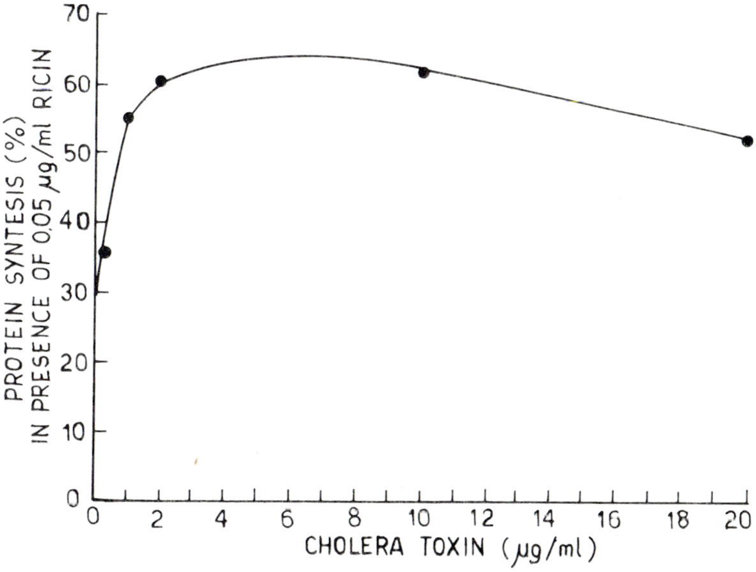

Fig. 2. Effect of cholera toxin on protein synthesis.

As previously described (Hollenberg and Cuatrecasas, 1973), cholera toxin does not contribute directly to the inhibition of protein synthesis but through a block of DNA synthesis. This is not surprising since there is an inverse correlation between the level of cyclic AMP, increased after incubation with cholera toxin, and the level of DNA synthetic activity. In this line, it should be also noted that the level of cyclic AMP reaches a maximum in about 3 h, while the protective effect of cholera toxin, after a 10 min lag period, increases and levels off in about 30 min (Fig. 3).

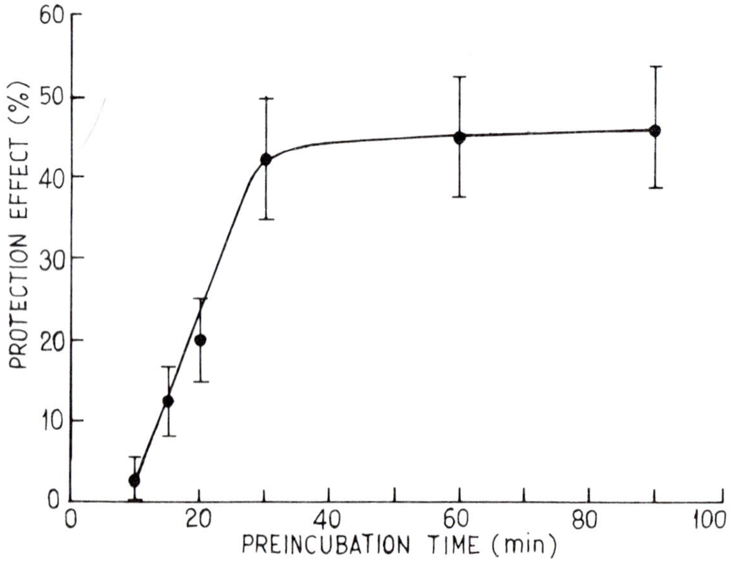

Fig. 3. Time dependence of protection effect.

The magnitude of protection appeared similar in HeLa cells that were pre-incubated, for 1 h, with ricin prior to the addition of cholera toxin. In addition incubation of HeLa cells with ricin decreases 2-fold their cyclic AMP level (Gasperi-Campani, personal communication). Although a direct comparison was not made, it appears from our data that there is no clear correlation between the protective effect of cholera toxin and time-dependent course of cyclic AMP concentration in cells treated with both toxin.

In order to verify if the amount of cholera toxin, associated to the cell surface, affects the protection from ricin inhibition of protein synthesis, experiments were performed with different cellular concentrations of gangliosides. When the cell membrane was supplemented with different amounts of GM1 or of a mixture of beef brain gangliosides, no effect on the protection from ricin activity was observed both before and after the addition of cholera toxin. The functional incorporation of gangliosides into the cells correlates well with the amount of bound cholera toxin. However, preliminary data show that cholera toxin treated cells bind substancially as much ricin as untreated ones. Moreover the binding of ricin is very fast reaching a final binding level in a few minutes both in presence and in absence of cholera toxin, these results show that cholera toxin does not inhibit the action of ricin by competing for ricin receptor sites.

Since the protective action of cholera toxin cannot be attributed to a block of ricin initial binding, its effects on longer incubation times were investigated. In fact, several changes in membrane structure and function have been described in cells exposed to cholera toxin for longer incubation times (Bennet and Cuatrecasas, 1976). These include redistribution phenomena, i.e. "patching" of cholera toxin-receptor complexes and modification of the membrane permeability to ions (Hansson, Holmgren and Svennerholm, 1977; Tosteson and Tosteson, 1978). Thus protection could result from the redistribution in the membrane of cholera toxin-receptor complexes, which may partially influence the affinity of ricin for its receptor sites. In order to verify this hypothesis we have determined the amount of ricin bound in cholera toxin treated cells. We found in cells exposed to cholera toxin an amount of ricin binding equivalent to that of untreated cells. However, experiments with fluorescein-labelled ricin showed that in control cells ricin is more homogeneously distributed on the cell surface than in cells preincubated with cholera toxin (Fig. 4).

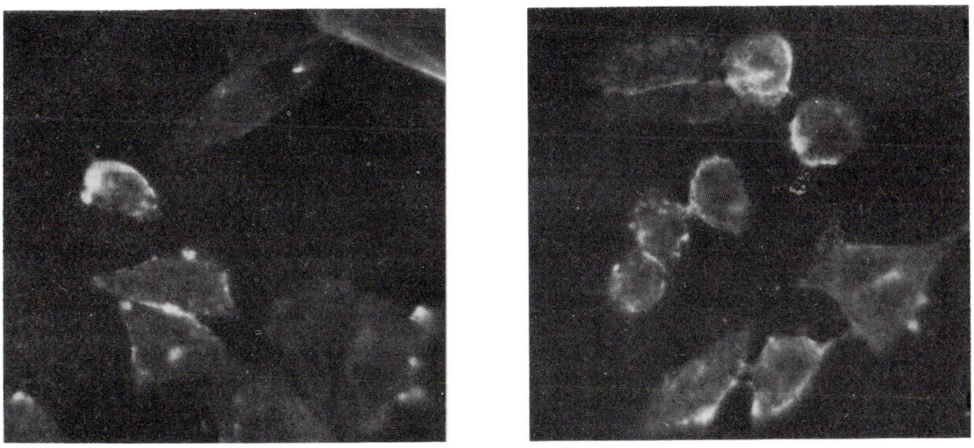

Treated Untreated

Fig. 4. Distribution of fluorescein-labelled ricin.

This suggests that the ability of cholera toxin to prevent ricin activity on protein synthesis is not directly related to its ability to induce "patching" and "capping" of the ganglioside receptors. A more likely explanation consistent with our data is that cholera toxin decreases the efficiency of ricin uptake mechanism into the cell.

REFERENCES

Benedetto, A., Delfini, C., Puledda, S., and A. Sebastiani (1972). Actinomycin D binding to 37 RC and HeLa cell lines. Biochim. Biophys. Acta, 287, 330-339.

Bennet, V., and P. Cuatrecasas (1977). Cholera toxin: membrane gangliosides and activation of adenylate cyclase. In P. Cuatrecasas (Ed.), The Specificity and Action of Animal, Bacterial and Plant Toxins, Chapman and Hall, London. pp. 3--65.

Callies, R., Schwarzmann, G., Radsak, K., Siegerd, R., and H. Wiegandt (1977). Characterization of the cellular binding of exogeneous gangliosides. Eur. J. Biochem., 80, 425-432.

Finkelstein, R. A. (1973). Cholera. CRC Crit. Rev. Microbiol., 2, 553-632.

Ghidoni, R., Tettamanti, G., and V. Zambotti (1974). An improved procedure for the in vitro labelling of ganglioside. Ital. J. Biochem., 23, 320-328.

Gill, D. M. (1976). The arrangement of subunits in cholera toxin. Biochemistry, 15, 1242-1248.

Goldstein, J. L., Anderson, R. G. W., and M. S. Brown (1979). Coated pits, coated vesicles, and receptor-mediated endocytosis. Nature (London), 279, 679-685.

Hansson, H. A., Holmgren, J., and L. Svennerholm (1977). Ultrastructural localization of cell membrane GM1 ganglioside by cholera toxin. Proc. Nat. Acad. Sci. USA, 74, 3782-3786.

Nicholson, G. L., and J. Blaustein (1972). The interaction of Ricinus comunis agglutinin with normal and tumor cell surfaces. Biochim. Biophys. Acta, 266, 543-547.

Olsnes, S., and A. Phil (1977). Abrin, ricin and their associated agglutinins. In P. Cuatrecasas (Ed.), The Specificity and Action of Animal, Bacterial and Plant Toxins, Chapman and Hall, London. pp. 129-173.

Riordan, J. F., and B. L. Vallee (1972). Acetylation. In C. H. W. Hirs, and S. N. Timasheff (Eds.), Methods in Enzymology, Vol. XXV, Academic Press, New York. pp. 494-499.

Sigler, P. B., Druyan, M. E., Kiefer, H. C., and R. A. Finkelstein (1977). Cholera toxin crystals suitable for X-ray diffraction. Science (Wash.), 197, 1277--1279.

Sperti, S., Montanaro, L., Mattioli, A., and F. Stirpe (1973). Inhibition by ricin of protein synthesis in vitro: 60 S ribosome subunits as the target of the toxin. Biochem. J., 136, 813-815.

Tomasi, M., Battistini, A., Ausiello, C., Roda, L.G., and G. D'Agnolo (1978). The role of environmental parameters on the stability of cholera toxin functional regions. FEBS Lett., 94, 253-256.

Tomasi, M., Battistini, A., Araco, A., Roda, L. G., and G. D'Agnolo (1979). The role of the reactive disulfide bond in the interaction of cholera toxin functional regions. Eur. J. Biochem., 93, 621-627.

Tosteson, M. T., and D. C. Tosteson (1978). Bilayers containing gangliosides develop channels when exposed to cholera toxin. Nature (London), 275, 142-144.

RECEPTOR-MEDIATED BINDING AND INTERNALIZATION OF *PSEUDOMONAS* EXOTOXIN A AND DIPHTHERIA EXOTOXIN BY MAMMALIAN CELLS

J. L. Middlebrook, R. B. Dorland, S. H. Leppla and J. D. White

United States Army Medical Research Institute of Infectious Diseases, Frederick, Maryland 21701, USA

ABSTRACT

The uptake of diphtheria toxin (DE) or Pseudomonas exotoxin A (PE) by toxin-sensitive cultured cell lines was studied. At 4C, DE binding increased with time to a steady state; autoradiographic studies demonstrated that the label was distributed randomly at or on the plasma membrane. At 37C, the binding kinetics followed a biphasic pattern, reaching a maximum at 1-2h and subsequently decreasing. Assays were developed to measure toxin internalization and degradation and the effects of drugs on these processes are described. Concanavalin A prevented DE internalization, while chloroquine, a potent lysosomotropic agent, blocked DE degradation and/or excretion. Both compounds protected cells from the cytotoxic effects of DE. At 4C, radiolabeled PE binding to L929 cells increased with time and was blocked 30-40 per cent by excess unlabeled PE. At 37C, uptake was much greater and more specific. Immunochemical and autoradiographic studies demonstrated that at 4C, PE was localized at or on the plasma membrane in regions identified as "coated pits".

KEYWORDS

Diphtheria toxin; Pseudomonas exotoxin A; receptor; binding; internalization; concanavalin A; chloroquine; coated pits; mammalian cells.

INTRODUCTION

Diptheria toxin (DE) and Pseudomonas exotoxin A (PE), protein exotoxins produced respectively by Corynebacterium diphtheriae and Pseudomonas aeruginosa, share a number of structural and biochemical properties. The toxins have identical enzymatic activities (Iglewski and Kabat, 1975). Both toxins are secreted in the form of proenzymes by the bacteria and undergo an activation process prior to expression of cytotoxicity in mammalian cells. Diphtheria toxin is converted to an active form by proteolytic cleavage or "nicking" followed by disulfide bond reduction (Collier, 1975). PE can be activated by either proteolytic cleavage or by simultaneous treatment with denaturing agent and reductant (Leppla, Martin and Muehl, 1978). In either case, these toxins (or their active fragments) must enter the cytoplasm in order to express their cytotoxic activity. All available evidence suggests that this is a receptor-mediated process. In this report, we present data on the binding of DE and PE to receptors on cultured cells.

MATERIALS AND METHODS

Cells and Reagents

Seed stocks of the L-929 and Vero cells were obtained from the American Type Culture collection and cultured as recommended. Concanavalin A was purchased from Pharmacia and "low pH" $Na^{125}I$, from New England Nuclear. All other chemicals were reagent grade obtained from commercial sources.

Toxins

Diphtheria toxin was purchased from Connaught Laboratories and purified by previously described methods (Middlebrook, Dorland and Leppla, 1978). Labeling with ^{125}I was carried out using Chloramine T (Middlebrook, Dorland and Leppla, 1978). Pseudomonas exotoxin was produced and purified in this laboratory (Leppla, 1976) and was labeled with ^{125}I employing lactoperoxidase (Marchalonis, 1969).

Assays

Total cell-associated radiolabeled toxin was measured by a previously described method (Middlebrook, Dorland and Leppla, 1978). Details on the assay employed to distinguish between cell surface-bound and internalized DE will be published elsewhere (Dorland, Middlebrook and Leppla, 1979). Briefly, after binding with radiolabeled toxin under the conditions stipulated, the cells were washed and incubated with a mixture of pronase (2.5 mg/ml) and inositol hexaphosphate (10 mg/ml) (PIHP) for 1 hr at 0C. The detached cells were then centrifuged and both pellet (internalized) and supernatant (cell surface) radioactivity were counted. Degradation and excretion of DE was measured by preincubating cells with radiolabeled DE, washing away unbound toxin and adding back fresh medium. At the indicated times, the culture medium was removed, mixed with an equal volume of 10 per cent trichloroacetic acid (TCA) and centrifuged. An aliquot of the resulting (TCA-soluble) supernatant was then assayed for radioactivity (Dorland, Middlebrook and Leppla, 1979). Effects of toxins on cellular protein synthesis were measured as previously described (Middlebrook, Dorland and Leppla, 1979).

Autoradiography was carried out by incubating radiolabeled PE or DE with cells as indicated, washing away unbound toxin and fixing with 2% gluteraldehyde. Samples were processed using the methods described by Gorden and co-workers (1978). After 21 days exposure, grids were developed and examined in a JEOL-JEM 100 B electron microscope at 10,000 magnification.

Immunochemical staining for electron microscopy was performed by the method of Sternberger (1973). After incubation of L-929 cells with PE, unbound toxin was washed away and the cells fixed with 2% gluteraldehyde. In succession, rabbit anti-PE, goat anti-rabbit and rabbit - PAP (Polysciences) were added followed by diaminobenzidine and H_2O_2. Preparation for microscopy was by standard procedures (Sternberger, 1973).

RESULTS

Figure 1 shows the kinetics of DE-cell association at 4 and 37C. At both

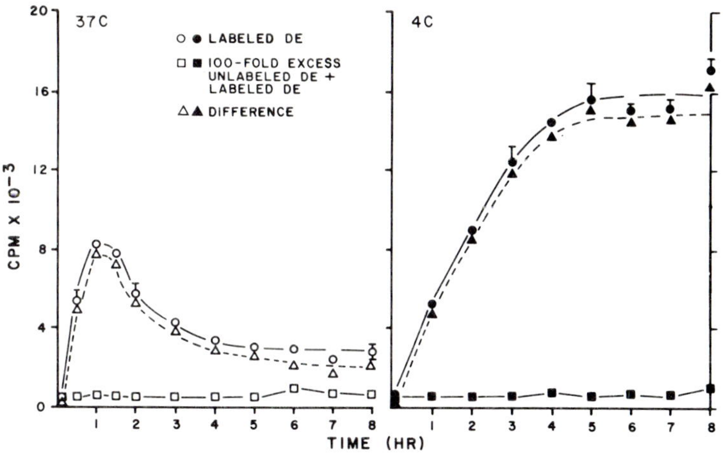

Fig. 1. Kinetics of ^{125}I-DE association with Vero cells (from Middlebrook, Dorland and Leppla, 1978).

temperatures, toxin-cell association was measured with and without an excess of unlabeled toxin, the difference of which is referred to as specific binding. At 4C, association increased with time to a steady state by 4-6h. It is generally believed that, at 4C, binding of DE takes place at the cell surface, but internalization does not proceed. This supposition was supported by an autoradiographic analysis. Figure 2 shows some representative autoradiographs of radiolabeled DE bound to Vero cells at 4C. A majority (60%) of the grains were found randomly distributed at or near the plasma membrane.

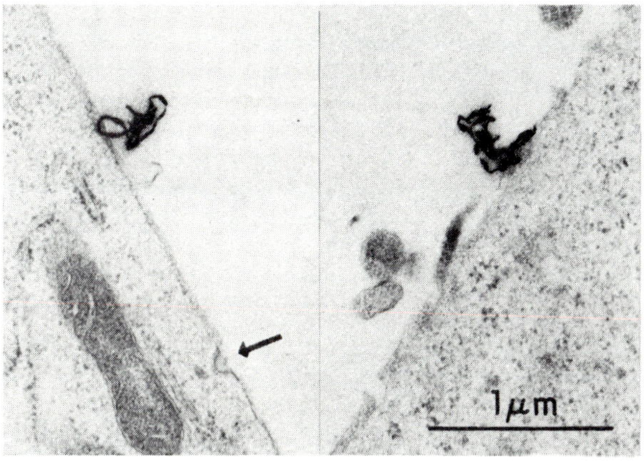

Fig. 2. Autoradiography of ^{125}I-DE bound to Vero cells at 4C. Arrow denotes a coated pit.

At 37C, the kinetics of DE-cell association were biphasic, increasing for 1-1 1/2h and decreasing thereafter (Fig. 1). At this temperature, DE binds to its receptor and is internalized. An assay was developed which allows a distinction between cell surface and internalized DE (Dorland, Middlebrook and Leppla, 1979). After washing away unbound toxin, cells were treated with PIHP (see Materials and Methods) a process which removes toxin bound at the cell surface. At 4C (Fig. 3),

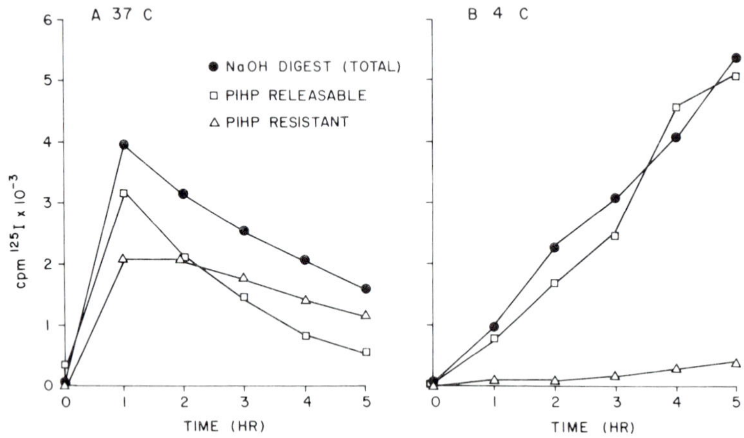

Fig. 3. Differentiation of cell surface bound from internalized DE (from Dorland, Middlebrook and Leppla, 1979).

little or no specific radioactivity was found in the PIHP resistant (pellet) fraction, i.e., no internalization. At 37C, even at early time points a significant portion of the total radioactivity was PIHP resistant; later on, the PIHP resistant fraction predominated (Fig. 3).

The PIHP assay proved useful in determining the mechanism of concanavalin A (Con A) protection from DE. Previous workers (Draper, Chin and Simon, 1978) had found that Con A protected Chinese hamster V79 cells from DE. However, there was some uncertainty as to whether Con A blocked the binding or internalization of DE. Using the PIHP assay, we were able to show that Con A has no effect on the binding of DE at 4C (Fig. 4A and B). However, at 37C the pattern of cell surface and internalized radioactivity was altered by Con A into essentially that seen at 4C (Fig. 4C and D). It appears, therefore, that Con A protects cells from DE by retarding internalization of the toxin. This conclusion was further supported by an autoradiographic study. We found only 10% of the cell-associated grains were plasma membrane localized after 2h incubation of Vero cells with radiolabeled DE at 37C; when Con A (100 μg/ml) was present, that figure increased to 61%.

At 37C, cell associated radiolabeled DE increases then decreases as a function of time (Fig. 1). One likely explanation for this pattern is a sequential binding, internalization and excretion of the toxin or toxin fragments. We examined the nature of radioactivity released from cells which had been bound with radiolabeled DE and found it to be primarily TCA soluble. Chromatography proved the radiolabel to be monoiodotyrosine, indicating extensive cellular degradation of DE (Dorland, Middlebrook and Leppla, 1979). The extent and rapidity of breakdown and excretion suggested lysosomal involvement so we examined the effects of chloroquine, a potent lysosomotropic drug, on this process. The results (Fig. 5) demonstrated that chloroquine markedly inhibits the excretion of TCA soluble radioactivity. When chloroquine was subsequently tested in a protein synthesis-based toxicity assay, the drug proved to be a potent protective agent from DE (Fig. 6).

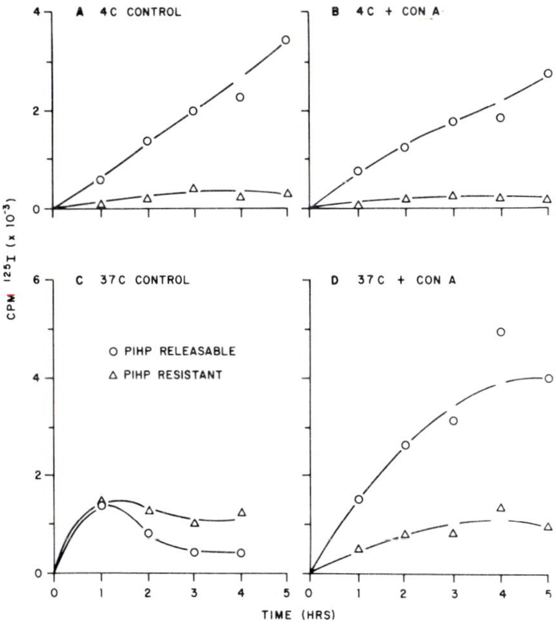

Fig. 4. Effect of Con A on DE internalization by Vero cells (from Middlebrook, Dorland and Leppla, 1979).

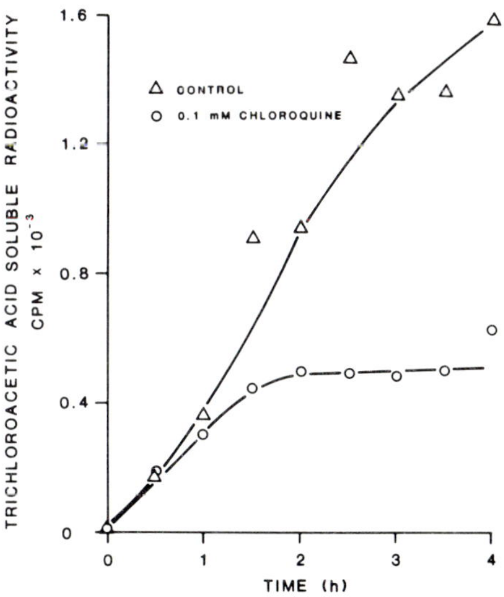

Fig. 5. Effect of chloroquine on DE degradation and excretion by Vero cells.

Figure 7 shows the kinetics of PE-L-929 cell association at 4 and 37C. Toxin-cell binding proceeded in the cold, but never achieved the levels observed with the DE-Vero cell system. Furthermore, specificity of the interaction, as judged by competition with a 100 fold excess of unlabeled PE, was low, at best only 30-40%. At 37C, the magnitude of association was much greater, as was the specificity, 60-70%.

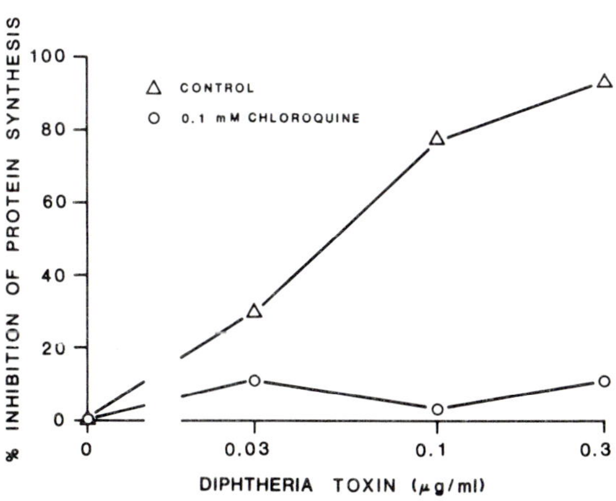

Fig. 6. Chloroquine protection of Vero cells from DE.

Autoradiography of PE bound to L-929 cells at 4C showed that most of the cell-associated grains were at the cell membrane usually in the region of membrane substructures called "coated pits" (Fig. 8). The localization of PE binding in coated pits was shown much more clearly by an immunochemical staining procedure developed by Sternberger (1973). The electron dense staining product can readily be seen concentrated in coated pits (Fig. 9).

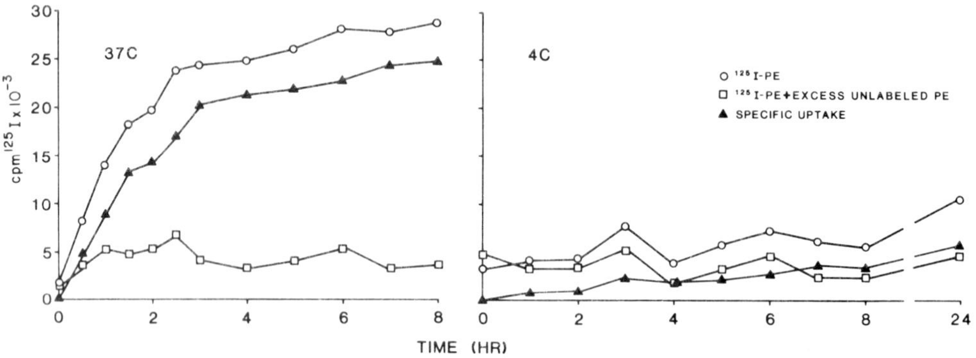

Fig. 7. Kinetics of ^{125}I-PE association with L-929 cells.

DISCUSSION

In these studies, investigation of the mechanism of cellular intoxication by diphtheria or Pseudomonas exotoxin was approached by a variety of biochemical and morphological methods. In the case of diphtheria toxin, a receptor-mediated internalization and degradation process was identified that appears to be directly

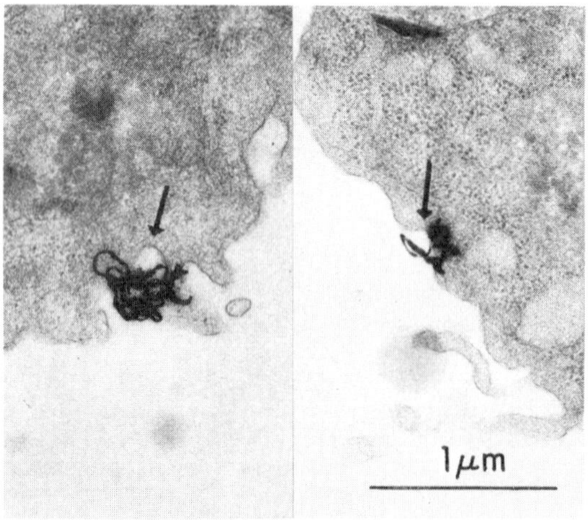

Fig. 8. Autoradiography of ^{125}I-PE bound to L-929 cells at 4C. Arrows denote coated pits.

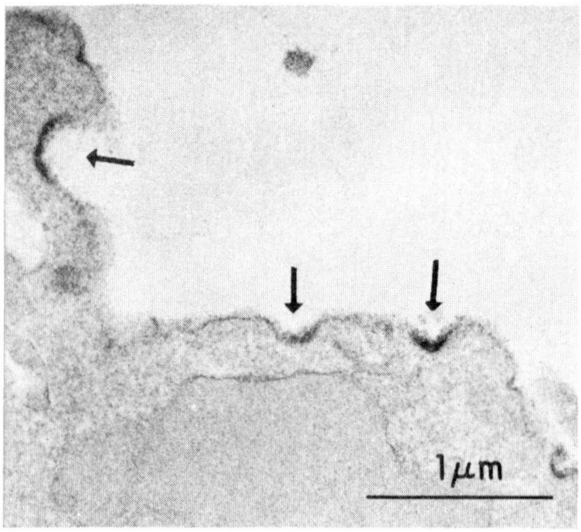

Fig. 9. Immunochemical staining of PE bound to L-929 cells at 4C. Arrows denote coated pits.

related to the expression of cytotoxicity. Binding of ^{125}I-labeled DE to highly sensitive Vero cells is specific (Fig. 1) and in previous studies (Middlebrook, Dorland and Leppla, 1978) has been shown to involve a biologically relevant receptor. We hypothesized that DE might parasitize receptors for some component normally taken up by the cell, such as a hormone or growth factor. Accordingly, we tested a number of hormones, growth factors, and related compounds for their ability to block diphtheria toxin-cell binding. No effect was observed with excess molar concentrations of insulin, glucagon, FSH, TSH, hCG, LH, ACTH, epidermal growth factor, somatostatin, thrombin, angiotensin, prolactin, growth hormone, placental lactogen, or PE (data not shown).

At 37C, the kinetics of DE binding are biphasic (Fig. 1), increasing to a peak at 1-2 hr and subsequently decreasing to a steady state. The basis for this pattern is unclear. One hypothesis is that the curve represents sequential binding, internalization, and degradation of radiolabeled toxin; the eventual decrease in cell-associated radioactivity results from excretion of degraded toxin fragments into the culture medium. Therefore, at physiological temperature, the measured cell-associated radioactivity presumably includes both surface receptor-bound and internalized toxin molecules. This is demonstrated in Fig. 3, using the PIHP assay which differentiates between surface-bound and internalized DE. At 4C, total cell-associated radioactivity increased with time but remained completely releasable by PIHP treatment, indicating that at this temperature essentially all the toxin molecules are on the cell surface. At 37C, however, the increase in PIHP-releasable radioactivity was accompanied by a substantial increase in PIHP-resistant radioactivity, indicating progressive internalization. Continued incubation at 37C resulted in a loss of radioactivity from the cells, as internalized toxin was degraded intracellularly and excreted into the culture medium.

The relevance of this internalization/degradation process to the expression of cytotoxicity was confirmed using drugs which appear to block specific steps in the uptake pathway. Concanavalin A (Con A) was found to effectively block the internalization of diphtheria toxin as determined by the PIHP assay (Fig. 4) and autoradiographic techniques. Since Con A at this concentration (100 μg/ml) protects cells from the cytotoxic effects of DE, it appears that the observed internalization process is required for cytotoxicity.

Similarly, intracellular degradation of internalized toxin is apparently related in some manner to expression of cytotoxic activity. It was found that the potent lysosomotropic agent, chloroquine, markedly protected cells from DE (Fig. 6). At the protective concentration, chloroquine did not affect either toxin-receptor binding or internalization, but blocked toxin degradation (Fig. 5). Since chloroquine acts as an inhibitor of lysosomal function, it appears that a degradation or processing step by the lysosomes is an essential stage in the cytotoxic pathway.

In general, the results obtained with DE are consistent with a receptor-mediated uptake process. In many respects, this process corresponds to receptor-mediated endocytosis, a mechanism by which a number of polypeptide hormones, growth factors, and other biologically active macromolecules are taken up by sensitive cells. One of the best documented instances of receptor-mediated endocytosis has been described by Goldstein, Anderson and Brown (1979) in their studies of low-density lipoprotein uptake. Low-density lipoprotein (LDL) was shown to bind to specific receptors localized in coated pit regions of the plasma membrane in human fibroblast or vascular endothelial cells. Coated pits containing LDL-receptor complexes regularly invaginate to form cytoplasmic coated vesicles which subsequently lose their coats and fuse with lysosomes. Degradation of LDL with concomitant release of free cholesterol occurred intralysosomally. While our autoradiographic study showed that the DE receptor was apparently not prelocalized in coated pits, this observation does not rule out localization of the DE-receptor complex in coated pits after binding. Indeed, that sequence of events has been reported for several hormones and macromolecules (Maxfield and others, 1979).

Results obtained with PE were somewhat less clear. Though an assay was developed to study the uptake of ^{125}I-labeled PE by sensitive mouse L-929 cells (Fig. 7), interpretation of results was complicated by a high level of nonspecific binding. Morphological methods, including immunochemical staining (Fig. 8) and autoradiography (Fig. 9) showed that PE bound to cells at 4C was localized in coated pits on the plasma membrane. This observation implies that cellular intoxication by PE may also proceed via receptor-mediated endocytosis.

REFERENCES

Collier, R. J. (1975). Diphtheria toxin: mode of action and structure. Bacteriol. Rev., 39, 54-85.

Dorland, R. B., J. L. Middlebrook, and S. H. Leppla (1979). Receptor-mediated internalization and degradation of diphtheria toxin by mammalian cells. J. Biol. Chem., 254, 11337-11342.

Draper, R. K., D. Chin, and M. I. Simon (1978). Diphtheria toxin has the properties of a lectin. Proc. Natl. Acad. Sci., 75, 261-265.

Goldstein, J. L., R. G. W. Anderson and M. S. Brown (1979). Coated pits, coated vesicles, and receptor-mediated endocytosis. Nature, 279, 679-685.

Gordon, P., J. L. Carpenter, S. Cohen and L. Orci (1978). Epidermal growth factor: Morphological demonstration of binding, internalization, and lysosomal association in human fibroblasts. Proc. Natl. Acad. Sci., 75, 5025-5029.

Iglewski, B. H., and D. Kabat (1975). NAD-dependent inhibition of protein synthesis by Pseudomonas aeruginosa toxin. Proc. Natl. Acad. Sci., 72, 2284-2288.

Leppla, S. H. (1976). Large-scale purification and characterization of the exotoxin of Pseudomonas aeruginosa. Infect. Immunity, 14, 1077-1086.

Leppla, S. H., O. C. Martin, and L. A. Muehl (1978). The exotoxin of P. aeruginosa: a proenzyme having an unusual mode of activation. Biochem. Biophys. Res. Commun., 81, 532-538.

Marchalonis, J. J. (1969). An enzymic method for the trace iodination of immunoglobulins and other proteins. Biochem. J., 113, 299-305.

Maxfield, F. R., M. C. Willingham, P. J. A. Davies and I. Pastan (1979). Amines inhibit the clustering of α_2-macroglobulin and EGF on the fibroblast cell surface. Nature, 277, 661-663.

Middlebrook, J. L., R. B. Dorland and S. H. Leppla (1978). Association of diphtheria toxin with Vero cells. Demonstration of a receptor. J. Biol. Chem., 253, 7325-7330.

Middlebrook, J. L., R. B. Dorland and S. H. Leppla (1979). Effects of lectins on the interaction of diphtheria toxin with mammalian cells. Exp. Cell. Res., 121, 95-101.

Sternberger, L. A. (1973). Enzyme Immunocytochemistry, Electron Microscopy of Enzymes, Principles and Methods. Van Nostrand/Reinhold Co., 150-192.

SHIGELLA SHIGAE CYTOTOXIN. ISOLATION, CHARACTERIZATION AND INTERACTION WITH CELLS

S. Olsnes*, K. Eiklid* and J. Jonsen**

**Norsk Hydro's Institute for Cancer Research, Montebello, Oslo 3, Norway*
***Department of Microbiology, Dental Faculty, University of Oslo, Norway*

ABSTRACT

A procedure was developed for isolation of a cytotoxin produced by Shigella shigae. Advantage was taken of the fact that the toxin binds strongly to a column of acid-treated chitin. The toxin was eluted with 1 M NaCl and further purified by chromatography on DE-52 and by sucrose gradient centrifugation. The toxin was found to consist of two kinds of peptide chains with molecular weights of 30,500 and 11,000. Different cell lines varied considerably in sensitivity to the toxin. Sensitive HeLa S_3 cells were found to bind about 10^6 molecules ^{125}I-labelled toxin per cell with a K_a of about 10^{10} M^{-1}. Resistant HeLa cells contained about 10^5 binding sites with the same affinity.

KEYWORDS

Shigella shigae, dysentery, toxin, receptors, chitin.

INTRODUCTION

In the pathogenesis of dysentery caused by Shigella shigae two properties of the bacterium are apparently involved, viz. its ability to enter epithelial cells of the colon and to produce a cytocidal toxin (van Heyningen and Gladstone, 1953, Rout and collegues, 1975). The toxin has been partially purified in several laboratories (van Heyningen and Gladstone, 1953, Vicari, Olitzki and Olitzki, 1960, McIver, Grady and Keusch, 1975) and there is evidence that it binds to receptors on sensitive cells. These receptors apparently involve 1-4-linked N-acetyl-D-glucosamine oligomers (Keusch and Jacewicz, 1977). We have purified the toxin and studied its properties and interaction with cells.

MATERIALS AND METHODS

A partially purified preparation of Shigella shigae toxin was a kind gift from dr. W.E. van Heyningen, Oxford (van Heyningen and Gladstone, 1953). This material had been stored in lyophilized state at -20° since 1953. It was dissolved in 5 mM Na-phosphate (pH 7.4), 0.14 M NaCl before use and undissolved material was removed by low speed centrifugation. Another sample was obtained by concentrating culture medium after growth of Shigella shigae. The concentration was carried out by pressure dialysis on Amicon PM 10 (Amicon Ltd., Oosterhout, Holland). The concentrated material was dialyzed against 5 mM Na-phosphate (pH 7.4) containing 50 mM NaCl.

Crab shell chitin (purified, obtained from Sigma Chemical Co., St. Louis, Mo.) was treated with 5% acetic acid and fine particles were removed. It was packed into small columns (2 ml of packed chitin each) and washed with 10 bed volumes of a solution containing 50 mM NaCl and 5 mM Na-phosphate (pH 7.4) before use.

Cells were maintained in monolayer cultures in Eagle's Minimum Essential medium containing 10% calf serum as described (Sandvig, Olsnes and Pihl, 1976). For toxicity tests the cells were seeded into Linbro tissue culture plates with 16 mm troughs and increasing amounts of toxin were added to the wells. The next day the medium was removed, replaced by medium containing reduced concentration of unlabelled leucine and 0.5 µCi/ml of $[^{14}C]$leucine and the incorporation of radioactivity into acid precipitable material was measured as earlier described (Sandvig, Olsnes and Pihl, 1976).

Partially purified Shigella shigae toxin was radioiodinated using the lactoperoxidase method (Marchalonis, 1969) or the Bolton-Hunter reagent (Bolton and Hunter, 1973).

To measure binding of labelled toxin to cells, increasing amounts of ^{125}I-labelled toxin were added to cells growing in Linbro tissue culture plates or to cells in suspension and after incubation for 60 min at 0°, the medium was removed, the cells rapidly washed with 1 ml Hanks' solution, dissolved in 0.1 M KOH and the radioactivity was measured.

Polyacrylamide gel electrophoresis was carried out in 10-20% exponential gradient gel slabs using the buffers of Laemmli (1970).

RESULTS

Crude toxin was first applied to a column of acid treated chitin at low salt concentration (50 mM NaCl). Most of the protein passed through the column, whereas some material was retained and could be eluted with 1 M NaCl (Fig. 1). This material contained about 60% of the toxic activity. The protein eluted from the chitin

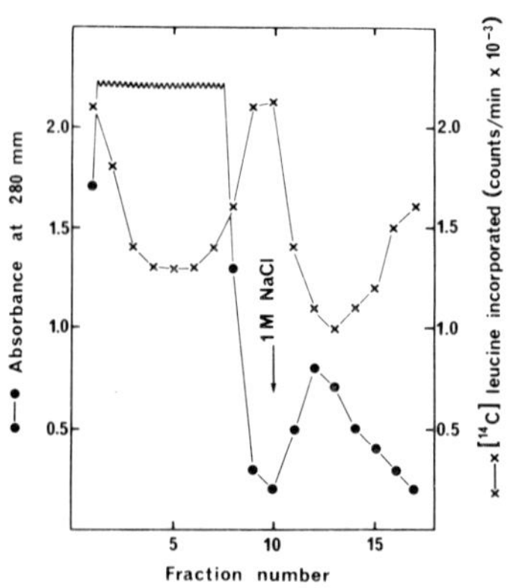

Fig. 1 Chromatography of crude Shigella toxin on a column

of acid treated chitin. Shigella toxin (50 mg), partially purified as described by van Heyningen and Gladstone (1953), was applied at room temperature to a 2 ml column of chitin, pretreated as described in Materials and Methods, and, after washing with 3 ml 5 mM Na-phosphate (pH 7.5), 50 mM NaCl, the adsorbed material was eluted with 1 M NaCl in the same buffer. The eluted material was transferred to a dialysis bag which was first incubated with dry polyethylene glycol to reduce the volume to about 0.3 ml and then dialyzed against 0.1 M Na-phosphate (pH 7.5 The material was labelled with ^{125}I using the lactoperoxidase method. The specific activity obtained was 500 counts/min/ng protein. The labelled material was once more applied to a chitin column and bound material was eluted with 1 M NaCl. Finally, 70 µg rabbit hemoglobin was added to each tube. To cells growing in Linbro FB 16-24 TC trays (10^5 cells/well) were added 1 µl of each fraction. The plates were incubated for 20 h, the medium was then removed and 0.5 ml of low leucine medium was added to each well together with 0.05 µCi [^{14}C] leucine and the incubation was continued for one hour more. Finally, the medium was removed, the cells were dissolved in 1 ml of 0.1 M KOH and the acid precipitable radioactivity was measured.

column with 1 M NaCl consisted of several protein species. Due to the small amounts of material it was radioiodinated and then mixed with unlabelled rabbit hemoglobin to protect the toxin during the further purification steps. The material was then resubmitted to affinity chromatography on a chitin column. About half of the labelled protein was bound to the column and was eluted with 1 M NaCl.

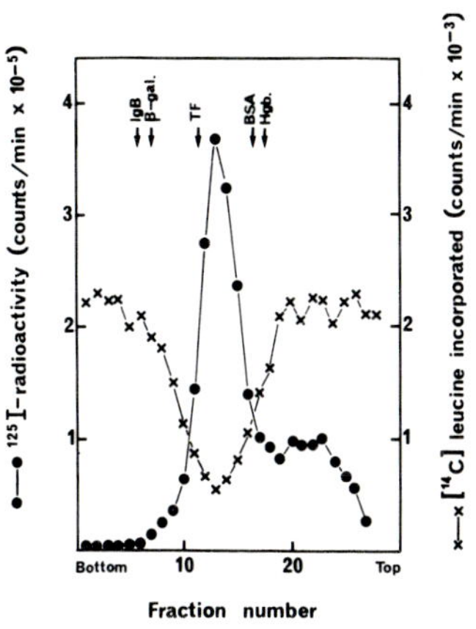

Fig. 2. Sucrose gradient centrifugation of ^{125}I-labelled Shigella toxin. Material eluted from the DE-52 column at NaCl concentrations between 0.08 and 0.12 M was concentrated and layered onto a 5 ml sucrose gradient (5-20% w/v) in 5 mM Na-phosphate (pH 7.4), 0.14 M NaCl and centrifuged at 230,000 x g_{av} for 14 hours.

Fractions were collected by puncturing the bottom of the tube. Aliquots (1 µl) were added to wells of Linbro plates containing HeLa S_3 cells and inhibition of protein synthesis was measured as described in Fig. 1. The arrows indicate the peak fractions of different marker proteins centrifuged under identical conditions. IgG: Human IgG (MW 150,000); β-gal: β-galactosidase (MW 130,000); TF: Human transferrin (MW 90,000); BSA: Bovine serum albumin (MW 67,000); Hgb: Rabbit hemoglobin (MW 65,000).

The labelled material eluted with 1 M NaCl was dialyzed against 10 mM Tris-HCl (pH 9.0), applied to a DE-52 column and eluted with a linear NaCl gradient. The major part of the toxic material appeared at a concentration of NaCl between 0.08 M and 0.12 M as a rather broad shoulder in the radioactivity profile (not demonstrated). When analyzed by polyacrylamide gel electrophoresis in the presence of sodium dodecyl sulfate, most of the labelled material was found in two bands migrating corresponding to molecular weights of 30,500 and about 11,000. Additional bands of varying intensity were also seen and the toxin was therefore further purified by sucrose gradient centrifugation (Fig. 2). The major peak of radioactivity sedimented slightly more slowly than transferrin and somewhat in front of hemoglobin and serum albumin. A shoulder of labelled material sedimented at a lower rate. Toxicity tests on HeLa S_3 cells clearly showed that toxic material was present in the same fractions as the major radioactivity peak. When the material in the main peak was analyzed by polyacrylamide gel electrophoresis in the presence of sodium dodecyl sulfate, bands of radioactivity (Fig. 3) corresponding to molecular weights of 30,500 and

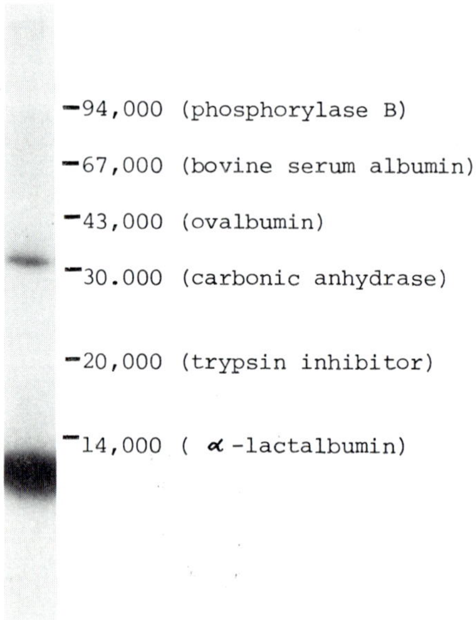

Fig. 3. Polyacylamide gel electrophoresis of Shigella toxin. Isolated Shigella toxin was analyzed by polyacrylamide gel electrophoresis in the presence of sodium dodecyl sulfate in 10-20% exponential gradient gels. The position and molecular weights of marker proteins are indicated by horizontal bars at the edge of the gel.

11,000 were found. In some experiments two additional bands corresponding to molecular weights of about 14,500 and 16,000 were found. There was no difference whether or not the sample had been pretreated with 2-mercaptoethanol. The data thus indicate that the intact toxin consists of 2 or more kinds of polypeptides joined by weak interactions.

To test if both of the two chains are indeed constituent parts of the toxin, labelled toxin was analyzed by polyacrylamide gel electrophoresis in the absence of sodium dodecyl sulfate as well as by gel filtration on Sephacryl 300 superfine. In both cases the material moved as one peak and there was good correlation between the radioactivity and toxic effect (data not shown). Upon gel filtration the toxin eluted in the same fractions as hemoglobin, whereas in sucrose gradients the toxin sedimented clearly in front of hemoglobin. The reason for this discrepancy is not clear. The fact that the heavy and the light chains of the toxins were present in the same relative amounts in all cases clearly demonstrates that both chains are constituent parts of the intact Shigella shigae cytotoxin.

When analyzed by isoelectric focusing Shigella shigae cytotoxin did not focus as one peak, but showed a rather broad distribution between pH 5.5 and 7.5. Two-dimensional gel electrophoresis of the toxin indicated that this is due to charge heterogeneity both in the large chain and in the small chain (A. Sundan, unpublished data).

We accidently observed that while HeLa S_3 cells are very sensitive to Shigella toxin, another strain of HeLa cells was highly resistant. For this reason we studied the sensitivity of various cell lines to the toxin. This was done either by measuring the ability of toxin to inhibit colony formation or by measuring its ability to inhibit the incorporation of $[^{14}C]$leucine into acid precipitable material. As shown in Fig. 4 similar results were were obtained with the two methods although the colony assay system was somewhat more sensitive.

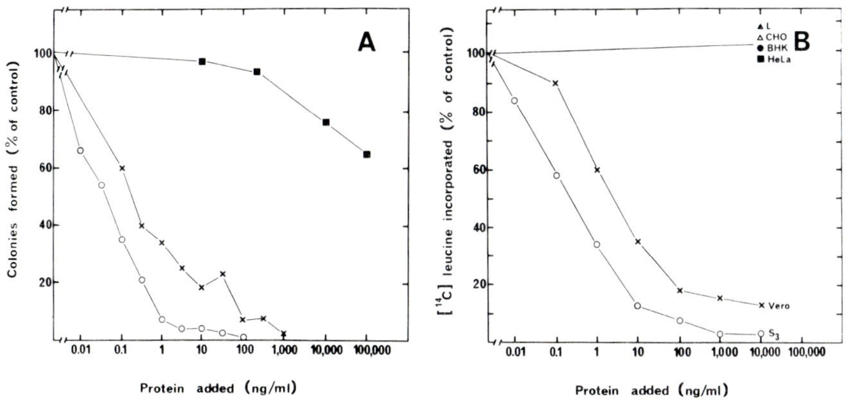

Fig. 4. Ability of crude Shigella toxin to inhibit colony formation (A) and protein synthesis (B) in different cell lines.
(A) Two hundred cells were plated out in the presence of increasing concentrations of toxin. After two weeks the medium was removed and the colonies were fixed and stained.
(B) Increasing amounts of crude Shigella toxin was

added to cells growing in Linbro plates and the ability to inhibit protein synthesis was measured as in Fig. 1. The results are expressed as per cent of the control value (no toxin present) which was about 10,000 counts/min.
(O), HeLa S_3 cells; (△), HeLa cells adapted to suspension culture; (X), Vero cells; (□), CHO-cells; (▲), L-cells; (●), BHK-cells; (■), human melanoma cells.

It is also clear from Fig. 4 that the cells can be classified into two groups, one where the protein synthesis is reduced 50% in the presence of less than 1 ng/ml of crude Shigella toxin and another group which is essentially unaffected in the presence of 10 ug/ml of the crude toxin. (Crude toxin here used contained about 1% pure toxin).

One possible explanation of the difference between different cells lines in their sensitivity to Shigella toxin could be the presence of different numbers of toxin receptors on the cell surface. To test this, we first measured the ability of the sensitive HeLa S_3 cells and the intensitive HeLa cells to absorb Shigella toxin out of solution. After sedimenting the cells we then gauged the amount of toxin remaining in the supernatant by adding increasing amounts to HeLa S_3 cells measuring its ability to inhibit protein synthesis. Is was found that toxin solution pretreated with HeLa S_3 cells had lost most of its toxicity, whereas toxin preincubated with the insensitive HeLa cells showed little reduction in toxicity (not demonstrated). This suggests that only the sensitive HeLa S_3 cells are able to efficiently absorb Shigella toxin out of solution. This is in accordance with earlier findings by Keusch and Jacewicz (1977).

To test in a more sensitive system the ability of cells to bind Shigella toxin increasing numbers of cells were added to a fixed amount of ^{125}I-labelled toxin and the amount of cell-bound radioactivity was measured. It was found that with increasing concentrations of the sensitive HeLa S_3 cells an increasing amount of radioactivity was bound and the curve rapidly levelled off (Fig. 5).

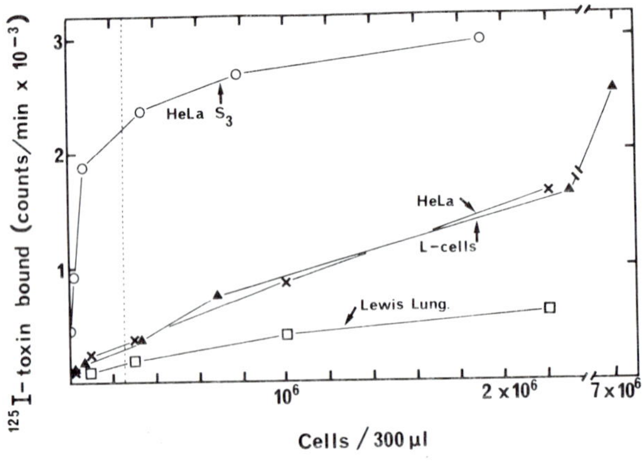

Fig. 5. Ability of different cell lines to bind ^{125}I-labelled Shigella shigae cytotoxin. Cells grown in monolayer

cultures were trypsinized and washed twice with Hanks' solution. To tubes containing 300 ul of Hanks' solution and 100 ug of rabbit hemoglobin were added increasing amounts of cells as indicated and then 6 ng (3,000 counts/min) of ^{125}I-labelled pure Shigella toxin. After mixing, the tubes were incubated for 1 hour at 0° with occasional shaking. Finally, the cells were sedimented by low-speed centrifugation, washed with 1 ml ice-cold Hanks' solution and the amount of radioactivity associated with the cell pellet was measured.
The dashed vertical line indicates for comparison the cell concentration used in Fig. 4 B.

In contrast with the insensitive HeLa cells, L-cells and "Lewis lung "murine carcinoma cells, much more cells must be added to bind the toxin. When binding date were plotted according to Scatchard (1949) it was found that a HeLa S_3 cell containes about 10^6 binding sites whereas an L-cell and a HeLa cell (insensitive) contains about 10^5 sites. In all cases the association constant, K_a, was found to be about 10^{10} M^{-1}.

DISCUSSION

The data presented clearly show that the cytotoxin from Shigella shigae consists of at least two kinds of polypeptides. It is, however, unclear how many chains are present in each molecule of intact toxin. The data obtained from sucrose gradient centrifugation experiments showed that the toxin sediments slightly behind transferrin. This indicates a molecular weight of about 80,000. In contrast to this, the data obtained from gel filtration experiments indicate a molecular weight of approximately 65,000. Attempts to obtain more reliable data on the molecular weight by treating the labelled material with formaldehyde or glutaraldehyde to form covalent linkages between the constituent peptide chains and then analyzing the material by polyacrylamide gel electrophoresis in the presence of sodium dodecyl sulfate, did not give unambiguous results. After this treatment several new bands occurred corresponding to complexes of small and large subunits. The largest complexes seen corresponding to a molecular weight of about 90,000, whereas the major part of the labelled material was found in a zone correponding to molecular weights between 60,000 and 70,000. Most likely the intact toxin consists of one heavy chain (molecular weight 30,500). and 4 or 5 copies of the light chains (molecular weight about 11,000). Obviously further work is required to establish the exact subunit composition of the toxin.

The reason for the great variability in sensitivity of different cell lines cells to the toxin is not clear. Although the sensitive cells contain about ten times more binding sites for the toxin than resistant cells, the affinity of the receptors for the toxin is the same in both groups of cells. This indicates that at least the toxin binding part of the receptors have the same structure. In spite of this the resistant cells tolerate about 10^4 times higher toxin concentrations than the sensitive cells. This indicates that other factors than difference in toxin binding must account for the difference in sensitivity of the cells to the toxin.

It is interesting that out of 15 human cell lines so far tested all sensitive lines are epithelial cells. Also a cell line derived from human cancer of the colon proved to be sensitive (unpublished data). This indicates that also the normal epithelial cells of the colon are sensitive and that the toxin is responsible for the necrosis of the epithelium seen in the colon of patients with *Shigella shigae* dysentery.

The fact that Shigella toxin is lethal to a small number of cell types makes the toxin an interesting candidate for treatment of tumors originating from these cells. Possibly Shigella toxin may have a sufficiently selective effect to be used to induce cell death in tumors of the colon without serious side effects on other cells in the organism.

ACKNOWLEDGEMENT

The authors are indebted to Prof. A. Pihl for his helpful discussion and suggestions. Mrs. Lill Næss provided excellent technical assistance.

This work was supported by The Norwegian Cancer Society.

REFERENCES

Bolton, A. E., and W. M. Hunter (1973). *Biochem. J., 133*, 529-539.
Keusch, G. T., and M. Jacewicz (1977). *J. Exp. Med., 146*, 535-546.
Laemmli, U. K. (1970). *Nature, 227*, 680-685.
Marchalonis, J. J. (1969). *Biochem. J., 133*, 299-305.
McIver, J., G. F. Grady, and G. T. Keusch (1975). *J. Infect. Dis., 131*, 559-566.
Rout, W. R., S. B. Romal, R. A. Gianella, and G. J. Dammin (1975). *Gastroenterology, 68*, 270-278.
Sandvig, K., S. Olsnes, and A. Pihl (1976). *J. Biol. Chem., 251*, 3977-3984.
Scatchard, G. (1949). *Ann. N. Y. Acad. Sci., 51*, 660-672.
van Heyningen, W. E., and G. P. Gladstone (1953). *Br. J. Exp. Pat., 34*, 202-216.
Vicari, G., A. L. Olitzki, and Z. Olitzki (1960). *Br. J. Exp. Pat., 41*, 179-189.

Structure and Function of Polypeptide Neurotoxins

CHEMICAL STRUCTURE, BIOLOGICAL AND PHARMACOLOGICAL ACTIVITIES OF APAMIN, AND THEIR RELATIONS

C. Granier and J. Van Rietschoten

Laboratoire de Biochimie, INSERM U 172, Faculté de Médecine Secteur Nord, Boulevard Pierre Dramard, 13326 Marseille Cedex 3, France.

ABSTRACT

The present knowledge of apamin, the bee-venom neurotoxin, is briefly reviewed : the main fields of investigation in progress are the elucidation of the spatial organization of this eighteen-membered polypeptide, and the understanding of its mode of action. In each domain, interesting but preliminary results are available : neither the exact peptide chain folding nor the true mechanism of poisoning of apamin are known.

Existence in rat brain homogenates of binding sites for apamin has been reported and synthetic analogs of apamin have been tested to find out a possible parallelism between their ability to bind to these sites and their neurotoxicity in mice.

KEYWORDS

Apamin ; neurotoxin ; peptide synthesis ; binding sites ; synthetic apamin analogs ; structure activity relationships.

Apamin, the shortest polypeptide neurotoxin known so far, was purified from bee venom by Habermann (Habermann and Reitz, 1965). Until the middle of the seventies relatively little attention has been drawn to this molecule. However, since 1975 apamin has been considered both as a nice model peptide to check the possibilities of powerful techniques such as peptide synthesis (van Rietschoten and colleagues, 1975) or high field N.M.R. spectroscopy (Bystrov and colleagues, 1978) and as interesting molecular tool, because of its specific action on central nervous system (Habermann and Cheng-Raude, 1975).

H-Cys-Asn-Cys-Lys-Ala-Pro-Glu-Thr-Ala-Leu-Cys-Ala-Arg-Arg-Cys-Gln-Gln-His-NH_2 (disulfide bridges: Cys1–Cys11, Cys3–Cys15; positions 13 and 14 marked)

Fig.1 : Covalent structure of apamin

The size of this relatively small peptide of 18 amino-acids crosslinked by two disulfide bonds (Callewaert and colleagues, 1968 ; Haux and colleagues, 1967 ; Shipolini and colleagues, 1967 ; see Fig. 1) together with its peculiar mode of action promoted this toxin as a challenging target for synthesis. Successful trials were achieved using either the solid phase method (Cosand and Merrifield, 1976 ; van Rietschoten and colleagues, 1975 ; Sandberg and Ragnarsson, 1978) or a fragment condensation approach (Nuriddinov and colleagues, 1978). Despite the large amounts thus available, attempts to crystallize synthetic or natural apamin have failed. Some knowledge of apamin's spatial structure in solution might be acquired by spectroscopic methods. Circular dichroism data of Miroshnikov and co-workers (1978) afforded the first experimental clues for the high stability of this neurotoxin : CD spectra of the peptide are not significantly modified either by large pH variations or by drastic changes in solvent's polarity. Proton N.M.R. study of Bystrov and colleagues (1978) enlarged the knowledge of apamin's conformation. From a complex 300 MHz NMR spectrum, and thanks to the use of sophisticated methods they were able to identify each amide and Cα linked proton, to determine their coupling constants, to study the influence of titratable groups of the molecule on their chemical shifts, and finally, to assess the rate of exchange of each N-H proton with deuterium atoms of surrounding heavy water. Conclusions were : i) apamin possesses a fixed, folded conformation ; ii) many amide protons are not readily exchangeable and are thought to be involved in intramolecular hydrogen bonds ; iii) most of the identified protons are sensitive to the ionization state of titratable groups and likely remained in the close vicinity of these groups. The side chain carboxylate group of Glu^7 seems to have a central position within the folded chain of polypeptide and to be involved in a salt linkage with α -NH_2 group. A schematic model of apamin's peptide backbone is proposed by Bystrov and colleagues, but quantitative data assessing the exact peptide chain folding are not yet available.

The direct action of apamin on central nervous system is now clearly established (Habermann and Cheng-Raude, 1975). When injected by a peripheral route into a test animal, large quantities of peptide are eliminated through the kidneys but trace amounts of apamin are able to cross over the blood-brain barrier and to interact with brain matter, thus inducing the typical symptoms of poisoning that lead to death. Direct, intraventricular injection into the mouse brain of, as little as, 10 picomoles of apamin elicits the same typical symptomatology of poisoning and death. However, attempts have failed to demonstrate an action of this peptide on known biochemical mechanisms of brain such as displacement of specifically bound brain neurotransmitters (Cavey and colleagues, 1979) or change in cAMP or cGMP content of brain slices or influence on Na^+, K^+ ATPase of bovine brain (Habermann and Fischer,

1979a). The first experimental evidence of a direct interaction of the neurotoxin with central nervous matter is the finding of sites, in various parts of mammal brain, able to bind radioactively (^{125}I) labeled apamin (Habermann and Fischer, 1979a,b). This binding seems to be specific for apamin, with a dissociation constant K_D between 10 and 20 pM and a maximum capacity of binding sites between 1 and 3 pmol/g of wet rat cortex.

However, the significance of this fixation in the mechanism of poisoning by the toxin had to be demonstrated. One way to do so, was to check for a direct relation between the various neurotoxicities of a series of synthetic analogs of apamin (Granier and colleagues, 1978) and their ability to compete with labeled natural peptide for binding to its specific sites. For each derivative, LD_{50}'s for mice both by subcutaneous and by intraventricular injections were assessed and compared to the corresponding IC_{50} (amount of peptide able to inhibit 50 % of the maximum binding of ^{125}I labeled apamin to rat brain membranes). The competition ability of each analog was assessed following the experimental conditions given in Fig. 2. In this figure are also given experimental results of the binding assay and table 1 summarizes the data obtained with synthetic analogs in the three available tests.

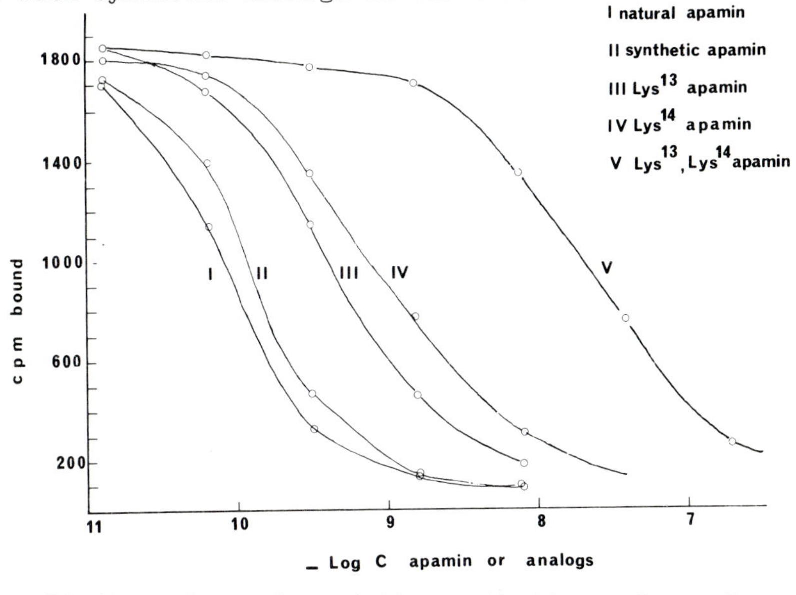

Fig. 2 : Binding of apamin and its synthetic analogs. Experimental conditions are as follows : in glass tubes 0.2 ml of the apamin or apamin derivatives dilutions in a solution containing 0.1 M Tris/HCl buffer, pH 7.5 and bovine serum albumin (1mg/1ml), was mixed with 0.1 ml of a dilution of labeled apamin (33 pg, 3390 counts / min ; specific radioactivity 82 mCi/mg) in the same diluent. Then 0.1 ml sucrose (0.32 M) containing 0.02 M KCl and 0.2 ml of the brain membranes in sucrose were added and the tube was kept for 60 min at 5°C. Thereafter 5 ml ice-cold Tris-saline was rapidly added, the mixture filtered at once under reduced pressure through a double layer of pre-wetted glass filter (GF-C) and quickly washed twice with each 5 ml of Tris -saline.

Table 1 : Relative activities of apamin analogs

Derivative	Origin	Relative toxicity[1] (subcutaneous route)	Relative toxicity[2] (intraventricular route)	Relative activity[3] in competition experiments
Apamin	Natural	1.00	1.00	1.00
Lys^{13} apamin	Synthetic	0.67	0.31	0.21
Lys^{14} apamin	Synthetic	0.59	0.50	0.11
Lys^{13},Lys^{14} apamin	Synthetic	0.07	0.03	0.004

1 Relative toxicity is the ratio LD_{50} of apamin/LD_{50} of the derivative. LD_{50} of analogs are those published by : Granier and colleagues (1978).

2 As in 1 except that the LD_{50} of each analog has been determined following the method described by Habermann and Cheng-Raude (1975).

3 Relative activity in competition experiments is the ratio IC_{50} of apamin/IC_{50} of analog. Values of IC_{50} are drawn from data shown in Fig. 2 .

Figure 2 shows clearly that all synthetic peptides bind to the specific sites of apamin with competition curves nicely parallel to the reference (curve I) , meaning that derivatives are competing with the same binding site. A striking fact is that any change in position 13 or 14 of the toxin induces a drastic loss of the affinity of the peptide for its fixation sites (table 1) : the most potent analog in the competition assay possesses only 21 % of the binding ability of the parent peptide. This low level of affinity contrasts, however, with the neurotoxicity of this derivative and the discrepancy remains to be explained. Nevertheless there seems to be a link between the changes of neurotoxicity and binding ability of the different apamin analogs, as it was suggested with the chemically modified derivatives of apamin or the synthetic analogs prepared by B. Sandberg (1979) (Habermann and Fischer, 1979a). More accurate results could be expected if one could correlate the binding assay to a pharmacological or biochemical effect of apamin. Recent discovery of some actions of this toxin on peripheral organs (smooth muscle, liver cells) (Banks et al,1979; Vladimirova and Shuba, 1978), probably involving ion transport phenomena, together with the known existence of binding sites in some peripheral organs (Habermann and Fischer, 1979a,b) provide the interesting possibility of using apamin, or apamin derivatives, in simple *in vitro* systems for a better understanding of its molecular action.

As a conclusion, apamin -the bee venom neurotoxin- possesses a rigid structure which can only be investigated in solution because of the inability of this peptide to give crystals. Preliminary results are consistent with a highly stable, hydrogen bonded structure but the exact polypeptide folding remains unknown. The mode of action of this neurotoxin is not clear : it acts on the central nervous system, but no biochemical event can be associated with its action. Sites for a specific fixation of apamin are present in various parts of the central nervous system, however, despite their neurotoxicity analogs of apamin seem to bind less to these sites than natural apamin. A promising field seems to be the use of simple in vitro preparations of the peripheral organs where apamin exhibits pharmacological activities.

ACKNOWLEDGEMENT

The authors wish to acknowledge Prof. Habermann for many discussions and careful reading of the manuscript. The binding assays and the intraventricular injections of synthetic derivatives have been performed in his Institute.

REFERENCES

Banks, B.E.C., C. Brown, G.M. Burgess, G. Burnstock, M. Claret, T. Cocks and D.H. Jenkinson (1979). Apamin blocks certain neurotransmitter-induced increases in potassium permeability. Nature, in press.

Bystrov, V.F., A.S. Arseniev and Yu. D. Gavrilov (1978). NMR spectroscopy of large peptides and small proteins. J. Magnetic Resonance 30, 155-184.

Callewaert, G.L., M. Shipolini and C.A. Vernon (1968). The disulfide bridges of apamin. F.E.B.S. Letters 1, 111-113.

Cavey, D., J.P. Vincent and M. Lazdunski (1979). A search for the apamin receptor in the central nervous system. Toxicon 17, 176-179.

Cosand, W.L. and R.B. Merrifield (1977). Concept of internal structural controls for evaluation of inactive synthetic peptide analogs : synthesis of $Orn^{13,14}$ apamin and its guanidination to an apamin derivative will full neurotoxic activity. Proc. Natl. Acad. Sci. USA 74, 2771-2775.

Granier, C., E. Pedroso-Muller and J. Van Rietschoten (1978). Use of synthetic analogs for a study on the structure activity relationship of apamin. Eur. J. Biochem. 82, 293-299.

Habermann, E. and K.G. Reitz (1965). Ein neues Verfahren zur Gewinnung der Komponenten von Bienengift, insbesondere des zentralwirksamen Peptids Apamin. Biochem. Z. 341, 451-466.

Habermann, E. and Cheng-Raude (1975). Central neurotoxicity of apamin, crotamin, phospholipase A and α-amanitin. Toxicon 13, 465-473.

Habermann, E. and K. Fischer (1979a). Apamin, a centrally acting neurotoxic peptide : binding and actions. In B. Ceccarelli and F. Clementi (Eds) Advances in Cytopharmacology, vol. 3, Raven Press, New York, pp. 387-393.

Habermann, E. and K. Fischer (1979b). Bee venom neurotoxin (apamin) : iodine labeling and characterization of binding sites. Eur. J. Biochem. 94, 355-364.

Haux, P., H. Sawerthal and E. Habermann (1967). Sequenzanalyse des Bienengift Neurotoxins (Apamin) ans seinen tryptischen und chymotryptischen Spaltstücken. Hoppe Seyler's Z. Physiol. Chem. 348, 737-738.

Miroshnikov, A.I., E.G. Elyakova, A.B. Kudelin and L.B. Senyavina (1978). Physico-chemical characteristics of apamin, a neurotoxin from honey-bee Apis mellifica. Bioorganicheskaya Khimiya 4, 1022-1028.

Nuriddinov, A.R., G.F. Zhukova, V.I. Tsetlin and V.T. Ivanov (1978). Synthesis of apamin, a bee venom neurotoxin. Bioorganicheskaya Khimiya 4, 1322-1333.

van Rietschoten, J., C. Granier, H. Rochat, S. Lissitzky and F. Miranda (1975). Synthesis of apamin, a neurotoxic peptide from bee venom. Eur. J. Biochem. 56, 35-40.

Sandberg, B.E.B. and U. Ragnarsson (1978). Solid phase synthesis of apamin, the principal neurotoxin in bee venom. Int. J. Pept. Prot. Res. 11, 238-245.

Sandberg, B.E.B. (1979). Solid phase synthesis of 13-Lysine-apamin, 14-Lysine-apamin and the corresponding guanidinated derivatives. Int. J. Pept. Prot. Res. 13, 327-333.

Shipolini, R., A.F. Bradbury, G.L. Callewaert and C.A. Vernon (1967). The structure of apamin. Chem. Commun., 679-680.

Vladimirova, A.I. and M.F. Shuba (1978). Strychnine, hydrastine and apamine effect on synaptic transmission in smooth muscle cells. Neirofiziologiya 10, 295-299.

STRUCTURE-FUNCTION RELATIONSHIPS IN *CEREBRATULUS* TOXIN B-IV

K. M. Blumenthal* and W. R. Kem**

**Department of Biological Chemistry, University of Cincinnati College of Medicine, Cincinnati, Ohio 45267, USA*
***Department of Pharmacology and Therapeutics, University of Florida, College of Medicine, Gainesville, Florida 32610, USA*

ABSTRACT

A series of experiments are described which probe structure-function relationships in *Cerebratulus* toxin B-IV, a small, crustacean-selective, polypeptide neurotoxin whose primary effect is to greatly prolong the repolarization phase of the action potential. Nitration of a specific tyrosine residue, or alkylation of a specific tryptophan, are shown to abolish toxicity without causing gross conformational changes in the protein. A highly radioactive, pharmacologically active derivative of B-IV has been prepared, and preliminary studies of the binding of this molecule to crustacean axon membranes are described.

KEYWORDS

Polypeptide neurotoxin; axon; action potential; chemical modification; binding

INTRODUCTION

The large Atlantic coast heteronemertine *Cerebratulus lacteus* has been shown to synthesize two groups of toxic polypeptides, the cytolytic A toxins and the neurotoxic B group (Kem, 1976; Kem and Blumenthal, 1976, 1978), the groups consisting of either three or four (B) structurally related proteins. The B toxins are all small, highly basic proteins having molecular weights of about 6,000. Pharmacologically, the primary effect of these toxins is a marked prolongation of the repolarization phase of the action potential in crustacean neurons. As a groundwork for structure-function studies, the covalent structure of toxin B-IV, the most abundant constituent of the B-group, has been determined (Blumenthal and Kem, 1976, 1977). The experiments discussed herein have utilized specific chemical modification to pursue our goal of a detailed molecular understanding of the mechanism of action of toxin B-IV.

STRUCTURE OF TOXIN B-II

The amino acid sequence of toxin B-II, the most highly toxic B-variant, has been determined by automated Edman degradation of the intact protein and of maleylated tryptic peptides derived therefrom (Blumenthal, Heinrikson, and Kem, in preparation). The protein is a single chain of 55 amino acid residues, 54 of which have been unambiguously assigned in this study. The residue occupying position 10 could not be identified, either as a PTH-derivative or as the free amino acid following

es, one of these residues is far more reactive than the other. It is thus possible, purely by manipulation of reagent excess, to prepare mono- and di-HNB-B-IV and to assay each for biological activity. Bioassay (Fig. 3) reveals that mono-HNB-IV has lost a small amount of activity, being 20-25% less active than the native material, while di-HNB-B-IV retains less than 5% the activity of the unmodified protein. As the secondary structures of both derivatives are virtually the same as that of native B-IV, these data suggest the involvement of the "second" tryptophan in toxin-receptor binding. Identification of the "first" and "second" tryptophans was done by comparison of tryptic peptide maps derived from the two proteins (Fig. 4). As shown, for the mono derivative only one yellow spot is observed upon exposure of the chromatogram to NH_3 vapors (diagnostic of HNB-Trp) while for di-HNB-B-IV two such spots are observed. Elution of peptide from each spot, followed by amino acid analysis (Table 3) reveals that the "fast" Trp is Trp-5 and the slower Trp-30. The absorption spectra of these two peptides indicate

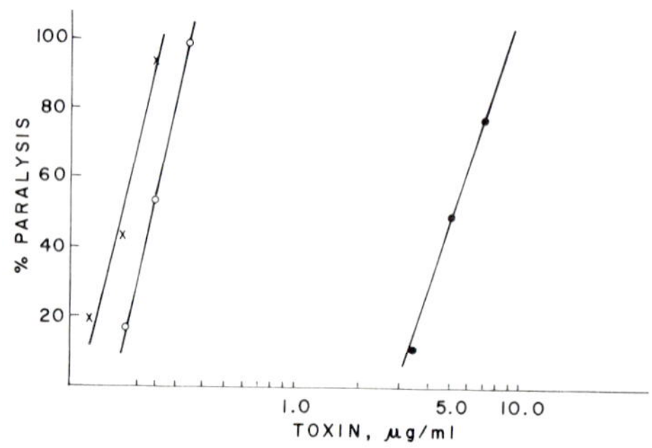

Fig. 3: Bioassay of native (x), mono-HNB (o), and di-HNB (•) toxin B-IV.

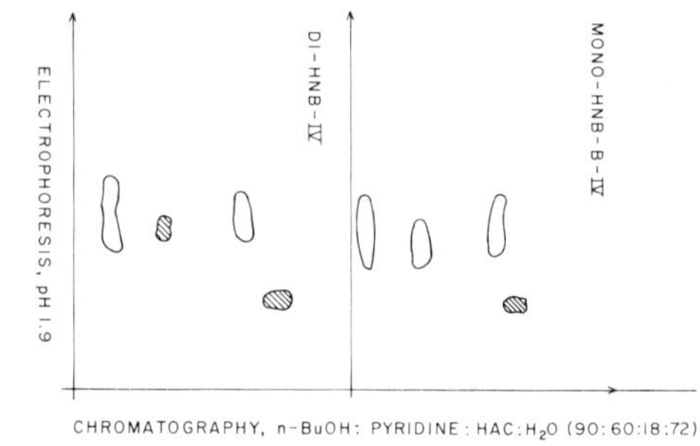

Fig. 4: Peptide maps of tryptic digests of mono- and di-HNB-B-IV. Circled spots were ninhydrin positive, hatched were yellow in NH_3 vapors.

that Trp-5 (MT-1) has been at least 80% converted to HNB-Trp in mono-HNB-B-IV while no HNB-Trp is detectable at Trp-30 (Peptide MT-3). The sensitivity of these determinations is such that a 10-15% level of HNB-Trp would most likely be undetected.

In summary, Tyr-9 and Trp-30 have both been implicated in the biological activity of toxin B-IV. Involvement of aromatic residues in the toxicity of such membrane active neurotoxins has been conclusively demonstrated in a number of other systems (Chang, *et. al.*, 1971; Seto, Sato, and Tamiya, 1970).

Table 3: Amino Acid Compositions of Tryptic Peptides from Mono-HNB-B-IV

Amino Acid	MT-1	MT-3
Aspartic acid	2.0(2)	
Threonine	0.9(1)	
Serine	1.2(1)	
Glutamic acid	1.1(1)	0.8(1)
Glycine	1.4(1)	1.9(2)
Alanine	3.9(4)	1.0(1)
Tyrosine	0.7(1)	
Lysine		2.3(2)
Arginine	1.1(1)	1.0(1)
Cm-Cysteine	1.8(2)	0.9(1)

TOXIN-RECEPTOR INTERACTION

A major goal of our research has been determination of the toxin-receptor dissociation constant and a measurement of receptor density. For this purpose, it has been essential to prepare a highly radioactive, pharmacologically active derivative of B-IV. Direct iodination did not seem promising, due to the involvement of tyrosine in toxin activity, so we turned our attention to an acylation system described by Bolton and Hunter (1972). In this instance, the major problem was to limit the extent of reaction since B-IV contains 11 amino groups per molecule. Figure 5 shows that this limitation was achieved by performing the reaction at pH 6.4 and a reagent:protein ratio of 5. Under these conditions, 1.0-1.3 moles of reagent are incorporated per mole protein. Virtually all of this incorporation must be at the α-amino group, since the derivatized protein is completely refractory to any N-terminal determination. Using this approach, it has been possible to prepare protein having specific radioactivities in the range $4\text{-}8 \times 10^5$ cpm/μg. Figure 6 shows that Bolton-Hunter modified B-IV is 70-75% as active as the native toxin. This specific toxicity appears to be independent of whether or not the

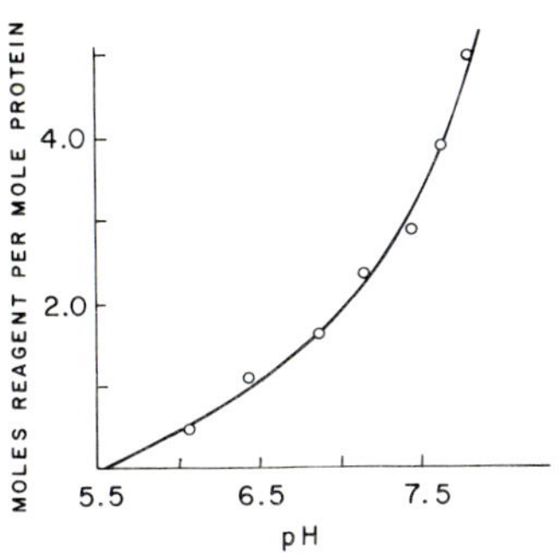

Fig. 5: Reaction of toxin B-IV with Bolton-Hunter reagent as a function of pH.

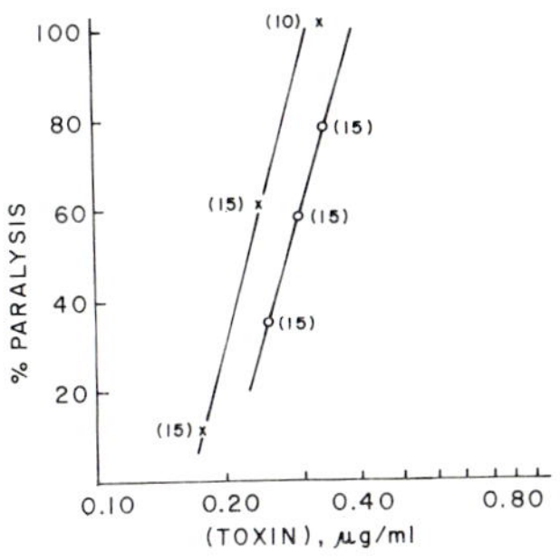

Fig. 6: Bioassay of native (x) and Bolton-Hunter (o) treated B-IV. Modified protein incorporated 1 hydroxyphenylpropionyl group per mole.

reagent has been iodinated. Preliminary studies have been carried out to measure the binding of this material to lobster axonal membranes (Fig. 7). Although no specific binding is detectable in membrane fragments prepared as described by others (Denburg, 1972; Barnola, Villegas, and Camejo, 1973), specific binding to vesicles prepared from lobster nerve has been observed (Toth and Blumenthal unpublished). The binding is saturated at toxin concentrations in excess of 1μ*M*, and the dissociation constant from these preliminary data is of the order of 80-100 nM. Presentation of the binding data as a Hill plot gives a straight line having a slope of 1.26, indicative of positive binding cooperativity. As positive cooperativity has not hitherto been observed in the binding of axonal toxins to their receptors (Catterall, 1977; Courad, Rochat and Lissitzky, 1978; Jover, *et. al.*, 1978; Ray, Morrow, and Catterall, 1978), we are currently engaged in confirming and refining these preliminary data.

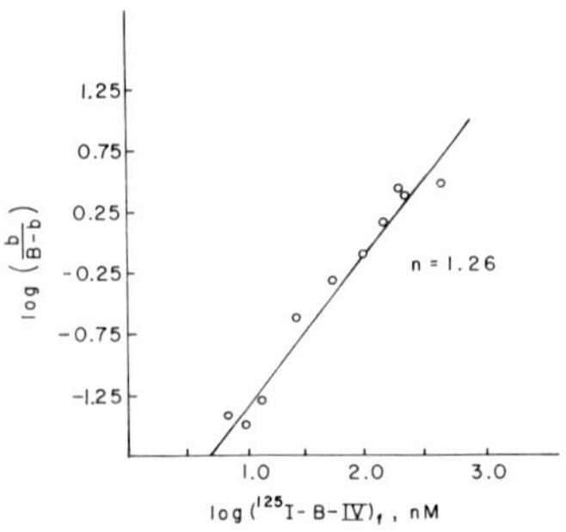

Fig. 7: Binding of ^{125}I-B-IV to lobster axon membrane vesicles.

ACKNOWLEDGEMENTS

These studies were aided by grants from the National Science Foundation (BNS 76-06266, W. R. K.) and the National Institutes of Health (NS-14368, K.M.B.). K.M.B. holds Research Career Development Award NS-00304 from the National Institutes of Health, and is indebted to Ms. Catherine Azar for her assistance in a number of the experiments described herein.

REFERENCES

1. Barnola, F. V., Villegas, R., and Camejo, G. (1973) *Biochim. Biophys. Acta 298*, 84-94.
2. Blumenthal, K.M., and Kem, W.R. (1976) *J. Biol. Chem. 251*, 6025-29.
3. Blumenthal,K.M., and Kem, W.R. (1977) *J. Biol. Chem. 252*, 3328-31.
4. Bolton, A.E., and Hunter, W.M. (1973) *Biochem. J. 133*, 529-38.
5. Catterall, W.A. (1977) *J. Biol. Chem. 252*, 8660-68.
6. Chang, C.C., Yang, C.C., Hamaguchi, K., Nakai, K., and Hayashi, K. (1970) *Biochim, Biophys. Acta 236*, 164-73.
7. Couraud, F., Rochat, H., and Lissitzky, S. (1978) *Biochem. Biophys. Res. Comm. 83*, 1525-30.
8. Denburg, J.L. (1972) *Biochim. Biophys. Acta 282*, 453-58.
9. Glazer, A.N., DeLange, R.J., and Sigman, D.S. (1975) "Chemical Modification of Proteins", Elsevier, New York, 95-99.
10. Jover, E., Martin-Moutot, N., Couraud, F., and Rochat, H. (1978) *Biochem. Biophys. Res. Comm. 85*, 377-82.
11. Kem, W.R. (1976) *J. Biol. Chem. 251*, 4184-92.
12. Kem, W.R., and Blumenthal, K.M. (1976) in "Toxins: Animal, Plant, and Microbial", P. Rosenberg, ed., Pergamon Press, New York, 509-16.
13. Kem, W.R., and Blumenthal, K.M. (1978) *J. Biol. Chem. 253*, 5752-57.
14. Ray, R., Morrow, C.S., and Catterall, W.A. (1978) *J. Biol. Chem. 253*, 7307-13.
15. Seto, A., Sato, S., and Tamiya, N. (1970) *Biochim. Biophys. Acta 214*, 483-89.

CONFORMATION OF PARDAXIN, THE PURIFIED POLYPEPTIDE FROM THE TOXIC SECRETION OF THE FLATFISH *PARDACHIRUS MARMORATUS* STUDIED BY LASER RAMAN SPECTROSCOPY AND CIRCULAR DICHROISM

N. Primor and A. T. Tu

Dept. of Biochemistry, Colorado State Univ., Ft. Collins, Colarado 80523, USA

ABSTRACT

Pardaxin, the toxic compound from the secretion of the Red Sea flatfish Pardachirus marmoratus has been examined by Raman and circular dichroism techniques. Conformational information regarding the peptide backbone, disulfide bond and tyrosine chromophores was obtained. The Amide I band appeared at 1658 cm^{-1} as a strong, discrete band and the Amide III appeared at 1280 cm^{-1}. Analysis of the Raman spectra by the method of Lippert and colleagues (1976) shows that the toxin consists of 39% α-helix, 23% β-structure and 39% random coil. The Lippert equation does not include the β-turn term; therefore, the content of β-reverse turn could not be obtained. The occurrence of a band at 510-512 cm^{-1} indicates the conformational geometry of the disulfide C-C-S-S-C-C linkages to be gauche-gauche-gauche. The lack of -SH stretching vibration in the region of 2500 ∿ 2700 cm^{-1} region indicates that all half-cystines are used in disulfide linkages. The far-UV CD spectrum showed the positive 196 and negative 208 and 222 nm bands. Pardaxin possesses quite unusual helical structure which does not fit the models based on the quantitatively estimated secondary structure. The best fit secondary structure based on CD ellipticity by the method of Chen and colleagues (1972) was found to be: 23% α-helix, 21% β-structure and 56% random. At the most acidic and alkaline pH the far-UV Pardaxin spectra showed extensive loss of its helical structure, which was found to be reversible. Examination of the near-UV CD spectrum showed the existence of phenylalanine and tyrosine bands. Since Pardaxin toxicity to fish is enhanced when the toxin is applied in media containing very high NaCl concentrations, the possible influence of salt on Pardaxin's secondary structure was tested. From the examination of the far-UV CD and Raman spectra it appears that salt does not alter the structural conformation. It is believed that the enhanced toxicity to fish in high NaCl medium concentration is due to the effect on the fish transport mechanism rather than a direct effect of the salt media on Pardaxin conformation.

---

*Present address: Department of Physiology and Biophysics, New York University Medical Center, School of Medicine, 550 First Ave., New York, N. Y. 10016

**To whom requests for reprints should be addressed.

KEY WORDS

Peptide conformation; fish toxin.

INTRODUCTION

Pardaxin is a purified toxin isolated from the venom of the Red Sea flatfish, Pardachirus marmoratus (Soleidae)(Primor and colleagues, 1978) and possesses a variety of pharmacological actions. It releases acetylcholine from the post-ganglionic nerve terminals when tested on the ileal smooth muscle preparation (Parness and Zlotkin, 1976). When the frog nerve-muscle preparation is used, an increase in spontaneous transmitter release occurs and pathological changes in the neuromuscular junction have been demonstrated by histological examination (Spira and colleagues, 1976). Pardaxin also inhibits Na^+, K^+-ATPase activity. When applied into the media, ichthyotoxicity of Pardaxin is dependent on external salt concentration (Primor and colleagues, 1979).

In the present investigation, the secondary structure of Pardaxin was extensively examined by two independent methods, laser Raman spectroscopy and circular dichroism. Effects of sodium chloride and hydrogen ion concentration were also investigated.

MATERIALS AND METHODS

The crude secretion of the Red Sea flatfish Pardachirus marmoratus (Pisces, Soleidae) was obtained as described by Clark and Chao (1973) and stored in a lyophylized form. The toxic component, Pardaxin, was isolated by Primor and colleagues (1978).

Laser Raman Spectroscopy. Raman spectra were obtained using a Spex Ramalog 5 Raman spectrometer with a spectrophysics SP-164 laser argon ion beam. The spectra over the range of 1700 to 450 cm^{-1} were obtained with a 515.5 nm excitation line and a 5 cm^{-1} spectra slit width. For sulfhydryl group vibration, the spectra were examined over the range of 2500-2700 cm^{-1}. For deuteration Pardaxin was dissolved in deuterium oxide and allowed to stand for one hour and then lyophilized. This procedure was repeated three times for completion of deuterium exchange. The final sample was dissolved in D_2O again to make a 9% solution for Raman spectroscopic observation.

Circular Dichroism. Circular Dichroism spectra were obtained on a JASCO Y-41C spectropolarimeter at 23 $\pm$ 2°C. Spectra from 190-250 nm (far-UV) were recorded using a scanning speed of 0.5 nm/s. and an instrumental time constant of 16 s. Pardaxin samples were approximately 0.04% protein (W/V) in 0.1 cm path-length cells with a spectral band width of 0.5 nm. Spectra from 250-300 nm (near-UV) were recorded using a scan speed of 2.5 nm/s. and an instrument time constant of 4 sec. Pardaxin samples were approximately 0.12% protein (W/V) in 1.0 cm path-length cells with a spectral band width of 1 nm. The instrument was calibrated using an aqueous solution of ($\pm$)-10 camphor sulfonic acid which is assumed to have a molar ellipticity at 290.5 nm of 7775 deg cm^2/d mole (Kreuger and Pschigoda, 1971). The ellipticity data were converted to molar ellipticity $[\theta]$ employing the relationship given by Adler and colleagues (1973). The α-helix content was calculated from the molar ellipticity at 208 nm using Equation (1) of Greenfield and Fasman (1969); from the ellipticity at 222 nm using the equation of Chen and colleagues (1972) and the computed program of Chen and colleagues (1972). Using the basic functions of Greenfield and Fasman (1969), we attempted to ascertain the distribution of the remainder of the molecule between β-sheet and unordered conformation. A value of 20% α-helix was assumed and theoretical CD curves were generated for various values of f_β and f_R at intervals of 0.05.

These theoretical curves were compared with the experimental curve by inspection. The calculated values of α-helix, β-structure and unordered conformation were also obtained using the computed program method of Chen and colleagues (1972). The mean residue weight was taken as 162 amino acid residues with an assumed molecular weight of 16,000. Protein concentrations were determined from the absorbance at 280 nm, using the previously reported extinction coefficient (Primor, Parness and Zlotkin, 1978). The aqueous Pardaxin samples were titrated with NaOH or HCl to the pH at which the spectra were taken.

RESULTS AND DISCUSSION

Peptide Backbone Conformation. Raman spectroscopy has been extensively used for the elucidation of the secondary structure of different proteins. For peptide backbone conformation analysis, both the Amide I and Amide III bands are extensively used. The Amide I band originates from in-plane vibration of the peptide bond but the main contribution is from the bending motion of an -NH of a peptide bond. Thus, deuteration of a protein will not significantly change the Amide I band but the Amide III has significant isotopic shift to lower the frequency by a factor of $\sqrt{2}$.

Normally the α-helix gives a sharp Amide I band at 1650-1657 cm^{-1}, random coil at 1664-1666 cm^{-1}, and β-sheet conformation in the region of 1665-1680 cm^{-1}. The β-reverse turn conformation has the Amide I band at 1663-1670 cm^{-1} (Tu and colleagues, 1978, 1979; Hruby and colleagues, 1978).

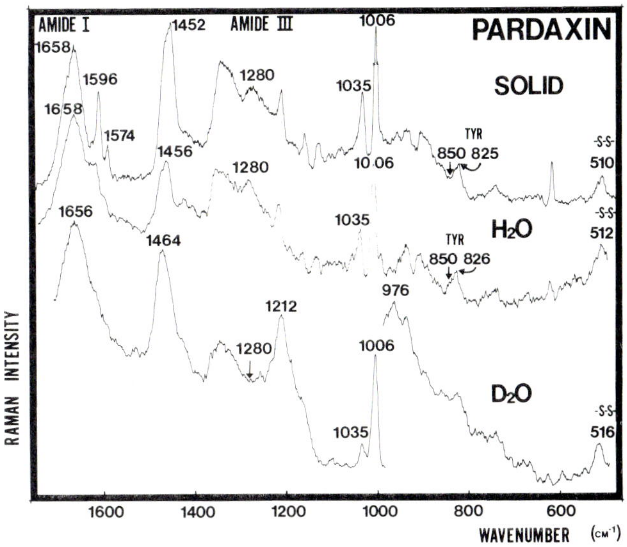

Fig. 1. Laser Raman spectra of Pardaxin in the solid state, in water, pH 4.9, and of deuterated form. Spectra were recorded as described in Materials and Methods.

Pardaxin shows a prominent Amide I band at 1658 for both solid and aqueous samples (Fig. 1). On deuteration, the Amide I band has very little change and appeared at 1656 cm^{-1}. The 1658 cm^{-1} is an extreme end of frequency range for α-helix. This frequency is also close to lower frequency ranges for random coil, β-sheet and β-turn structure. It is, therefore, not possible to assess quantitatively different conformations by mere inspection although the Raman spectra clearly suggest the presence of α-helix. Recently Lippert and colleagues (1976) introduced a method to quantitatively determine different conformations. This method was applied to carbonic anhydrase B (Craig and Gaber, 1977), sea snake neurotoxin (Fox and Tu, 1979) and Myotoxin a (Bailey and colleagues, 1979). Consequently, this method was used for more quantitative analysis of Pardaxin conformation. Lippert and colleagues (1976) set up four simultaneous equations using the relative intensities of the Amide I and Amide III bands at three specific frequencies:

$$C^{protein}_{1240} \quad I^{protein}_{1240} = f_\alpha I^\alpha_{1240} + f_\beta I^\beta_{1240} + f_R I^R_{1240}$$

$$C^{protein}_{1632} \quad I^{protein}_{1632} = f_\alpha I^\alpha_{1632} + f_\beta I^\beta_{1632} + f_R I^R_{1240}$$

$$C^{protein}_{1660} \quad I^{protein}_{1660} = f_\alpha I^\alpha_{1660} + f_\beta I^\beta_{1660} + f_R I^R_{1660}$$

$$f_\alpha + f_\beta + f_R = 1$$

The I^α_ν, I^α_ν, I^R are Raman intensities previously determined for polylysine in the various secondary structural forms. A scaling constant, $C^{protein}$, represents the relative intensity of the methylene band in the protein.

Since the equation uses the Raman intensities of particular frequencies at the Amide I and Amide III bands, it is essential to establish that the band observed at 1280 cm^{-1} is indeed the Amide III band. The deuterated Pardaxin shows that the original 1280 cm^{-1} band disappears completely and shifts to 976 cm^{-1} (Fig. 1). The frequency ratio of 1280/976 is 1.31, which is very close to the theoretical value of 1.41 or $\sqrt{2}$. This indicates that the broad band observed at 1280 cm^{-1} is the Amide III band.

By solving these equations, Pardaxin appears to contain 38.6% α-helix, 22.8% β-sheet, and 38.6% random coil. The equations developed by Lippert and colleagues (1976) do not include a term for β-reverse turns. The high content of α-helix of 38.6% as compared to 17.8%, 18.5% and 23% by CD methods of Greenfield and Fasman (1969) and Chen and colleagues (1972) presumably include β-reverse turn content in the percentage of α-helix. As mentioned before, the Amide I of 1658 cm^{-1} is rather high to be accounted for solely by α-helix. The Amide I frequency for β-sheet, β-reverse turn and random coil are all above 1660 cm^{-1}. Therefore, it is not possible to determine what conformation besides α-helix may be involved by inspecting only the Amide I band. The broad band at 1280 cm^{-1} for the Amide III clearly indicates the presence of α-helix. The Amide III for β-reverse turn structure usually appears in the range of 1266 to 1278 cm^{-1} (Tu and colleagues, 1978; Hruby and colleagues, 1978; Bandekar and Krimm, 1979) or as high as 1690 cm^{-1}. Therefore, the high Amide III value of 1280 cm^{-1} may suggest the coexistence of both α-helix and β-reverse turn structure. The CD methods of Chen and colleagues (1972) and Greenfield and Fasman (1969) do not provide the information of β-turn content. Pardaxin is a toxin isolated from a fish secretion; however, it seems that Pardaxin's peptide backbone conformation is quite different from other marine toxins. Sea snake toxins consist mainly of β-sheet and β-reverse turn with little α-helix (Fox and Tu, 1979). Comparisons of the amino acid compositions and molecular weights of sea snake toxins and Pardaxin are indeed quite different.

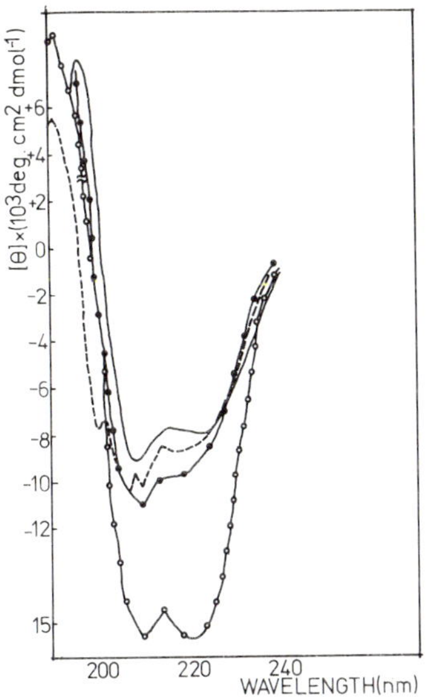

Figure 2. Comparison of observed Pardaxin far-ultraviolet circular dichroism spectra with the predicted models. (——) the measured pardaxin spectra in water, pH 4.9. (----) predicted from Greenfield and Fasman (1969) using the following structure contributions: 20% α-helix, 30% β-structure and 50% random. (●——●) predicted from the computed method of Chen and colleagues (1972), using the following structure contributions: 23% α-helix, 21% β-structure and 50% random. (○——○) predicted from Lippert and colleagues (1976), using the following structure contributions: 38.6% α-helix, 22.8% β-structure and 38.6% random.

The far-UV CD spectrum of proteins can reveal information concerning the secondary structure (Greenfield and Fasman, 1969; Chen and colleagues, 1972). Examination of the far-UV CD spectrum of Pardaxin in water (pH 4.9) showed a positive band at 196 nm, ($[\theta]_{MRW}$ = 8000) and negative bands at 208 nm, ($[\theta]_{MRW}$ = 9160) and 222 nm, ($[\theta]_{MRW}$ = 8040) (Fig. 2). The overall Pardaxin spectrum qualitatively resembles model spectra of α-helical polypeptides which give a characteristic double minimum at 222 and 208 nm and a positive peak between 190-192 nm (Greenfield and Fasman, 1969). However, the Pardaxin spectrum contains two features which appear to be unusual. These are relatively high magnitude with λ_{max} at 208 nm and the position of the positive band at 196 nm (Fig. 2).

The one point equation methods (Greenfield and Fasman, 1969; Chen and colleagues, 1972) gave values in good agreement of about 18% α-helix. By use of the Greenfield and Fasman (1969) method the secondary structure of native Pardaxin (in water) is best approximated as 20% α-helix, 30% β-structure and 50% random coil. Percentages of different conformations calculated by 3 different methods based on CD ellipticity agreed very well (Table I). For instance, 17.8% α-helix by Greenfield and Fasman's (1969) method, 18.5% and 23% by the method of Chen and colleagues (1972). A higher percentage of α-helix, 38.6% was obtained by the Raman method of Lippert and colleagues (1976). None of the methods used give the percentage of β-turn structure. The fact that CD methods give fairly consistent results suggests that the content of α-helix is most likely in the range of 18 to 23%. When the method of Chen and colleagues (1972) was used for Myotoxin a (Bailey and colleagues, 1979) and Anthopleurin A which are rich in β-reverse turn, the equation was not applicable (Ishizaki and colleagues, 1979) due to negative values being obtained. Another reason for the failure of the method of Chen and colleagues (1972) may be due to the fact that these are relatively small molecules with high disulfide bond content. Myotoxin a and Anthopleurin A consist of 42 and 49 amino acid residues only, whereas Pardaxin is much larger with 162 amino acid residues. It seems the method developed by Chen and colleagues (1972) is more applicable for larger molecules or with less β-reverse turn content. The far-UV CD spectrum predicted for this conformation should exhibit a positive 191 nm band and negative 207-210 and 217 nm bands. The predicted curve using the estimated values of α-helix, β-structure and random coil from the computed method of Chen and colleagues (1972) resulted in the best fit to the observed Pardaxin spectra. The 208 nm ellipticity, with accordance to the measured Pardaxin spectra, is found to have higher ellipticity than the 222 nm band. This indicates that the Pardaxin secondary structure is best approximated by 23% α-helix, 21% β-structure and 56% random. On the other hand, the spectra predicted for the conformation inferred from Figure 2 should contain extrema of nearly equal magnitude at 210 and 222 nm and a peak of 191 nm. The discrepancy between the above models and the actual spectra pointed out the unusual conformation of Pardaxin.

The UV Pardaxin spectra resemble those of Parvalbumins (a peculiar group of muscle proteins) in view of their high relative phenylalanine content. In addition, there is a general similarity based on amino acid composition (Primor, Parness and Zlotkin, 1978). Examination of the far- as well as near-UV CD spectra of Parvalbumins from fish muscle (Parello and Pechere, 1971) shows that no similarity with the CD of Pardaxin exists. Parvalbumins, in contrast to Pardaxin, show a positive band at 190 nm. The near UV CD spectra are also different, showing bands at 268 and 262 and a shoulder at 255 nm. Compared to Parvalbumins, Pardaxin appears to comprise a completely different structure. This conclusion is further supported by the most recent findings concerning the Pardaxin sequence. The N-terminal of Pardaxin in contrast to the Parvalbumins (Demaille and colleagues, 1974) is not acetylated and the sequence of its amino acids is different (Zlotkin, in preparation). Comparing the far-UV CD spectra, Pardaxin shows a great resemblance to insulin. Insulin at pH 3.0 possesses extrema at 222, 208 and 196 nm (Ettinger and Timasheff, 1971). It resembles Pardaxin in that the 209 nm extremum shows considerably greater magnitude than the 222 nm band. Furthermore, rather than containing an extremum at 191-192 nm, as is found in the α-helical polypeptide spectra, Pardaxin and insulin possess an extremum at 196 nm, i.e., at the position of β-structural polypeptides (Townend and colleagues, 1967).

In spite of the curious resemblance in the far-UV CD spectrum to insulin, the CD of Pardaxin shows no such similarity to any toxin studied thus far. Crotoxin, a toxic compound from the venom of Crotalus durissus terrificus (Tropical rattlesnake) possesses 37.5% α-helix and 45% β-structure at pH 4.0 and the magnitude of the 220 nm extremum is higher than that of the 208 nm (Hanley, 1979). A similar state exists with the toxic phospholipase A_2 from the venom of Bitis gabonica (Gaboon viper) which contains 22% α-helix (Viljoen and colleagues, 1976). Neurotoxins from cobra venom (Elapidae) or sea snakes (Hydrophiidae) contain little or no α-helix (Menez and colleagues, 1976; Tu, 1977; Fox and Tu, 1979). The far-UV and Raman spectra of the sea anemone Anthopleurin A (Ishizaki and colleagues, 1979) show also no similarity to Pardaxin. It should be pointed out that in spite of the toxicity of the Pardachirus marmoratus secretion (from which Pardaxin was isolated) no definite information is known concerning the biological function of this secretion. Additional biological functions should be considered too. Although the Raman and CD methods used gave qualitatively similar results, they do not give absolute conformation of protein molecules. In the estimation of α-helix composition from CD based on calculated ellipticity at 222 nm, it should be considered that this wavelength is based on the existence of good agreement between globular proteins and ideal α-helices (Madison and Schellman, 1972).

Disulfide Bonds and Amino Acid Side Chains

In addition to peptide backbone conformation, Raman spectroscopy has been extensively used for the conformation of disulfide bonds (Yu and colleagues, 1975; Tu and colleagues, 1976; Maxfield and Scheraga, 1977). The disulfide bond stretching vibration of Pardaxin shows 510 cm^{-1} for solid samples, 512 cm^{-1} for aqueous samples and 516 cm^{-1} for deuterated sample. This indicates clearly the gauche-gauche-gauche conformation for each of the C-C-S-S-C-C of two half-cystine residues in the disulfide bridges. By using a number of disulfide compounds, Sugeta and colleagues (1972, 1973) showed that gauche-gauche-gauche conformation gives ν_{S-S} (stretching vibration at 510 cm^{-1}, trans-gauche-gauche at 525 cm^{-1}, and trans-gauche-trans at 540 cm^{-1}. Apparently the gauche-gauche-gauche conformation represents the most stable conformation since proteins and/or polypeptides usually give ν_{S-S} at 510 cm^{-1}. It is of interest in this regard that some synthetic peptides with oxytocin antagonists, penicillamine-oxytocin, penicillamine, and leucyl-oxytocine show different disulfide conformations of trans-gauche-gauche and trans-gauche-trans conformation (Tu and colleagues, 1978, 1979; Hruby and colleagues, 1978).

Lack of sulfhydryl vibrational band in the 2500-2700 cm^{-1} region suggests that all 8 half-cystine residues in Pardaxin must be involved in disulfide bond formation. Raman spectroscopy is also extensively used for the analysis of the microenvironment of the tyrosine side chain by comparing the Raman intensities of 850 and 830 cm^{-1} lines. It has been found that these lines originate from Fermi resonance between the ring-breathing and out-of-plane vibration of the para-substituted benzene (Siaminza and colleagues, 1975). Yu and colleagues (1973) used a dipeptide, Gly-Tyr, as a model of exposed tyrosines. From this it was found that exposed tyrosines give a high I_{850}/I_{830} intensity ratio. Judging from the intensity ratio of Pardaxin at 850 cm^{-1} and 825 cm^{-1}, the tyrosine side chains are exposed. Pardaxin has two residues of tyrosine; therefore, the judgement is not as clear as a protein containing one residue. Therefore, the data reflect "average information," but do not indicate that at least one residue is exposed.

The near-UV region has contributions from tryptophan, tyrosine, phenylalanine side chains and disulfide bonds (Strickland, 1974). The near-UV CD spectra were expected to indicate changes in local structure around dichroic chromophores. Examination of the near-UV CD spectra of Pardaxin in water, pH 4.9 (Fig. 3) showed bands with maxima at 259, 265 and 271-3 nm and a shoulder at 284 nm. The region from 250-270 nm possesses only very weak tyrosyl transitions. Phenylalanine side chains produce sharp CD fine structure between 270-255 nm, a region where other amino acid side chains give only broad bands. In proteins with a number of phenylalanines, such as Pardaxin, the CD fine structure is more complex. CD and absorption spectra of model compounds confirm that tyrosyl and phenylalanyl moieties have fine structure, whereas the disulfide does not (Horwitz and colleagues, 1970). The region between 270-290 nm is dominated by tyrosine, tryptophan and disulfides (Strickland, 1974). The identification of tyrosyl bands is less complicated in the case of Pardaxin, which is devoid of tryptophan and possesses only 2 tyrosyls. Pardaxin possesses 13 phenylalanines, representing 8% of the amino acid content of the whole molecule, and two tyrosines (Primor, Parness and Zlotkin, 1978). However, the rotational strength of the tyrosine L_b transition is considerably larger than that of the phenylalanine L_b band (Horwitz and colleagues, 1970). The identification of the tyrosyl L_b bands should be possible on

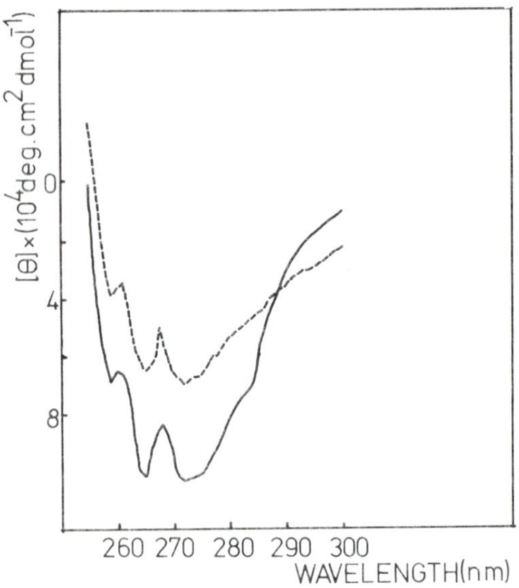

Fig. 3. Near-ultraviolet circular dichroism spectra of Pardaxin in pH 4.9 and 10. Spectra were recorded as described in Materials and Methods. (——) pH 4.9, (----) pH 10.

the basis of fine structure occurring between 275-290 nm. Each of the tyrosyl residues may have its 0-0 transition located at a different wavelength. Based on the interpretation of tyrosyl side chains in different proteins such as Ribonuclease-A (Horwitz and colleagues, 1970) and insulin (Ettinger and Timasheff, 1971), the 271-3 peak and 284 shoulder (Fig. 3) appears to result from the tyrosyl moiety, but some contribution from the four disulfide bonds is also possible. This conclusion is further supported by the near-UV spectra of Pardaxin at pH 10. Raising the pH from 4.9 to 10 causes two major changes: loss of CD intensity and removal of the 284 nm shoulder. These alterations probably reflect ionization of the tyrosyl as well as other conformational effects (Fig. 3).

Effect of NaCl Concentration

As mentioned previously, ichthyotoxicity of Pardaxin is highly dependent on salt concentration, and it is enhanced at very high NaCl concentrations. The toxicity in a 9% salt solution is 30 times higher than in 0.9% NaCl. The explanation of this medium-dependent toxicity involves two possible mechanisms: 1) interaction between NaCl and Pardaxin molecules resulting in activation of Pardaxin, 2) interaction between the medium (salt + Pardaxin) and the fish target organ.

In order to clarify these hypotheses, the effect of sodium chloride concentration was examined both by Raman spectroscopy and CD.

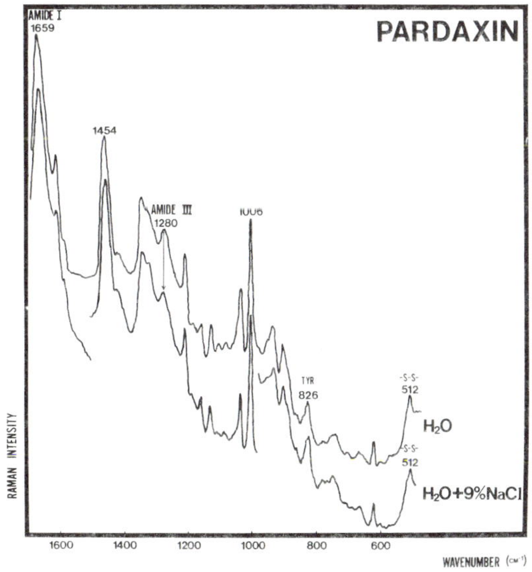

Fig. 4. Laser Raman spectra of Pardaxin in pH 4.9 in water and in 9% NaCl. Spectra were recorded as described in Materials and Methods.

The Raman spectra of a 9% NaCl solution show the Amide I and III bands appearing at 1659 cm^{-1} and 1280 cm^{-1} (Fig. 4). Apparently there is no substantial change in the peptide backbone conformation whether Pardaxin is in a salt free medium or a high salt medium (Fig. 4). Examination of the Raman spectra of Pardaxin in water and in 9% NaCl (Fig. 4) show no apparent differences in the major peaks (Amide I, Amide III, disulfide band). It is therefore obvious that the enhanced toxicity to fish at high salt concentrations is not due to a conformational change of the Pardaxin molecule.

pH Perturbation Studies

The Pardaxin far-UV CD spectra at various pHs are shown in Figure 5. At pH 3.45 and 8.7 Pardaxin shows the double minimum at 223 and 208 nm and a positive 196 nm peak indicating the presence of α-helix. However, the α-helix fraction is reduced compared to that at pH 4.9 (Table 1). On the other hand, at pHs of 2.8, 9.4, and 10.2, Pardaxin did not show the positive 190-196 nm peak, the 208 nm band was shifted to 205-6 nm and the 223 nm band was much weaker. In order to clarify if the loss of α-helical structure is reversible, Pardaxin at pH 10.2 (showing loss of α-helical structure) was titrated to pH 4.9. The titrated Pardaxin shows the recovery of α-helical structure (Fig. 5 and Table I), indicating the reversible nature of the transformation between these two different conformations. Increasing the pH of proteins may alter the conformation of aromatic side chains, of disulfide bridges or of the peptide backbone due to the ionizing tyrosyl or other groups (Strickland, 1974). The utility of CD in studying the conformation depends upon the possibility of correlating specific structures with characteristic CD spectra. It is not possible at present to give a detailed accounting of the origin of the pH dependent conformational changes in Pardaxin. At the most acidic pH, nor at the most alkaline pH, did the CD curve resemble the CD of unordered structure (Greenfield and Fasman, 1969).

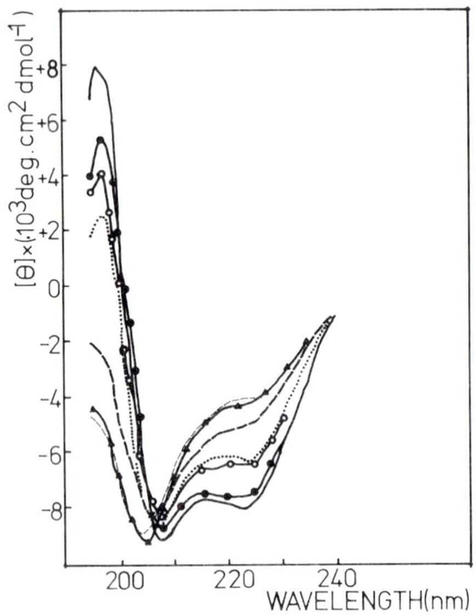

Fig. 5. Far-ultraviolet circular dichroism spectra of Pardaxin as a function of pH. In order to obtain a final pH Pardaxin in appropriate pH was incubated for 3 h at 20°C. (——) pH 4.9, (●——●) titrated 10.2 pH to pH 4.9, (— —) pH 10.2, (----) pH 2.8, (····) pH 3.4, (▲——▲) pH 9.4, (○——○) pH 8.7.

ACKNOWLEDGEMENTS

We would like to acknowledge the valuable assistance of Dr. Robert W. Woody, Mr. G. Shimer, Dr. Jay Fox, and Dr. Robert Hendon. This work was supported by NIH grant R01 GM 19172, by grant 1739 from the U.S.-Israel Binational Science Foundation (BSF), Jerusalem, Israel, and grant 14-75-C-0766, ONR, U. S. Navy.

Table I: Secondary Structure Estimations of Pardaxin from Far-Ultraviolet CD and Raman Spectroscopy.

Raman				CD						
Lippert et al. (1976)				Greenfield and Fasman (1969) (208 nm)			Chen et al. (1972) (222 nm)	Chen et al. (1972) (computed)		
α-helix (%)	β-structure (%)	Random (%)	pH	α-helix (%)	β-structure (%)	Random (%)	α-helix (%)	α-helix (%)	β-structure (%)	Random (%)
38.6	22.8	38.6	4.9	17.8	30[a]	50[a]	18.5	23	21	56
			4.9[a]	15.2			17.2			
			3.45	15.7			12.5			
			8.7	14.7			13.1			

[a]Pardaxin in pH 10.2 was titrated to pH of 4.9.

REFERENCES

Adler, A. J., Greenfield, N. Y., and Fasman, G. D. (1973). In Methods in Immunology, Colowick, S. P., and Kaplan, N. O., eds., Academic Press, XXVII, p. 689.
Bailey, G. S., Lee, J., and Tu, A. T. (1979). J. Biol. Chem., in press.
Bandekar, J., and Krimm, S. (1979). Proc. Nat. Acad. Sci. USA 76, 774-777.
Chen, Y. H., Yang, J. T., and Martinez, H. M. (1972). Biochemistry 11, 4120-4131.
Clark, F., and Chao, S. (1973). Sea Fish Res. Stn. Haifa Bull. 60, 53-56.
Craig, W. S., and Gaber, B. P. (1977). J. Am. Chem. Soc. 99, 4130-4134.
Demaille, J., Dutruge, F., Capony, Y. P., and Pechere, J. F. (1974). In Calcium Binding Proteins, Drabinowski, W., Stszelecka-Galaszewska, E., and Carafoli, E., eds., Elsevier, p. 643.
Ettinger, M. J., and Timasheff, S. N. (1971). Biochemistry 10, 824-831.
Fox, J., and Tu, A. T. (1979). Arch. Biochem. Biophys. 193, 407-414.
Greenfield, N., Fasman, G. D. (1969). Biochemistry 8, 4108-4126.
Hanley, M. R. (1979). Biochemistry 18, 1681-1688.
Horwitz, J., Strickland, E. H., and Billups, C. (1970). J. Amer. Chem. Soc. 92, 2119, 2129.
Hruby, V. M., Deb, K. K., Fox, J., Bjarnason, J., and Tu, A. T. (1978). J. Biol. Chem. 253, 6060-6067.
Ishizaki, H., McKay, R. H., Norton, T. R., Yasunobu, K. T., Lee, J., and Tu, A. T. (1979). J. Biol. Chem., in press.
Kreuger, W. C., and Pschigoda, L. M. (1971). Anal. Biochem. 43, 675-677.
Lippert, J. L., Tyminski, D., Desmeules, P. J. (1976). J. Am. Chem. Soc. 98, 7075-7080.

Madison, V., and Schellman, J. (1972). Biopolymers 11, 1635-1643.
Maxfield, F. R., and Scheraga, H. A. (1977). Biochemistry 16, 4443-4449.
Menez, A., Bouet, F., Tamiya, N., and Fromageot, P. (1976). Biochim. Biophys. Acta 543, 121-132.
Parello, J., and Pechere, J. F. (1971). Biochimie 53, 1079-1083.
Parness, J., and Zlotkin (1976). Toxicon 14, 85-91.
Primor, N., Parness, J., and Zlotkin, E. (1978). In Toxins: Animal, Plant and Microbial, Rosenberg, P., ed., Pergamon Press, pp. 539-547.
Primor, N., Sabnay, I., Lavie, V., and Zlotkin, E. (1979). J. Exp. Zool., in press.
Siamwiza, M. N., Lord, R. C., and Chen, M. C. (1975). Biochemistry 14, 4870-4876.
Spira, M. E., Klein, M., Hochner, B., Yarom, Y., and Castel, M. (1976). Neuroscience 1, 117-124.
Strickland, E. N. (1974). CRC Crit. Rev. Biochem. 2, 113-175.
Sugeta, H., Go, A., and Miyazawa, T. (1973). Bull. Chem. Soc. Japan 46, 3407-3411.
Sugeta, H., Go, A., and Miyazawa, T. (1972). Chem. Lett. 38, 83-86.
Townend, R., Kumosinski, T. F., and Timasheff, S. N. (1967). J. Biol. Chem. 242, 4538-4545.
Tu, A. T. (1977). Venoms: Chemistry and Molecular Biology, Wiley, 560 pages.
Tu, A. T., Bjarnason, J., and Hruby, V. J. (1978). Biochim. Biophys. Acta 533, 530-533.
Tu, A. T., Lee, J., Deb, K. K., and Hruby, V. J. (1979). J. Biol. Chem. 254, 3272-3278.
Tu, A. T., Jo, B. H., and Yu, N. (1976). Int. J. Peptide and Prot. Res. 8, 337-343.
Viljoen, C. C., Visser, L., and Bobes, D. P. (1976). Biochim. Biophys. Acta 438, 424-436.
Yu, N., Lin, T., and Tu, A. T. (1975). J. Biol. Chem. 250, 1782-1785.
Yu, N., Jo, B. H., and O'Shea, D. C. (1973). Arch. Biochem. Biophys. 156, 71-76.

STRUCTURE-FUNCTION RELATIONSHIPS IN POSTSYNAPTIC SNAKE NEUROTOXINS

B. W. Low

Department of Biochemistry, College of Physicians and Surgeons, Columbia University, 630 West 168 Street, New York, N.Y. 10032, USA

ABSTRACT

Detailed information about the three-dimensional structure of the protein, erabutoxin b, (Low and others, 1976) provides a recognized and recognizable stereochemical prototype (Low and others, 1976; Low, 1979a) or model for the whole class of more than 50 curaremimetic postsynaptic neurotoxins from both land and sea snakes. Homology of structure and function in this class has a broad base defined by the whole spectrum of chemical, physicochemical, and toxicological, etc. studies: in particular, amino acid primary sequence determinations establish extensive homologies expressed as multiple positions of residue invariance and conservative substitution. Toxicities (LD_{50}) lie within a very narrow range; in some instances direct evidence has shown that these neurotoxins bind to the acetylcholine receptor at the neuromuscular junction. Most of the principal main-chain features of this remarkably open structure have been described earlier; (Low and others, 1976; Sato, 1977). They will be reviewed and discussed here in terms of their role in maintaining structural and, therefore, functional integrity (Kimball and others, 1979). The structural role of the four invariant disulfide linkages has been established chemically:- a role evident in the molecular stereochemistry; they form a stabilizing central core.

The reactive site, that is the region of binding interactions with the acetylcholine receptor, asserts itself. Most positions of residue invariance or conservative substitution fall within the sequence range 25—>53 (K60) and thus within the shallow cupped region bounded by 32-49...32 (K33-K56...K33) which this sequence forms in three dimensions. The key 'structural' role of some residues is evident. Other residues have been designated 'functional'. These all point essentially up from or into the sweeping hollow of the loop region 32-49...32. Replacement of some 'functional' residues in deviant toxins and/or their chemical modification results in reduced toxicity. Details of the inter-residue packing in this region led to the characterization of 5 discrete reactive interactive groupings (Low, 1979 a and b).

Recent studies (Kimball and Low, 1979) have provided an alternative view of the reactive site, that is the topographical features of this concavity. The striking distribution of charged polar and hydrophobic residues which characterizes the reactive site surface, as well as the molecule as a whole, will be discussed, and a secondary structure/function role for the whole proposed (Low and others, in preparation). Thus, a new and, to date, unique reactive surface and general molecular stereochemistry has been defined which may be appropriate, not only to these neurotoxins, but to other membrane active proteins of this general type. All the principal structure/function relationships considered here (determined from erabutoxin b, a short series toxin) can easily be adapted to long series toxins without fundamental alterations.

REFERENCES

Kimball, M. R., and B. W. Low, (1979). Structure and Function in the Snake Venom Postsynaptic Neurotoxins - A Three-Dimensional View of the Reactive Site. XIth International Congress of Biochemistry, Toronto, Canada, Poster Abstract, p. 557. Based on results obtained using the GRIP-75 Molecular Graphics System (University of North Carolina) and on shaded-surface plots made on this system.

Kimball, M. R., A. Sato, J. S. Richardson, L. S. Rosen, and B. W. Low, (1979). Molecular Conformation of Erabutoxin b; Atomic Coordinates at 2.5A Resolution. Biochem. Biophys. Research Comm., 88, 950-959.

Low, B. W., H. S. Preston, A. Sato, L. S. Rosen, J. E. Searl, A. D. Rudko, and J. S. Richardson, (1976). The Three Dimensional Structure of Erabutoxin b Neurotoxic Protein: Inhibitor of Acetylcholine Receptor. Proc. Nat. Acad. Sci., USA 73, 9, 2991-2994.

Low, B. W. (1979a). In Chen-Yuan Lee (Ed.), Snake Venoms - Handbook of Experimental Pharmacology, Vol. 52. Springer-Verlag, Berlin. Pp. 213-257.

Low, B. W. (1979b). In B. Ceccarelli and F. Clementi (Eds.), Advances in Cytopharmacology, Vol. 3. Raven Press, N. Y. Pp. 141-147.

Sato, A. (1977). Ph.D. thesis, Tohoku University, Japan.

THREE-DIMENSIONAL STRUCTURE OF α-COBRATOXIN

M. D. Walkinshaw*[1], W. Saenger* and A. Maelicke[2]**

**Max Planck-Institut für experimentelle Medizin, Abteilung Chemie, Hermann-Rein-Str. 3, D-3400 Göttingen, Federal Republic of Germany*
***Rockefeller University, New York, N.Y. 10021, USA*

ABSTRACT

The three-dimensional structure of the principal neurotoxin of the cobra, Naja naja siamensis, has been determined at 2.8 Å resolution. Crystals were grown by microdialysis of toxin solutions against a mixture (3:1) of 2-methyl-2,4-pentanediol and buffer (0.05 M glycine.HCl, pH 2.0). The hexagonal needles had the space group $P6_522$ with unit cell dimensions a=b=74.59 Å, c=42.89 Å. Two heavy atom derivatives were prepared by cocrystallization.

The polypeptide chain folds into three major loops and one tail emerging from a globular head. The protuding long central loop (residues 21-40) is flanked on either side by two shorter loops (residues 4-13 and 44-55); the C-terminal tail (residues 63-71) hangs behind this loop. The molecular conformation is determined by four disulfide bridges in the head and one at the tip of the long loop, by a triple standed ß-pleated sheet involving the long loop, and by hydrophobic interactions stabilizing the other two loops.

KEYWORDS

x-ray; crystal structure; neurotoxin; snake venom; cobra.

INTRODUCTION

The neurotoxins of elapid (cobra and krait) and hydrophid (sea) snakes produce non-depolarizing neuromuscular block by acting at the nicotinic receptors of postsynaptic membranes. Their powerful curarizing effects (Chang and Lee, 1963) and the slow rates of dissociation of receptor-toxin complexes have made the neurotoxins outstandingly useful as labeling reagents for isolation, purification and assay of nicotinic receptors (Klett and colleagues, 1973; Maelicke and colleagues, 1977).

---

[1]present address: Department of Chemistry, Edinburgh University, West Mains Road, Edinburgh, Scotland

[2]present address: Max-Planck-Institut für Ernährungsphysiologie, Rheinlanddamm 201, D-4600 Dortmund

While all other cholinergic ligands have low molecular weights, the snake neurotoxins are macromolecules with polypeptide structure. To aid in understanding their mode of action, many attempts were made to elucidate their three-dimensional structure. Although the first neurotoxin crystals were reported as early as 1938 (Slotta and Fraenkel-Conrat), the first crystal structure has only been solved in 1976 (Tsernoglou and Petsko; Low and colleagues). While this sea snake toxin belongs to the group of small neurotoxins (with 4 disulfide bridges and 60-62 amino acids), we now have succeeded in obtaining the three-dimensional structure of a long neurotoxin (with 5 disulfide bridges and 71 aminoacids). Together with the results of biochemical, immunological and physiological studies the three-dimensional structures of the two archetype toxins may open the way to a better understanding of both the subtle structure-function differences between the two families of neurotoxins and the nature of neurotoxin-receptor interaction.

TOXIN PREPARATION AND CRYSTALLIZATION

For the purpose of growing crystals, more than 45 g of cobra venom (Naja naja siamensis), obtained from Miami Serpentarium, Florida (batches NS44-1, NS2S and NS5-B7) and Biologicals Unlimited, Baltimore, were purified and characterized. Two different purification procedures were employed. The first one (Karlsson, Arnberg and Eaker, 1971, Karlsson and Sundelin, 1976) did not yield material of sufficient purity. Chromatography on sulphopropyl Sephadex at pH 9 and two dimensional polyacrylamide gels revealed up to six different impurities, totaling 8 to 30% (depending on source and batch of the venom). They could not be separated by gel filtration on Sephadex G-50 as suggested by Karlsson (1971) but, instead, appeared to have either identical or closely similar molecular weights. We do not know whether this heterogeneity in the α-toxin region of cobra venom reflects the existence of isotoxins in the venom or whether it was due to venom collection from several snake subspecies. These impurities affected growth and diffraction properties of crystals and, hence, further purification was required. We therefore developed an alternative procedure based on the method of Cooper and Reich (1972). It involved ion exchange chromatography employing successively (1) phosphocellulose eluted with a gradient of 0.01 to 0.3 M potassium phosphate, pH 6.0, (2) Biorex 70 eluted with a shallow gradient of 0.08-0.18 M ammonium acetate, pH 6.5 and (3) carboxymethyl cellulose, eluted with a gradient of 0.08-0.18 NaCl in 0.01 M TrisHCl, pH 6.8. In some preparations CM-cellulose was replaced by SP-Sephadex, eluted with a gradient of 0.05-0.15 M sodium borate buffer, pH 9.0. In the final two chromatographic steps we generally employed a Gilson Mixograd gradient former with peak detector. The best results were obtained with linear gradient profiles. The major toxin obtained by this way displayed a single band of protein in polyacrylamide gradient gel electrophoresis (Rüchel, 1976) and isoelectric focussing on microgels (Rüchel, 1977). The ratios of toxicity (determined by intravenous injection into female NMRI/80 mice (Kang and Maelicke, 1980) and of binding affinity (determined as described by Maelicke and colleagues, 1977) to protein concentration remained constant across the peak. Antibodies raised in rabbits against highly purified material of one preparation reacted specifically with the major purified fraction of other preparations but had lower reactivity towards the other fractions in the α-toxin region. Fingerprint pattern and aminoacid analysis were in agreement with the aminoacid sequence determined by Karlsson and colleagues (1972). Depending on source and batch of venom, total α-toxin comprised 6-18% of weight of lyophilized venom. Yield of highly purified α-toxin was 2-5%. A detailed account of preparation and purification of α-toxin will be published in a separate paper.

Crystallization of the toxin was achieved under a variety of conditions using as precipitants sodium or ammonium sulfate, n-propanol or 2-methyl-2,4- pentanediol (MPD) at pH-ranges from 2 to 8. Of the five crystal forms obtained by vapor diffusion or microdialysis techniques (Dattagupta and colleagues, 1975), those grown from a 1.5 % (w/v) protein/water solution dialyzed against 75 % (v/v) MPD/0.05 M glycine·HCl in water, pH 2 (final pH 2.83) exhibited the best properties for X-ray diffraction work. These crystals grew within a few days as hexagonal needles up to 3 mm long and 0.5 mm wide.

X-RAY DIFFRACTION ANALYSIS

For X-ray experiments the crystals were sealed in thin walled quartz capillaries. Diffraction patterns of the crystals displayed symmetry and systematic extinctions consistent with the hexagonal space group $P6_122$ or its enantiomorph $P6_522$. Cell constants are a = b = 74.59 (4) Å, c = 42.89 (3) Å. In order to solve the inherent phase problem, two heavy atom derivatives were prepared by crystallising the toxin from 1 mM solutions of HgI_2 and of $Hg(Acetate)_2$ in the above described MPD/buffer system.
X-ray intensity data were collected on a four circle diffractometer in the ω-scan mode using Ni-filtered CuKα-radiation. For the native crystal, 2800 unique reflections to 2.5 Å resolution were measured and for derivative crystals, 4200 anomalous data (Friedel mates hkl, h>k and h<k) were collected to 2.8 Å. Crystal decay was monitored by four reference reflections and in no case exceeded 27 %. Data were corrected for background (Pähler and Saenger, 1979), for Lorentzpolarization factors, for crystal decay and for absorption (North and colleagues, 1968). Native and derivative data were put on a common scale by analyzing them in ranges of $\sin^2\theta/\lambda^2$.

According to Matthew's (1966) formula, lower estimates of heavy atom contributions (F_{HLE}) were calculated. These data were used in MULTAN (1977) as well as in Patterson techniques to obtain heavy atom locations. Refinement by conventional full matrix least squares led to R-indices of 38.2 % for HgI_2 but to only 54.7 % for $Hg(Acetate)_2$, probably due to non-isomorphism of native and derivative unit cells.

In both derivatives, Hg atoms are in nearly identical positions and located on a diad passing through z = 0.25. Final atomic parameters are:

HgI_2		x	y	z	occupancy	B(Å²)
	Hg	0.5961	1.1922	0.2500	0.4947	7.8
	I	0.5727	1.1823	0.2949	0.9894	10.3
$Hg(Acetate)_2$						
	Hg	0.609	1.198	0.267	0.55	7.6

For phase determination (Blow and Crick, 1959), only the HgI_2 derivative was used and the phase ambiguity was resolved by utilizing anomalous data. The 2161 reflections to 2.8 Å resolution yielded a mean figure of merit (m) of 73.8 % and were used to compute an electron density map with "best" centroid phases and $|F_P|$ weighted by m.

Decision between the two enantiomorphic space groups $P6_122$ and $P6_522$ was made in favour of the latter on the basis of difference Fourier maps calculated with native phases in both space groups and coefficients $||F_P|-|F_{Hg(Acetate)_2}||$. In $P6_522$, the Hg-peak showed up stronger than in $P6_122$ and the electron density map of the protein calculated in $P6_522$ was more clearly defined than a map in $P6_122$. Interpretation of the $P6_522$ map was done by means of a Richard's box (1968) using Kendrew's wire models, scale 2 cm = 1Å to build a model according to the density, with the known sequence shown in Fig. 1.

3-DIMENSIONAL STRUCTURE OF α-COBRATOXIN

The overall molecular shape of α-cobratoxin can be described as a well defined ellipsoidal disk of dimensions 40 x 30 x 20 Å. The main topological features of the electron density map are a triple stranded antiparallel ß-pleated sheet, disulfide groups bridging density belonging to the main chain and aromatic side groups showing up strongly. The tail region of the molecule (residues 62 to 71) is not as well defined as other parts but it is still clear enough to allow definite chain tracing. The molecule appears as a globular head from which a long central loop hangs down as a nose (residues 21 to 40), flanked on both sides by two shorter loops (residues 4 to 13 and 44 to 55) reminiscent of floppy ears (Fig. 2). The tail piece hangs down behind the nose. The main structural feature is the antiparallel triple stranded ß-pleated sheet formed by (A) residues 20 to 25, (B) residues 36 to 40 and (C), residues 53 to 57, with the arrangement (B)↑(A)↓(C)↑. Further, four of the five disulfides are located in the globular head tightening the three loops together. Going along the chain, Fig. 2, the first short loop (4-13) is stabilized entirely by hydrophobic interactions of side groups pointing to each other. Coming up to the globular head, a ß-turn formed by Pro 15 and His 18 reverses the chain direction down into the long central loop which, providing two antiparallel strands of the triple ß-pleated sheet, displays two ß-turns at the lower tip involving Asp 27, Cys 30 and Cys 30, Arg 33. This intricate structure is further stabilized by the fifth disulfide Cys 26-Cys 30. Going up the central loop, the chain falls gently into the second short loop (residues 45-56) which, as described for the first short loop, is stabilized by hydrophobic interactions involved in the triple ß-pleated sheet via residues 53 to 57. The prolongation of this loop is directed towards and "behind" the globular head and is forced by a ß-turn between Thr 59 and Cys 62 to fall down to form the long tail which is tightened to the core of the molecule by hydrophobic interactions between Phe 64, Pro 65 and Phe 4, Thr 9, Val 37, Leu 39.

Within the hexagonal unit cell the α-cobratoxin molecules are packed such that Phe 29 of one molecule is in hydrophobic contact with the tail residues (63-68) and the "back side" of the first loop (residues 3-10). Further intermolecular interactions are provided by carboxyls of Asp 8, Asp 60 and Pro 71, which are located near diads and, since they are protonated at the pH of crystallization, allow for strong carboxyl - carboxyl hydrogen bonds. It is interesting to note the heavy atom group HgI_2, located on a diad, is in 3.5 Å vicinity of a hydrophobic cage formed at the globular head by the bridge Cys 14-Cys 41 and by Pro 15, Asn 16, Gly 17, Ala 42 and 43. This special location indicates why the HgI_2 derivative displays a fully occupied heavy atom site.

DISCUSSION

Comparing the three-dimensional structure of the "long" α-cobratoxin with that of the "short" erabutoxin b (Tsernoglou and Petsko, 1976; Low and colleagues, 1976), one finds that both have a similar overall shape. There are, however, a number of significant structural differences. (1) The first hydrophobic loop is 3 residues shorter in the "long" toxin compared to the "short" one, and therefore is less prominent. It protects a side section (residues 38-41) of the long central loop and allows the long tail (absent in the "short" toxin) to hang down over the "back side" of this loop. (2) The protuding tapered neck region of the "short" toxin is reduced in the "long" structure. (3) The lower tip of the long loop in the "long" toxin shows a much broader, more complicated structural feature compared to that of the "short" toxin. (4) The third hydrophobic loop in the "long" toxin is more planar than in the "short" toxin and its plane is nearly vertical to the plane formed by the triple stranded ß-pleated sheet.

Looking at amino acid sequences of "long" and "short" neurotoxins aligned in register with sequences of cardiotoxins, we conclude that homologous amino acids in all three types of toxins are likely to have a structural role. There are, in the "long" series, Cys 3, 14, 20, 41, 45, 56, 57; Gly 17, 40,; Pro 46; Asn 63 and Tyr 21. Those amino acids common to "long" and "short" neurotoxins but not to cardiotoxins may be called functional with respect to neurotoxicity and involve Trp 25; Arg 33; Gly 34. Homologous in "long" neurotoxins" only are residues Cys 26, 30; Lys 35; Ala 43; Thr 44; Ser 58 and Asp 60. A recent review (Low, 1979) points out residues likely to be involved in the binding of neurotoxin to the acetylcholine receptor. These are, in the "long" toxin series, Trp 25; Asp 27; Arg 33; Gly 34 and Lys 49. Four of these are located on the lower tip and on the "upper" surface of the long central loop (Fig. 2). Lys 49 is on the outer rim of the third, hydrophobically centered loop (residues 45-56).

One of the most striking differences between "long" and "short" toxins is their specific binding to antibodies. Antibodies raised against "long" neurotoxins do not complex with "short" ones and _vice versa_ (Menez and colleagues, 1979; Tamiya and Abe, 1979). It has been established that most of the neurotoxin aminoacids involved in antibody binding are located on the "tail-side" of the toxin molecules where, according to the three-dimensional studies, major structural differences are observed.

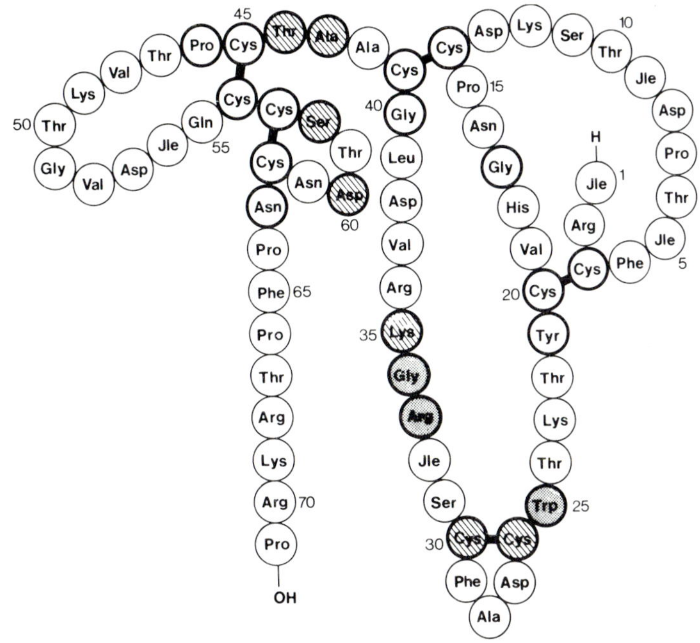

Fig. 1

Primary structure of α-cobratoxin from _Naja naja siamensis_. As described by Karlsson (1979), heavy circles indicate invariant residues in the long, short and cardiotoxin families, hatched circles represent residues invariant only in the long toxin family and stippled circles correspond to residues which are invariant in long and short toxin families but not in cardiotoxins.

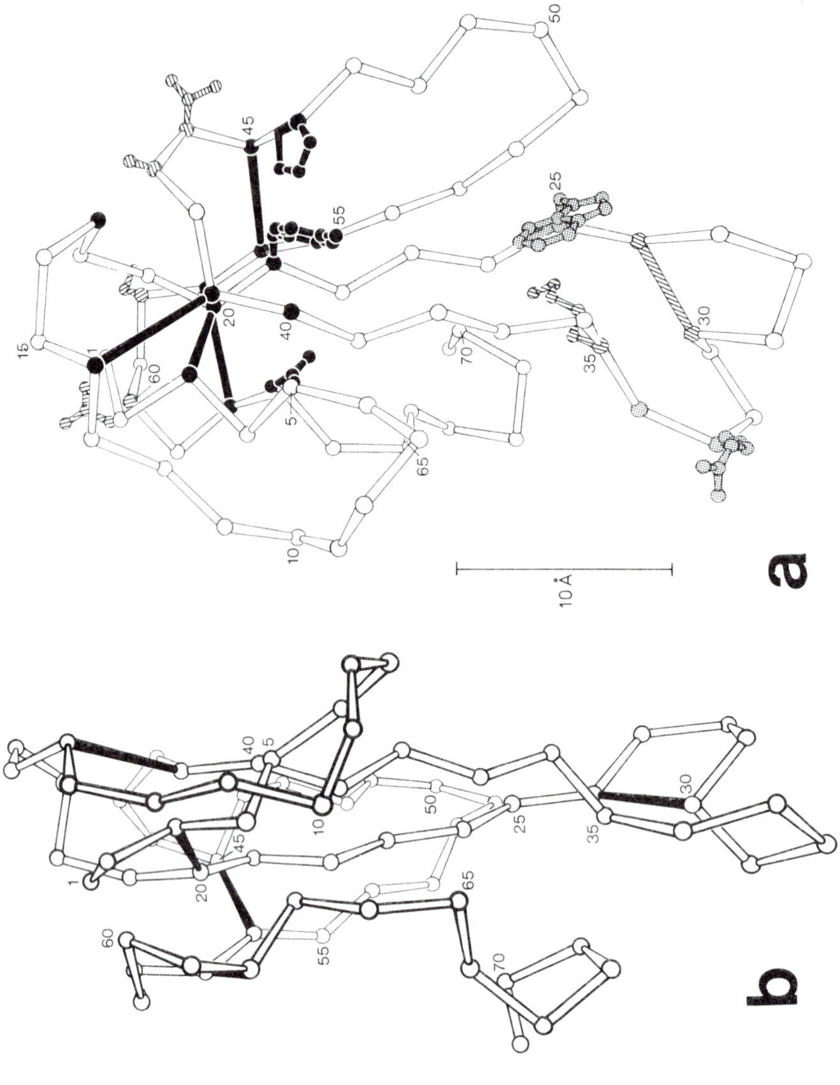

Fig. 2

Front (a) and side (b) view of the α-cobratoxin molecule, showing the folding of the peptide chain. Only C_α-positions are shown and, in (a), some side groups are indicated. Those drawn black are invariant in long, short and cardiotoxins, those drawn hatched are invariant in long neurotoxins only and stippled side groups are invariant in long and in short toxins but not in cardiotoxins.

REFERENCES

Blow, D. M., and F. H. C. Crick (1959). Acta Cryst.,12, 794-802.
Chang, C. C. and C.-Y. Lee (1963). Arch Int. Pharmacodyn., 114, 241-257.
Cooper, D., and E. Reich (1972). J. Biol. Chem., 247, 3008-3013.
Dattagupta, J. K., T Fujiwara, E. V. Grishin, K. Lindner, P. C. Manor, N. J. Pieniiazek, W. Saenger, and D Suck (1975). J. Mol. Biol., 97, 267-271.
Kang, S., and A. Maelicke (1980). J. Biol. Chem., in press.
Karlsson, E. (1979). Handbook of Experimental Pharmacology, Ed. C.-Y. Lee (Springer-Verlag, Berlin, Heidelberg) 52, 159-212.
Karlsson, E., H. Arnberg, and D. Eaker (1971). Eur. J. Biochem., 21, 1-16.
Karlsson, E., D. Eaker, and G. Ponterius (1972). Biochim. Biophys. Acta, 257, 235-248.
Karlsson, E., and J. Sundelin (1976). Toxicon, 14, 295-306.
Klett, R. P., B. W. Fulpius, D. Cooper, M. Smith, E. Reich, and L. D. Possani (1973). J. Biol. Chem., 248, 6841-6853.
Low, B. W. (1979). Handbook of Experimental Pharmacology, Ed. C.-Y. Lee (Springer-Verlag, Berlin, Heidelberg) 52, 213-257.
Low, B. W., H. S. Preston, A. Sato, L. S. Rosen, J. E. Searl, A. D. Rudko, and J. S. Richardson (1976). Proc. Natl. Acad. Sci. USA, 73, 2991-2994.
Maelicke, A., B. W. Fulpius, R. P. Klett, and E. Reich (1977). J. Biol. Chem., 252, 4811-4830.
Main, P., L. Lessinger, M. M. Woolfson, G. Germain and J. P. Declercq (1977). MULTAN. A System of Computer Programs for the Automatic Solution of Crystal Structures from X-Ray Diffraction Data. Univ. of York, England and Louvain, Belgium.
Matthews, B. W. (1966). Acta Cryst., 20, 230-239.
Menez, A., J. C. Boulain, and P. Fromageot (1979). Toxicon, 17, Suppl. 1, 123.
North, A. C. T., D. C. Phillips, and F. S. Matthews (1968). Acta Cryst. A24, 351-359.
Pähler, A., and W. Saenger (1979). Z. Krist., 149, 192.
Richards, F. M. (1968). J. Mol. Biol., 37, 225-230.
Rüchel, R. (1976). J. Histochem. Cytochem., 24, 773-791.
Rüchel, R. (1977). J. Chromatog., 132, 451-468.
Slotta, K. H., and H. Fraenkel-Conrat (1938). Ber. Dtsch. Chem. Ges.,71, 1076-1081.
Tamiya, N., and Abe, T. (1979). Toxicon, 17, Suppl. 1, 186.
Tsernoglou, D., and G. A. Petsko (1976). FEBS Lett., 68, 1-4.

THE STRUCTURE OF THE REACTIVE SITE IN ELAPIDAE NEUROTOXINS

R. C. Hider and M. J. Dufton

Dept. of Chemistry, Univ. of Essex, Wivenhoe Park, Colchester, Essex, UK

ABSTRACT

There is now extensive sequence and chemical modification data regarding Elapid neurotoxins and, with the availability of X-ray crystallographic structures of the two major types, the undertaking of structure activity relationships has become highly feasible. Comparison of these X-ray structures with relevant solution studies reveals facets of these molecules which are not evident from the former in isolation and thus have a great bearing on the manner by which structure-activity relationships can be approached. It is hypothesised that under physiological conditions there is a conformational equilibrium between two defined states, one of which could be a close stereochemical mimic of curare-like alkaloids.

KEYWORDS

Venom; neurotoxin; structure-activity relationships; circular dichroism; alkaloid mimic.

INTRODUCTION

Many workers have accepted the challenge of trying to understand how Elapid neurotoxins achieve their toxicity, but, to date, a comprehensive explanation has proved elusive. Although these protein toxins are relatively small in size (60-70 residues), stable to denaturant conditions and relatively easy to isolate and analyse, it is their "target" - the nicotinic cholinergic receptor - that preserves the mystery through its resistance to many characterisation techniques. The researcher, therefore, must make use of the extensive structural information that is now available on neurotoxins and combine this with the limited knowledge of the receptor and established precedent for possible protein-protein interactions.

In outline, experiment has so far shown that the neurotoxins can form a very stable complex with the receptor, but without the formation of covalent bonds as such. Amongst the remaining attractive forces, hydrophobicity would appear to be the most important. In addition, some kind of conformational change, either in the toxin, target or both, may be a prerequisite of binding (Maelicke and co-workers, 1977). As suggested by Chicheportiche and co-workers (1975), this binding could be similar to that of an enzyme and its appropriate protein inhibitor, involving hydrogen bonding, electrostatic attraction, Van der Waals forces and a gross complementation of the architecture of the two molecules.

Toxin Structure

Numerous sequences of neurotoxins from different Elapids have been obtained and it is clear that they are all homologous and thus related through evolution. There are some distinct features, however, and on the basis of these, the sequences can be divided into two groups - the "short" neurotoxins (60-62 residues, 4 disulphide bridges) and "long" neurotoxins (67-70 residues, 5 disulphide bridges). There are other homologous toxins (e.g. the cytotoxins), but here the differences in sequence are associated with distinct pharmacological properties (Karlsson, 1979).

Sequence information is especially useful when it can be appraised relative to the 3-D conformation that the polypeptide chain as a whole adopts. Significant advances were thus the deductions of the crystallographic backbones of a short and long neurotoxin. These are portrayed in Fig. 1 and it can be seen that the molecular organisation of the two toxin types is essentially the same. Since amino acid sequences are expected to inherently code the 3-D conformation, many

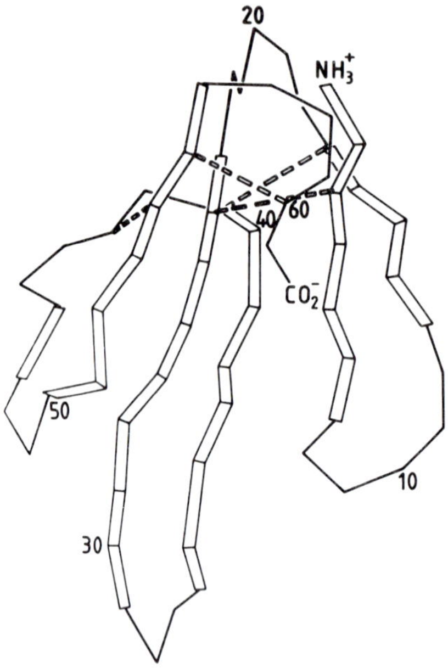

(erabutoxin *b*)
Short Neurotoxin

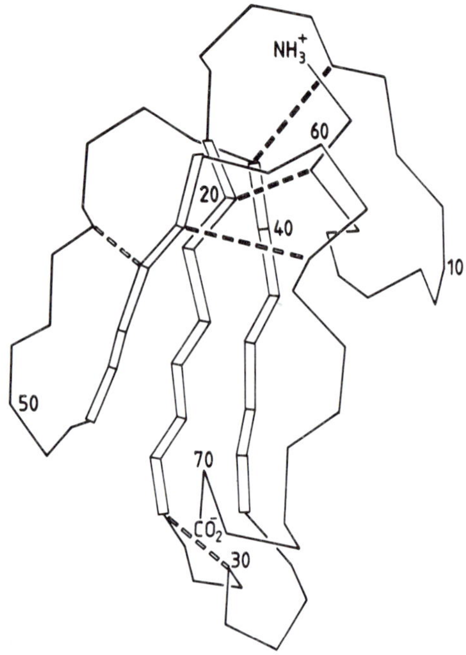

(α-cobratoxin)
Long Neurotoxin

Fig. 1. Peptide backbone structures of a short neurotoxin (Kimball and co-workers, 1979) and a long neurotoxin (Walkinshaw and co-workers, 1980) as determined by X-ray crystallography. The plate sections indicate β-sheet, the dashed lines indicate disulphide bridges.

workers have attempted to predict toxin structure from the sequences alone. With the advent of the X-ray crystallographic structure of erabutoxin *b* some of these have proved to be more accurate than others (Dufton and Hider, 1977; Menez and co-workers, 1978). Figure 2 shows aggregate β-sheet predictions for short and long neurotoxins as derived from a modified Chou and Fasman analysis (Dufton and Hider, 1977). The most consistently predicted segments show close approximation to the areas of β-conformation as detected by the crystallography, so to regard the experimentally derived structures as representative of their particular groups appears justified. Predictions for β-turns similarly show much agreement with the crystallography and also complement the β-sheet predictions. Interestingly, although no helical conformation is expected in these molecules, it has been found that most helix potential occurs in distinct domains that are very similar to those of the βsheet. The C-terminal "tail" unique to long neurotoxins is shown by the crystallography not to contribute significantly to the β-sheeted network of the molecule and thus it has a certain independence. Predictions (Dufton and Hider, 1977) suggest that it has a "random coil" nature in all such toxins and also that its positioning along the central loop may be defined by certain conserved residues in the latter.

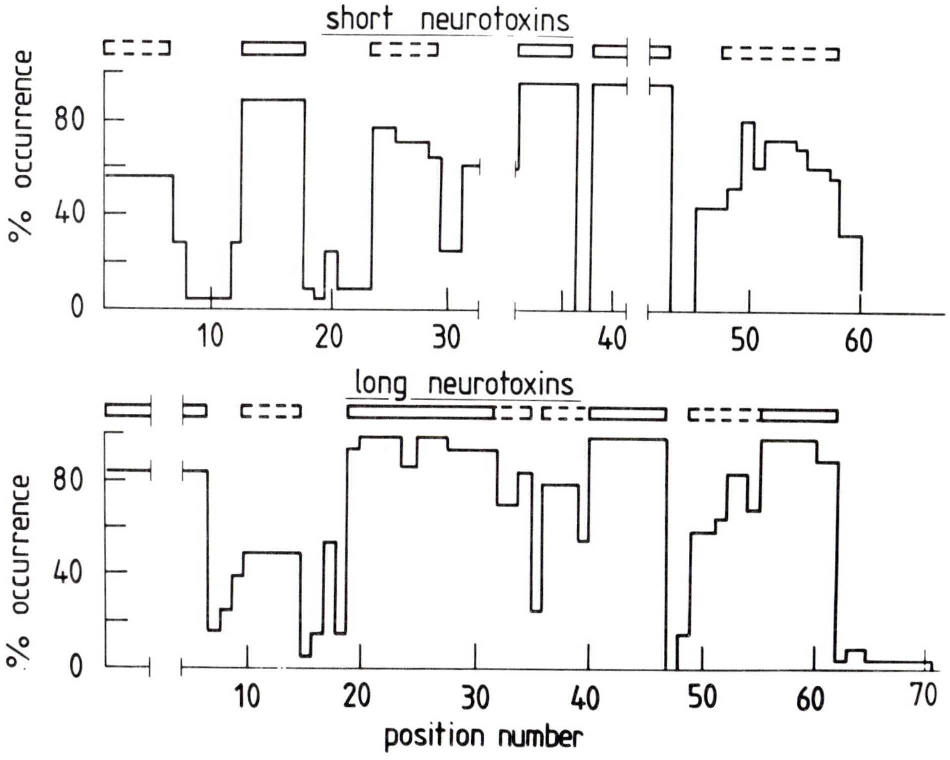

Fig. 2. Aggregate β-sheet predictions (Dufton and Hider, 1977) for short neurotoxins (24) and long neurotoxins (20).

TOXIN STRUCTURE IN SOLUTION

Given the X-ray crystallographic conformation and extensive sequence and chemical modification data, one can pick out those residues that have been conserved through evolution and those that have the most effect on toxicity when chemically altered. Such residues may be termed "essential" and so it remains to interpret the juxtaposition of these as revealed by the crystallography. This kind of approach has been pursued by several workers, including the authors, but it can be criticised on several counts, the most important being the question of how relevant a crystal structure can be to a solution structure.

It is often the case that indicators of molecular organisation such as CD, NMR and Laser Raman spectroscopy are regarded as "interim" until the advent of the crystallographic map, and that once the latter has been obtained, information from the former may be neglected. However, as crystallisation is difficult - the toxins required high salt media and organic solvents - there is a greater risk of deducing a structure that has been perturbed from its conformation in physiological media. This is because the dielectric changes involved can give preference to otherwise unfavourable conformations. For the short neurotoxins, disagreements between solution studies and the crystallography centre on the molecular environment of tryptophan-29 (Lauterwein and co-workers, 1978) and histidine 7 (Inagaki and co-workers, 1978). It has been shown by Drake and co-workers (1977) that the CD spectrum of a similar short neurotoxin can be perturbed by the crystallising media, the change appearing to involve tryptophan-29 and its vicinity independently of the overall content of β-conformation. In addition, erabutoxin *b* was solved by two groups of workers using different crystallising media, and close examination of the respective structures reported (Tsernoglou and co-workers, 1978; Kimball and co-workers, 1979) reveals that they are not identical. Similarly, long neurotoxins have also been found to be sensitive to such media.

Figure 3 shows the response of the CD spectrum of a short neurotoxin to temperature variation, and from this one can deduce that under physiological conditions, a conformational equilibrium independent of the β-content exists. Such conformational changes were first reported by Menez and co-workers (1976). The presence of the isosbestic point in this spectrum shows that the change proceeds between defined initial and final states. Again, identical changes can be observed in the response of long neurotoxin CD spectra to temperature increase.

EXTENT OF CONFORMATIONAL LABILITY

Inspection of the crystal structure of erabutoxin *b* suggests that the prominence of the central loop is extremely exposed to the solvent (Fig. 1). In solution, this would necessarily mean that the associated peptide chain and residues are extensively solvated. In essence, a hydrogen bonded structure similar to that of a "Schwyzer-form" cyclic hexapeptide is formed by this extremity. Many such hexapeptides are known to favour two transannular hydrogen bonds in the solid state, but according to NMR, they become more randomised in aqueous solution with much less propensity to form these bonds (Llinás and co-workers, 1972). Thus, the behaviour of these peptides provides a suitable model with which to appreciate the kind of conformational balance that may exist in neurotoxins and to understand how it could be perturbed by different media.

In terms of actual residues, the conformational change is envisaged to involve the relatively exposed aromatic side chain at position 32 (Fig. 4A) moving towards tryptophan-29 (Fig. 4B). This reorientation could explain the findings of several workers that the latter residue is partially buried in aqueous solution. The NMR data obtained by Bystrov and co-workers (1978) from short neurotoxins provides

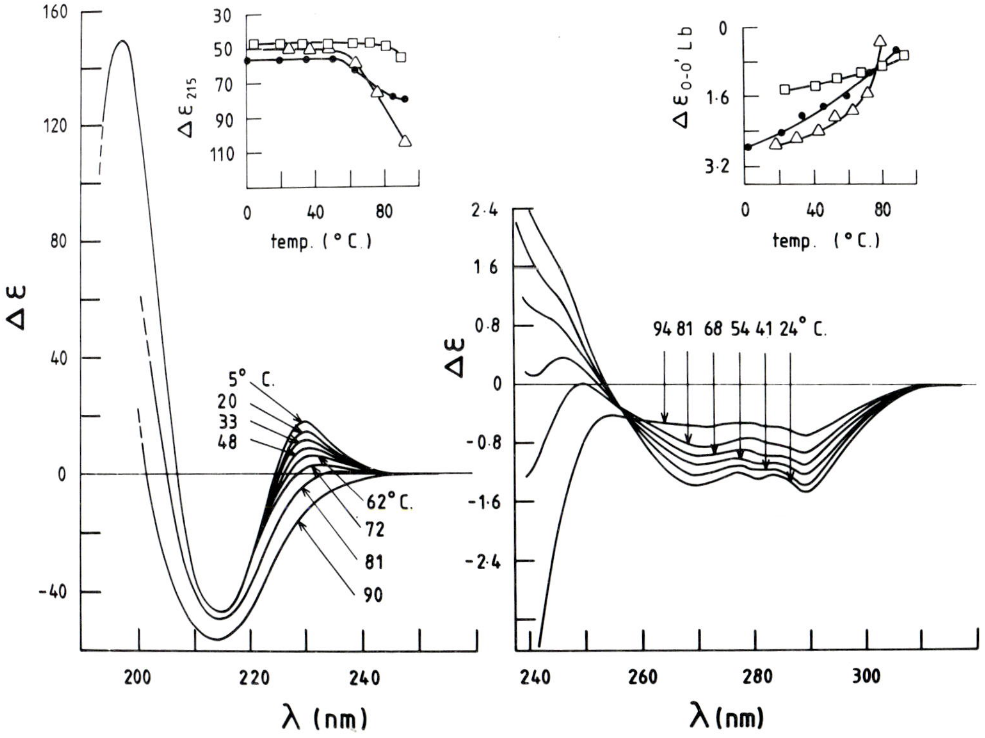

Fig. 3. Response of the CD spectrum of 4.11.3 to temperature variation. The insets show melting curves for the β-sheet structure ($\Delta\varepsilon_{215}$) and the temperature dependence of a conformational change ($\Delta\varepsilon_{0-0}{}^{1}Lb$) for two long and one short neurotoxin. □, 4.11.3; Δ, 3.9.4; and ●, 4.9.3.

further evidence for the proximity of positions 29 and 32.

Under physiological conditions, therefore, it appears that short and long neurotoxins can exist in an equilibrium of two conformers, which in the case of short neurotoxins, may be essentially as shown in Fig. 4. The crystallisation process is expected to perturb this equilibrium and thus give an indication of only one of these conformers after X-ray analysis. An interesting possibility is that this equilibrium is also perturbed as a neurotoxin approaches its membrane associated target and so has a rôle in specificity.

STRUCTURE-ACTIVITY RELATIONSHIPS

Bearing in mind the crystal structure and that in solution there may be some inherent flexibility it becomes possible to undertake a more realistic 'structure-activity' study. Comparison of the homologous sequences of neurotoxins and cytotoxins (95) has highlighted a number of residues likely to be directly involved in neurotoxicity (Karlsson, 1979; Low, 1979). By virtue of chemical modification studies and the invariant or conservative nature of certain positions (SN:LN); tryptophan (29:25), aspartate (31:27), arginine (33:33), acidic amino acid (38:38) and basic aminoacid (47:50) are generally considered to be essential for neurotoxicity. The conservative aromatic residue (32:29) has also been in-

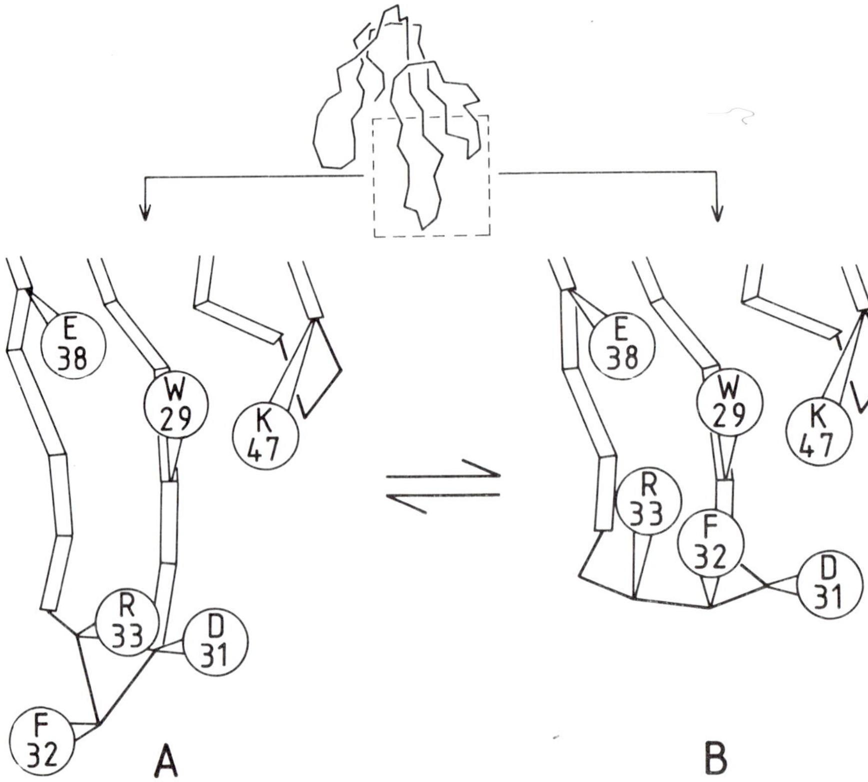

Fig. 4. Possible local conformation equilibrium of short neurotoxins. Conformation A corresponds to the X-ray crystallographic structure. The circles indicate the general orientation of the bulk of the side chain.

cluded in this group by Dufton and Hider (1977). The pK_a of histidine-32 is 5.6-5.8, so at pH 7.4 over 95% of the imidazole nuclei will not be protonated, and consequently can be regarded as hydrophobic. In both short and long neurotoxins these residues are localised on one face of the extensive β-sheet. Low (1979) has postulated that this region forms the reactive site of neurotoxins, so essentially it consists of a hydrophobic area containing two aromatic residues, two positive charges and two carboxylic acid functions. The finding that the carboxylic acid functions at positions 31 and 38 on cobrotoxin can be amidated and still retain much of the neurotoxicity (Chang and co-workers, 1971) implies that the negative charge of the group is not essential and that these residues probably act as hydrogen bond acceptors. Given the probable extremes of short neurotoxin conformation present in solution (Fig. 4) it becomes possible to compare the relative positions of the essential residues in each of these conformations with the orientation of functional groups within typical cholinergic agonists and antagonists.

Tsernoglou and co-workers (1978) and Low (1979) have compared the salt link between aspartate-31 and arginine-33 (Fig. 4A) with acetylcholine and have suggested that these residues mimic acetylcholine by binding to the agonist site. This concept is difficult to extrapolate to the long neurotoxins since, in contrast to erabutoxin *b*, where the distance between the C_α atoms of aspartate-31 and arginine-

33 is 6.2 Å (Kimball and co-workers, 1979), the analogous distance in α-cobratoxin is closer to 10 Å.

An alternative explanation suggested by Dufton and Hider (1977) groups the "essential" residues together in such a manner as to form a nicotinic antagonist mimic. The most potent alkaloid antagonists are isolated from the South American plants *Chondodendron* and *Strychnos*. As d-tubocurarine is a flexible molecule (Reynolds and co-workers, 1975) the conformation which binds to the receptor is not known. In contrast, C-Alkaloid E (I) is rigid (Grdinic and co-workers, 1964)

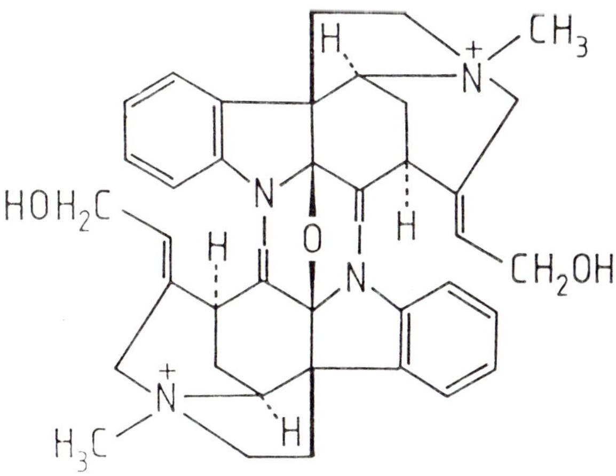

I

and thus the conformation present in solution must also be the one which binds to the receptor. Significantly, this molecule contains 2 aromatic nuclei, two positive charges and two hydroxyl groups capable of acting as hydrogen bond acceptors. The relative juxtaposition of these residues is very similar to the corresponding essential functional groups in one of the proposed short neurotoxin conformations (Fig. 4B). C-Curarine, a structural homologue of C-alkaloid E, lacking both hydroxyl functions, is much less toxic than C-alkaloid E.

PHARMACOLOGICAL PROPERTIES OF NEUROTOXINS

The neuromuscular blocking action of the postsynaptic toxins mimics d-tubocurarine closely, except that the onset of action and the rate of dissociation are both slower (Vyskocil and Magazanik, 1972). It is clear from a variety of studies that both agonists and antagonists influence neurotoxin binding; indeed, under certain conditions excess d-tubocurarine completely displaces neurotoxin from eel electroplax (Weber and Changeux, 1973). These results fit with a reversible and mutually exclusive toxin-cholinergic ligand competition for a common binding site. Careful analysis of this effect shows that agonists produce a slower rate of inhibition when compared to d-tubocurarine; in fact, the time constant is far slower than would be expected for simple receptor occupancy. Thus in the case of agonist inhibition the apparently simple competitive behaviour may be misleading. In contrast, no delay is observed with d-tubocurarine indicating that the interaction between the alkaloid and the toxin may be one of simple competition

(Colquhoun and Rang, 1976). Thus the initial interaction between neurotoxins and the receptor may be centred on the reactive site of the toxin in a conformation similar to that depicted in Fig. 4B.

ACKNOWLEDGEMENT

The authors would like to express their gratitude to Dr. R.A. Shipolini who generously donated samples of 4.11.3 and 4.9.3 isolated from *Dendroaspis viridis* venom and a sample of 3.9.4 isolated from *Naja melanoleuca* venom.

REFERENCES

Bystrov, V. F., A. S. Arseniev and Y. D. Gavrilov (1978). J. Mag. Resonance, 30, 151-181.
Chang, C. C., C. C. Yang, K. Nakai and K. Hayashi (1971). Biochim. Biophys. Acta, 251, 334-344.
Chicheportiche, R., J. Vincent, C. Kopeyan, H. Schweitz and M. Lazdunski (1975). Biochemistry, 14, 2081-2091.
Colquhoun, D. and H. P. Rang (1976). Mol. Pharmacol., 12, 519-535.
Drake, A. F., M. J. Dufton and R. C. Hider (1977). FEBS Letters, 83, 202-206.
Dufton, M. J. and R. C. Hider (1977). J. Mol. Biol., 115, 177-193.
Grdinic, M., D. A. Nelson and V. Boekelheide (1964). J. Am. Chem. Soc., 86, 3357-3363.
Inagaki, F., T. Miyazawa, H. Hori and N. Tamiya (1978). Eur. J. Biochem., 89, 433-442.
Karlsson, E. (1979). Handbook of Experimental Pharmacol., 52, 159-204.
Kimball, M. R., A. Sato, J. S. Richardson, L. S. Rosen and B. W. Low (1979). Biochem. Biophys. Res. Comm., 88, 950-959.
Lauterwein, J., M. Lazdunski and K. Wüthrich (1978). Eur. J. Biochem., 92, 361-371.
Llinás, M., M. P. Klein and J. B. Neilands (1972). Int. J. Peptide Protein Res., 4, 157-166.
Low, B. W. (1979). Handbook of Experimental Pharmacol., 52, 213-254.
Maelicke, A., B. W. Fulpius, R. P. Klett and E. Reich (1977). J. Biol. Chem., 252, 4811-4830.
Menez, A., F. Bouet, N. Tamiya and P. Fromageot (1976). Biochim. Biophys. Acta, 453, 121-132.
Menez, A., G. Langlet, N. Tamiya and P. Fromageot (1978). Biochimie, 60, 505-516.
Reynolds, C. D., R. A. Palmer, B. A. Gorinsky and C. Gorinsky (1975). Biochim. Biophys. Acta, 404, 341-344.
Tsernoglou, D., G. A. Petsko and R. A. Hudson (1978). Mol. Pharmacol., 14, 710-716.
Vystočil, F. and L. G. Magazanik (1972). Experientia, 29, 158-160.
Walkinshaw, M. D., A. Maelicke and W. Saenger (1980). This publication.
Weber, M. and J. P. Changeux (1974). Mol. Pharmacol., 10, 1-34.

SPIN AND FLUORESCENCE LABELED NEUROTOXIN II. CONFORMATIONAL STUDIES AND INTERACTION OF THE TOXIN WITH THE ACETYLCHOLINE RECEPTOR

V. T. Ivanov*, V. I. Tsetlin*, E. Karlsson, A. S. Arseniev*, Yu. N. Utkin*, V. S. Pashkov*, A. M. Surin*, K. A. Pluzhnikov* and V. F. Bystrov***

**Shemyakin Institute of Bioorganic Chemistry, USSR Academy of Sciences, Moscow, USSR*
***Institute of Biochemistry, Uppsala, Sweden*

ABSTRACT

Fifteen *Naja naja oxiana* neurotoxin II derivatives mono and di spin-labeled on Lys-15, Lys-25, Lys-26, Lys-44 and Lys-46 have been prepared and the position of the label(s) identified. Spin label distances to a number of the side chains were determined by ^{1}H NMR for the mono-labeled species and interlabel distances were determined by EPR for the di-labeled residues. Binding of the mono spin-labeled derivatives to solubilized acetylcholine receptor protein (AChR) from *Torpedo marmorata* was followed by EPR. By means of a spin probe technique, it was found that spin labels on Lys-15, Lys-25, Lys-46 and, especially Lys-26, are less accessible in the AChR complexes than in the free toxins. Involvement of the dansyl labels on Lys-26 and Lys-46 in the binding was demonstrated by fluorescence spectroscopy. The data obtained yielded evidence of a β-structure of the toxin and allowed preliminary characterization of the neurotoxin binding surface.

KEYWORDS

Snake venom neurotoxins; conformation; spin and fluorescence labels; ^{1}H NMR; EPR; fluorescence; acetylcholine receptor protein; neurotoxin binding site.

INTRODUCTION

For a number of years we have been engaged in studying solution conformations of cobra venom neurotoxins by the approach which relies upon a combined use of various spectroscopic techniques. Along with native toxins, their chemically modified derivatives (for example, trifluoroacetylated analogs) were also analyzed. By means of ^{1}H NMR and ^{19}F NMR procedures the folding of the polypeptide backbone of neurotoxin II (NT-II) from *Naja naja oxiana* was elucidated to a first approximation (Ivanov and others, 1978; Tsetlin and others, 1979a, and references therein). The present report deals with the results obtained from the insertion of spin labels into the NT-II molecule. The resultant compounds, along with the fluorescence labeled analogs obtained earlier (Utkin and others, 1978), have proved useful in studying structural aspects of the interaction of neurotoxins with their nicotinic AChR target, as well as aids in solving purely conformational problems.

CONFORMATIONAL STUDIES OF NT-II

Synthesis of NT-II Mono and Di Spin-labeled Derivatives

As the lysine acylated derivatives of NT-II partially retained its biological activity and spatial characteristics (Tsetlin and others, 1979a) we made use of the acylation reaction to attach spin labels to the lysine residues of the molecule. Mono-labeled derivatives were prepared by treating NT-II with one equivalent of 2,2,6,6,-tetramethyl-4-carboxymethylpiperidyl-1-oxyl N-hydroxysuccinimide ester. The reaction preferentially yielded mono spin-labeled (SL) derivatives, but contaminated with a good proportion of higher substituted products and also unreacted toxin. The individual products were separated by ion-exchange chromatography (Fig. 1).

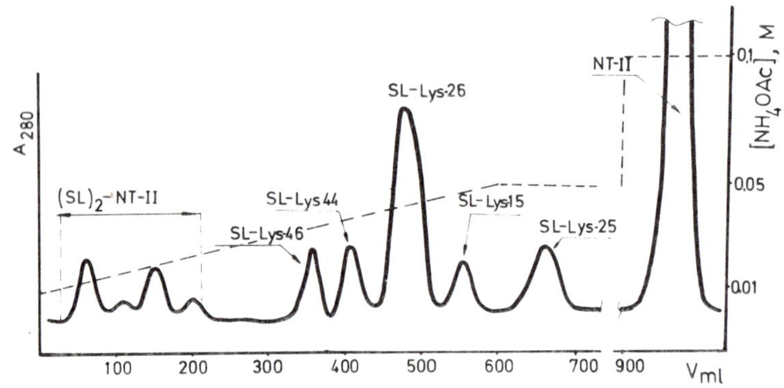

Fig. 1. Bio Rex-70 column chromatography of the products of NT-II spin labeling.

In order to locate the position of the label in each of the mono-substituted derivatives, it was reduced, carboxymethylated, and subjected to tryptic hydrolysis. After separation of the hydrolyzate components on Sephadex G-25 in 0.1 M acetic acid the spin-labeled peptide was identified by EPR and its amino acid composition and in some cases N-termini were determined.

The di spin-labeled derivatives were prepared by treating the toxin with 4.5 equivalents of 2,2,5,5-tetramethyl-3-carboxypyrrolin-1-oxyl N-hydroxysuccinimide ester. Larger reagent excess was found to considerably augment the proportion of compounds with 3 or more spin labels (SL') per molecule. Chromatography on Bio Rex-70 in dilute (0.005 M to 0.05 M) NH_4OAc pH 7.0 yielded ten fractions each containing 2 spin labels per mole toxin and corresponding to one of the ten possible di-labeled derivatives with labels on Lys-15 and Lys-25, Lys-15 and Lys-26, etc. All the fractions were found to be homogeneous excepting one consisting of a mixture of Lys-26, Lys-46 (70%) and Lys-15, Lys-46 (30%) labeled derivatives.

The spin labeled compounds preserved 10-60% of the initial toxicity. CD and ^1H NMR data indicated that their structures were closely similar to that of the native toxin.

^{1}H NMR Studies of Mono Spin-labeled NT-II Derivatives.

The unpaired electron of the spin label contributes considerably to the relaxational processes causing line broadening of a number of proton signals depending on their distance from the unpaired electron. For the SL-Lys-26 compound calculation showed that there is a relatively short distance from the spin label to the Trp-28, Tyr-24, and Ile-35 side chains, whereas it is far from the sequentially adjacent Trp-27 (Fig. 2). Differences in the spacings between the label and the individual Tyr-24 and His-31 protons give an idea of the orientation of the aromatic rings of the residues with respect to the unpaired electron. Broadening of the His-31 C_2H signal is pH-dependent, i.e. protonation of the imidazole ring is accompanied by change of its orientation. The ^{1}H NMR data also showed that the Lys-25 spin label was close to the Trp-27 and Ile-36 side chains and far from the Trp-28 and Ile-35 residues, thereby substantiating the β-structure of the central loop.

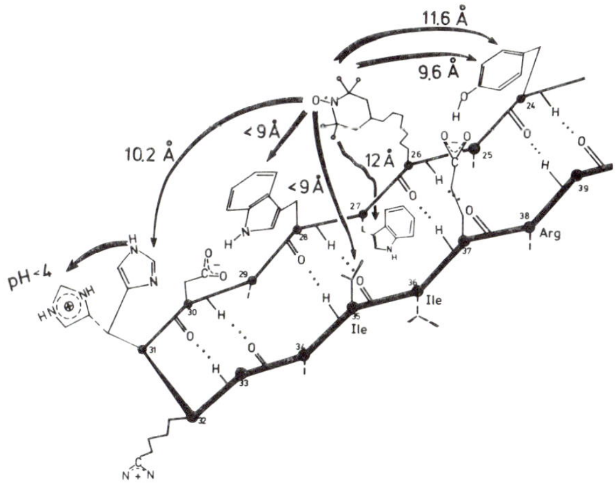

Fig. 2. Conformation of the central fragment of the NT-II molecule.

Moreover, the Lys-26 spin label broadens the methyl signals of the Val-45 and Val-49 residues located in the loop confined by the Cys-42 - Cys-53 disulfide bridge, evidence of closeness of this loop to the central loop. Along with some inter-residue interactions as revealed by the ^{1}H NMR data on SL-Lys-46 it permitted definition of the mutual arrangement of the two loops.

EPR Studies of NT-II Di Spin-labeled Derivatives.

The distances between the spin labels were determined essentially by the technique described in (Likhtenstein, 1976). The EPR spectra were recorded in 50% aqueous glycerol at 77°K (Fig. 3). To obtain the distances given in Table 1 use was made of a calibration curve plotted for vitrified solutions of N-(2,2,5,5-tetramethyl-3-carbonylpyrrolin-1-oxyl)glycine. The short distance (13 Å) between the spin labels on Lys-26 and Lys-46 confirms an earlier qualitative conclusion regarding the proximity of the two side chains (Tsetlin and others, 1979a); the distances between Lys-25 and Lys-26, or Lys-44 and Lys-46 are in accord with β-structure of the respective segments of the polypeptide chain. A model (Fig. 4) of the NT-II spatial structure constructed with aid of the coordinates found for crystalline erabutoxin *b* (Kimball and others, 1979), under the assumption that the residue side chains of the two neurotoxins are similarly oriented, displayed inter spin-label distances

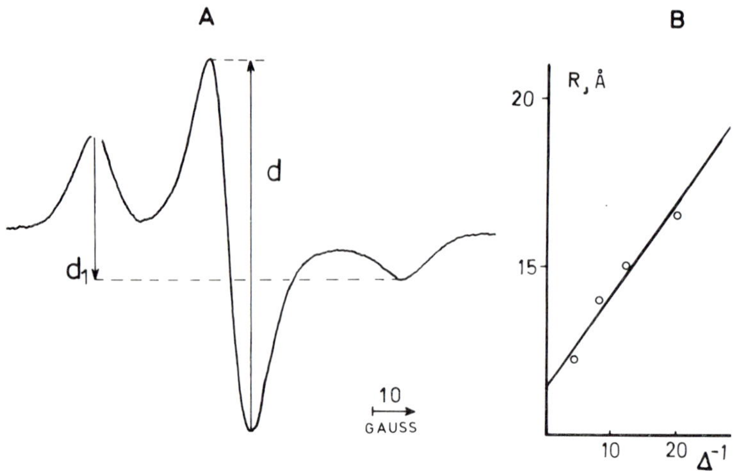

Fig. 3. EPR spectrum of frozen solution of SL'-Lys-26, SL'-Lys-44 NT-II (A) and calibration plot (B); $\Delta = d_1/d - (d_1/d)_0$, where $(d_1/d)_0$ is taken from the spectrum of frozen monoradical.

close to those found experimentally, with the exception of Lys-15 SL' to the other labels. The discrepancy can be explained by differences in the Lys-15 side chain orientation or in relative position of the Lys-15 containing loop with respect to other loops in erabutoxin *b* and NT-II.

TABLE 1 Interspin Distances

Spin-labeled residues	Δ	Distance R, Å
Lys-15, Lys-25	0.02	>20
Lys-15, Lys-26	0.10	14.2
Lys-15, Lys-44	0.04	18.5
Lys-15, Lys-46	0.05	17.0
Lys-15, Lys-26	0.07	15.3
Lys-25, Lys-44	0.04	18.5
Lys-25, Lys-46	0.02	>20
Lys-26, Lys-44	0.09	14.5
Lys-26, Lys-46	0.17*	13.0
Lys-44, Lys-46	0.04	18.5

*corrected for the presence of Lys-15, Lys-46 labeled derivative

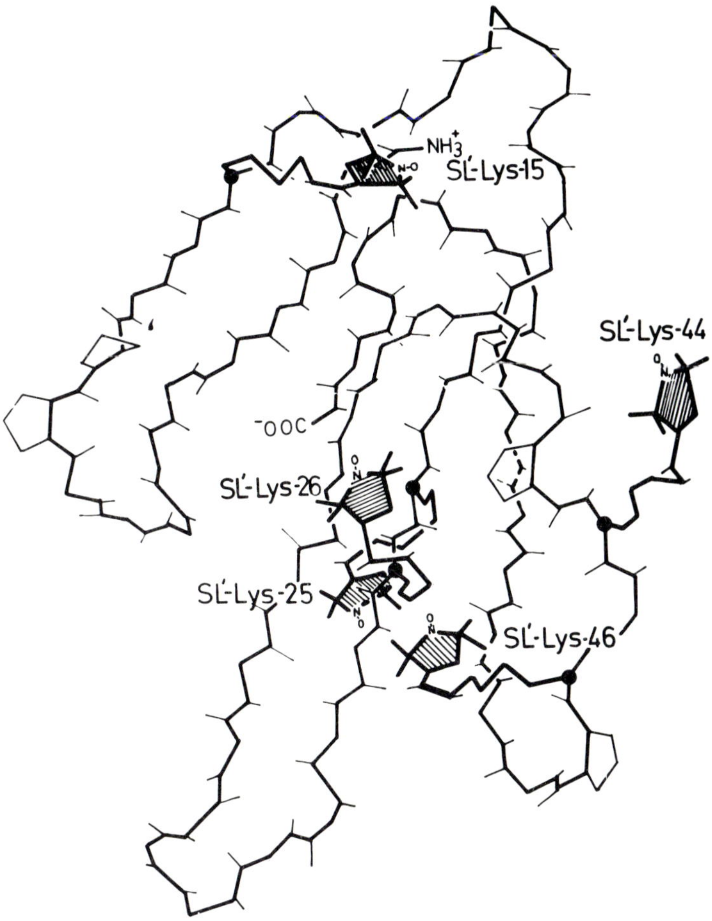

Fig. 4. Location of spin labels in the polypeptide chain of NT-II

EPR AND FLUORESCENCE STUDIES OF THE NEUROTOXIN - ACETYLCHOLINE RECEPTOR BINDING

Despite extensive studies on both the AChR and the snake venom neurotoxins, recently reviewed by Heidmann and Changeux (1978) and Karlsson (1979), direct evidence is lacking as to what regions of the neurotoxin molecule bind to the AChR. The availability of a series of NT-II derivatives carrying spin or fluorescence labels in various known positions of the molecule provides the means for outlining the topography of the neurotoxin binding to AChR.. The study was carried out on Triton X-100 solubilized AChR from *Torpedo marmorata*. The isolation procedure essentially according to Karlsson and colleagues (1976) yielded a preparation binding ~10000 nmol [^{3}H]-NT-II or *Naja naja siamensis* toxin 3 per g receptor protein.

Binding of Lys-26 dansylated NT-II to the AChR caused a blue shift (562→544 nm) in the emission fluorescence band together with an increase in the quantum yield, evidence of augmented hydrophobicity of the dansyl chromophore environment in the complex as compared to the free toxin. Similar spectral changes occur if a dansyl-glycyl group is attached to the Lys-46 side chain. Titration of AChR with these derivatives revealed a saturable binding process. From Fig. 5 it follows that 2 moles of toxin are bound to 1 mole of AChR, assuming the molecular weight of the latter to be ~250000 (Reynolds and Karlin, 1978).

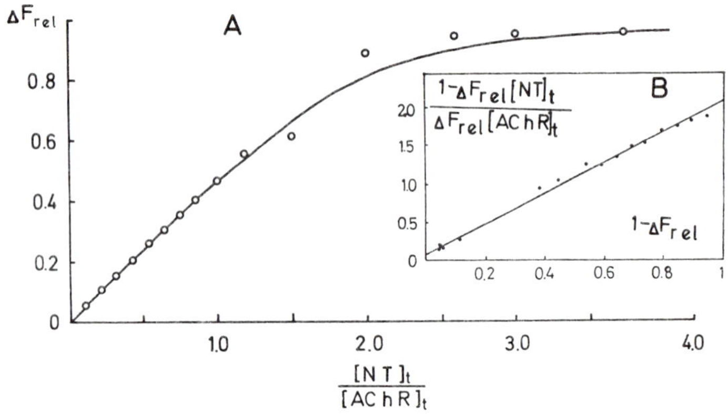

Fig. 5. AChR titration with Lys-26 dansylated NT-II. In A circles are experimental values, solid line - a theoretical curve calculated for K_d=7.3·10^{-8}M and n=2 found from plot B.

Binding of the Lys-26 dansylated NT-II affects the tryptophan fluorescence of the AChR: there is a ~10% drop in fluorescence intensity and a concomitant blue shift (329→327 nm, λ_{max} in the difference spectrum at 332 nm). This effect could be due to the possibility that the earlier observed (Tsetlin and others, 1979b) energy transfer to the dansyl group occurs from only part of the AChR tryptophan residues, apparently from those located in the toxin-binding site; another possibility could be a neurotoxin induced conformational change in the AChR.

Binding of the spin-labeled derivatives is accompanied by line broadening in the EPR spectra (Fig. 6). Calculation of the rotational correlation times of the spin label motion independent of the motion of the toxin globule or of the toxin-receptor complex, in terms of an isotropic rotation mode shows that mobility is hindered most noticeably in the AChR complex with SL-Lys-25 and with SL-Lys-26 derivatives (Tsetlin and others, 1979b).

The spin-labeled analogs formed complexes with AChR of the same 2:1 stoichiometry as the dansyl analogs. High binding specificity is evidenced by displacement of the labeled compounds by excess native NT-II. They may also be totally displaced by the earlier synthesized NT-II acetyl derivatives, the displacing capacity of which paralleled the toxicity. Even in high excess nontoxic hexa(trifluoroacetyl)-NT-II (Tsetlin and others, 1979a) displaces only about half of the spin or dansyl analogs

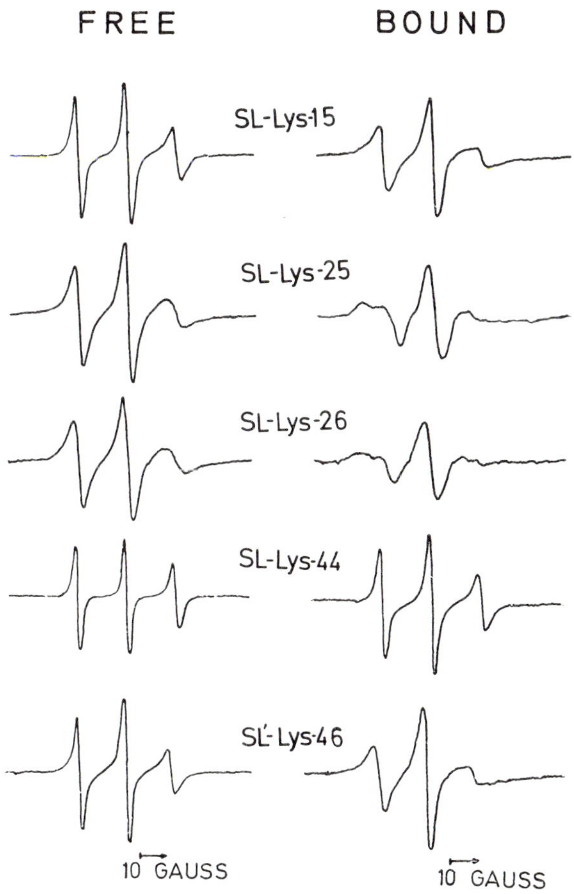

Fig. 6. EPR spectra of NT-II spin-labeled derivatives.

bound to the receptor and thus may prove a useful tool for studying differences between neurotoxin binding sites of the AChR.

By means of spin-probe technique (Likhtenstein, 1976) with $K_3(Fe(CN)_6)$ as the paramagnetic probe we have been able to determine whether and what spin labels are extracted from aqueous environment in the formation of the toxin-receptor complex, i.e. participate directly in the binding. The Lys-44 spin label undergoes almost no change in accessibility on formation of the toxin-AChR complex, i.e. it apparently does not contact the receptor. With all other lysine spin labels binding diminishes accessibility of the label by the paramagnetic probe. The labels undergoing the most screening proved to be those on Lys-46 and especially on Lys-26.

Considering the apparent close similarity of the solution spatial structure of NT-II to that of crystalline erabutoxin *b*, we made use of the crystalline structure to illustrate the binding of a neurotoxin molecule to AChR (Fig. 7).

The results obtained show that the toxin binding site of the AchR must be quite

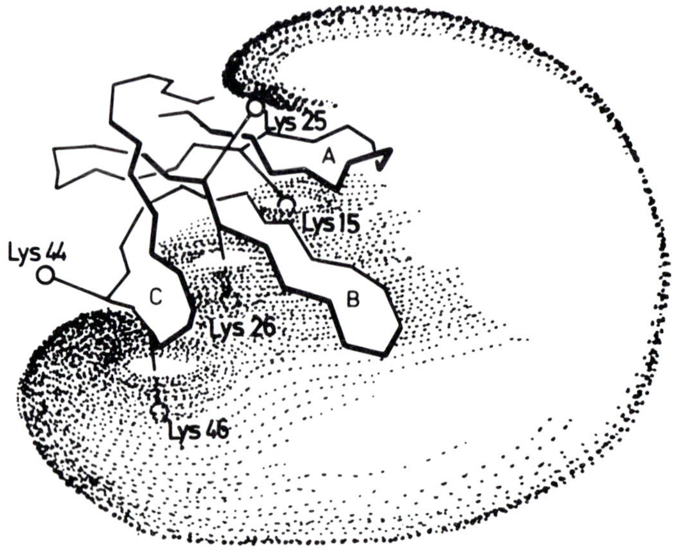

Fig. 7. Scheme for neurotoxin-AChR binding

extensive and the binding itself must be multiple, involving segments from at least three loops (A,B,C) bridged by disulfide bonds. Participation of the B and C loops had been earlier inferred from solution studies on NT-II (Tsetlin and others, 1979a) and from analysis of erabutoxin *b* X-ray structure and sequence homologies in neurotoxins (Kimball and others, 1979).

REFERENCES

Heidmann, T., and J.-P. Changeux (1978). In E.E. Snell (Ed.), Annual Rev. Biochem., Vol. 47, Annual Reviews Inc., Palo Alto, pp. 317-357.

Ivanov, V.T., V.I.Tsetlin, I.I. Mikhaleva, O.M. Volpina, A.R. Nuriddinov, Yu.N. Utkin, A.S. Arseniev, V.S. Pashkov, E. Karlsson, A.M. Surin and V.F. Bystrov (1978). Proceedings of the XVth European Peptide Symposium, Gdansk.

Karlsson, E. (1979). In C.Y. Lee (Ed.), Handbook of Experimental Pharmacology, Vol. 52 Springer-Verlag, Berlin-Heidelberg-New York, pp. 159-212.

Karlsson, E., J. Fohlman, and M. Groth (1976) Bull. Inst. Pasteur, 74, 11-22.

Kimball, M.R., A. Sato, J.S. Richardson, L.S. Rosen, and B.W. Low (1979). Biochem. Biophys. Res. Commun., 88, 950-959.

Likhtenstein G.I. (1976) Spin Labeling Methods in Molecular Biology. John Wiley, New York.

Reynolds, J.A., and Karlin (1978) Biochemistry 17, 2035-2038.

Tsetlin, V.I., A.S. Arseniev, Yu.N. Utkin, A.Z. Gurevich, L.B. Senyavina, V.F.Bystrov, V.T.Ivanov, and Yu.A.Ovchinnikov (1979a). Eur. J. Biochem., 94, 337-346.

Tsetlin, V.I., E. Karlsson, A.S. Arseniev, Yu.N. Utkin, A.M. Surin, V.S. Pashkov, K.A. Pluzhnikov, V.T. Ivanov, V.F. Bystrov, and Yu.A. Ovchinnikov (1979b) FEBS Lett., 106, 000.

Utkin, Yu.N., V.S. Pashkov, A.M. Surin, V.I. Tsetlin, and V.T. Ivanov (1978). Proceedings of the XVth European Peptide Symposium, Gdansk.

MUSCARINIC ACETYLCHOLINE RECEPTOR

T. Bartfai*, B. Hedlund*, J. Järv and Ö. Nordström***

**Department of Biochemistry, Arrhenius Laboratory, S-106 91 Stockholm, Sweden*
***Department of Organic Chemistry, Tartu University, Estonian SSR, USSR*

ABSTRACT

Muscarinic acetylcholine receptors from rat cerebral cortex and small intestine were studied by the high affinity and high specific activity antagonists ^{3}H-3-quinuclidinyl benzilate (3-QNB) (29.4 Ci/mmol) and ^{3}H-N-methyl-4-piperidinyl benzilate (4-NMPB) (55.4 Ci/mmol). Equilibrium binding data combined with studies on association and dissociation rates of the receptor·antagonist complex are compatible with the reaction sequence:

$$A + R \rightleftarrows AR \rightleftarrows AR^{*}$$

where R and A stand for receptor and antagonist, respectively. For both antagonists of benzilate class the equilibrium constant of the isomerization step was 0.15 in phosphate buffer (Järv and co-workers, 1979). The results of agonist binding studies carried out under equilibrium conditions can be described as if there were two classes of agonist binding sites with affinities 100 µM and 0.05 µM for carbamylcholine (Hedlund and Bartfai, 1979). It appears that it is the low affinity binding site that is associated with muscarinic activation of cyclic GMP synthesis in cortical slices and in N1E 115 neuroblastoma cells. In the latter the low affinity muscarinic receptor controls a non-voltage dependent Ca^{2+} channel (Study and co-workers, 1978).

Calcium channel blocking agents such as D600 and Co^{2+} inhibit the receptor mediated rise in cyclic GMP levels. Experiments with the cardiotoxin V^{II}_{2} from *N.m. mossambica* (supplied by Dr. L. Visser) indicate that the cardiotoxin and D600 may share some common site on the receptor-coupled Ca^{2+} channel, or on the muscarinic receptor itself.

KEYWORDS

Muscarinic acetylcholine receptor, Ca^{2+} channel, D600, cardiotoxin, agonist binding, cyclic GMP.

INTRODUCTION

The physiological actions of acetylcholine that are mediated via muscarinic receptors are crucially dependent on the presence of Ca^{2+} ions in the extracellular medium (cf. Triggle, 1979; Heilbronn and Bartfai, 1978). This fact has often been neglected since it is possible to study the binding of radiolabeled antagonists and agonists to muscarinic receptor sites in Ca^{2+} free medium (Yamamura and Snyder, 1974).

The biochemical events that follow muscarinic receptor occupancy with agonist are also Ca^{2+} dependent with the exception of increased phosphatidylinositol turnover (Michell and co-workers, 1976). The present study examines the possibility that the muscarinic receptor is coupled to a calcium channel or pump whose occupancy with Ca^{2+}, or blockade by Ca^{2+} antagonists could be reflected in the ligand binding properties of the receptor. Among the muscarinic receptor ligands examined is a cardiotoxin from *N.m. mossambica* (V_2^{II}) that appears to interact with sites similar to those blocked by the Ca^{2+} antagonist D600.

MATERIALS AND METHODS

^{3}H-3-Quinuclidinyl benzilate (29.4 Ci/mmol) was purchased from New England Nuclear, Boston, Mass., USA. ^{3}H-N-methyl-4-piperidinyl benzilate (55.4 Ci/mmol) was prepared and generously donated by Drs. Yoel Kloog and Mordechai Sokolovsky, Tel Aviv University, Tel Aviv, Israel. Purified cardiotoxin from *N.m. mossambica* (V_2^{II}) was generously donated by Dr. Leon Visser, National Chemical Research Laboratory, Pretoria, South-Africa. All other chemicals were of reagent grade.

Membranes from rat (Sprague-Dawley, male) cerebral cortex and from rat heart were prepared as described previously (Hedlund and Bartfai, 1979).

Ligand binding studies were carried out by filtration method (as described previously, Hedlund and Bartfai, 1979) in Ca^{2+}-free medium (phosphate buffer 50 mM, phenylmethylsulfonyl fluoride 0.1 mM, pH 7.4) or in Krebs-Ringer´s buffer (NaCl 137 mM, KCl 2.68 mM, $CaCl_2$ 1.8 mM, $MgCl_2$ 1.05 mM, Hepes 1 mM, phenylmethylsulfonyl fluoride 0.1 mM, pH = 7.4).

RESULTS AND DISCUSSION

Antagonist Binding

Kinetic studies on the binding of the benzilate based muscarinic antagonists N-methyl-4-piperidinyl benzilate (4-NMPB) (Kloog and Sokolovsky, 1977) and 3-quinuclidinyl benzilate (3-QNB) (Yamamura and Snyder, 1974) have shown that in Ca^{2+}-free medium the binding of these antagonists can be described by a two-step scheme (eqn. 1).

$$A + R \underset{k_{-1}}{\overset{k_1}{\rightleftharpoons}} AR \underset{k_{-2}}{\overset{k_{+2}}{\rightleftharpoons}} AR^* \qquad (1)$$

where A stands for the antagonist and R for the receptor. k_1-k_{-2} are kinetic constants.

The first step of binding of both benzilates is fast, followed by a slower isomerization of the receptor-ligand complex (Järv and co-workers, 1979). The equilibrium constant of the isomerization reaction was identical for both antagonists.

The total number of specific binding sites is 15-20 % lower in Ca^{2+} free medium: phosphate buffer (+ EDTA) than in Krebs-Ringer´s buffer. This difference could be due to Ca^{2+} specifically or to the different ionic composition and ionic strengths of the two buffers. Experiments carried out in Krebs Ringer´s buffer (0.4 ± 0.03 picomoles ^{3}H-QNB bound/mg protein) and in Krebs Ringer´s buffer devoid of Ca^{2+} and supplemented with 1 mM EGTA (0.3 ± 0.04 picomoles ^{3}H-QNB bound/ mg protein) suggest that the difference in the measured number of binding sites is dependent on Ca^{2+} rather than on differences in other ions or on ionic strength.

Not only the total number of antagonist binding sites, but also the kinetics of binding and dissociation are affected by the presence and absence of Ca^{2+}. The equilibrium binding constants (the product of the equilibrium constants for the two reactions in equation 1) are identical in phosphate buffer and in Krebs-Ringer´s buffer. The rate constants for dissociation (k_{-2}) are closely identical whereas the rate constant for isomerization (k_{+2}) is much lower in the presence of Ca^{2+} ($1.25 \cdot 10^{-3}$ sec^{-1}). (In phosphate buffer (+ EDTA) k_{+2} was $8.8 \cdot 10^{-3}$ sec^{-1}). This implies that the first rapid binding step also has to be affected by change of buffer as to produce the same overall equilibrium binding constant.

The known blocker of Ca^2-movements D600 (Fleckstein and co-workers, 1971) inhibits binding of the muscarinic antagonist 3-QNB to membranes from rat heart when measured in Tris buffer 50 mM, pH = 7.4 (Cavey and co-workers, 1977). In our hands, when Ca^{2+} is removed by 2 mM EDTA (phosphate buffer, 50 mM), D600 in 10 μM concentration had no effect on 3-QNB binding in the 0.1 to 5 nM concentration range. In Krebs-Ringer´s buffer D600 (10 μM) inhibited ^{3}H-3-QNB binding to 50 %. This suggests that the presence of Ca^{2+} is required for the inhibitory action of D600 on antagonist binding to the receptor. In higher concentration D600, a lipophilic compound, can of course inhibit receptor-ligand interactions through a "nonspecific" blockade of the membrane-bound receptor. However, it should be born in mind that even 10 μM is a higher concentration than that usually used to block Ca^{2+} movement by D600 (Fleckstein and co-workers, 1971).

The inhibition pattern observed with D600 reflects that it is a noncompetitive inhibitor with respect to 3-QNB and therefore it is likely that D600 and 3-QNB do not bind to identical sites on the receptor. More likely is that D600 binds to a Ca^{2+} channel that is somehow connected to the receptor.

Previous studies by us (Study and co-workers, 1978) have indicated that in N1E 115 neuroblastoma cells D600 has blocked both the muscarinic receptor and the K^+ depolarization mediated increases in cyclic GMP concentrations. The 50 % blockade of both of these Ca^{2+}-dependent processes required ∿ 10 μM concentration of D600.

The cardiotoxin (V_2^{II}) from *N.M. mossambica* that has molecular weight 6800 ($E_{280}^{1\%}$:12.96) inhibited in 10^{-5} M concentration antagonist binding to muscarinic receptor from rat heart and from rat cerebral cortex to 60 %. The inhibition by cardiotoxin and by D600 in the presence of Ca^{2+} was not additive despite the fact that submaximal doses of both agents were used; rather the same inhibition was found as by cardiotoxin V_2^{II} alone (Figure 1). Whether binding of cardiotoxin V_2^{II} and D600 are mutually exclusive or only partially exclusive cannot be concluded without examining the cardiotoxin V_2^{II} concentration dependence of inhibition of 3-QNB binding at different D600 concentrations. Cardiotoxin V_2^{II}, because of limited supply, could not be used at higher concentrations. Increase in D600 concentration or application of D600 and cardiotoxin V_2^{II} together did not increase the inhibition despite the fact that ∿ 30 % of the sites were not yet inhibited by the cardiotoxin (10^{-5} M). This suggests that neither D600 nor cardiotoxin V_2^{II} may be able to fully inhibit antagonist binding to the receptor. Previous studies on agonist binding, modification of receptors, etc. suggested the presence of two receptor populations (cf. Birdsall and Hulme, 1976) at least with respect to agonist binding. It is possible that only one of these is sensitive to D600 and cardiotoxin V_2^{II}.

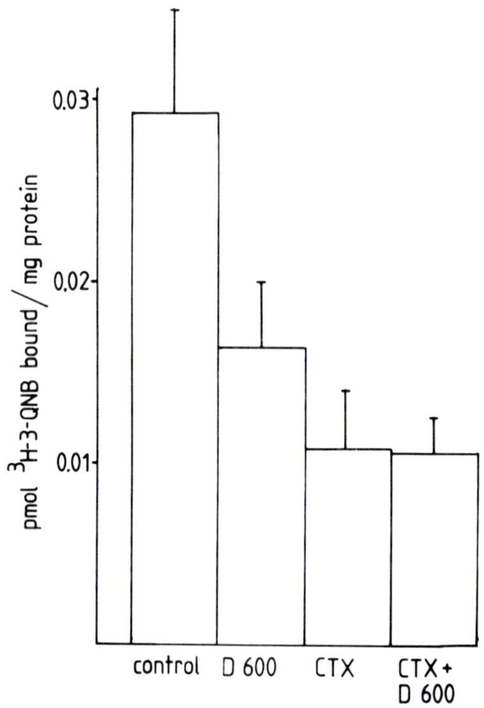

Fig. 1. Inhibition of ^{3}H-3-QNB (0.1 nM) binding to cerebral cortical membranes by cardiotoxin V_2^{II} *N.m. mossambica* (10 μM) and by D600 (10 μM).

Furthermore, the finding in Figure 1 suggests that cardiotoxin V_2^{II} and D600 may share a common site of action. This site could be at the receptor coupled Ca^{2+} channel.

To examine this possibility, the effects of D600 and cardiotoxin V_2^{II} were studied on agonist binding since it is agonist binding that should operate the receptor coupled Ca^{2+} channel. (Direct measurements on Ca^{2+} fluxes in N1E 115 neuroblastoma cells are in progress.) D600 was a noncompetitive inhibitor of agonist binding (not shown) in Krebs-Ringer´s buffer whereas in Ca^{2+} free medium D600 (10 μM) had no effect on the efficacy of carbachol in competing with ^{3}H-3-QNB. Cardiotoxin V_2^{II}, like D600, was a noncompetitive inhibitor of agonist binding in Krebs-Ringer´s buffer (Figure 2) causing a change both in the number of receptor sites that are available and in their affinity.

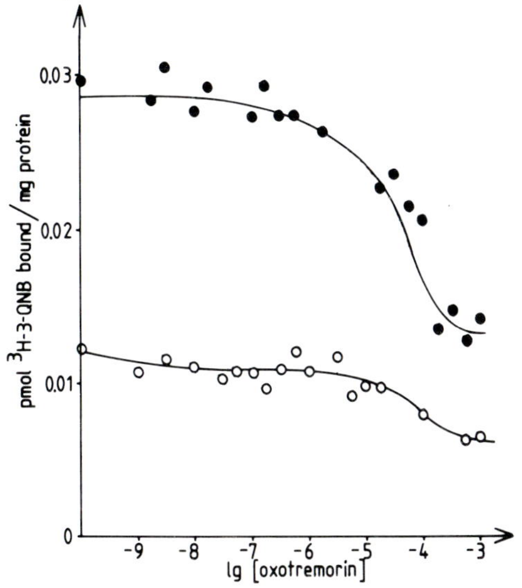

Fig. 2. Inhibition of oxotremorine-^{3}H-3-QNB (0.1 nM) competition by cardiotoxin *N.m. mossambica* V_2^{II} (10 μM). Note that cardiotoxin must bind to several "nonspecific sites" too since the residual ^{3}H-3-QNB binding at high oxotremorine concentrations is lowered by the cardiotoxin. Control (-●-●-), CTX (-o-o-).

Lack of more purified cardiotoxin prevented studies on additivity of the inhibitory effects of D600 and cardiotoxin V_2^{II} on agonist binding.

On the basis of the present data, it may be suggested that D600 and cardiotoxin V_2^{II} share a common site that may relate to the receptor coupled Ca^{2+} channel whose existence is suggested by previous experiments (Triggle, 1979; Study and co-workers, 1978) in which involvement of Ca^{2+} in the receptor mediated smooth muscle contraction or in receptor mediated increases in cyclic GMP levels were studied.

ACKNOWLEDGEMENTS

This work was supported from grants from the Swedish Medical Research Council, Harald och Greta Jeanssons Stiftelse and from Magnus Bergvalls fond. The authors are indebted to Dr. Leon Visser for the supply of the purified cardiotoxin V_2^{II} and for discussions.

REFERENCES

Birdsall, N.J.M. and E.C. Hulme (1976). Biochemical studies on muscarinic receptors. J. Neurochem., 27, 7-16.

Cavey, D., J.P. Vincent and M. Làzdunski (1977). The muscarinic receptor of heart cell membranes. FEBS Lett., 84, 110-114.

Fleckstein, A., G. Gruen, H. Tritthart, K. Byon, and P. Harding (1971). Uterus relaxation induced by highly potent calcium-antagonistic inhibitors of electromechanical coupling such as isoptin, D600 and segontin. Experiments on the isolated virgin rat uterus. Klin. Wochenschr., 49 (1) 23-41.

Hedlund, B. and T. Bartfai (1979). The importance of thiol- and disulfide groups in agonist and antagonist binding to the muscarinic receptor. Mol. Pharmacol., 15, 531-544.

Heilbronn, E. and T. Bartfai (1978). Muscarinic acetylcholine receptor. Progress in Neurobiol., 11, 171-188.

Järv, J., B. Hedlund and T. Bartfai (1979). Isomerization of the muscarinic receptor-antagonist complex. J. Biol. Chem., 254, 5595-5599.

Kloog, Y. and M. Sokolovsky (1977). Muscarinic acetylcholine receptor interactions: competition binding studies with agonists and antagonists. Brain Res., 134, 167-172.

Michell, R.H., S.S. Jafferji, and L.M. Jones (1976). Receptor occupancy dose-response curve suggests that phosphatidylinositol breakdown may be intrinsic to the mechanism of the muscarinic cholinergic receptor. FEBS Lett., 69, 1-5.

Study, R.E., X.O. Breakefield, T. Bartfai, and P. Greengard (1978). Voltage-sensitive calcium channels regulate guanosine 3',5'-cyclic monophosphate levels in neuroblastoma cells. Proc. Natl. Acad. Sci., 75, 6295-6299.

Triggle, D.J. (1979). The muscarinic receptor: structural, ionic and biochemical implications. In F. Gualtieri, M. Giannella, and C. Melchiorre (Eds.), Recent Advances in Receptor Chemistry, Elsevier, Holland, pp. 127-146.

Yamamura, H.I. and S.H. Snyder (1974). Muscarinic cholinergic binding in rat brain. Proc. Natl. Acad. Sci., 71, 1725-1729.

Venom Toxins Affecting Neurotransmitter Release

PHARMACOLOGY OF PRESYNAPTIC NEUROTOXINS FROM SNAKE VENOMS

C. Y. Lee and C. L. Ho

Pharmacological Institute, College of Medicine, National Taiwan University and Institute of Biological Chemistry, Academia Sinica, Taipei, Taiwan, Republic of China

ABSTRACT

A number of snake venom toxins with phospholipase A_2 (PLA) activity, such as β-bungarotoxin, taipoxin and crotoxin, act presynaptically at the motor nerve ending to produce a triphasic change in the transmitter release; an initial transient inhibition followed by facilitation of acetylcholine (ACh) release and then progressive depression leading to an irreversible blockade of transmission. The initial decrease in ACh release may result from the toxin binding to a specific presynaptic site, which appears unrelated to the PLA activity, while the facilitation followed by eventual failure of transmission has been attributed to the toxin's PLA activity. Besides presynaptic effects, most of these toxins have more or less postsynaptic and/or musculotropic (myotoxic) effects. A notable example is notexin. The postsynaptic site of action may be on the cholinergic ionophore and the fish electroplaque appears particularly sensitive to the PLA activity of these toxins at the postsynaptic site. The musculotropic action of notexin, as well as the basic PLA from *Naja nigricollis*, can be protected by pretreatment with heparin, whereas the presynaptic effect of these toxins remains little affected. Some autonomic motor transmissions are also affected by these toxins. While the cholinergic transmission of the guinea-pig or rat ileum is resistant, the inhibitory effect of the vagus nerve on the guinea-pig atrium is abolished by β-bungarotoxin. The non-cholinergic transmission of the guinea-pig vas deferens is also inhibited by notexin as well as by β-bungarotoxin. So far, no sympathetic (adrenergic) transmission has been found to be affected by these toxins.

KEYWORDS

Presynaptic neurotoxins; phospholipase A; transmitter release; β-bungarotoxin; crotoxin; taipoxin; notexin.

I. INTRODUCTION

A number of presynaptically active toxins have been isolated from certain snake venoms which may prove useful as specific pharmacological tools to study the mechanisms of synaptic transmitter release (for reviews see Chang, 1979; Eaker, 1978; Karlsson, 1979; Lee, 1979). The best known of these toxins are β-bungarotoxin from the many-banded krait, *Bungarus multicinctus* (Chang and Lee, 1963), notexin from the Australian tiger snake, *Notechis scutatus scutatus* (Karlsson, Eaker and Rydén, 1972), taipoxin from the Taipan, *Oxyuranus scutellatus scutellatus* (Fohlman and co-workers, 1976), and crotoxin from the South American rattlesnake, *Crotalus durissus terrificus* (Slotta and Fraenkel-Conrat, 1938). Although crotoxin was isolated more than two decades before any other toxin of the same type, its presynaptic action was not definitely demonstrated until recently (Vital Brazil and Excell, 1971; Chang and Lee, 1977). Among these four toxins, only notexin is a single peptide chain, while β-bungarotoxin has two covalently linked subunits (Kelly and Brown, 1974; Kondo, Narita and Lee, 1978), crotoxin has two non-covalently linked subunits (Breithaupt, Rübsamen and Habermann, 1974; Hendon and Fraenkel-Conrat, 1971), and taipoxin is a non-covalent complex of three subunits (Fohlman and co-workers, 1976). Notexin is a strongly basic phospholipase A_2 (PLA) and the other three toxins also contain a basic polypeptide with marked PLA activity. Besides the β-bungarotoxin with two chains (β_1-bungarotoxin of Kondo, Narita and Lee, 1978), a single chain toxin with a molecular weight of 11,000, having similar biological activities, has also been isolated from the same venom (Livengood and co-workers, 1978). Two presynaptic neurotoxins, toxins III-A and III-B, were purified from the Indian krait *Bungarus caeruleus* (Lee, Chen and Mebs, 1976). Ceruleotoxin from the same venom has been reported to be an acidic neurotoxin with several subunits which blocks the electrogenic action of acetylcholine (ACh) on the postsynaptic membrane without binding to the cholinergic receptor site (Bon and Changeux, 1975; 1977). A recent study has revealed that this toxin behaves pharmacologically just like notexin (Lee and Ho, 1978a). The Mojave toxin from the Mojave rattlesnake *Crotalus scutulatus scutulatus*, originally reported as an acidic cardiotoxin (Bieber, Tu and Tu, 1975), has turned out to be a presynaptic neurotoxin similar to crotoxin (Gopalakrishnakone and co-workers, 1979).

Although the principal mode of action of these toxins is to modify transmitter release at the motor nerve terminal, most of them also have more or less postsynaptic and/or musculotropic (myotoxic) actions. The best known examples are notexin (Harris, Johnson and Karlsson, 1975; Lee, Chen and Karlsson, 1976) and taipoxin (Harris, Johnson and MacDonell, 1977). More recently, the PLAs from *Naja naja oxiana* venom (Magazanik and co-workers, 1979) and *Bitis caudalis* venom (Lee, Ho and Botes, 1979) have been shown to be presynaptically active neurotoxins. It is predictable that most of the toxic PLAs, if not all, will be eventually proven to affect transmitter release at the motor nerve terminal, although some of them may be more myotoxic rather than neurotoxic. Thus, the classification of these toxic PLAs as presynaptic neurotoxins or myonecrotic toxins indicates only their most conspicuous characteristic (Karlsson, 1979).

II. LETHALITY AND SPECIES DIFFERENCES

There is a great difference in lethality among various PLAs obtained from snake venoms. Several of the most potent snake toxins are either basic PLA or contain a subunit which is a basic PLA while most of acidic PLAs have little or very low toxicity (Lee and Ho, 1978b). Although the enzyme activity appears to be essential for their toxicity, there is apparently no parallelism between the lethality and their PLA activity. On the other hand, there is a good correlation between the lethality and their potency in causing neuromuscular (N-M) blockade of skeletal muscles (Lee and Ho, 1978b). Indeed, the selectivity of toxins to act at the presynaptic site of the motor nerve ending seems to be responsible for the high lethality of these presynaptic neurotoxins.

Pigeons, chicks, and their isolated nerve-muscle preparations are much more sensitive than mice to β-bungarotoxin (Lee and Tseng, 1969) and crotoxin (Chang and Lee, 1977; Vital Brazil, Franceschi and Waisbich, 1966) but not to notexin and taipoxin (Chang and co-workers, 1977a). Taipoxin is more potent in blocking the mouse diaphragm but much less potent in the chick muscle than β-bungarotoxin and crotoxin. On the other hand, the rat diaphragm is more resistant than the mouse diaphragm to crotoxin and taipoxin but is more sensitive to β-bungarotoxin (Chang and co-workers, 1977a).

III. PRESYNAPTIC EFFECTS ON VERTEBRATE SKELETAL MUSCLES

Presynaptic neurotoxins have many features in common in their action on the N-M transmission in vertebrate skeletal muscles; i.e., the sensitivity of the endplate to ACh is not significantly decreased when the N-M transmission is blocked with a lower toxin concentration, the N-M block occurs after a latency, especially in the rat and mouse diaphragm preparations, but continues to progress after washout of the toxin, and the block is accelerated by increasing the rate of nerve stimulation. The release of ACh is severely depressed, as revealed by the decrease in the frequency of miniature endplate potentials (mepps) and the quantal contents of evoked endplate potentials (epps). The depression of transmitter release is usually preceded by an initial facilitation in most of these presynaptic toxins.

A. Electrophysiological Studies

All of the presynaptic neurotoxins so far studied produce phasic changes in the frequency of spontaneous mepps and in the quantal contents of epps leading to the final blockade of transmitter release. The failure of transmitter release is usually preceded by a period of facilitation as revealed by an increase in the frequency of mepps and the quantal content of epps (Abe, Limbrick and Miledi 1976; Alderice and Volle, 1975; Chang, Chen and Lee, 1973; Chang and Lee, 1977; Lee and Chang, 1966; Oberg and Kelly, 1976; Strong, Heuser and Kelly, 1977). The amplitude of mepps is not reduced and occasionally giant mepps are observed. Bursts of mepps occur spontaneously and can be also evoked by high K^+ immediately after N-M block (Chang, Chen and Lee, 1973; Chang and Lee, 1977; Chang and co-workers, 1977a). By contrast, high K^+ has no effect on the muscle paralysed by notexin and taipoxin *in vivo* (Harris, Karlsson and Thesleff, 1973; Kamenskaya and Thesleff, 1974), probably due to depletion of the synaptic vesicles at the advanced stage of toxin effects. As manifested in the frog or mammalian nerve-muscle preparations exposed to Sr^{2+} or a low Ca^{2+} medium, the initial facilitation of these toxins is still preceded by an immediate and transient depressant effect (Abe, Limbrick and Miledi, 1976; Chang and Lee, 1977; Chang and co-workers, 1977b; Kelly, von Wedel and Strong, 1979; Livengood and co-workers, 1978). The latter effect remains unaffected when the enzyme is inactivated either directly by chemical modification with p-bromophenacyl bromide (Kelly, von Wedel and Strong, 1979), or by boiling it at pH 8.6 for 3 min (Livengood and co-workers, 1978).

B. Ultrastructural Changes in the Motor Nerve Terminals

Morphological changes of the motor nerve terminals in the diaphragm of mouse injected with a lethal dose of β-bungarotoxin were first described by Chen and Lee (1970). One hour after injection, the number of synaptic vesicles was decreased and numerous Ω-shaped indentations similar in size to synaptic vesicles were found on the axolemma. Two to 4 hours after the toxin administration, the synaptic vesicles were almost completely depleted and the mitochondria became swollen and vacuolized. By contrast, the structures of muscle fibers, Schwann cells and myelinated axons were unaffected. Similar ultrastructural changes of motor nerve terminals were observed in the diaphragm of mice poisoned with taipoxin, notexin (Cull-Candy and co-workers, 1976) and crotoxin (Tsai and Chang, unpublished). A more detailed account of β-bungarotoxin effects on frog nerve-muscle preparations, using both freeze-fracture replicas and conventionally fixed thin sections in the electron microscope was given by Strong, Heuser and Kelly (1976). These authors also found that β-bungarotoxin labeled with horseradish peroxidase bound selectively not only to the axolemma of the nerve terminals, but also to some of their internal membranes, including the membrane of synaptic vesicles and of mitochondria. The decrease of synaptic vesicles may be due to an inhibition of the recycling of synaptic vesicle membrane as suggested by Cull-Candy and co-workers (1976) for notexin and taipoxin. It is unlikely, however, that the inhibition of transmitter release by these toxins is due to the depletion of synaptic vesicles, since at the time of failure of transmitter release, mepps still persist and high K^+ still can increase the frequency of mepps (Chang, Chen and Lee, 1973; Chang and Lee, 1977; Chang and co-workers 1977a). Moreover, electron microscopic examination at this stage of intoxication revealed that the structure of the nerve terminal of the diaphragm was still quite normal, except the appearance of Ω-shaped indentations in the axolemma; most of the ultrastructual changes of the nerve terminal were seen only after complete paralysis of the diaphragm (Tsai, Chang and Lee, 1976). Therefore, the depletion of synaptic vesicles may be regarded as an advanced effect of these toxins, rather than the cause of their N-M blocking action.

C. Mode of Action-Relation with Phospholipase A Activity

It is now generally accepted that the PLA activity of these presynaptic toxins is responsible for their neurotoxicity. First, all of the presynaptic toxins so far isolated from snake venoms are basic PLAs, or at least contain a subunit which is a basic PLA. Second, inhibition of catalytic activity either by replacement of Ca^{2+} with Sr^{2+} in the medium or by direct chemical modification of the toxins results in a corresponding diminution in or abolition of neurotoxicity. Third, the ultrastructural changes of axonal organelles, synaptic vesicles and mitochondria, induced by these toxins also suggest that the membrane of these organelles are affected, probably by direct PLA action within the axon.

Nevertheless, why these presynaptic toxins should attack selectively the motor nerve terminals, whereas other enzymatically more active PLAs are almost without effect on the presynaptic site, remains a question to be answered. It has been postulated that β-bungarotoxin acts in two functionally separate steps: (i) by binding to a specific presynaptic site, which is unrelated to the toxin's PLA activity, and (ii) by perturbing the presynaptic membrane by its enzyme action, which results in an increase and then a failure in transmitter release (Abe, Limbrick and Miledi, 1976; Kelly and co-workers, 1975; Livengood and co-workers, 1978; Strong, Heuser and Kelly, 1977). They also suggest that the toxin possesses a site in addition to its enzymatic locus which permits it to recognize and selectively bind to the specific presynaptic site. As pointed out by I.H. Tsai (unpublished), some of the basic amino acid residues which are exposed on the surface of the toxin molecule may be essential for such specific binding. All of the non-neurotoxic PLAs so far sequenced do not have such basic amino acid residues at the strategic positions and therefore lack the features responsible for the specific binding. The finding that β-bungarotoxin is converted from a neurotoxic PLA to a PLA without neurotoxic activity by treatment with ethoxyformic anhydride (EOFA) in the presence of Ca^{2+} or dihexanoyllecithin (Howard and Truog, 1977) seems to lend support to this contention. EOFA alters at least two sites on the toxin: the PLA active site (histidine residue) and another site also required for neurotoxicity. Only the PLA active site could be protected by Ca^{2+} and dihexanoyllecithin. Previously, we have also found that both acetylation of lysine residues and N-terminal amino group and modification of arginine residues with glyoxal in β-bungarotoxin completely abolish its toxicity (S.L. Chang and C.Y. Lee, unpublished).

The initial transient decrease in transmitter release after applying the toxin has been attributed to the binding of the toxin to a specific presynaptic site, which is unrelated to the PLA activity (Abe, Limbrick and Miledi, 1976; Abe, Alema and Miledi, 1977; Kelly, von Wedel and Strong, 1979; Livengood and co-workers, 1978), but the exact mechanism of action remains to be elucidated. The second facilitatory phase of the toxin effects has been attributed to the subsequent PLA action after the toxin binding and explained in various ways. The simplest explanation is that the enzymatic activity produces transient holes in the axon membrane and that calcium ions moving in through the holes would cause the massive release of transmitter responsible for the bursts of mepps, while the increase in spontaneous release of transmitter quanta may be caused by a build-up of the intracellular level of ionized calcium (Abe, Limbrick and Miledi, 1976). Secondly, the toxin inhibition of Ca^{2+} removal by mitochondria may be responsible for the increase in the level of ionized calcium inside the terminal (Wagner, Mart and Kelly, 1974). Thirdly, the PLA action of the toxin may also activate the release process through the production of fatty acids and lysophospholipids (Abe, Limbrick and Miledi, 1976; Kelly and co-workers, 1975; Strong, Heuser and Kelly, 1977), both of which are known to promote membrane fusion (Kantor and Prestegard, 1975; Poole, Howell and Lucy, 1970). However, not all of presynaptic toxins show initial facilitation. No initial facilitatory phase was noted with notexin (Harris, Karlsson and Thesleff, 1973; Cull-Candy and co-workers, 1976). In view of the recent finding that the facilitatory phase observed with β-bungarotoxin, crotoxin and taipoxin was still prominent in the nerve muscle preparation bathed in Sr^{2+}-Tyrode solution, in which the PLA activity was inhibited (Chang and co-worker, 1977b), the role played by the PLA in the facilitatory effect of these toxins needs further investigation.

The final phase of eventual failure of transmitter release is apparently due to the progressive enzymatic hydrolysis of phospholipids within the nerve terminal, resulting in an inactivation of the release mechanism. The transmission failure has been attributed to a depletion of energy stores, resulting from the uncoupling of mitochondrial oxidative phosphorylation (Wernicke, Vanker and Howard, 1975). Kelly and co-workers (1975), however, have argued against this hypothesis, pointing out that known mitochondrial uncouplers cause the mepp frequency to increase to a rate of several hundred per second in calcium-free media (Glagoleva, Liberman and Khashayev, 1970), which does not resemble the effects of β-bungarotoxin. On the other hand, an inhibition of high-affinity choline uptake has also been proposed as the primary cause of transmission blockade (Sen, Grantham and Cooper, 1976). However, there is no correlation between inhibitory potency and presynaptic neurotoxicity among various toxins with PLA activity tested (Dowdall, Fohlman and Eaker, 1977). Moreover, the transmission blockade is apparently not due to depletion of transmitter stores, as mentioned above. These toxins may cause some general perturbation of the presynaptic membrane which upsets membrane-associated processes including choline transport. Finally, whether the transmission blockade by these toxins is due to a rise in the axoplasmic Ca^{2+} to excessively high levels as suggested by Abe, Limbrick and Miledi (1976) remains to be confirmed.

The role played by crotapotin of crotoxin complex, β- and γ-subunits of taipoxin and B-chain of β_1-bungarotoxin, respectively, in the neurotoxicity of these presynaptic toxins remains to be clarified. Fohlman and co-workers (1976) have suggested that these subunits may function as "chaperones", protecting the basic PLA against non-specific tissue binding and increasing its stability so as to minimize distraction and destruction en route to the site of action at the nerve terminal. This speculation was experimentally confirmed in the case of crotoxin complex (Chang and Su, 1978). The function of B-chain in β_1-bungarotoxin has been speculated to recognize and combine at the specific presynaptic site (Abe, Limbrick and Miledi, 1976; Kondo, Narita and Lee, 1978). However, since the 11,000-dalton β-bungarotoxin has been shown to be a single chain polypeptide with similar presynaptic activity (Donlon and co-workers, 1975; Livengood and co-workers, 1978), there is no reason to suppose that B-chain in β_1-bungarotoxin has any essential function at the target level.

IV. POSTSYNAPTIC AND MUSCULOTROPIC EFFECTS -- MYOTOXIC EFFECTS

Besides presynaptic effects, most of the snake toxins with PLA activity exhibit postsynaptic and direct musculotropic effects, decreasing the sensitivity of the motor endplate to ACh or carbamylcholine and producing a contracture of the muscle, especially at higher toxin concentrations (Lee and Ho, 1978b). The chick biventer cervicis muscle is more susceptible than the rat or mouse diaphragm in this respect. One μg/ml notexin induces marked contracture of chick muscle and the response to ACh is significantly decreased even at 0.1 μg/ml of notexin (Lee, Chen and Karlsson, 1976). Ceruleotoxin, like notexin, increases the tone of chick muscle and decreases the response to ACh at higher toxin concentrations, while at a lower concentration (10^{-6} g/ml), the toxin abolishes the twitch response to indirect stimulation without affecting the response to ACh (Lee and Ho, 1978a). The postsynaptic site of action of these toxins may be the cholinergic ionophore as suggested by Bon and Changeux (1977) for ceruleotoxin, since unlike postsynaptic toxins, this toxin does not interfere with the binding of [^{3}H]ACh and of *Naja nigricollis* α-[^{3}H]toxin to the cholinergic receptor site. The contracture induced by these toxins is apparently due to depolarization of muscle membranes (Lee and Ho, 1978b).

In the muscle preparation pretreated with heparin (10^{-3} g/ml), notexin as well as the basic PLA from *Naja nigricollis* venom does not produce contracture, whereas their presynaptic N-M blocking action remains little affected (Ho and Lee, unpublished). This finding strongly suggests that the basic amino acid residue(s) in the toxin molecule responsible for the binding to muscle membrane may be quite different from those for the specific binding to the axolemma of the nerve terminal.

Some presynaptically active neurotoxins cause severe myonecrosis when injected into the skeletal muscle. The notable example is notexin (Harris, Johnson and Karlsson, 1975). Taipoxin when applied locally has the same kind of myotoxic effect *in vivo* as notexin (Harris, Johnson and MacDonell, 1977). Myonecrosis appears to be the end result of direct musculotropic effect of these toxins. However, the presynaptic neurotoxicity of these toxins is so potent that animals are usually killed before myonecrotic changes become manifest, if injected intravenously or intraperitoneally.

There are also some toxic PLAs in other snake venoms, which show myonecrotic action with low or negligible presynaptic neurotoxicity. For example, both the basic and neutral PLAs isolated from *Naja nigricollis* venom cause myonecrosis in the injected leg of mice, the former being far more potent than the latter (Lee and Ho, 1978b). The myotoxin VI: 5 isolated from *Enhydrina schistosa* venom is also a basic PLA and causes myonecrosis and myoglobinuria in mice (Fohlman and Eaker, 1977) and in guinea pigs (Geh and Toh, 1978).

V. POSTSYNAPTIC EFFECTS ON FISH ELECTROPLAQUES

Recently, Bon and Changeux (1975, 1977) reported that ceruleotoxin, a toxin component with PLA activity isolated from *Bungarus caeruleus* venom, blocks *in vivo* the depolarisation caused by carbamylcholine on the isolated electroplaque from *Electrophorus electricus* and *in vitro* the increase of $^{22}Na^+$ and $^{42}K^+$ efflux caused by cholinergic agonists on excitable receptor-rich microsacs prepared from *Torpedo marmorata* electric organ. Since this toxin does not interfere with the binding of [^{3}H]ACh and of α-[^{3}H]toxin from *Naja nigricollis* venom to the cholinergic receptor site, these authors suggest that ceruleotoxin may interact specifically with the cholinergic ionophore. As mentioned above, however, in avian and mammalian nerve-muscle preparations, ceruleotoxin has been shown to exhibit presynaptic effects at a lower concentration than that required for postsynaptic effects (Lee and Ho, 1978a). More recently, Bon and co-workers (1979) have found that crotoxin, as its isolated PLA subunit (CB), also acts postsynaptically on fish electroplaque, by blocking the electrogenic action of cholinergic agonists. These postsynaptic effects of crotoxin have been observed even at lower concentrations than those used by Chang and Lee (1977) to demonstrate the presynaptic effect of crotoxin in birds and mammals. Like ceruleotoxin, crotoxin does not interfere with the binding of α-toxin from *Naja nigricollis* to the nicotinic receptor site. Apparently, the postsynaptic membrane, possibly the cholinergic ionophore, in fish electroplaques is particularly sensitive to the PLA activity of these toxins. However, there appears no parallelism between the postsynaptic effect on fish electroplaques and the neurotoxicity among various PLA preparations (Bon, personal communication). For example, as observed by Andreasen and McNamee (1977), a PLA isolated from the venom of *Naja naja siamensis* which is apparently non-toxic (Karlsson, Arnberg and Eaker, 1971), inhibits the increase of sodium efflux caused by cholinergic agonists from *Torpedo californica* membrane vesicles at a concentration 10 to 50 times lower than the concentration required for α-neurotoxin inhibition. It remains to be elucidated whether these toxins with PLA activity have any presynaptic effect on fish electroplaques as on the N-M junction of vertebrate skeletal muscle.

VI. EFFECTS ON THE AUTONOMIC TRANSMISSION

Presynaptic toxins from snake venoms have been generally considered to be inactive on the autonomic neurotransmission. For example, the twitch response of the guinea-pig ileum elicited by co-axial stimulation (Chang and Lee, 1963) and the contraction of the cat nictitating membrane to sympathetic preganglionic nerve stimulation (F.L. Lee and C.Y. Lee, unpublished) are not affected by β-bungarotoxin even at a concentration 100 times higher than that for neuromuscular blockade. Recently, however, Kato and co-workers (1977) reported that β-bungarotoxin increased spontaneous ACh release and decreased ACh release evoked by preganglionic nerve stimulation in the cat superior cervical ganglion and suggested that the toxin affects preganglionic and motor nerve terminals, but not postganglionic cholinergic nerve. In contrast, Muramatsu and co-workers (1979) have demonstrated that β-bungarotoxin abolishes the negative inotropic and chronotropic responses of guinea-pig atria to either pre- or postganglionic stimulation of the vagus nerve at a concentration as low as 0.01 μg/ml, while it fails to block the excitatory responses to either pre- and postganglionic sympathetic nerve stimulation. The release of noradrenaline from the adrenergic nerve terminals of a nictitating membrane preparation is also unaffected by β-bungarotoxin (Kato and co-workers, 1977).

On the other hand, the contractile response of the guinea-pig vas deferens to transmural stimulation has been shown to be inhibited transiently by notexin (Harris and Zar, 1978). Recently, we have also found that β-bungarotoxin as well as notexin causes a triphasic change in the motor transmission of the guinea-pig vas deferens, similar to that observed in the skeletal muscle preparation bathed in a low Ca^{2+} medium (Ho and Lee, to be published). The motor transmission in the vas deferens has been claimed to be neither cholinergic nor adrenergic (Ambache and Zar, 1971). The vas deferens preparation is unique in that its non-cholinergic motor transmission can be inhibited by presynaptic toxins.

REFERENCES

Abe, T., S. Alema and R. Miledi (1977) *Eur. J. Biochem.*, 80, 1-12.
Abe, T., A.R. Limbrick and R. Miledi (1976) *Proc. R. Soc. Lond. B.* 194, 545-553.
Alderice, M.T. and R.L. Volle (1975) *Neuroscience Abstract*, p. 967, New York Society Neuroscience.
Ambache, N. and M.A. Zar (1971) *J. Physiol.* (London) 216, 359-389.
Andreasen, T.J. and M.G. McNamee (1977) *Biochem. Biophys. Res. Commun.* 79, 958-965.

Bieber, A.L., T. Tu and A.T. Tu (1975) *Biochim. Biophys. Acta* (Amst.) 400, 178-188.
Bon, C. and J.-P. Changeux (1975) *FEBS Letters* 52, 212-216.
Bon, C. and J.-P. Changeux (1977) *Eur. J. Biochem.* 74, 43-51.
Bon, C., J.-P. Changeux, T.-W. Jeng and H. Fraenkel-Conrat (1979) *Eur. J. Biochem.* 99, 471-481.
Breithaupt, H., K. Rübsamen and E. Habermann (1974) *Eur. J. Biochem.* 49, 333-345.
Chang, C.C. (1979) The action of snake venoms on nerve and muscle. In: C.Y. Lee (Ed.), *Snake Venoms, Handb. Exp. Pharm.* vol. 52, Springer,Heidelberg, pp. 309-376.
Chang, C.C., T.F. Chen and C.Y. Lee (1973) *J. Pharmacol. Exp. Ther.* 184, 339-345.
Chang, C.C. and C.Y. Lee (1963) *Arch. Int. Pharmacodyn.* 144, 241-257.
Chang, C.C. and J.D. Lee (1977) *Naunyn-Schmiedebergs Arch. Pharmacol.* 296, 159-168.
Chang, C.C., J.D. Lee, D. Eaker and J. Fohlman (1977a) *Toxicon* 15, 571-576.
Chang, C.C., M.J. Su, J.D. Lee and D. Eaker (1977b) *Naunyn-Schmiedebergs Arch. Pharmacol.* 299, 155-161.
Chang, C.C. and M.J. Su (1978) *Toxicon* 16, 402-405.
Chen, I.-L. and C.Y. Lee (1970) *Virchows Arch. Abt. B. Zellpath.* 6, 318-325.
Cull-Candy, S.G., J. Fohlman, D. Gustavason, R. Lullmann-Ramch and S. Thesleff (1976) *J. Neurosci.* 1, 175-180.
Delori, P.J. (1971) *Biochimie* 53, 941-942.
Donlon, M.A., G.S. Tobias, W.G. Shain, and G.N. Catravas (1975) Abstracts, *Society for Neuroscience, 5th Annual Meeting*, vol. 1, 649.
Dowdall, M.J., J.P. Fohlman and D. Eaker (1977) *Nature* 269, 700-702.
Eaker, D. (1978) Studies of presynaptically neurotoxic and myotoxic phospholipase A_2. In: C.H. Li (Ed.), *Versatility of Proteins*, Academic Press, New York, pp. 413-431.
Fohlman, J. and D. Eaker (1977) *Toxicon* 15, 385-393.
Fohlman, J., D. Eaker, E. Karlsson and S. Thesleff (1976) *Eur. J. Biochem.* 68, 457-469.
Glagoleva, I.M., Y.A. Liberman and Z.K.M. Khashayev (1970) *Biofizika* 15, 76.
Geh, S.L. and H.T. Toh (1978) *Toxicon* 16, 633-643.
Gopalakrishnakone, P., B.J. Hawgood, S.E. Holbrooke, N.A. Marsh, S. Santana de Sa and A.T. Tu (1979) Abstracts, *6th Internat. Symposium on Animal, Plant and Microbial Toxins*, Uppsala, p. 56.
Halpert, J. and D. Eaker (1976) *J. Biol. Chem.* 251, 7343-7347.
Harris, J.B., M.A. Johnson and E. Karlsson (1975) *Clin. exp. Pharmacol. Physiol.* 2, 383-404.
Harris, J.B., M.A. Johnson and C. MacDonell (1977) *Br. J. Pharmacol.* 61, 133 p.
Harris, J.B., E. Karlsson and S. Thesleff (1973) *Br. J. Pharmacol.* 47, 141-146.
Harris, J.B. and M.A. Zar (1978) *Br. J. Pharmacol.* 62, 349-358.
Hendon, R.A. and H. Fraenkel-Conrat (1971) *Proc. Natl. Acad. Sci. USA* 68, 1560-1563.
Howard, B.D. and R. Truog (1977) *Biochemistry* 16, 122-125.
Kamenskaya, M.A. and S. Thesleff (1974) *Acta Physiol. Scand.* 90, 716-724.
Kantor, H.L. and J.H. Prestegard (1975) *Biochemistry* 14, 1790-1795.
Karlsson, E. (1979) Chemistry of protein toxins in snake venoms. In: C.Y. Lee (Ed.) *Snake Venoms, Handb. Exp. Pharm.* vol. 52, Springer, Heidelberg, pp. 159-212.
Karlsson, E., H. Arnberg and D. Eaker (1971) *Eur. J. Biochem.* 21, 1-16.
Karlsson, E., D. Eaker and L. Rydén (1972) *Toxicon* 10, 405-413.
Kato, A.C., J.E.B. Pinto, M. Glavinovic and B. Collier (1977) *Can. J. Physiol. Pharmacol.* 55, 574-584.
Kelly, R.B. and F.R. Brown (1974) *J. Neurobiol.* 5, 135-150.
Kelly, R.B., S.G. Oberg, P.N. Strong and B.M. Wagner (1975) *Cold Spring Harbor Symp. Quant. Biol.* 40, 117-125.
Kelly, R.B., R.J. von Wedel and P.N. Strong (1979) β-Bungarotoxin: Evidence for direct binding to nerve terminals: Separation of binding and enzymic action. In: B. Ceccarelli and F. Clementi (Eds.) *Neurotoxins: Tools in Neurobiology*, Raven Press, New York, pp. 77-85.
Kondo, K., K. Narita and C.Y. Lee (1978) *J. Biochem. (Tokyo)*, 83, 91-99.

Lee, C.Y. (1979) Recent advances in chemistry and pharmacology of snake toxins. In: B. Ceccarelli and F. Clementi (Eds.) *Neurotoxins: Tools in Neurobiology,* Raven Press, New York, pp. 1-16.
Lee, C.Y. and C.C. Chang (1966) *Mem. Inst. Butantan* 33, 555-572.
Lee, C.Y., Y.M. Chen and E. Karlsson (1976) *Toxicon* 14, 493-494.
Lee, C.Y., Y.M. Chen and D. Mebs (1976) *Toxicon* 14, 451-457.
Lee, C.Y. and C.L. Ho (1978a) Abstracts, *7th Internatl. Congress Pharmacol.* p. 571.
Lee, C.Y. and C.L. Ho (1978b) Pharmacology of snake toxins with phospholipase A_2 activity. In: C.H. Li (Ed.) *Versatility of Proteins,* Academic Press, New York, pp. 433-446.
Lee, C.Y., C.L. Ho and D.P. Botes (1979) Abstracts, *6th Internat. Symp. on Animal Plant and Microbial Toxins*, Uppsala, P. 101.
Lee, C.Y., C.L. Ho and D. Eaker (1977) *Toxicon* 15, 355-356.
Lee, C.Y. and L.F. Tseng (1969) *Toxicon* 7, 89-93.
Livengood, D.R., R.S. Manalis, M.A. Donlon, L.M. Masukawa, G.S. Tobias and W. Shain (1978) *Proc. Natl. Acad. Sci. USA* 75, 1029-1033.
Magazanik, L.G., I.M. Gotgilf, T.I. Slavnova, A.I. Miroshnikov and U.R. Apsalon (1979) *Toxicon* (in press)
Muramatsu, I., M. Fujiwara, A. Miura, K. Hayashi and C.Y. Lee (1979) Submitted to *J. Pharmacol. Exp. Ther.*
Oberg, S.G. and R.B. Kelly (1976) *Biochim. Biophys. Acta* 433, 662-673.
Poole, A.R., J.I. Howell and J.A. Lucy (1970) *Nature* 277, 810-812.
Ravdin, P.M. and D.K. Berg (1969) *Proc. Natl. Acad. Sci. USA* 76, 2072-2076.
Sen, I., P.A. Grantham and J.R. Cooper (1976) *Proc. Natl. Acad. Sci. USA* 73, 2664-2668.
Slotta, K. and H. Fraenkel-Conrat (1938) *Ber. Dtsch. Chem. Ges.* 71, 1076-1081.
Strong, P.N., J.E. Heuser, and R.B. Kelly (1977) Selective enzymatic hydrolysis of nerve terminal phospholipids by β-bungarotoxin: biochemical and morphological studies. In: Z. Hall, R. Kelly and C.F. Fox (Eds.) *"Cellular Neurobiology"* Alan R. Liss, Inc., New York, pp. 227-273.
Tsai, M.C., C.C. Chang and C.Y. Lee (1976) The relation between the blockade of transmitter release and the ultrastructural changes of the motor nerve terminals caused by β-bungarotoxin. *Memorial Volume to President Chang Kai-Shek, Academia Sinica.* pp. 289-305.
Vital Brazil, O. and B.J. Excell (1971) *J. Physiol. (Lond.)* 212, 34-35 p.
Vital Brazil, O., J.P. Franceschi and E. Waisbich (1966) *Mem. Inst. Butantan* 33, 973-980.
Wagner, G.H., P.E. Mart and R.B. Kelly (1974) *Biochem. Biophys. Res. Commun.* 58, 475-481.
Wernicke, J.F., T. Oberjat and B.D. Howard (1974) *J. Neurochem.* 22, 781-788.
Wernicke, J.F., A.D. Vanker, and B.D. Howard (1975) *J. Neurochem.* 25, 483-496.

INTERACTION OF β-BUNGAROTOXIN WITH SYNAPSES IN THE MAMMALIAN CENTRAL NERVOUS SYSTEM

J. O. Dolly*, J. V. Halliwell and J. W. Spokes***

**Dept. of Biochemistry, Imperial College, London SW7, UK*
***Dept. of Pharmacology, The School of Pharmacy, University of London WC1, UK*

ABSTRACT

β-Bungarotoxin, which was purified to homogeneity from the venom of Bungarus multicinctus by ion-exchange chromatography and isoelectric focussing, was shown to affect release of acetylcholine, glutamate and γ-aminobutyrate from rat cortex synaptosomes. In slices of rat olfactory cortex, the toxin irreversibly blocked neurotransmission by inhibiting transmitter release; in addition, it reduced the amplitude of the presynaptic action potential but at a slower rate. Inhibition of the toxin's phospholipase A_2 activity, by replacement of Ca^{2+} with Sr^{2+}, only attenuated its action on release of transmitters but abolished effects on the action potential. Irreversible binding of β-bungarotoxin occurred in Sr^{2+} and subsequent addition of Ca^{2+} restored its full neurotoxicity. Two pure phospholipases A_2 were much less potent than toxin in mediating effects on transmitter release from the synaptosomes and slices. It is concluded that under certain conditions β-bungarotoxin can specifically inhibit transmitter release at a central synapse and appears, therefore, to be a useful probe for studying this process.

KEYWORDS

β-Bungarotoxin, synaptosomes, transmitter release, phospholipase A_2, olfactory cortex slice, action potential, N- wave.

INTRODUCTION

At present the molecular mechanism(s) for release of neurotransmitters are not understood. Biochemical characterisation of nerve membrane components which are concerned with the process is, therefore, important. Neurotoxins that specifically interfere with the release of neurotransmitters may enable such studies to be performed, just as α-neurotoxins facilitated characterisation of nicotinic cholinoreceptors (Dolly, 1979). Although a number of toxins that act in this manner have been identified (D. Eaker; C.Y.Lee and others, this volume) their exact site(s) of action and specificities towards synapses with different transmitters have not been established. Of all the snake venom neurotoxins, β-bungarotoxin (β-BuTX) is one of the most lethal (Chang, 1979) and probably the most specific in that it acts solely on the presynaptic nerve membrane of the neuromuscular junction without any detectable postsynaptic effects (C.Y.Lee, this volume). It produces an initial decrease in the amplitude of the endplate potentials in a frog nerve-muscle preparation, followed by a transient increase and eventually a complete blockade (Abe, Alema and Miledi, 1977); the toxin also gives a similar triphasic effect on spontaneous release of transmitter (Abe, Limbrick and Miledi, 1976). β-BuTX exhibits phospholipase A_2 activity in presence of Ca^{2+} (Strong and others, 1976); removal of enzymic activity by chemical modification greatly reduces its lethality when injected into mice (Abe, Alema and Miledi, 1977: Strong, Heuser and Kelly, 1977). Likewise, the modified toxin or native toxin in which the phospholipase activity is inhibited by replacement of Ca^{2+} with Sr^{2+} show greatly diminished neurotoxicity. Moreover, in the latter cases only the initial decrease in amplitude of the endplate potential or frequency of miniature endplate potentials is observed (Abe, Alema and Miledi, 1977). Relative to β-BuTX, phospholipases A_2 when injected into mice are less toxic (Chang, 1979); they do not act preferentially on the presynaptic nerve membrane and are usually unable (but see Lee, Ho and Botes, 1979) to produce the initial inhibition of acetylcholine release (Abe and Miledi, 1978). Therefore, it appears that the toxin's phospholipase activity may give rise to the last two phases of its action (Strong, Heuser and Kelly, 1977). However, it cannot be wholly responsible for its specificity of action on the presynaptic membrane; in fact, the latter authors have proposed that the toxin has a site,in addition to the enzymatic locus,that enables it to bind selectively to a structure located on the nerve terminal membrane. The initial decrease in transmitter release produced by native or enzymically inactive toxins may result from its binding to a component concerned with the release process (Abe and Miledi, 1978). β-BuTX may, therefore, prove to be a useful probe for studying the release process in this system.

In certain respects,biochemical studies on molecular components of the release system can be more readily performed on preparations from the central nervous system such as synaptosomes and their purified membranes. However, β-BuTX has not yet been shown by electrophysiological procedures to affect neurotransmission at central synapses. In this report, a method is described for the purification of homogeneous β-BuTX and this has been shown to affect rat central synapses by both biochemical and electrophysiological techniques.

PURIFICATION AND CHARACTERISATION OF β-BuTX

The venom of Bungarus multicinctus was fractionated on a column of CM-Sephadex C-50 as previously described (Dolly and others, 1978; Spokes and Dolly, 1980); analytical isoelectric focussing of the major β-toxin peak obtained revealed three contaminants while gel electrophoresis showed only one extraneous protein band. Further purification by preparative isoelectric focussing in a narrow pH gradient separated at least four proteins from the β-BuTX which was then homogeneous on analytical focussing (Fig.1) and electrophoresis under native or denaturing conditions (Spokes and Dolly, 1980).

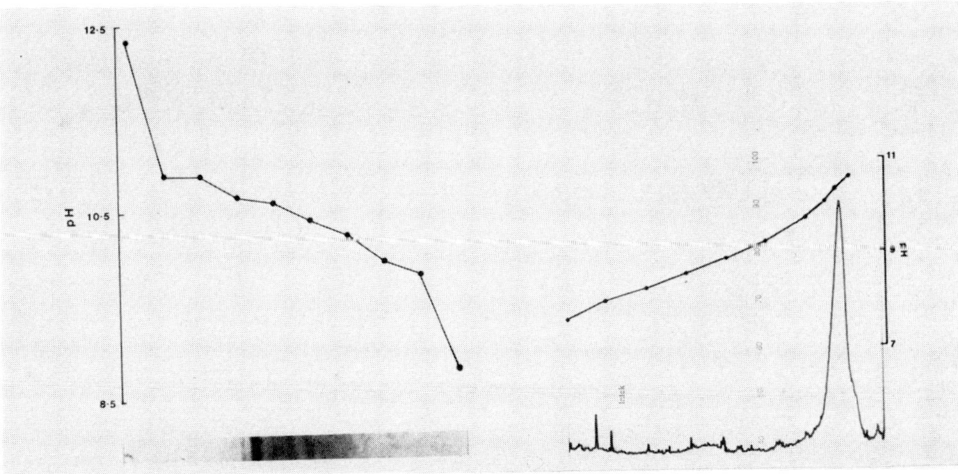

Fig.1. Isoelectric focussing of β-BuTX. Left: Preparative isoelectric of β-BuTX, obtained by chromatography on CM-Sephadex, was performed at 8 W constant power for 16 h in a flat bed of Sephadex G-75 containing 1% ampholytes (pH 8 - 10). The pH gradient was measured; a paper print of the bed was fixed in 10% TCA and stained with Coomassie R-250. Right: Analytical focussing of pure β-BuTX in a polyacrylamide gel, using pH 7 - 9 and 9 - 11 ampholytes. The protein was fixed with 40% TCA, washed and the gel scanned at 450 nm.

We could not remove the contaminants by chromatography on CM-cellulose (Strong and others, 1976), SP-Sephadex (MacDermot, Westgaard and Thompson, 1978) or Sephadex G-75 (Hanley and others, 1977); they may be 'isotoxins'. On gel filtration the toxin had a molecular weight of 21,000; after reduction it was shown by electrophoresis in SDS to consist of two subunits with molecular weights of about 11,400 and 9,000, similar to those reported (C.Y.Lee, this volume). The pure β-BuTX was highly toxic when injected into mice (LD_{50} = 10 ng/g body wt) and irreversibly inhibited neurotransmission in a frog nerve-muscle preparation. In the presence of Ca^{2+} and deoxycholate it exhibited phospholipase activity (at 37° C 63 μmole of egg yolk phosphatidylcholine were hydrolyzed min^{-1} mg^{-1} of protein) but this was less than one-twentieth of that observed with pure phospholipase A_2 from bee venom. On removal of Ca^{2+} or its substitution with Sr^{2+}, the toxin's enzyme activity was reduced by 100 and 96% respectively. With the inclusion of Ca^{2+} but omission of deoxycholate very little (less than 1% of the maximum) or no activity (Dolly and others, 1978) was detectable. β-BuTX stimulated O_2 uptake by synaptic mitochondria; pretreatment with ADP prevented this effect and β-BuTX inhibited the stimulatory effect normally seen with ADP alone (Tse, Dolly and Diniz, 1980). This action of the toxin may be related to its complete blockade of transmitter release (see below).

EFFECTS OF β-BuTX ON RELEASE OF NEUROTRANSMITTERS FROM BRAIN SYNAPTOSOMES

For studies on transmitter release, synaptosomes purified from rat cortex were preloaded with radiolabelled choline (Spokes and Dolly, 1980) glutamate (Glu) and γ-aminobutyrate (GABA) (Tse, Dolly and Diniz, 1980) by incubation at 37° C for 20 min. After washing, the synaptosomes were resuspended in Krebs medium and incubated with low and high K^+ concentrations in the absence and presence of toxin; the amounts of transmitter released into the supernatants were measured by scintillation counting. High-voltage paper electrophoresis was employed to separate choline and acetylcholine (ACh) and also to check the proportion of released radioactivity which was due to metabolites of the amino acids used.

Depolarisation of the synaptosomes by raising the external concentration of K^+ increased the release of ACh (Table 1) and the two putative neurotransmitters, Glu and GABA (Table 2); it also increased the rates of lactate production and oxygen uptake by the synaptosomes, important criteria of their viability.

TABLE 1 Effects of β-BuTX on the release of ACh and choline from synaptosomes

	ACh	Choline	ACh	Choline
Series a			$-Ca^{2+}$ / +5mM EGTA	
Control	86 ± 46	22 ± 12	70 ± 124	1 ± 25
23 mM K^+	293 ± 104	60 ± 95	113 ± 14	82 ± 20
Series b			$-Ca^{2+}$ / +0.74 mM Sr^{2+}	
Control	417 ± 61	61 ± 4	253 ± 16	39 ± 38
β-BuTX(10^{-7}M)	882 ± 67	372 ± 33	473 ± 54	128 ± 58
23 mM K^+	595 ± 142	90 ± 6	776 ± 128	162 ± 34

Synaptosomes which had been preloaded with [^{3}H]choline were incubated at 25°C for 20 min and the amounts of [^{3}H]ACh and [^{3}H]choline released into the supernatant determined. The values are the mean (± S.D.) of those obtained from two separate incubations using a single synaptosome preparation. Incubations contained 10 mM eserine sulphate to inhibit hydrolysis of ACh. Data are in dpm released/mg of protein.

TABLE 2 Effects of β-BuTX on synaptosomal release of previously accumulated Glu and GABA

	Glu		GABA		GABA	
	$+Ca^{2+}$	$-Ca^{2+}$	$+Ca^{2+}$	$-Ca^{2+}$	$+Ca^{2+}$	$-Ca^{2+}/+Sr^{2+}$
Control		(0.87)		(1.15)		(1.63)
	1.00±0.06	1.00±0.07	1.00±0.05	1.00±0.17	1.00±0.01	1.00±0.07
55 mM K^+	1.41±0.10	1.29±0.12	1.49±0.16	1.13±0.08	1.28±0.20	1.85±0.10
1μM β-BuTX	2.22±0.18	1.18±0.11	2.31±0.15	1.82±0.14	2.94±0.02	1.27±0.01

Synaptosomal suspensions were loaded with [^{14}C]GABA or [^{14}C]Glu, washed once and incubated at 37°C for 25 min. The amounts of radioactivity released are expressed relative to the appropriate controls (no additives). Numbers in parenthesis are the control values obtained in the absence of Ca^{2+} with EGTA or Sr^{2+} present, expressed as a ratio to those measured in the presence of Ca^{2+}.

With the three transmitters the presence of Ca^{2+} in the medium was necessary to obtain the maximum degree of K^+ - stimulated release. Thus, this synaptosome system exhibits many important characteristics of the physiological release process.

Incubation of synaptosomes with β-BuTX stimulated release of ACh, Glu and GABA (Tables 1 and 2) and the concentrations which gave 50% of the maximum effect were 50 (Fig.2) 20 and 30 nM, respectively.

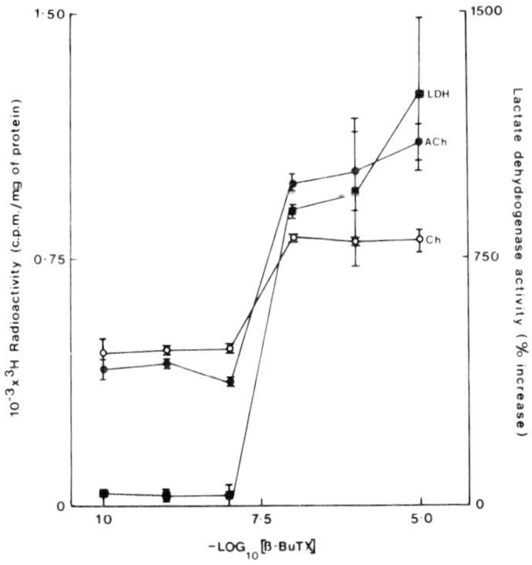

Fig.2. Concentration dependence of β-BuTX-stimulated release from synaptosomes of ACh, choline and lactate dehydrogenase. The amounts of [^{3}H]ACh (●) and [^{3}H]choline (o) released after incubation of preloaded synaptosomes for 20 min at each toxin concentration are shown. Released lactate dehydrogenase activity (■), which was measured spectrophotometrically, is expressed as a percentage increase of that in the supernatants of control samples not treated with toxin. Mean values (± S.D.) obtained for two separate incubations using a single synaptosome preparation are given. It was previously demonstrated that release of ACh and choline was linear with time, for 40 min, at the highest toxin concentration used.

The toxin caused a smaller efflux of choline but it had a similar concentration dependence. At high K^+ concentration β-BuTX also increased release of transmitters (Spokes and Dolly, 1980; Tse, Dolly and Diniz, 1980). Ca^{2+} was required for the toxin to exert its maximum effects; Sr^{2+} was unable to substitute for it. As β-BuTX possesses Ca^{2+}-dependent phospholipase activity, the possibility was examined that toxin-induced lysis of the synaptosomes is responsible for its effects on release. Figure 2 shows that β-BuTX increases the release of lactate dehydrogenase, a cytoplasmic marker, with equal potency to its effects on efflux of ACh and choline. As in the case of the three transmitters studied, when Ca^{2+} was replaced by Sr^{2+}, toxin-induced release of lactate dehydrogenase (Tse, Dolly and Diniz, 1980) and choline (Table 1) was inhibited; in Ca^{2+}-free Sr^{2+} medium K^+-stimulated efflux of transmitters was observed, consistent with results of electrophysiological experiments (see below). Collectively, these results are consistent with the proposal that phospholipase activity of β-BuTX is at least partly responsible for its action on transmitter release from brain synaptosomes. However, purified bee venom phospholipase A_2, which is about 20 times more enzymatically active than β-BuTX, was nevertheless four times less effective in causing synaptosomal efflux of Glu. Furthermore, incubation of synaptosomes with 1μM β-BuTX for 20 min at 37°C did not produce observable ultrastructural changes (Tse, Dolly and Diniz, 1980). Much higher concentrations of toxin, however, are known to give rise to structural damage of synaptosomes (Sen, Grantham and Cooper, 1976).

EFFECTS OF β-BuTX ON CENTRAL SYNAPTIC TRANSMISSION

As β-BuTX increases the release of transmitters from rat cortex synaptosomes, it seemed worthwhile to investigate electrophysiologically the toxin's actions at a cortical synapse. The preparation used was the rat olfactory cortex slice; briefly, the reasons for selecting this were the ease of drug administration and ionic control, the capability of simultaneous pre- and post- synaptic measures and the probable involvement of the excitatory amino acids, Glu and aspartate, as neurotransmitters at the synapse studied (Harvey and others, 1975; Bradford and Richards, 1976; Collins, 1979a).

Slices were cut from rat brain, with a bow-cutter and guide, to a thickness of ca 400 μm (McIlwain and Rodnight, 1962) and comprised the outer layers of the piriform cortex down to and including the sheet of cortical cells. Running across the surface of such a slice is the major afferent input to the piriform area, the lateral olfactory tract (LOT), fibres of which spread out and make synaptic contact in the most superficial layer with the distal dendritic portions of underlying cortical neurons (Price, 1973) (Fig. 3A).

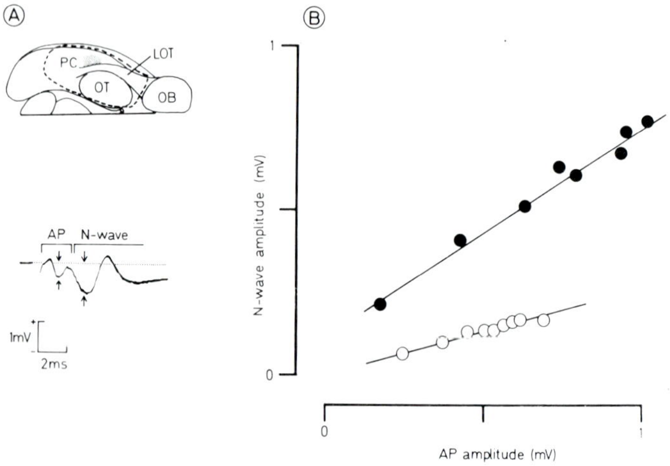

Figure 3. A diagram of the ventral view of the rat brain is given in A. The dotted line indicates the area removed when taking an olfactory cortex slice. The stippled region denotes the recording site typically used in the present experiments. Abbreviations used are: LOT; lateral olfactory tract; OB: olfactory bulb; OT: olfactory tubercle; PC: piriform cortex. Also in A is a typical evoked potential showing the presynaptic volley (AP) and the postsynaptic negative wave (N-wave) and the points of measurement. The positive deflection superimposed on the N-wave occurring at a latency of about 4 ms represents the synchronous discharge of many cortical cells to the excitatory input (Richards and Sercombe, 1968, Andersen, Bliss and Skrede, 1971). The linear relationship between the presynatic volley and postsynaptic response amplitudes determined in a typical experiment is shown in B. A range of stimuli from 100-500 μA, 100 μs pulse width were delivered to the LOT at 0.2 - 0.5 Hz; the amplitude of the AP is plotted (abscissa) against the height of the N-wave measured at a fixed latency before the N-wave peak (ordinate). Plots are given for responses in normal Krebs solution (filled circles) and in modified medium when 2.5 mM Ca^{2+} was replaced by 5 mM Sr^{2+} (open circles).

The slices were perfused in an incubation chamber at 28°C with a modified Krebs solution which had been pre-equilibrated with 95% O_2/5% CO_2. Conventional stimulating and recording techniques were used to investigate the electrophysiological properties of the slices. Unstimulated olfactory cortex slices are normally electrically silent; however, when brief (50 - 100 µs) electrical pulses above a threshold amplitude are delivered to the anterior end of the LOT, the earliest components of the surface wave-form evoked in the piriform cortex are (i) a di- or tri-phasic complex followed by (ii) a slower negative potential (N-wave) (See Fig.3A). These represent respectively the arrival of the LOT-fibre action potential volley and the extracellular current flow during the synaptic activation of the olfactory cortical neurons. Reasons for identifying these electrical responses with pre- and postsynaptic events include differential sensitivities of the two components to (amongst other things) stimulation frequency, anoxia, divalent cation concentration and barbiturate administration (Yamamoto & McIlwain, 1966; Richards & Sercombe, 1968; 1970; Richards, 1972; see Fig.3B and 4).

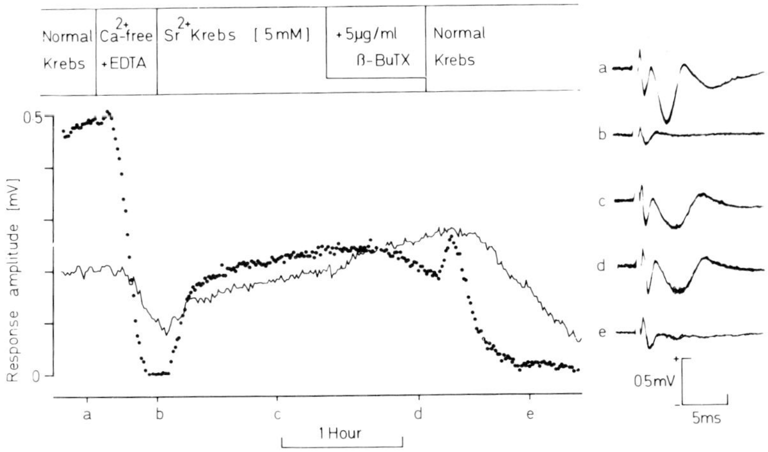

Fig.4. Effects of β-BuTX on neurotransmission in the absence of Ca^{2+}. Presynaptic (—) and postsynaptic responses (•) were measured as in Fig.3 during the indicated solution changes: 230 nM β-BuTX was administered when 2.5 mM Ca^{2+} in the bathing medium had been replaced by 5 mM Sr^{2+} after removing Ca^{2+} from the tissue with 50 µM EDTA. Responses a - e on the right were recorded at the times indicated on the abscissa.

Over a range of stimulus intensities between threshold and maximal the size of the postsynaptic response is linearly related to the amplitude of the presynaptic volley (Fig.3B). Changing the divalent cation content of the bathing medium alters the slope of the post:presynaptic response relationship but the latter remains linear. The size of the presynaptic volley indicates the number of LOT fibres being excited by the electrical stimulus; the postsynaptic response amplitude, being related to the synaptic currents flowing in the population of excited cortical neurons, is a measure of the effectiveness of the transmitter released; hence the post:presynaptic ratio may be regarded as a measure of relative synaptic efficiency. β-BuTX abolished electrical activity evoked in slices by stimulation of the LOT; the initial effects of the toxin normally resulted in a monotonic decline in the N-wave after a latent period of 5 - 10 min, although on three out of twelve occasions a clear potentiation of the N-wave preceded the depression. The LOT action potential also decreased after exposure to β-BuTX but with a slower time-course than that of the postsynaptic component. In accord with the action of the toxin at the neuromuscular junction,continuous perfusion was not necessary to produce blockade and typically, exposure to 230 nM β-BuTX for 20 min was sufficient to abolish electrical activity completely within 90 min. No recovery of either pre-or postsynaptic components was observed after washing the tissue for up to 18 h after the toxin application; in contrast a control slice which had not been exposed to β-BuTX displayed widespread synaptic activity at a comparable time (ca 24 h) after cutting. The rate of synaptic blockade was dose dependant between 46 and 460 nM as was the rate of the action potential decline, but the half-time of the latter was 2 - 3 times longer than that for the synaptic response. Replacement of Ca^{2+} in the bathing medium with 5 mM Sr^{2+} sustains synaptic transmission at a reduced level (Figs. 3B and 4) and prevents the phospholipase A_2 activity of the toxin (see above). β-BuTX (230 nM) was much less effective in Sr^{2+} -medium; the half-time for N-wave depression was prolonged from 27-43 min (n = 4) to more than 60 min (range: 60 - 110 min; n = 4) with no depressive effect on the LOT action potential. Restoration of Ca^{2+} to the medium produced a transient recovery of the synaptic response followed by its rapid decline which was accompanied by a slower decline in the presynaptic action potential (Fig.4). A similar effect of restoring Ca^{2+} was observed when the tissue was washed with toxin-free Sr^{2+} -medium for 20 min prior to Ca^{2+} replacement. The effects of Sr^{2+} -containing medium alone on the evoked responses were reversible. As the abolition of its enzyme activity reduced the neurotoxicity of β-BuTX at the central synapse, the effectiveness of two pure phospholipases(PLA_2) were assessed. Bee venom PLA_2, at a concentration (10 nM) showing equivalent enzyme activity to 230 nM β-BuTX, was ineffective and even at a concentration of 500 nM was less potent than the toxin in depressing synaptic transmission.

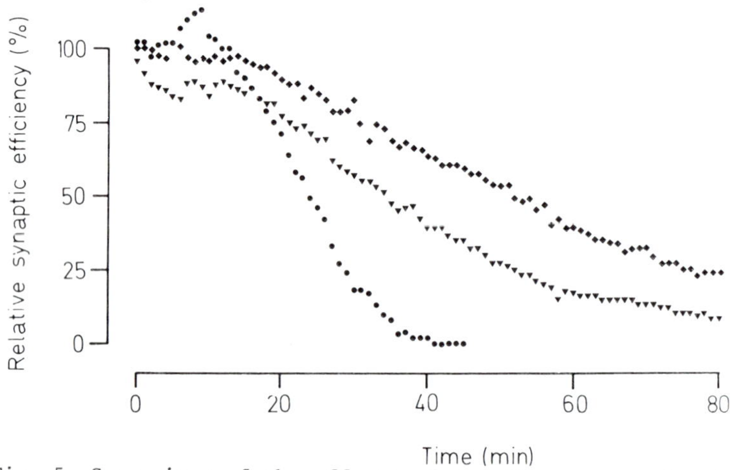

Fig. 5. Comparison of the effects of β-BuTX and pure phospholipases A_2 on central neurotransmission. The graphs show the effect of 230 nM β-BuTX (●), 500 nM bee venom PLA_2 (▼) and 500 nM Naja melanoleuca PLA_2 (◆) on synaptic efficiency. The latter was determined as the ratio of post:presynaptic response amplitudes measured as in previous figures and is the slope of the function plotted in Fig.3; it is expressed as a percentage of the average pre-toxin response ratio. The 95% confidence limits for the average are 97 - 103%. β-BuTX and PLA_2 from bee venom and Naja melanoleuca were applied to the tissue at time zero and removed at 20 min, 50 min and 70 min, respectively.

PLA_2 from venom of Naja melanoleuca,which was ineffective at 50 nM,depressed synaptic transmission at 500 nM but with lower potency than the bee enzyme; the specific activity of the snake PLA_2 was about 10-fold greater than that of β-BuTX. In contrast to β-BuTX, the two enzymes had no depressive effects on the presynaptic action potential: in fact, 500 nM bee venom PLA2 produced a sustained

48% increase in this measure (cf Abe & Miledi ,1978).

These results demonstrate that β-BuTX exerts an action at an intact synapse in the central nervous system. Demonstrations of the toxin's electrophysiological action have hitherto been confined to preparations of the peripheral nervous system; presynaptic blockade at the vertebrate neuromuscular junction (discussed above),at nicotinic synapses in autonomic ganglia (Kato and others, 1977; D.A. Brown, S.J.Marsh, J.O.Dolly & J.V. Halliwell, unpublished observations) but not at muscarinic or noradrenergic autonomic effectors (Kato and others, 1977) nor at the glutamatergic myoneural junction of the locust (Tse, Dolly and Diniz, 1980), suggests a specificity of the toxin for non-central sites where ACh mediates nicotinic effects. In contrast, effects of β-BuTX on rat cortex synaptosomes appear to lack neurotransmitter specificity (see above; also Sen, Grantham and Cooper, 1976; Wernicke, Vanker and Howard, 1975). The electrophysiological findings agree with these latter observations in that LOT terminals probably release Glu and/or aspartate (discussed above). β-BuTX affected both pre- and postsynaptic responses. However, the postsynaptic response was more sensitive to the toxin than was the presynaptic volley; thus the ratio of post: presynaptic responses declined after the administration of β-BuTX, suggesting that, initially, the efficiency of transmission across the synapse was impaired and that block of conduction in the LOT fibres was not solely responsible for the observed reduction in postsynaptic activity. Failure of action potentials to invade the actual terminal regions of the LOT fibres remains a possibility which cannot be entirely excluded as an initial mode of toxin action but this appears unlikely since conduction along unmyelinated vagal C-fibres is not affected by β-BuTX (S.J.Marsh, unpublished observations). Ultimately though, block of the LOT compound action potential was experienced following exposure to β- BuTX. A possible explanation for this particular susceptibility may lie in the presence of terminal boutons and short branches along the length of the LOT fibres (Westrum,1969; Stevens, 1969); by presenting many sites at which the toxin might act, LOT fibres could possess a vulnerability not shared by the C-fibres. This is consistent with the observation of Abe, Limbrick and Miledi (1976) that β-BuTX causes rapid withdrawal and degeneration of the motor nerve terminal. Chronic neurotoxic effects of β-BuTX , not confined to presynaptic structures, have recently been demonstrated in the mammalian central nervous system (Hanley & Emson, 1979) following discrete injections of toxin that could produce local concentrations comparable with those used in the present study.

By themselves, the present data do not allow the distinction to be drawn between pre- or postsynaptic effects as the cause of the reduced synaptic efficacy. However, preliminary experiments have shown that depolarisations recorded intracellularly in olfactory cortical neurons in vitro in response to bath applied Glu and aspartate are unimpaired at a time when a prior exposure to β-BuTX has abolished any trans-synaptic activity (J.V. Halliwell & C.N.Scholfield, unpublished observations); β-BuTX, therefore, appears not to cause a postsynaptic blockade of Glu or aspartate receptors. In all probability the initial toxic effects on synaptic efficacy described above reflect an alteration of the release process as has been demonstrated in the periphery (Kato and others, 1977). Our most common finding was that β-BuTX produced a simple and rapid decline in neurotransmission, although on occasion a clear potentiation of synaptic efficiency was observed (Fig. 5). Thus, it is not obvious whether the peripheral triphasic response to toxin has an easily distinguishable central analogue. Administration of β-BuTX in Ca^{2+} -free medium markedly attenuated the blockade exerted by the toxin; a slow decline in the postsynaptic measure alone was observed in Sr^{2+} -medium. A low level of Ca^{2+} -dependent PLA_2 activity may have been responsible for this but it seems unlikely since Ca^{2+} -removal in these experiments was to a very low level (as evidenced by conduction failure in the LOT fibres: Frankenhaeuser & Hodgkin, 1957) and, in addition, any remaining Ca^{2+} would be antagonised by the excess of Sr^{2+}. The Sr^{2+} -resistant slow synaptic depression may be akin to the first phase of the peripheral response, although the experiments in Sr^{2+} -medium were not continued long enough to determine whether this effect was similar to the partial neuromuscular blockade in Sr^{2+} -medium described by Abe and Miledi (1978) or the transient blockade by enzymically-inactive toxin (Abe and others, 1977). However, in our present study the rapid decline in electrical activity on return to Ca^{2+} -containing medium, after toxin exposure and subsequent wash-out in Sr^{2+} -solution, suggests that irreversible β-BuTX binding takes place in the absence of Ca^{2+}. In view of this, Sr^{2+} -medium would not be predicted to protect the slice preparation from ultimate irreversible blockade. Further experiments are required to examine this hypothesis. Nevertheless, the correlation between PLA_2 activity of the toxin and the different rates of synaptic blockade described above, suggests that its enzymic actions are important for the expression of all the toxic effects of β-BuTX in the central nervous system.

The Ca^{2+} -dependent rapid decline of the postsynaptic activity reported here probably represents a state analagous to the third phase of toxin's action at the neuromuscular junction. The enhanced release of putative transmitters from rat brain synaptosomes by β-BuTX, a PLA_2 -dependent effect, has been equated with the second phase of its action in the periphery. In contrast with these results, marked increases in postsynaptic activity or synaptic efficacy in the slices were not regularly (but see Fig.5) observed sequelae to β-BuTX administration. The reasons for this remain obscure but the fact that responses are averaged over many synaptic loci, offering different degrees of accessibility to toxin, may be a partial answer. While β-BuTX appears to require PLA_2 activity for the expression of its rapid action, it is far more effective in depressing evoked activity in the slices than pure PLA_2 from other sources (Fig.5). Hanley and Emson (1979) have also found a differential toxicity when assessing neuronal damage following local injections of β-BuTX or PLA_2 into the central nervous system. A site on the β-BuTX molecule that binds specifically to presynaptic nerve terminals has been proposed (see Introduction) as a mechanism whereby the toxin's PLA_2 activity may be made more effective. The description above of β-BuTX action on conduction along presynaptic fibres, not shared by pure PLA_2's of much greater enzymic activity even when applied at high molar concentrations, suggests that the toxin exhibits a specificity which is not the property of pure PLA_2's This notion accords with the relative ineffectiveness of pure PLA_2's in releasing neurotransmitters from synaptosome preparations (see above).

β-BuTX, then, initially blocks neurotransmission in the olfactory cortex slice, probably primarily by affecting transmitter release, but eventually exerting a conduction block in the presynaptic LOT fibres. A rapid component of the toxin's effect on synaptic efficiency and the conduction block in presynaptic fibres may be abolished in Ca^{2+} -free medium, implying that both effects result from a PLA_2 activity. These actions have been likened to the third phase of β -BuTX effects at the vertebrate neuromuscular junction. It is concluded that the PLA_2 activity is an important factor in the toxic action of β-BuTX at this central synapse but even without enzymic activity the toxin depresses synaptic transmission; this appears to result from irreversible binding to an, as yet unidentified, site and could cause complete blockade if exposure were long enough. In comparison with the enzyme activity of pure PLA_2's β-BuTX appears inordinately toxic; it is concluded that the toxin possesses a specificity which is not the property of the pure phospholipases tested.

ACKNOWLEDGEMENTS

This work was supported by MRC and SRC. The authors thank C.K.Tse for valuable contributions and Dr.R.Shipolini for generous gifts of phospholipases A_2 purified from *Naja melanoleuca* and bee venom.

REFERENCES

Abe, T., S. Alema and R.Miledi (1977). *Eur.J.Biochem.*, *80*, 1-12.
Abe, T., A.R.Limbrick and R.Miledi (1976). *Proc.R.Soc.Lond.B.*, *194*, 545-553.
Abe, T. and R. Miledi (1978). *Proc.R.Soc.Lond.B.*, *200*, 225-230.
Andersen,P., T.V.P.Bliss and K.K.Skrede (1971) *Exp.Brain Res.*, *13*, 208-221.
Bradford, H. and C.D.Richards (1976). *Brain Res.*, *105*, 168-172.
Chang, C.C. (1979). In C.Y. Lee (Ed.), *Handbook of Experimental Pharmacology*, Vol. 52. Springer-Verlag, Berlin, Heidelberg, New York. Chap.10, pp.309-376.
Collins, C.G.S. (1979a). *J.Physiol.*, *291*, 51-60.
Collins, C.G.S. (1979b). *Brain Res.*, *171*, 552-555.
Dolly, J.O. (1979). In K.F.Tipton (Ed.), *International Review of Biochemistry*, Vol.26. University Park Press, Baltimore. Chap.6, pp.257-309.
Dolly, J.O., C.K.Tse, J.W.Spokes and C.R.Diniz (1978). *Biochem.Soc.Trans.*, *6*, 652-654.
Frankenhaeuser,B. and A.L.Hodgkin (1957). *J.Physiol.*, *137*, 218-244.
Hanley, M.R. and P.C.Emson (1979). *Neuroscience Letts.*, *11*, 143-148.
Hanley, M.R., V.A.Eterovic, S.P.Hawkes, A.J.Hebert and E.L.Bennett (1977). *Biochemistry*, *16*, 5840-5849.
Harvey, J.A., C.N.Scholfield, L.T.Graham, Jr. and M.M.Aprison (1975). *J. Neurochem.*, *24*, 445-449.
Kato, A.C., J.E.B.Pinto, M.Glavinovic and B.Collier (1977). *Can.J.Physiol. Pharmacol.*, *55*, 574-584.
Lee, C.Y., C.L.Ho and D.P.Botes (1979). *Toxicon*, *17*, suppl.No.1, 101.
MacDermot, J., R.H.Westgaard and E.J.Thompson (1978). *Biochem.J.*, *175*, 271-279.
McIlwain, H. and R.Rodnight (1962). *Practical Neurochemistry*. J.A.Churchill Ltd., London, pp.109-133.
Price, J.L. (1973). *J.Comp.Neurol.*, *150*, 87-108.
Richards, C.D. (1972). *J.Physiol.*, *227*, 749-767.
Richards, C.D. and R.Sercombe (1968). *J.Physiol.*, *197*, 667-683.
Richards, C.D. and R.Sercombe (1970). *J.Physiol.*, *211*, 571-584.
Sen, I., P.A.Grantham and J.R.Cooper (1976). *Proc.Natl.Acad.Sci. U.S.A.*, *73*, 2664-2668.
Spokes, J.W. and J.O.Dolly (1980). *Biochim.Biophys.Acta*, *596*, 81-93.
Stevens, C.F. (1969). *J.Neurophysiol.*, *32*, 184-192.
Strong, P.N., J.Goerke, S.G.Oberg and R.B.Kelly (1976). *Proc.Natl.Acad.Sci.U.S.A.* *73*, 178-182.
Strong, P.N., J.E.Heuser and R.B.Kelly (1977). In *Cellular Neurobiology*. A.R. Liss, Inc., New York. pp 227-249.
Tse, C.K., J.O.Dolly and C.R.Diniz (1980). *Neuroscience*, *5*, 135-143.
Wernicke, J.F., A.D.Vanker and B.D.Howard (1975). *J.Neurochem.*, *25*, 483-496.
Westrum, L.E. (1969). *Z.Zellforsch.*, *98*, 157-187.
Yamamoto, C. and H.McIlwain (1966). *J.Neurochem.*, *13*, 1333-1343.

BIOLOGICAL ACTIVITIES OF CROTOXIN AND AMINO ACID SEQUENCE OF CROTOXIN B

H. Fraenkel-Conrat*, T-W. Jeng* and M. Hsiang**

**Dept. of Molecular Biology*
***Dept. of Biochemistry, University of California, Berkeley, California 94720, USA*

ABSTRACT

The history of crotoxin research and theories about its mode of action are reviewed. Its biochemical properties, such as phospholipase activity, indirect hemolytic activity, binding to membranes, and toxicity resemble those of taipoxin more than those of β-bungarotoxin. On several grounds it is suggested that crotoxin has both pre- and post-synaptic action. The sequence of the 123 amino acids of crotoxin B is reported, further establishing that this protein of M.W. 14,350 belongs to the family of phospholipase A2 proteins.

KEYWORDS

Snake venom; neurotoxin; crotoxin; indirect hemolysis; amino acid sequence; membrane binding; phospholipase A2; presynaptic action; postsynaptic action; isotoxins.

PART I: BIOLOGICAL AND BIOCHEMICAL ACTIVITIES OF CROTOXIN AND ITS COMPONENTS

H. Fraenkel-Conrat and T-W. Jeng

The Brazilian rattlesnake, Crotalus durissus terrificus has the rare feature of producing a venom that contains a single very predominant active protein component which is a neurotoxin. This enabled Slotta and Fraenkel-Conrat to isolate and crystallize crotoxin in the early days of protein purification methodology (Slotta and Fraenkel-Conrat, 1938; Slotta and Fraenkel-Conrat, 1939). It was then noted that the neurotoxic principle was associated and purified together with the indirect hemolytic activity of that venom, and a functional interrelation between neurotoxicity and phospholipase action was suggested. Although crotoxin behaved as a homogeneous protein in the ultracentrifuge (Gralen and Svedberg, 1938), as well as in the Tiselius electrophoresis apparatus (Li and Fraenkel-Conrat, 1942), treatment with dinitrofluorobenzene yielded two DNP derivatives, one water-soluble and the other water-insoluble, which showed quite different amino acid compositions (Fraenkel-Conrat and Singer, 1956). Modification with less bulky acylating agents confirmed the presence of these two proteins (Hendon and co-workers, 1970) and indicated that for neurotoxicity the presence of both was required. Since one of these proteins was quite acidic (pI about 3.8) and the other basic (pI about 8.7) both types of ion exchange chromatography in the presence of 6 M urea became the methods of choice for the separation of these proteins (Hendon and Fraenkel-Conrat, 1971; Rübsamen and co-workers, 1971; Horst and co-workers, 1972).

Chemical and biological characterization of these two proteins was then taken up in several laboratories and our findings along those lines will now be reviewed. The basic component, crotoxin B, showed only about one-fortieth of the lethality of the complex (A+B), yet fully retained the indirect hemolytic activity of the complex. It also showed similar phospholipase A2 activity as the complex when tested on egg yolk or purified phospholipids. Attempts to replace A as an activator of the neurotoxicity by other poly-peptides showed partial positive effect with volvatoxin A2, one of the two neutral components of a mushroom synergistic cardiotoxin (Jeng and Fraenkel-Conrat, 1976).

All known phospholipases A2 that have been isolated from a great variety of species and organs show considerable similarities in size, high cystine content, and properties of the active center. Particularly, they all contain a single histidine that is very reactive towards p-bromophenacyl bromide, a reaction resulting in inactivation. Crotoxin B was found to share these properties, including the reactive and essential histidine. Interestingly, in the crotoxin complex that histidine is not reactive and no loss of any biological activity results from treatment of the complex with p-bromophenacyl bromide (Jeng and Fraenkel-Conrat, 1978). Ultracentrifugation studies (Paradies and Breithaupt, 1975) and spectroscopic studies (Hanley, 1979) came to the same conclusion that drastic conformational changes happened during complex formation.

Acylation of more than two and three amino groups progressively inactivates B and the complex, respectively, but of the three amino groups of A only one becomes acylated, and that without effect on its synergizing activity (Jeng and Fraenkel-Conrat, 1978).

The relatedness of crotoxin B to the phospholipases is borne out by its amino acid sequence which is reported as Part II of this paper.

As far as the mode of crotoxin's neurotoxicity is concerned, some of its properties suggests similarity to the classical prototype for presynaptic action, β-bungarotoxin, and various experiments were therefore carried out, comparing these two neurotoxins with one another as well as with taipoxin and with the non-neurotoxic phospholipase A2 of *Crotalus adamanteus*.

The results, some of which are illustrated by a few examples in Table I and summarized in Table II, may be summarized as follows:

1. Crotoxin at high dosages kills mice slower than a typical postsynaptic neurotoxin, α-bungarotoxin, but faster than β-bungarotoxin (Hendon and Fraenkel-Conrat, 1976).

2. Taipoxin is considerably more lethal than β-bungarotoxin which is slightly more so than crotoxin.

3. Taipoxin hemolyses indirectly at much lower concentrations than crotoxin, but β-bungarotoxin lacks this activity, being less active even than *C. adamanteus* phospholipase.

4. Phospholipase activity in the absence of detergents is very high for the *C. adamanteus* enzyme, similarly lower for crotoxin and taipoxin, and almost nil for β-bungarotoxin.

5. Crotoxin B is bound nonspecifically and in non-saturable manner by erythrocytes and ghosts, with release of A if the complex is used; β-bungarotoxin is bound very much less and the *C. adamanteus* enzyme not at all (Jeng and co-workers, 1978).

6. Collaborative studies with Drs. Bon and Changeux (Bon and co-workers, 1979) have demonstrated conditions for saturable binding of crotoxin B to receptor-rich membranes from *Torpedo marmorata*, again releasing A, and being of the same order but not competitive with α-bungarotoxin binding.

Footnote to Fig. 1

*Peptides resulting from cyanogen bromide cleavage are designated as CN-1, CN-2 and CN-3. Not all the thermolytic peptides (Th) or N-bromosuccinimide peptides (NBS) are purified to homogeneity.

→ : Manual Edman degradation and dansyl chloride method.

⇀ : Automatic Edman degradation in sequencer; PTH-amino acid identified by GC or amino acid analyzed after HI hydrolysis.

⇢ : Ambiguity in the identity of the residue. Peptide CN-2 was specifically cleaved at tryptophan by a mixture of cyanogen bromide and heptafluorobutyric acid (CN-HFBA). The resulting mixture of four peptides was sequenced without further separation. Since the sequences of three of the four peptides are known and the first thirteen residues of the fourth peptide are also known the sequence of the fourth peptide from residue number 14 to 24 was deduced. The results from the first 13 Edman degradations also served to confirm the previously determined sequences. The data concerning the order of residues 50 and 51 are ambiguous, and we have chosen the one that is in agreement with other phospholipases.

of the octapeptide was determined by the Edman degradation-dansyl chloride method (Gray, 1972) and confirmed to be his-leu-leu-gln-phe-asn-lys-met. The isotoxins of crotoxin B (Hendon and co-workers, 1970; Breithaupt and co-workers, 1975) were not separated before sequence analysis and this probably accounts for the presence of two N-terminal amino acids in this octapeptide, showing a histidine to serine molar ratio of 3:1.

After reduction and carboxymethylation of the cyanogen bromide cleaved large fragments of crotoxin B, an oligopeptide containing 14 amino acids and shown to be from the C terminus of the molecule was separated from the large polypeptide chain. The sequence of this oligopeptide was determined by the Edman degradation method as phe-tyr-pro-asp-ser-arg-cys-arg-gly-pro-ser-glu-thr-cys, confirming the sequence reported by Omori-Satoh and co-workers (1975).

The large polypeptide chain with 101 amino acids and homoserine as C terminal obtained as described above, was then further fragmented by thermolysin digestion and also by N-bromosuccinimide cleavage. The peptides obtained were separated by DEAE-cellulose column chromatography in 0.1 M Tris-HCl (pH 6.0) with 8 M deionized urea, followed by Sephadex G-25 (fine) column filtration to remove urea and salt; the peptides were then sized by Sephadex G-50 (fine) gel filtration in 10% formic acid. When needed, peptides were further purified by high-voltage paper electrophoresis in pyridine acetate buffer (pH 3.5) and by paper chromatography with the n-butanol-pyridine-acetic acid-water (v/v 15:10:3:13) system. The purified peptides were sequenced with a Beckman automatic sequencer 890-C and the Beckman DMAA peptide program. The PTH-amino acid released was quantitatively identified by gas-liquid chromatography on a Varian gas chromatograph 1840A, and by amino acid analysis (Smithies and co-workers, 1971). The aligned sequence was further checked by direct sequencing of the large polypeptide as described above for the first 50 residues, and also by analyzing the amino acid composition of purified tryptic peptides obtained from carboxymethylated crotoxin B. The sequence of crotoxin B thus established is presented in Fig. 1 with major overlapping peptides indicated. Isotoxin variants of valine to isoleucine at position 18, leucine to tyrosine at position 27 and glutamic acid to glycine at position 107 are also noted.

On Fig. 2 we compare the amino acid sequence of crotoxin B with one of the typical presynaptic neurotoxic phospholipase A2 sequences, the larger of the two polypeptide chains of β-bungarotoxin (Kondo and co-workers, 1978), and with the sequence

Fig. 2. Comparison of amino acid sequences of three phospholipase A2-active proteins

	5 10 15 20 25 30
Crotoxin B:	H L L Q F N K M I K F Z T R - K B A I P F Y A F Y G C Y C G
β-Bungarotoxin:	N L I N F M E M I R Y T I P C E K T W G E Y A D Y G C Y C G
Porcine pancreatic phospholipase A2:	A L W Q F R S M I K C A I P G S H P L M D F N N Y G C Y C G

	35 40 45 50 55 60
Crotoxin B:	W G G Z G R P K B A T B R C C F V H B C C Y G K L A K C B T
β-Bungarotoxin:	A G G S G R P I D A L D R C C Y V H D N C Y G D A E K K H K
Porcine pancreatic phospholipase A2:	L G G S G T P V D E L D R C C E T H D N C Y R D A K N L D S

	65 70 75 80 85 90
Crotoxin B:	K Y W B I Y R - Y S - - L K - S G Y - - - I T C - G K - G T
β-Bungarotoxin:	C N P K T S Q - Y S - - Y K L - - T K R T I I C Y G A A G G
Porcine pancreatic phospholipase A2:	C K F L V D N P Y T E S Y S Y S C S N T E I T C N S K N N A

	95 100 105 110 115 120
Crotoxin B:	W C Z Z Z I C Z C B R V A A Z C L R R B L S T Y K B G Y M F
β-Bungarotoxin:	T C - R I V C D C D R T A A L C F G Q S D Y I E E H K N I D
Porcine pancreatic phospholipase A2:	- C E A F I C N C D R N A A I C F S K A P Y N K E H K N L D

	125 130
Crotoxin B:	Y P D S R C R G P S E T C
β-Bungarotoxin:	T A R F - C Q
Porcine pancreatic phospholipase A2:	T K K Y - C

of the non-toxic phospholipase A2 of porcine pancreas (Puyk and co-workers, 1977). Considerable homology among these is obvious in the N-terminal 40%, as well as from residues 97 to 106. Most of the half-cystine residues can be aligned (11 out of 14) assuming a small number of deletions and insertions, as well as the essential histidine residue at position 48 (homology numbering). The most variable part is located in the middle of the sequence and would be on the surface of the molecule based on the X-ray model of the bovine pancreatic phospholipase A2 presented by Dijkstra and co-workers (1978). However, whether this stretch actually represents a binding domain for crotoxin B to crotoxin A awaits further investigation.

ACKNOWLEDGEMENT

This work was supported NIH research grant No. ES 00 700 from the National Institute of Environmental Health Sciences.

REFERENCES

Bon, C., J.-P. Changeux, T.-W. Jeng. and H. Fraenkel-Conrat (1979). Eur. J. Biochem., 99, 471.
Breithaupt, H., T. Omori-Satoh and J. Lang (1975). Biochim. Biophys. Acta, 403, 355.
Chang, C., and J. Lee (1977). Naunyn-Schmiedeberg's Arch. Pharmacol. 296, 159.
Dijkstra, B. W., J. Drenth. K. H. Kalk, and P. J. Vandermaelen (1978) J. Mol. Biol. 124, 53.
Fraenkel-Conrat, H., and B. Singer (1956). Arch. Biochem. Biophys., 60, 64.
Gralén, N., and T. Svedberg (1938). Biochem. J., 32, 1375.
Gray, W. R. (1972). Methods Enzymol. 25, 333.
Hanley, M. R. (1979). Biochemistry, 18, 1681.
Hawgood, B. J., and J. W. Smith (1977). Brit. J. Pharmacol., 61, 597.
Hendon, R., D. Roy, and H. Fraenkel-Conrat (1979). Toxicon, 8, 135.
Hendon, R., and H. Fraenkel-Conrat (1971). Proc. Natl. Acad. Sci. USA, 68, 1560.
Hendon. R., and H. Fraenkel-Conrat (1976). Toxicon, 14, 283.
Horst, J., R. A. Hendon, and H. Fraenkel-Conrat (1972). Biochem. Biophys. Res. Commun., 46, 1042.
Jeng, T.-W., and H. Fraenkel-Conrat (1976). Biochem. Biophys. Res. Commun., 70, 1324.
Jeng, T.-W., and H. Fraenkel-Conrat (1978). FEBS Lett., 87, 291.
Jeng, T.-W., R. A. Hendon, and H. Fraenkel-Conrat (1978). Proc. Natl. Acad. Sci. USA, 75, 600.
Kondo, K., K. Narita, and C.-Y. Lee (1978). J. Biochem., 83, 91.
Li. C.-H., and H. Fraenkel-Conrat (1942). J. Am. Chem. Soc. , 64, 1586.
Omori-Satoh, T., J. Lang, H. Breithaupt, and E. Habermann (1975). Toxicon, 13, 69.
Paradies, H. H., and H. Breithaupt (1975). Biochem. Biophys. Res. Commun., 66, 496.
Puijk, W.C., H.M. Verheij, and G. H. de Haas (1977). Biochim. Biophys. Acta, 492, 254.
Rübsamen, K., H. Breithaupt, and E. Habermann (1971). Naunyn-Schmiedeberg's Arch. Pharmacol., 270, 274.
Slotta, K. H., and H. Fraenkel-Conrat (1938). Nature, 142, 213.
Slotta, K. H., and H. Fraenkel-Conrat (1939). Nature, 144, 290.
Smithies, O., D. Gibson, E. M. Fanning, R. M. Goodfliesch, J. G. Gilman, and D. L. Ballantyne (1971). Biochemistry, 10, 4912.

MUSCLE NECROSIS INDUCED BY SOME PRESYNAPTICALLY ACTIVE NEUROTOXINS

J. B. Harris, M. A. Johnson and C. A. MacDonell

Muscular Dystrophy Group Laboratories, Regional Neurological Centre, Newcastle General Hospital, Newcastle upon Tyne, UK

ABSTRACT

In this brief review the myotoxic activity of a few snake-venom toxins is discussed. The discussion is limited to those toxins which are normally classified as presynaptically active neurotoxins. Particular attention is paid to the characteristics of the damage caused to the muscle and to its ultimate regeneration.

KEYWORDS

Muscle necrosis; myotoxicity; necrotising myopathy; neurotoxins; neurotoxicity.

TOXINS DISCUSSED

This review is primarily concerned with the toxins notexin and notechis II-5 from the venom of the Australian tiger snake Notechis scutatus, taipoxin from the venom of the Australian taipan Oxyuranus scutellatus, and B-bungarotoxin from the venom of the banded krait Bungarus multicinctus. The toxin crotoxin from the venom of the South American rattlesnake Crotalus durrissus terrificus and the myotoxic toxin from the sea snake Enhydrina schistosa are mentioned briefly.

THE ADMINISTRATION OF TOXIN

Although muscle necrosis may be seen following the intravenous injection of some toxins, it is the practice of this laboratory to use the subcutaneous route of injection, such that the underlying muscle is exposed to the toxin, but not physically damaged by the insertion of the hypodermic needle. Provided little or no evidence of systemic poisoning is seen, the muscle(s) from the contralateral limb may be used as controls. The subcutaneous route of injection probably resembles most closely the injection of venom into the victim following a bite by the elapidae, most of which carry short, fixed fangs.

WHICH TOXINS ARE MYOTOXIC?

Of the toxins with demonstrable neurotoxicity, notexin, notechis II-5, taipoxin and crotoxin have well documented myotoxic properties (Harris, Johnson and Karlsson, 1975; Harris, Johnson and MacDonell, 1977; Harris and Johnson, 1978; Gopalakrishnakone and Hawgood, 1979). B-bungarotoxin, probably the most widely studied of the presynaptically active neurotoxins from snake venom, does not appear to be myotoxic in rats even at doses exceeding the LD_{50}. Some toxins, such as fraction VI from the venom of the sea snake Enhydrina schistosa which is certainly myotoxic in mice and guinea pigs (Fohlman and Eaker, 1977; Geh and Toh, 1978), may only be slightly neurotoxic. It should be noted, however, that this list is almost certainly incomplete, and also that preparing a ranking order to compare the myotoxicity of the various toxins is, for several reasons, very difficult. For example, in this laboratory we concentrate on the effects of subcutaneous injections of toxins into rats. Fohlman and Eaker (1977) and Gopalakrishnakone and Hawgood (1979) administer the toxins to mice by intravenous injection and Geh and Toh (1978) to guinea-pigs by intraperitoneal injection. The use of the intravenous route for the administration of fairly high doses of notexin (Harris, Karlsson and Thesleff, 1973) and taipoxin (Kamenskaya and Thesleff, 1974) led to the identification of neurotoxicity in these toxins but not of myotoxicity; clearly both the dose and the route of administration of toxin is of importance. Furthermore little is known about possible species variability in response to the toxins. This may be important since although Fohlman and Eaker (1977) characterise the myotoxin from Enhydrina schistosa as being strongly myotoxic in mice, experiments utilising rats suggested that it was 20-40x less potent on a weight for weight basis than notexin (Harris unpublished). If species differences do exist, then the suggestion that β-bungarotoxin, for example, is not myotoxic may need some qualification.

Not all of the toxins have been studied for their possible myotoxic effects on isolated muscle, but it is now known that notexin, originally considered to be virtually inactive in vitro (see Harris, Johnson and Karlsson, 1975), is capable of causing damage to adult rat muscle maintained in a suitable medium (Harris and MacDonell, unpublished observation) and Hawgood and Smith (1977) have come to the same conclusions regarding crotoxin. However, it is necessary to use large doses of the toxins and/or to allow contact with the muscles for prolonged periods (that is, 1-6 hrs).

THE INDUCTION AND CHARACTERISTICS OF NECROSIS

The first signs of necrosis are the pale and oedematous appearance of the skeletal muscle. This is evident within 3 hrs of the injection of either notexin (2.0 µg) notechis II-5 (2.0 µg) or taipoxin (2.0 µg). The wet weight of the injected muscle is increased, reaching a peak at about 12 hrs when the injected muscle may weigh almost twice the unaffected contralateral muscle. Some typical data are illustrated in fig. 1. From 12 hrs the wet weight of the injected muscle begins to decline, and maximum loss of muscle weight is usually seen during the period 3-5 days post injection (Pluskal and colleagues, 1978). During this time, the loss in weight of the muscle closely parallels the loss of non-collagen protein (Pluskal and colleagues, 1978). Serum creatine kinase levels are elevated within 6 hrs after the administration of notexin (Pluskal and colleagues, 1978).

Morphological changes in the muscle may be seen as early as 1-3 hrs after the administration of the myotoxic toxins. The appearance of the muscle at this stage (fig. 2) typically includes the oedematous separation of floccular and hypercontracted muscle fibres and the extensive infiltration of the perivascular spaces by phagocytic cells of various types. By 6 hrs most necrotic fibres are invaded by phagocytic cells and by 24 hrs there is a clear distinction between the damaged areas and the undamaged areas of muscle. Muscle degeneration is complete by 2-3 days, and regeneration may have started by 3 days (Harris, Johnson and Karlsson, 1975). By 7 days, numerous small regenerating fibres may be recognised in the skeletal muscle, and these appear to become fully mature by 21 days (see Harris,

Johnson and Karlsson, 1975 for details).

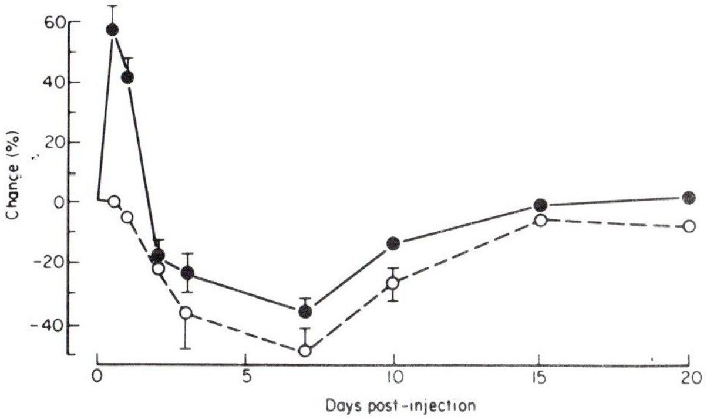

Fig. 1. Changes in the wet weight (solid points) and non-collagen protein (open points) of rat EDL muscles at various times after the injection of notexin (2.0 μg). Each point expresses then mean change (± s.e.m.) of 6 injected muscles relative to the controls (from Pluskal and colleagues, 1978; reproduced with the permission of the publishers).

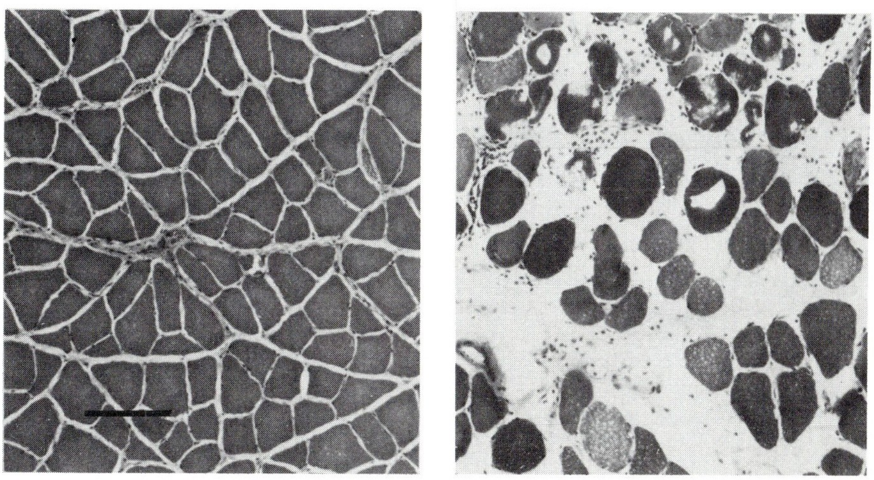

Fig. 2. Control (left) and damaged (right) soleus muscles of the rat, 6 hrs after injection of taipoxin (2.0 μg) into one hind limb. Calibration bar: 100 μ; frozen sections; H & E.

The underlying features of the process of degeneration may be followed using electron microscopy. Within 1–3 hrs, lesions in the plasma membrane are readily identified. At the same time, many fibres exhibit hypercontraction (fig. 3) of the myofilaments and (rather uncommonly) disorganization of the sarcomeres. By 3–6 hours the necrotic fibres are invaded by a variety of phagocytic cells and the muscle fibre cytoplasm develops an amorphous appearance (fig. 4). The basal lamina appears to be undamaged by the myotoxic toxins, although as a result of the demise of the necrotic fibre, the membrane routinely takes on a ruffled appearance (fig. 4).

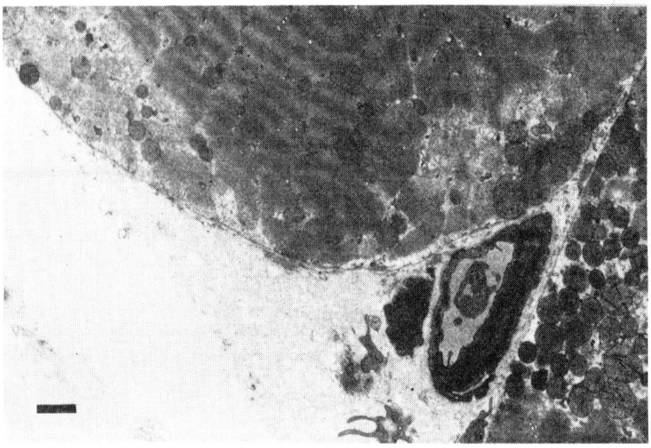

Fig. 3 Hypercontraction of filaments in rat soleus muscle fibre 1 hr after injection of taipoxin (2.0 μg). Calibration bar: 1 μ

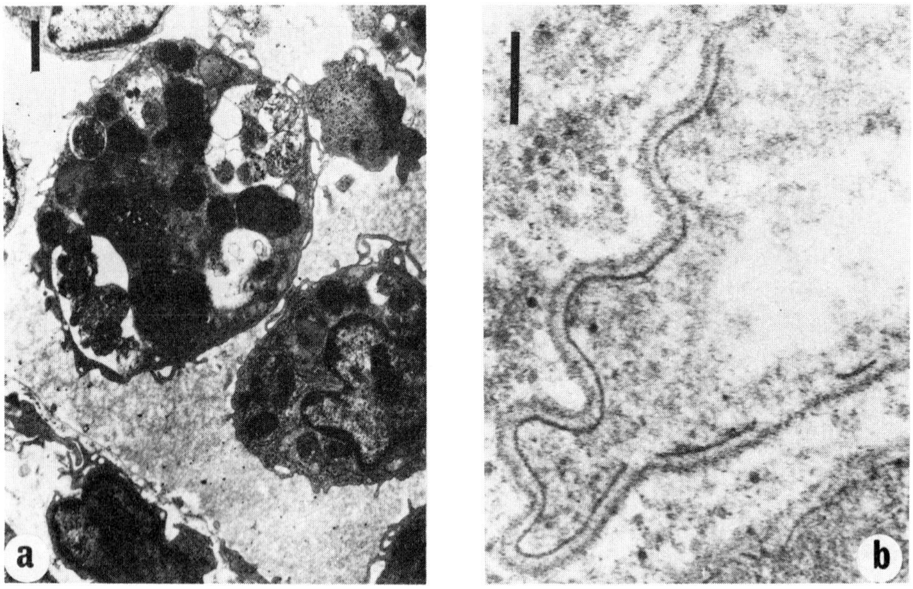

Fig. 4(a). Invasion of necrotic rat soleus muscle fibre by phagocytic cells 3 hrs after injection of taipoxin (2.0 μg). Calibration bar: 1 μ. (b) Portion of collapsed, necrotic soleus muscle fibre, 3 hrs after injection of taipoxin (2.0 μg). Note the intact but folded basal lamina, and the broken plasma membrane. Calibration bar: 1 μ.

The onset of necrosis in the skeletal muscle is accompanied by a rapid and precipitous loss of resting membrane potential in the damaged fibres. For example, in rat soleus muscles damaged by notexin, the mean resting membrane potential falls from a control level of −77.6 mV ± s.e.m. 0.46 (n = 90) to −27.8 mV ± 3.89 (n = 50) at 1 hr and −4.9 mV ± 0.38 (n = 93) at 6 hrs. The muscles are, of course, quite inexcitable at this stage.

During the early stages of necrosis, the activity of the 'lysosomal enzymes' Cathepsin B_1 and Acid proteinase, increases. It seems most probable that the enzymes are located within the invading cells rather than in the muscle fibres themselves (Pluskal and colleagues, 1978) and are involved in the digestion of the debris accumulated by the phagocytic cells.

MUSCLE STRUCTURES RESISTANT TO THE TOXINS

The distribution of damaged and undamaged fibres in muscles exposed to the toxins varies according to the type of muscle under examination. In soleus, which in the rat consists almost exclusively of Type I (slow oxidative), Type IIa (fast oxidative/glycolytic) and 'intermediate' (Type IIc) fibres, there is a sharp dividing line between the cuff of damaged fibres and the deeper undamaged fibres. In the case of extensor digitorum longus (EDL) which is a true 'mixed' muscle consisting of Type I, IIa and IIb (fast glycolytic) fibres, the toxins leave undamaged the latter, fast glycolytic fibres resulting in a 'chequerboard' of damaged and undamaged fibres.

Also resistant to the toxins is immature muscle growing either in tissue culture or developing in vivo (MacDonell, unpublished), muscle spindles and blood vessels (Harris and Johnson, 1978) and the satellite cells (MacDonell, 1979).

It is not clear why such structures should be resistant. On teleological grounds one may argue that immature muscle, blood vessels and probably satellite cells are resistant because such an arrangement might be expected to be beneficial to a tissue that is attempting to regenerate. Whatever the consequences of resistance however, it seems not unreasonable to suggest that the resistant structures are lacking either a suitable binding site or a relevant substrate for interaction with the toxins.

It should be noted that the nerve terminals are not spared the actions of the toxins. MacDonell (1979) has clear evidence that nerve terminals are damaged by taipoxin for example, and that such damage extends for several nodes. However, functional reinnervation of the regenerating muscle occurs between 3–5 days post-injection, thus allowing the muscle to differentiate normally during the process of regeneration.

THE RELATIONSHIP BETWEEN NEUROTOXICITY AND MYOTOXICITY

Since the toxins notexin, taipoxin and β-bungarotoxin are usually considered to be good examples of presynaptically active neurotoxins, it is relevant to ask whether or not the muscle damage caused by some of the toxins might be causally related to neurotoxicity. The question is particularly important when it is considered that immature muscle growing in vitro in tissue culture is devoid of any form of innervation and is also resistant to both notexin and taipoxin. However, several experiments and observations make it unlikely that myotoxicity is either directly or indirectly the result of neural damage. The evidence is enumerated below.

1) Acutely denervated muscle (i.e. muscle surgically denervated immediately prior to toxin administration) is damaged by the toxins to the same degree as related normal muscles (Harris, Johnson and Karlsson, 1975). From this it might be inferred that neurally mediated electrical and mechanical activity in the muscle is not

relevant to the development of myotoxicity.

2) Chronically denervated muscle (surgically denervated 10 days before toxin administration) is susceptible to the myotoxic toxins (Harris and MacDonell, unpublished observation). Since it is known that the nerve terminals in soleus muscle are totally lost by 24 hrs following axotomy (Slater, C.R., personal communication to J.B. Harris), it is inconceivable that myotoxicity in this case is causally related to neurotoxicity.

3) At the interface between those soleus muscle fibres damaged by the toxins and those fibres undamaged by the toxins it is not uncommon to find muscle fibres that are, according to ultrastructural criteria, completely spared the effects of the toxins, but in which the nerve terminals have been totally destroyed (fig. 5).

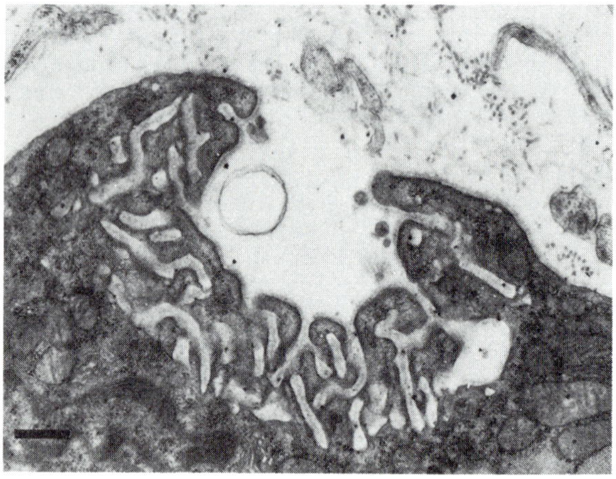

Fig. 5. End-plate region of a rat soleus muscle fibre 24 hrs after the injection of taipoxin (2.0 μg). Note the loss of the nerve terminal but preservation of both sub-synaptic region of the end-plate, and the intracellular organisation of the muscle fibre. Calibration bar: 1 μ.

4) Although β-bungarotoxin is a potent neurotoxin, capable of destroying nerve terminals in frog and rat nerve-muscle junctions (Abe, Limbrick and Miledi, 1976), the toxin is either devoid of myotoxicity or has very low levels of such activity.

None of the evidence presented above would be considered definitive in its own right, but taken en masse, it seems difficult to believe that myotoxicity merely reflects some aspects of neurotoxicity.

INTERACTIONS BETWEEN THE MYOTOXIC NEUROTOXINS AND THE TOXIN SUBUNITS

There are few data presently available on the interactions between the various myotoxic toxins, and those that are available are incomplete and involve only notexin and taipoxin and its subunits. Of the 3 subunits of taipoxin, only the basic α-subunit is myotoxic in its own right, neither the acidic γ- nor the neutral β-subunits exhibiting any significant activity at all. Moreover, the activity of the α-subunit appears to be only 1/10th as active in isolation as it is when present in the entire complex (taipoxin). Recombination experiments have shown that $\alpha+\beta$ and $\beta+\gamma$ are inactive, but that the recombination of $\alpha+\gamma$ results in the full expression of activity. In view of this, and of the close chemical similarity between α-taipoxin and notexin (see Eaker, this volume) it was of interest to note that a low, marginally active dose of notexin could not be rendered 'fully' active by combination with γ-taipoxin.

PROTECTION AGAINST MYOTOXICITY

A variety of drugs has been used in an attempt to control the muscle necrosis that follows the injection of notexin and taipoxin. The list includes anti-inflammatories of various types, cytotoxic drugs and the mast cell degranulator 48/80 (see table 1). Although some drugs - notably the cytotoxic drugs - prevented the elevation of the enzymes Cathepsin B_1 and Acid proteinase, none of the drugs had any effect on the development of necrosis. Neither was necrosis prevented by the

TABLE 1 Drugs used to Modify Action of Notexin and Taipoxin

Drug	Classification	Dose Schedule
Mepyramine	Anti-histamine	5 mg/kg i.p. daily
Hydrocortisone	Anti-inflammatory	50 mg/kg s.c. daily*
Indomethacin	Anti-inflammatory	40 mg/kg i.p. 12 hrly*
Cycloheximide	Cytotoxic	See Pluskal and colleagues (1978)
Actinomycin	Cytotoxic	
Methotrexate	Cytotoxic	
48/80	Mast-cell degranulator	

* Treatment started 24 hrs before toxin administered. All muscles removed 24 hrs after toxin administration.

administration of the relevant specific anti-venom after the injection of toxin. This seems to be due to the extreme rapidity of the onset of necrosis rather than the low antigenicity of either notexin or taipoxin (compare with the low molecular weight myotoxin from *Crotalus viridis viridis* discussed by Cameron and Tu, 1977), since pre-incubation of notexin with *Notechis scutatus* antivenom and of taipoxin with *Oxyuranus scutellatus* antivenom respectively renders the toxins inactive. Of some interest is the observation that *Notechis scutatus* antivenom will inactivate taipoxin and conversely that *Oxyuranus scutellatus* antivenom will inactivate notexin. This might be expected in view of the similarities between notexin and the active α-subunit of taipoxin, but it is not easily reconciled with the findings of Ramlau, Bock and Fohlman (1979) who reported that there was no cross reactivity between anti-taipoxin antibodies and notexin.

THE ROLE OF PHOSPHOLIPASE ACTIVITY

All of the presynaptically active neurotoxins discussed in this article have measurable phospholipase activity. It is not easy to 'rank' them in order of potency as phospholipases because different workers have used different conditions when assaying the toxins but there do not seem to be major differences in activity.

All of the toxins have an absolute requirement for Ca^{2+}, and in all cases, any chemical modification that causes a loss of phospholipase activity also causes a loss of myotoxicity. However, the possession of phospholipase activity does not necessarily confer marked myotoxicity on a toxin. Thus B-bungarotoxin is as active a phospholipase as notexin (when assayed against either bacterial membranes or synthetic phosphatidyl choline) but is not myotoxic. At the present time it is difficult to know how to interpret these data. It seems clear that phospholipase activity is essential for the expression of myotoxicity, and it also seems probable that the non-myotoxic phospholipases are either unable to bind to the target tissue or are unable to undergo the appropriate conformational change to allow the active site to accommodate the substrate or are unable to find the right substrate in the tissue. These various alternatives will only be accepted or excluded when it becomes possible to make the appropriate competition experiments.

RECOVERY FROM NECROSIS

In spite of the rapid and extensive necrosis caused by the toxins, recovery is similarly rapid. The process has been studied in detail only for notexin and taipoxin, but probably applies to the other myotoxic neurotoxins as well. Briefly, the muscles form primitive myotubes by 3-5 days (fig. 6), immature muscle fibres by 7-10 days, differentiated muscle fibres by 14 days and functionally normal muscles by 21 days. Some details of the process of regeneration are presented in work published by Harris, Johnson and Karlsson (1975); Harris and Johnson (1978); Harris, Johnson and MacDonell (1977); Cullen, Harris and MacDonell (1978) and in MacDonell (1979).

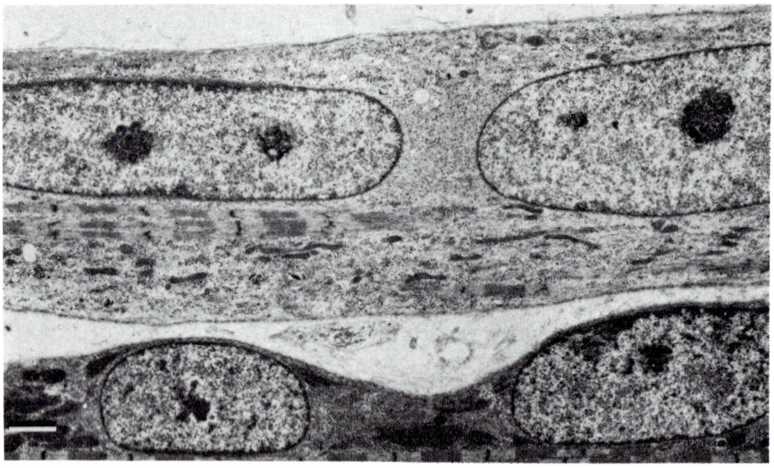

Fig. 6. Longitudinal section through a regenerating myotube (top) in a rat soleus muscle 3 days after the injection of taipoxin (2.0 µg). Note the row of centrally located nuclei, and the organisation of sarcomeres in the regenerating structure. The adjacent (lower) muscle fibre has not been damaged by the toxin. Calibration bar: 1 µ.

The regenerated muscle is to all intents and purposes completely normal the only evidence of damage being the persistence of central nucleation of the regenerated fibres and the existence of a considerable number of 'split' fibres in the regenerated muscle.

CLINICAL IMPLICATIONS

It is commonly held that experiments such as those described in this short article are scarcely relevant either to the expression of evenomation or intoxication in the human, or to the management of the evenomated patient. This belief is derived partly from the observation that often the results of laboratory experiments do not correlate with experience in the field, and partly from the prejudice that the rodent and the human cannot be considered sufficiently closely related to warrant comparison. However at least one cause of difficulty can now be recognised. Thus, the administration of large doses of venom or toxins to isolated preparations or by intravenous injection into the the intact animal may emphasize the activity of one component of the venom concerned, or of one mode of activity of the toxin at the expense of another which may be preferentially expressed when the snake or the biologist delivers a dose of venom or toxin to an intramuscular or subcutaneous site.

This particular analysis may be seen in the case of notexin and the venom of *Notechis scutatus*. Prior to 1975, it was believed that evenomation by the Australian tiger snake caused neurotoxic poisoning with no local tissue damage, and this was apparently borne out by experiments in the laboratory. In 1975 however, Hood and Johnson reported the myotoxic effects of the venom in man and Harris, Johnson and Karlsson the myotoxic effects of notexin on rat muscle following the subcutaneous injection of sublethal doses of the toxin. Since then, muscle necrosis has been recognised as a major feature of evenomation by the snake (Sutherland and Coulter, 1977) and it is probable that the offending venom constituents are the "presynaptically active neurotoxins" notexin and notechis II-5. It will be of interest to see whether or not evenomation by the taipan *Oxyuranus scutellatus* will be found to be accompanied by muscle damage.

CONCLUSIONS

Several toxins, isolated from the crude venoms of various species of snake, and generally considered to be presynaptically active neurotoxins are potent myotoxins. There is no direct relationship between neurotoxicity and myotoxicity, although it seems probable that both forms of activity are dependant upon the phospholipase activity that characterises all of these toxins. Recognition of the fact that animal toxins may not fit neatly into one category or another complicates the interpretation of many experimental observations, but may help to clarify some of the differences that appear to exist between the evenomated patient and the evenomated laboratory animal.

ACKNOWLEDGEMENT

This work was supported by the M.D.A. Inc., M.D.G.B., S.K.F. Foundation and the M.R.C. All the toxins used were supplied by Dr. D. Eaker and colleagues, University of Uppsala. We acknowledge the assistance of the technical staff of the Regional Neurological Centre.

REFERENCES

Abe, T., A. R. Limbrick and R. Miledi (1976). Proc. Roy. Soc. Lond. B., 194, 545-553.

Cameron, D. L. and A. T. Tu (1977). Biochemistry (U.S.), 16, 2546-2553.

Cullen, M. J., J. B. Harris and C. A. MacDonell (1978). Necrosis and rapid regeneration in rat skeletal muscle following taipoxin administration. Abstract 231, IVth Int. Congress on Neuromuscular Disease, Montreal, Canada.

Fohlman, J. and D. Eaker (1977). Toxicon, 15, 385-394.
Geh, S. L. and H. T. Toh (1978). Toxicon, 16, 633-644.
Gopalakrishnakone, P. and B. J. Hawgood (1979). J. Physiol. (Lond.), 291, 5-6P.
Harris, J. B. and M. A. Johnson (1978). Clin. exp. Pharmac. Physiol., 5, 587-600.
Harris, J. B., M. A. Johnson and E. Karlsson (1975). Clin. exp. Pharmac. Physiol., 2, 383-404.
Harris, J. B., M. A. Johnson and C. MacDonell (1977). Br. J. Pharmac., 61, 133P.
Harris, J. B., E. Karlsson and S. Thesleff (1973). Br. J. Pharmac., 47, 141-146.
Hawgood, B. J. and J. W. Smith (1977). Br. J. Pharmac., 61, 597-608.
Hood, V. L. and J. R. Johnson (1975). Med. J. Aust., 2, 638-641.
Kamenskaya, M. A. and S. W. Thesleff (1974). Acta physiol. scand., 90, 716-724.
MacDonell, C. A. (1979). Ph.D. Thesis, University of Newcastle upon Tyne, England.
Pluskal, M. G., J. B. Harris, R. J. Pennington and D. Eaker (1978). Clin. exp. Pharmac. Physiol., 5, 131-141.
Ramlau, J., E. Bock and J. Fohlman (1979). Toxicon, 17, 43-54.
Sutherland, S. K. and A. R. Coulter (1977). Med. J. Aust., 2, 177-180.

BLACK WIDOW SPIDER TOXIN: EFFECT ON CATECHOLAMINES RELEASE AND CATION PERMEABILITY IN A NEUROSECRETORY CELL LINE (PC12)

A. Grasso, S. Alemà, S. Rufini and M. I. Senni

Laboratory of Cell Biology, C.N.R., 00196 Rome, Italy

ABSTRACT

Black widow spider toxin (BWSTx), isolated from the venom of the spider Latrodectus mactans tredecimguttatus, acts as a presynaptic agent, stimulating transmitter release from several mammalian and amphybian preparations. PC12 cells, derived from a rat pheochromocytoma, appear to provide a suitable model for a better understanding of BWSTx effect at the molecular level. BWSTx greatly stimulates the release from PC12 cells of previously taken up ^3H -dopamine or ^3H -norepinephrine. When PC12 cells are incubated in a medium containing EGTA no increase in dopamine release in response to toxin treatment is observed. By substitution of the Ca^{++}-free medium with a Ca^{++}containing one, the response is restored. Addition of toxin to PC12 cells results in a massive and rapid increase in Ca^{++}influx. The toxin action is prevented by pretreatment of the cells with Concanavalin A but is not modified by the presence of agents known to interfere with Na^+channels or voltage-dependent Ca^{++}channels. These results seem to suggest that BWSTx acts in PC12 cells by binding at a specific site. Binding is followed by a sequence of events (e.g. Ca^{++}entry) reproducing naturally occurring exocytosis.

KEYWORDS

Black widow spider toxin; pheochromocytoma cells; neurotransmitter secretion; catecholamines; calcium channels; lectins.

INTRODUCTION

Black widow spider toxin (BWSTx) is an acidic polypeptide of mol.wt. 125,000 which is purified as the major component from the venom of the italian spider Latrodectus mactans tredecimguttatus (Frontali and others, 1976; Grasso, 1976). By electrophysiological techniques it has been shown that BWSTx main effect consists in a massive stimulation of transmitter release from the neuromuscular junction of vertebrates which eventually leads to block of transmission (Frontali and others,

1976; Gorio, Rubin and Mauro, 1978). More recently BWSTx was shown to induce release of a variety of transmitter substances from rat brain synaptosomes (Grasso, Rufini and Senni, 1977; Grasso and Senni, 1979) and cerebral cortex slices (Tzeng, Cohen and Siekevitz, 1978).

PC12 cells, derived from a rat pheochromocytoma, express several differentiative characteristics of sympathetic neurons, notably the property of responding to Nerve Growth Factor and the ability of synthesizing and releasing transmitters under different stimuli (Greene and Tischler, 1976; Greene and Rein, 1977). They therefore offer distinct advantages for a deeper understanding of the toxin mode of action in molecular terms, which so far has been hampered by the complexity or cellular heterogeneity of the preparations used.

RESULTS

Effect of BWSTx on Catecholamines Release

For uptake and release experiments PC12 cells are grown as monolayers on collagen-coated tissue culture dishes. Cultures are then exposed to Hepes-buffered Krebs-Ringer saline, and tritiated dopamine or norepinephrine uptake carried out at 37°C (Greene and Rein, 1977). Release experiments are performed either at 25° or 37°C essentially as described by Greene and Rein (1977). Highly purified BWSTx (Grasso, 1976) added for a 5 min period induces a large release of previously accumulated ^3H -dopamine into the external medium (see Fig. 1). Such release occurs very rapidly and concomitantly with release induced by depolarizing concentrations of K^+ (Fig.1). At variance with K^+ cells continue to release dopamine after toxin is washed out. The effect of toxin is concentration-dependent in the range 0.5 to 5.0 nM. At low toxin concentrations, however, the release of catecholamines is delayed and elicited only if toxin is maintained in the perfusing medium for several 5 min time intervals.

Several lines of evidence point to BWStx-elicited release of catecholamines reflecting an exocytotic process: 1) release seems to be calcium as well as 2) temperature dependent; 3) no appreciable stimulation over background is observed for a non-compartmentized, non-transmitter substance such as 2-deoxy-glucose or 4) in PC12 cells treated with reserpine; moreover 5) it is associated with a 60-70 per cent decrease in the total amount of labelled vesicles, as evaluated by the radioactivity pattern after density gradient centrifugation of lysed cells.

Inhibition by Concanavalin A

The effect of toxin is completely abolished by pretreating PC12 cells with micromolar concentrations of Concanavalin A (Con A) or other lectins such as *Lens Culinaris*, *Ricinus communis* or wheat germ agglutinins (Fig. 1). In Fig. 2 a concentration-effect curve for Con A shows that 50 per cent inhibition is obtained with amounts as low as 5×10^{-8} M. Interestingly succinyl-Con A, a dimeric derivative which induces much less crosslinking of surface glycoproteins than tetrameric Con A, is also able to inhibit dopamine release at comparable concentrations (Fig. 2). It should be noted that cells exposed to Con A fully respond to stimulation by K+ (Fig. 1).

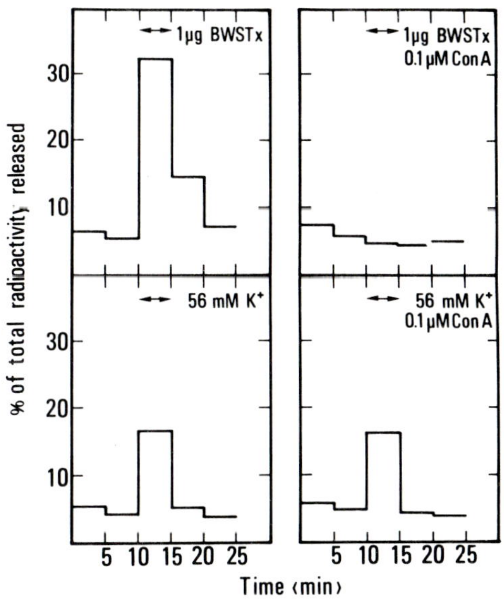

Fig. 1. Dopamine release from PC12 cells stimulated by BWSTx and 56 mM K^+ and effect of cell pretreatment with Concanavalin A. Release is expressed as per cent of total radioactivity present in the cells at the beginning of the experiments.

Calcium Dependence

As shown in Fig. 3 BWSTx is unable to stimulate dopamine release from PC12 cells when tested in Ca^{++}-free conditions obtained by the presence of 1 mM EGTA in the medium. That calcium ions do not affect toxin binding but its ability to stimulate release is deduced from the fact that after extensive washing of the cells the sole addition of physiological concentrations of Ca^{++} to the medium causes BWSTx effect to become apparent. The experimental conditions so obtained i.e. inactive toxin bound to the cells, represent an ideal system for studying the very early events triggered by the toxin after the primary step (binding) has occurred. The kinetic complications arising from toxin diffusion and binding to cells may in fact be avoided. An example is shown in Fig. 4 where the time course of ^{45}Ca uptake and dopamine release from PC12 cells preincubated in EGTA is contemporaneously measured in twin cultures. A massive influx of Ca^{++} ions lasting for several minutes follows superfusion of the cells with 1.8 mM Ca^{++}, the rate being dependent on toxin concentration. Stimulated dopamine release over background seems to be closely associated with Ca^{++} uptake, at least within the limits of the experimental conditions.

Voltage-dependent Ca^{++} channels have been recently described by Stallcup (1979) and Ritchie (1979) in PC12 cells. Typical blockers of these channels, like cobalt and verapamil, while fully inhibiting K^+-induced Ca^{++} influx and dopamine release, were scarcely active when tested on BWSTx action (Table 1). Specific Na^+ channels blockers like tetrodotoxin and sea anemone toxins were also inactive. On the whole

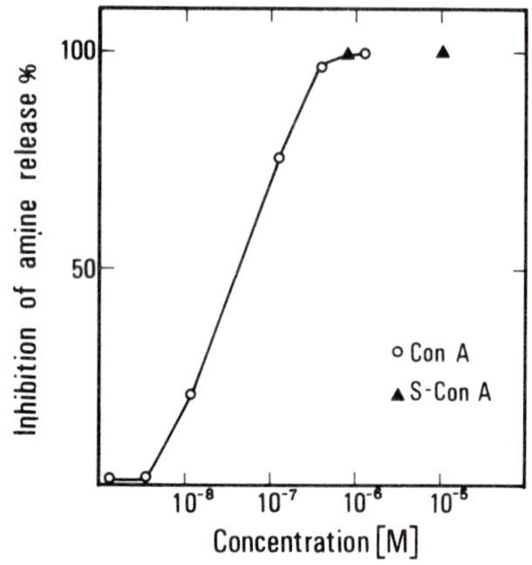

Fig. 2. Inhibition of dopamine release induced by 6 nM BWSTx as a function of Concanavalin A and its succinylated derivative concentrations.

these results suggest that the major part of BWSTx effect does not directly involve activation of voltage-dependent channels. An interesting observation is that pre-treatment of cells with low concentrations of Con A totally blocks toxin-induced Ca^{++} uptake (Table 1). On the contrary addition of lectins, or monospecific antibodies against BWSTx,, to PC12 cells sensitized to the toxin in EGTA (see Fig. 3), did not prevent the subsequent stimulation of dopamine release triggered by Ca^{++}.

Labelling of BWSTx and Binding Studies

Attempts to iodinate BWSTx by two different methods have ended up with labelled derivatives of low specific activity and devoid of appreciable biological activity in vitro. On the contrary BWSTx can be successfully tritiated by reductive methylation of lysine residues according to Rice and Means (1971). The labelled product (10-15 Ci/mmole) fully maintains its toxic activity both in vivo and in vitro. Moreover when run on SDS-gel electrophoresis (Fig. 5), it does not give rise to bands attributable to degradation products. Preliminary binding studies carried out with ^{3}H -BWSTx and PC12 cells grown in monolayer demonstrate saturable specific binding in the toxin concentration range $10^{-10} - 10^{-9}$ M. Specificity of binding was assessed by competition with a large excess of cold toxin. Binding was largely prevented by pretreatment of cells with micromolar concentrations of Con A.

CONCLUSIONS

The results reported here demonstrate the utility of the model we have adopted to analyze the properties and mode of action of BWSTx on target cells. Exposure of PC12 cells to the toxin releases the major portion of previously accumulated radioactive catecholamines, this process appearing to be exocytotic in nature. Two aspects of toxin action call for discussion.

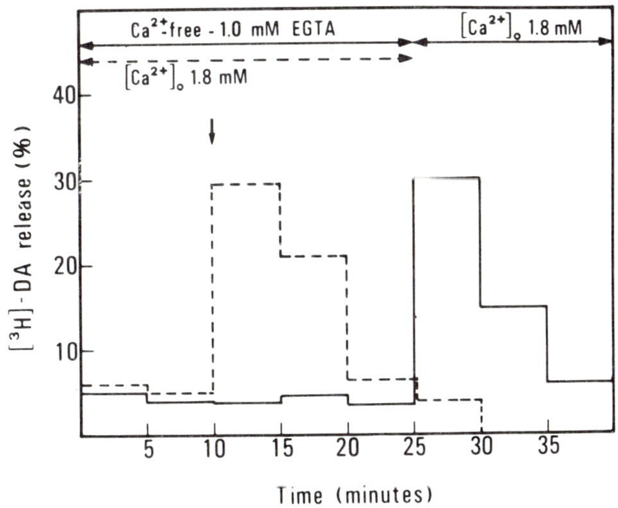

Fig. 3. Ca^{++} dependence of dopamine release in response to BWSTx. Arrow indicates addition of toxin (5 n-moles) to both sets of cultures. Toxin was present only in the following 5 min interval. Dashed lines refer to culture in the presence of standard medium. Continuous line refers to culture in EGTA medium.

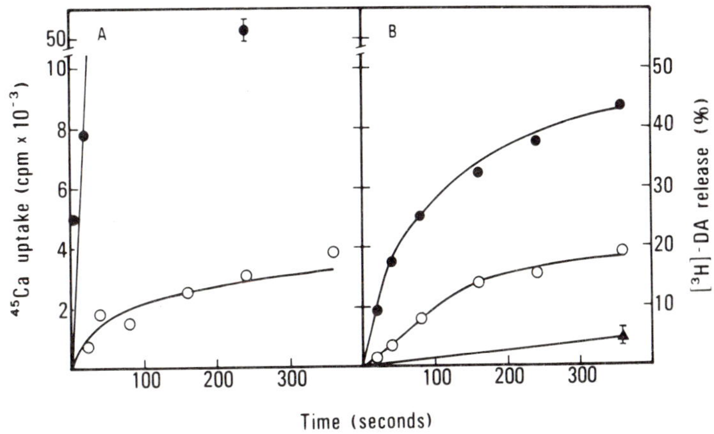

Fig. 4. Time course of ^{45}Ca uptake and ^{3}H -dopamine release induced by 0.7 (O) and 7.0 (●) nM BWSTx. a Ca^{++} uptake substracted of background; b dopamine release; (▲) refers to background release of tritiated dopamine. Release is expressed as in Fig. 1.

A considerable degree of uncertainty still exists in the literature as to the cation dependence of venom action. Depletion of synaptic vesicles in nerve terminals treated with BWSVenom has been observed either in the presence or absence of Ca^{++} ions (Gorio,Rubin and Mauro, 1978; Misler and Hurlbut, 1979; Smith, Clark and Kuster 1977). On the other hand discrete conductancies to several cations were induced by pure BWSTx on lipid bilayer membranes (Finkelstein, Rubin and Tzeng, 1976). The earliest detectable event after toxin treatment of PC12 cells seems to be a massive increase of cytosolic calcium. The major part of Ca^{++} entry induced by toxin is not inhibited by conventional blockers of voltage-dependent Na^{+} or Ca^{++} channels. The moderate reduction in Ca^{++} influx observed in 2 mM Co^{++} might be due to Co^{++} permeating through toxin-induced "channels", but being unable to stimulate release (Ritchie, 1979). Although we have no direct evidence for other cations beside Ca^{++} permeating the plasma membrane as a consequence of toxin action, neither Na^{+} nor Mg^{++} alone seem to be able to substitute for Ca^{++} in inducing transmitter release.

It has been suggested that lectins, by capping surface glycoproteins, interfere with a BWSTx-induced redistribution of membrane components. This process would in its turn be responsible for at least part of the toxin effect (Gorio, Rubin and Mauro, 1978). An alternative explanation would be a direct competition by Con A for the toxin "receptor". The present experiments confirm and extend previous observations on the antagonistic effect of Con A (Grasso, Rufini and Senni, 1978; Rubin, Gorio and Mauro, 1978) by showing that the lectin also inhibits toxin-induced Ca^{++} uptake. Thus, we may postulate that binding to a Con A sensitive membrane component is an obligatory step for the formation of the previously discussed Ca^{++} "channels"

TABLE 1 Effect of several agents on Ca^{++} flux and dopamine release induced by BWSTx and K^{+}.

Condition	Inhibition of maximum effect (%)			
	^{45}Ca flux		DA release	
	BWSTx	K^{+}	BWSTx	K^{+}
TTX ($1x10^{-6}$M)	0	0	0	0
Sea anemone Tx II (10^{-6}M)	0	0	0	0
Co^{++} ($1x10^{-3}$M)	0	80	0	75
($2x10^{-3}$M)	35	98	30	95
Cd^{++} ($2x10^{-3}$M)	n.d*	n.d.	0	90
Verapamil ($5x10^{-5}$M)	32	70	10	75
Concanavalin A (10^{-7}M)	100	0	100	0

Experimental conditions were similar to those described in Fig. 4, except that BWSTx and K^{+} were directly added to cells in standard medium.

* n.d. , not determined.

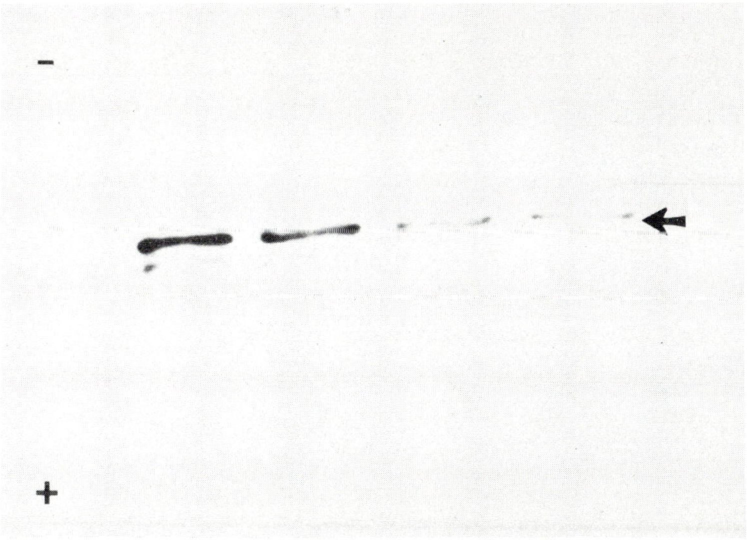

Fig. 5. Autoradiography of tritiated BWSTx run at different concentrations on SDS-slab gel electrophoresis. Toxin was labelled by reductive methylation with formaldehyde and tritiated sodium borohydride. Arrow on the right refers to mobility of β-galactosidase (mol.wt. 130,000).

BWSTx seems to have no definite specificity for any type of terminal, since it stimulates the release of different transmitters even from the same cell. It seems therefore reasonable to suppose that the toxin binds to some ubiquitous membrane constituent which is involved in neurotransmitter release. The availability of a labelled toxin with intact biological and binding abilities should make feasible the identification of such a component.

ACKNOWLEDGMENT

The female spiders used in this study were collected during summer 1978 and obtained through the courtesy of the late Mr. B.Capparella. The authors would like to thank Dr. A.Levi for comments and discussion and Mr. M.Pelliccia who assisted in the purification of the toxin and in antibody production.

REFERENCES

Finkelstein, A., Rubin, L.L. and M. C. Tzeng (1976). Science, 193, 1009-1011.
Frontali, N., B. Ceccarelli, A. Gorio, A. Mauro, P. Siekevitz, M.C. Tzeng, and W. P. Hurlbut (1976). J. Cell Biol., 68, 462-479.
Gorio, A., L. Rubin, and A. Mauro (1978). J. Neurocytol., 7, 193-205.
Grasso, A. (1976). Biochim. Biophys. Acta, 439, 406-412.

Grasso, A., S. Rufini, and M. I. Senni (1978). FEBS Lett., 85, 241-244.
Grasso, A., and M. I. Senni (1979). Eur. J. Biochem., 102, 337-344.
Greene, L. A., and A. S. Tischler (1976). Proc. natn. Acad. Sci. U.S.A., 73, 2424-2428.
Greene, L. A., and G. Rein (1977). Brain Res., 129, 247-263.
Misler, S., and W. P. Hurlbut (1979). Proc. natn. Acad. SCI. U.S.A., 75, 4016-4020.
Rice, R. H., and Means, G. I. (1971). J. Biol. Chem., 246, 831-832.
Ritchie, A. K. (1979). J. Physiol. Lond., 286, 541-560.
Rubin, L. L., A. Gorio, and A. Mauro (1978). Brain Res., 143, 107-124.
Smith, J., A. N. Clark, and T. A. Kuster (1977). J. Neurocytol., 6, 519-539.
Stallcup, W. B. (1979). J. Physiol. Lond., 286, 525-540.
Tzeng, M. C., R. S. Cohen, and P. Siekevitz (1978). Proc. natn. Acad. Sci. U.S.A., 75, 4016-4020.

Botulinum and Tetanus Toxins

BOTULISM: CLINICAL AND ELECTRICAL OBSERVATIONS

M. Cherington

University of Colorado Medical Center, Denver, Colorado 80220, USA

ABSTRACT

The treatment of botulism requires intensive medical and respiratory care. Guanidine hydrochloride has helped 70 percent of the patients treated with this drug. Corticosteroid treatment has little value.

KEYWORDS

Clostridium botulinum; botulism; guanidine therapy; corticosteroids; Lambert-Eaton syndrome; post-tetanic facilitation.

INTRODUCTION

Botulism is a paralyzing disease caused by the most toxic substance known to man. The toxin is produced by the bacterium, Clostridium botulinum. The toxin has been estimated to cause death in man in doses as small as 0.1 - 1.0 micrograms (Schantz and Sugiyama, 1974; Smith, 1977). Eight immunologically distinct toxins have been identified (A, B, C_1, C_2, D, E, F and G). Human cases are almost always due to type A, B or E. When contaminated sea food is found to be the responsible food, the toxin present is often type E.

Botulism toxin is heat-labile and thus is often destroyed by the cooking process. By contrast, the spores of Clostridium botulinum are heat resistant. When spores are present in food, actively multiplying bacilli produce the toxin at room temperature under anaerobic conditions at a pH of 6 or above (Finegold, 1977).

SYMPTOMS AND TREATMENT

The clinical symptoms of botulism usually occur within 12-36 hours after ingestion of contaminated food. The signs and symptoms begin in the cranial nerve territory (blurred vision, dysarthria, dysphagia) and then descend (Cherington, 1979). This distinguishes botulism from the Guillain-Barre syndrome, which is characterized by ascending paralysis.

In botulism, respiratory paralysis can follow quickly and is often fatal unless treated. Alertness, mentation and the sensory system remain normal. The pupils are usually normal, particularly early in the disease. Patients with severe botulism almost always have marked extraocular muscle weakness, including ptosis. Weakness of the face, tongue, pharynx, neck and sometimes, to a lesser degree, of the limbs, occurs. Weakness progresses until it reaches a plateau at about four or five days. Although the weakness is bilateral, it is often asymmetric. The patients may have more severe ptosis or limb weakness on one side than on the other. Severe respiratory paralysis can occur within the first day. Symptoms of parasympathetic dysfunction may include dryness of the mouth and eyes and gastrointestinal ileus. Deep tendon reflexes are reduced in proportion to the degree of muscular weakness.

Recovery, if it occurs, is prolonged but nearly total (Cherington, 1974). Laboratory confirmation usually requires the detection of toxin in the patient's serum, stool, or in the contaminated food. Mouse toxicity tests with antiserum neutralization are most useful. Specimens that should be examined include serum, gastric contents, feces, exudates from wounds and contents of the suspected jars or cans. Radioimmuneassay tests may be practical in the future.

The major treatment of botulism is good medical care. This consists of providing artificial ventilation for patients with respiratory paralysis. Tracheotomy and a positive pressure respirator are usually required. Mechanical assistance to respiration may be needed for as long as weeks or months. Early administration of antitoxin may be of value in cases of type E botulism. The literature and our experience seem to suggest that antitoxin is less effective in types A and B botulism. Corticosteroid treatment has not been beneficial (Cherington and Schultz, 1977).

The role of guanidine in the treatment of botulism remains that of an adjunct to therapy and not that of a cure. It has helped some, but not all patients. Guanidine was introduced in the treatment of botulism in 1968. Since that time it has been beneficial in 43 cases (39 previously reported plus four recent cases) and of little or no benefit in 19 cases (Puggliari and Cherington, 1979; Kaplan and others, 1979). In the cases of treatment failure, 18 of 19 patients recovered anyway. So far, no serious side effect has occured with short-term therapy, although there have been serious side effects when guanidine has been given for long periods in disorders such as the Lambert-Eaton syndrome.

Although guanidine therapy results in notable eye and limb muscle improvement, there often is minimal improvement in vital capacity or pulmonary function. Increasing the dose of guanidine may result in considerable epigastric distress and nausea. This is a problem, because guanidine has not been approved for parenteral administration and must be given orally. Another problem in treatment with guanidine is failure of its adsorption because of ileus.

The expected electrophysiological findings in botulism may be summarized as follows: (1) There is almost always a small evoked muscle action potential in response to single supramaximal nerve stimulation.

(2) Posttetanic facilitation is similar to but less notable than that seen in the Lambert-Eaton syndrome (Cherington, 1971; Gutman and Pratt, 1976). (3) Postactivation exhaustion is not prominent. (4) The decremented response of muscle action potential to slow rate of stimulation is absent or not notable. (5) Evoked action potential to single-nerve stimulation is increased after guanidine therapy. (6) Single-fiber EMG studies reveal increased jitter and blocking. Jitter is frequency-dependent and decreases with higher innervation frequency. Fiber density values are lowered (Schiller and Stålberg, 1978; Stålberg and Trontelj, 1979).

REFERENCES

Cherington, M. (1979). Acute muscle weakness. In: H. Klawans and S. Ringel (eds.), Handbook of Clinical Neurology, Vol 41, in press.

Cherington, M.(1971). Botulism: electrophysiologic and therapeutic observations. In: J. E. Desmedt (ed.), New Developments in Electromyography and Clinical Neurophysiology, Vol 1, S. Krager, Basel, pp. 375-397.

Cherington, M. (1974). Botulism: ten years experience. Arch Neurol. (Chicago), 30, 432-437.

Cherington, M. and D. Schultz (1977). Effect of guanidine, germine and steroids in a case of botulism. Clin Toxicol., 11, 19-25.

Finegold, S. F. (1977). Intoxications due to anaerobic bacteria. In: Anaerobic Bacteria in Human Disease. Academic Press, New York, pp. 472-487.

Gutmann, L. and L. Pratt (1976). Pathophysiologic aspects of human botulism. Arch. Neurol. (Chicago), 33, 175-179.

Kaplan, J. E., L. E. Davis, V. Narayan, J. Koster, and D. Katzenstein (1979). Botulism, Type A, and treatment with guanidine. Ann. Neurol., 6, 69-71.

Puggiari, M., and M. Cherington (1979). Botulism and guanidine. J. A. M. A., 21, 2276-2277.

Schantz, E. J., and H Sugiyama (1974). Toxic proteins produced by Clostridium botulinum. J. Agr. Food Chem., 22, 26-90.

Schiller, H. M., and E. Stålberg (1978). Human botulism studies with single-fibre electromyography. Arch. Neurol., 35, 346-349.

Smith, L. C. (1977). The toxins of Clostridium botulinum. In: Botulism., Ch. Thomas, Springfield, Ill., pp. 113-141.

Stålberg, E., and J. V. Trontelj (1979). Single-fiber Electromyography. The Mirvalle Press, Surrey, U. K., p. 131.

BOTULINUM A AND TETANUS TOXIN: EFFECTS ON NEUROTRANSMISSION TO STRIATED AND SMOOTH MUSCLES

E. Habermann, H. Bigalke, F. Dreyer and P. Streitzig

Pharmacological Institute, Justus Liebig-Universität Giessen, Federal Republic of Germany

ABSTRACT

1. Tetanus and botulinum A toxin inhibit the cholinergic transmission in both the phrenic-nerve diaphragm preparation and the guinea-pig myenteric plexus strip incubated in vitro. A close similarity, if not identity of the mode of action of both toxins on either system is indicated by the following observations:
   a) In any case, the course of poisoning can be divided into a period of latency, followed by a period of paralysis.
   b) Washing or antitoxin are effective during the latency period only.
   c) Transmission can be restored partially with substances increasing intracellular free Ca^{2+} directly or indirectly.
   d) Both toxins leave the total acetylcholine content of the myenteric plexus strip intact. They decrease release and formation of radioactive acetylcholine from ^{3}H choline.
2. In contrast, the adrenergic transmission in the cat nictitating membrane, the mouse vas deferens and the m.anococcygeus of the rat appears to be resistant against either toxin.

Further studies should show if the parallelism between the toxins holds true with other, preferentially central synapses.

KEYWORDS

Tetanus; botulism; cholinergic; synapses; muscarinic; nicotinic; adrenergic.

Both tetanus and botulinum A toxin are known to react with peripheral synapses. In botulism, death occurs by presynaptic block of the endplates whereas central effects are of minor importance. Conversely in tetanus, many clinical and experimental observations indicate that, besides, and hidden by the prominent symptoms of central origin, a botulinum-like neuromuscular paralysis takes place in the periphery. Both toxins can migrate intraaxonally (for botulinum toxin see Wiegand and others, 1976) albeit tetanus toxin (for review see Habermann, 1978) takes this way to a more pronounced and clinically relevant extent. Despite of the grossly different clinical manifestations one is tempted to assume a common mode of action for both toxins, whereas the quantitative differences might be due to pharmacokinetic peculiarities. The data to be presented for both nicotinic and muscarinic nerve endings can be interpreted in favour of this hypothesis. It is supported by the chemical similarity of both toxins (Das Gupta, 1979).

1. The neuromuscular junction as an example of a nicotinic synapse.

Under various clinical or experimental conditions paralysis due to tetanus toxin becomes manifest (for references see Habermann, 1978; Habermann and others, 1979). Preparations from in situ poisoned muscles essentially resemble those from botulinum-poisoned muscles. The number but not the size of m.e.p.p.'s decreases (Mellanby and Thompson, 1972), and axonal sprouting (Duchen and Tonge, 1973) indicates long-lasting impairment of the motor nerve endings. We have studied the course of tetanus poisoning in vitro, and some influences thereupon (Habermann and others, 1979). Because of its longevity and its size the mouse phrenic nerve-diaphragm preparation is particularly suitable for studying slow-acting toxins. It responds to tetanus toxin with paralysis preceded by a latency period. By weight, crystalline botulinum A toxin is about 500 times more potent. Contaminants, instead of tetanus toxin itself have been thought to be responsible for paralysis (see Feigen and others, 1963). However, there is a striking parallelism between paralyzing power in vitro and toxicity in vivo with respect to inactivation by antitoxin or brain homogenate, and with toxin preparations of different toxicities.
Tetanus and botulinum A toxin paralysis share many properties (for botulinum toxin see Simpson, 1977). In both cases, an asymptomatic latency period precedes the phase of manifest paralysis. Already during the former period, the efficacy of the toxins becomes progressively resistant first against washing, then against antitoxin. With both toxins, survival time of the diaphragm is shortened with increasing temperature. The Q_{10} is 2.7 in the case of tetanus toxin. The action of tetanus and botulinum toxin depends on synaptic activity. This may be the reason why raising temperature is so effective. Increasing the stimulation frequency shortens the survival time, and lowering the frequency, or rest, prolongs it. Accordingly, survival time is also prolonged in low Ca^{++} or high Mg^{++} medium, conditions known to inhibit transmitter release. Conversely, paralysis due to tetanus toxin, like that due to botulinum toxin, is temporarily restored by 4-aminopyridine (10^{-5} M) or guanidine (10^{-3} M). Like botulinum toxin, tetanus toxin diminishes the number, but not the size of miniature endplate potentials, which also proves its presynaptic attack.
Taken altogether, the findings (Habermann and others, 1979) allow the statement that tetanus toxin and botulinum A toxin are indistinguishable with respect to their neuromuscular effects.

2. The junctions in the myenteric plexus strip as examples of muscarinic synapses.

Like the endplates, the muscarinic nerve endings in various organs are sensitive to botulinum A toxin. Pupillary paralysis and obstipation belong to the clinical features of botulism. Accordingly, botulinum toxin has been reported to inhibit the sphincter iridis in vivo (Ambache, 1949), and the field stimulated guinea pig ileum in vitro (Harry, 1962).
Locally applied, tetanus toxin paralyzes the sphincter pupillae of the rabbit (Ambache and others, 1948; Fedinec, 1973). So far, in vitro studies with tetanus toxin on muscarinic cholinergic systems

are lacking.
Our comparative studies (Bigalke and Habermann, 1980) were performed with the myenteric plexus strip of the guinea-pig ileum which survives many hours in vitro. On appropriate field-stimulation, the contraction depends on the function of the muscarinic nerve endings but not of the muscle or the preganglionic nerve endings (Cowie and others, 1978). As with the indirectly stimulated diaphragm, the decrease of contraction amplitude may be taken as a measure of presynaptic actions of tetanus or botulinum toxin. Moreover, we have shown that tetanus toxin does not decrease the sensitivity to acetylcholine externally applied, and that the electrically elicited contractions are not diminished by the ganglionic blocker hexamethonium.
Both tetanus and botulinum A toxin diminish the amplitude of the electrically stimulated preparation, tetanus toxin being about 5 times less potent. The course of poisoning can be subdivided into a latency and a paralytic period, and is indistinguishable with both toxins. Moreover, the muscarinic synapses behave principally similar to the nicotinic neuromuscular synapses. Dependent on time after poisoning, the strip becomes progressively less sensitive to washing or antibody treatment. The velocity of the paralytic process can be enhanced by raising the stimulation frequency, and slowed by periods of no stimulation, high Mg^{2+}, or lower Ca^{2+}. Synaptic activity therefore appears to be important, but not indispensable for paralysis.
By weight, the myenteric plexus strip contains more acetylcholine than the phrenic nerve-diaphragm preparation which allows the measurement of total concentrations, uptake and release of the transmitter. There was no difference between the total acetylcholine contents of poisoned and not poisoned strips. However, when the strips were pretreated with tetanus or botulinum toxin and then loaded with ^{3}H-choline, less acetyl-^{3}H-choline was formed in the poisoned strips. Moreover the release of the labeled transmitter by depolarization with veratridine (5 μg/ml) was diminished by poisoning with either toxin.
The changes in transmitter metabolism closely resemble those found in other systems. As early as in 1949, Burgen and others reported that the acetylcholine release from rat diaphragm was severely depressed by botulinum toxin. Measurement of the m.e.p.p.'s indicates that the release process is impeded in nerve-muscle preparations poisoned with tetanus toxin in vitro or in vivo (see Habermann and others, 1979). Acetylcholine release due to potassium depolarization was also inhibited in synaptosomal preparations (Wonnacott and Marchbanks, 1976) and, by both tetanus and botulinum A toxin, in primary cultures from rat central nervous system (Bigalke and others, 1978). All the observations together make it obvious that both toxins prevent the acetylcholine release in the same way from both nicotinic and muscarinic nerve endings.

3. Botulinum A and tetanus toxin are not antisympathotonic.
Several authors reported on the adrenergic blockade by botulinum toxin (Rand and Whaler, 1965; Westwood and Whaler, 1968; Holman and Spitzer, 1973) whereas others had negative results (Ambache, 1951; Vincenci, 1967). In order to resolve the contradictory statements we tested botulinum A toxin at the cat nictitating membrane by local unilateral injection. No difference to the control side was evident within up to 22 hours after toxin treatment (Fig. 1). In vitro, the indirectly stimulated nictitating membrane was poisoned with up to 3 μg/ml botulinum toxin A. Within more than 6 hours no differences in contraction amplitude occurred against the contralateral control. To get a more direct measure, the nictitating

membrane was loaded with ^{3}H-noradrenaline according to Langer and Enero (1974), and the fractional release of radioactivity upon indirect stimulation was compared between poisoned and not poisoned muscles. Again, in only one out of four groups the difference was statistically significant (Fig. 2). Finally, we applied botulinum A toxin (0.7 μg/ml) to the isolated indirectly stimulated vas deferens preparation (Huković, 1961) of the mouse and to the isolated field-stimulated m. anococcygeus (Gillespie, 1972) of the rat. The contraction amplitude of both poisoned preparations, the vas deferens (Fig. 3a) and the m. anococcygeus (not shown) did not differ from the controls for up to 5 hours.- Tetanus toxin (10 μg/ml) was tested at the field-stimulated mouse vas deferens (Fig. 3b) and at the field-stimulated m. anococcygeus without any effect on the contraction amplitude. The indirect character of stimulation was established by complete depression of the systems by enkephalin (10^{-7} M), phenoxybenzamine or phentolamine (both 10 μg/ml). In summary, there was no evidence for any effect of the two clostridial toxins on sympathetic transmission. This is especially remarkable because tetanus toxin ascends also via the sympathetic nerves (Stöckel and others, 1975).

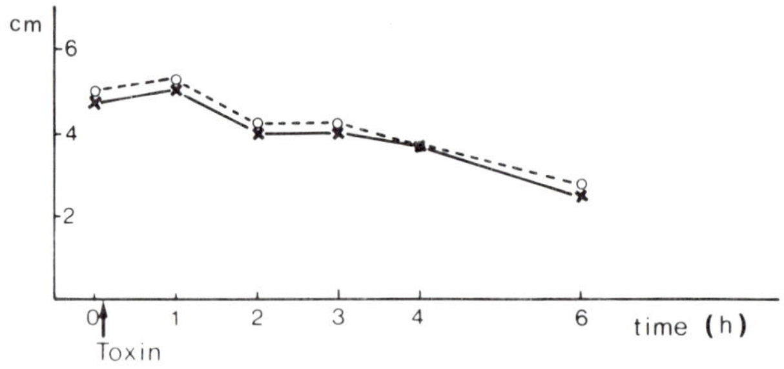

Fig. 1. Failure of locally injected botulinum A toxin (10 μg) to alter the response to postganglionic sympathetic stimulation of the third eyelid of the cat in situ.
Ordinate: Height of contraction (cm) of the poisoned (o) and the control (x) side. Abscissa: Time of registration (hours). Cats were anesthetized with chloralose. The postganglionic sympathetic nerves were stimulated in the neck region by trains of square wave impulses (1 ms, 36/s) of increasing duration (16 ms to 2 s) and supramaximal voltage.

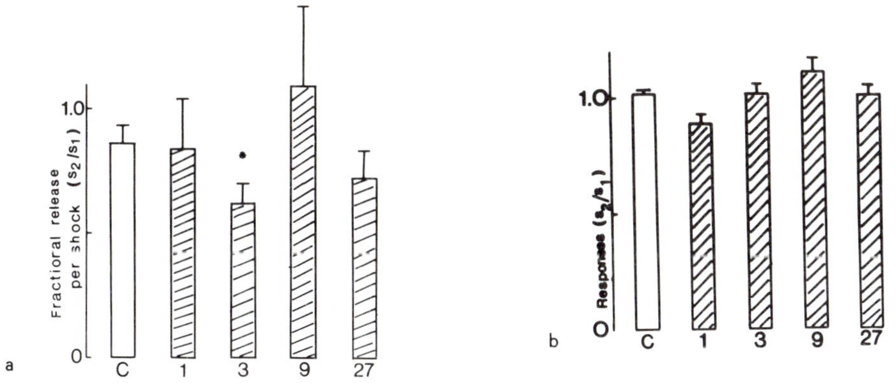

Fig. 2. Failure of botulinum A toxin to influence a) the fractional release of ^{3}H noradrenaline from the cat nictitating membrane after indirect stimulation in vitro, and b) its response to indirect stimulation in vitro. The bars represent controls (C) and experiments with different concentrations of toxin (1-27 µg/ml). Given are the ratios of ^{3}H noradrenaline release (a) or of the mechanical responses (b) per train between periods after (S_2) and before (S_1) 2 hours of incubation with toxin.
The organ was incubated for 30 min with 10 µCi/ml of ± 7-^{3}H noradrenaline. The tissue was then washed 8 times for 1 min each with fresh Krebs solution, subsequently 6 times for 10 min each before the stimulation was started. Two periods of nerve stimulation were applied in each experiment, the second period (S_2) 144 min after the first one (S_1). Toxin was kept in contact with the diaphragm for this time. The outflow was measured in 5 samples (1 ml each) before, 1 during and 7 after the periods of nerve stimulation (see Langer and Enero, 1974).

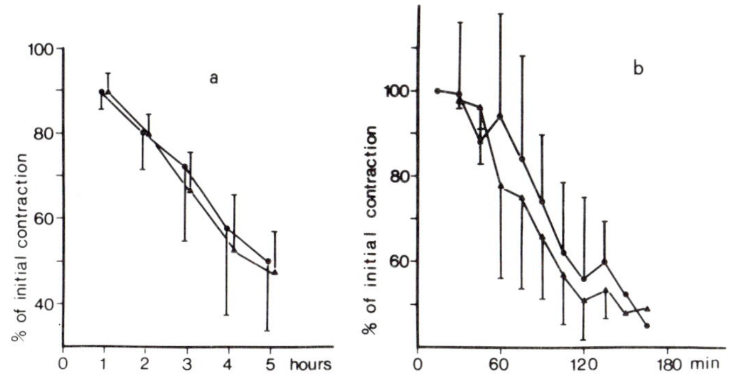

Fig. 3. Failure of botulinum A (a) and tetanus (b) toxin to alter the sensitivity of the indirectly stimulated vas deferens of the mouse.
a) Botulinum toxin (0.6 µg/ml; n = 4)
b) Tetanus toxin (10 µg/ml; n = 3).

REFERENCES

Ambache, N. (1949). The peripheral action of clostridium botulinum toxin. J. Physiol. (Lond.), 108, 127-141.
Ambache, N. (1951). A further survey of the action of clostridium botulinum toxin upon different types of autonomic nerve-fibres. J. Physiol. (Lond.), 113, 1-17.
Ambache, N., R.S. Morgan, and G.P. Wright (1948). The action of tetanus toxin on the rabbits iris. J. Physiol. (Lond.), 107, 45-53.
Bigalke, H., W. Dimpfel, and E. Habermann (1978). Suppression of ^{3}H-acetylcholine release from primary nerve cell cultures by tetanus and botulinum-A toxin. Naunyn-Schmiedebergs Arch. Pharmacol., 303, 133-138.
Bigalke, H., and E. Habermann (1980). Effects of tetanus and botulinum-A toxin on muscarinic nerve endings as studied with the myenteric plexus preparation. Naunyn-Schmiedebergs Arch. Pharmacol., (in press).
Burgen, A.S.V., F. Dickens, and L.J. Zatman (1949). The action of botulinum toxin on the neuromuscular junction. J. Physiol. (Lond.), 109, 10-24.
Cowie, A.L., H.W. Kosterlitz, and A.A. Waterfield (1978). Factors influencing the release of acetylcholine from the myenteric plexus of the ileum of the guinea-pig and rabbit. Brit. J. Pharmacol., 64, 565-580.
Das Gupta, B.R. (1979). Botulinum neurotoxin: Studies on the structure and structure-biological activity relation. Toxicon Suppl. 1, 17, 33.
Duchen, L.W., and D.A. Tonge (1973). The effects of tetanus toxin on neuromuscular transmission and on the morphology of motor-endplates in slow and fast skeletal muscle of the mouse. J. Physiol., 228, 157-172.
Fedinec, A.A. (1973). Antitoxin's effect on tetanus toxin-induced spincter pupillae paralysis in the rabbit. Naunyn-Schmiedebergs Arch. exp. Path. Pharmak., 276, 311-320.
Feigen, G.A., N.S. Peterson, W.W. Hofman, G.H. Genther, and W.E. van Heyningen (1963). The effect of impure tetanus toxin on the frequency of miniature endplate potentials. J. gen. Microbiol., 33, 489-495.
Gillespie, J.S. (1972). The rat anococcygeus muscle and its response to nerve stimulation and to some drugs. Br. J. Pharmacol., 45, 404-416.
Habermann, E. (1978). Tetanus. In P.J. Vinken and G.W. Bruyn (Eds.), Handbook of Clinical Neurology, 33 (I), North Holland Publ. Comp., Amsterdam. pp. 491-547.
Habermann, E., F. Dreyer, and H. Bigalke (1979). Tetanus toxin blocks the neuromuscular transmission in vitro like botulinum A toxin. Naunyn-Schmiedebergs Arch. Pharmacol. (in press).
Harry, J. (1962). Effect of cooling, local anaesthetic compounds and botulinum toxin on the responses of and the acetylcholine output from the electrically transmurally stimulated isolated guinea-pig ileum. Brit. J. Pharmacol., 19, 42-55.
Holman, E., and N.C. Spitzer (1973). Action of botulinum toxin on transmission from sympathetic nerves to the vas deferens. Brit. J. Pharmacol., 47, 431-433.
Huković, S. (1961). Responses of the isolated sympathetic nerve - ductus deferens preparation of guinea-pig. Brit. J. Pharmacol., 16, 188-194.

Langer, S.Z., and M.A. Enero (1974). The potentiation of response to adrenergic nerve stimulation in the presence of cocaine: its relationship to the metabolic fate of released norepinephrine. J. Pharmacol. exp. Ther., 191, 431-443.

Mellanby, J., and P.A. Thompson (1972). The effects of tetanus toxin at the neuromuscular junction of the goldfish. J. Physiol., 224, 407-419.

Rand, M.C., and B.C. Whaler (1965). Impairment of sympathetic transmission by botulinum toxin. Nature (Lond.), 206, 588-590.

Simpson, L.L. (1977). Presynaptic actions of botulinum toxin and β-bungarotoxin. The specificity and action of animal, bacterial and plant toxins. In Cuatrecasas (Ed.) Chapman and Hall. pp. 271-295.

Stöckel, K., M.Schwab, and H. Thoenen (1975). Comparison between the retrograde axonal transport of nerve growth factor and tetanus toxin in motor, sensory and adrenergic neurons. Brain Res., 99, 1-16.

Vincenzi, F.F. (1967). Effect of botulinum toxin on autonomic nerves in a dually innervated tissue. Nature (Lond.), 213, 394-395.

Westwood, D.A., and B.C. Whaler (1968). Postganglionic paralysis of the guinea-pig hypogastric nerve-vas deferens preparation by clostridium botulinum type D toxin. Brit. J. Pharmac. Chemother., 33, 21-31.

Wiegand, H., G. Erdmann, and H.H. Wellhöner (1976). ^{125}I-labelled botulinum A neurotoxin. Pharmacokinetics in cats after intramuscular injection. Naunyn-Schmiedebergs Arch. Pharmacol., 292,161-165.

Wonnacott, S., and R.M. Marchbanks (1976). Inhibition by botulinum toxin of depolarization evoked release of ^{14}C-acetylcholine from synaptosomes in vitro. Biochem. J., 156, 701-712.

ACKNOWLEDGEMENT

The experiments on the isolated nictitating membrane were performed by one of us (P.S.) in the laboratory of Dr. S.Z. Langer (Paris) in cooperation with Dr. Dubocovich. We are very much indebted to them.

STUDIES ON THE PROPHYLAXIS AND TREATMENT OF BOTULISM

G. E. Lewis, Jr. and J. F. Metzger

United States Army Medical Research Institute of Infectious Diseases
Frederick, Maryland 21701, USA

ABSTRACT

The efficacy of heterologous and homologous antitoxins was evaluated for the prophylaxis and treatment of botulism in guinea pigs. Botulism Immune Plasma (Human) was shown to be efficacious for the prophylaxis and treatment of botulism in guinea pigs. The effective half-life of heterologous (horse) antitoxin was 5 to 7 days in a human patient treated for Type A botulism. A half-life of 21 days is anticipated for homologous antitoxin in man.

KEYWORDS

Botulism; antitoxin; prophylaxis; therapy; toxoid; anamnestic response; immune plasma.

INTRODUCTION

The treatment of botulism is directed primarily towards the neutralization of cirulating botulinal neurotoxin by the administration of specific antitoxin and intensive medical supportive care. Heterologous antitoxins are less than desirable, but are often necessary for both prophylaxis and treatment. An adverse reaction rate of 21 per cent has consistently been reported for the equine-derived botulinum antitoxins used in man (Merson *et al.*, 1974). Therefore, the production of a homologous (human) specific antitoxin for the prophylaxis and treatment of botulism in man is highly desirable.

The efficacy of specific antitoxins in the prophylaxis and treatment of botulism in various animal models has been demonstrated repeatedly as reviewed by Cooper (1964). In a comparison study of the persistence of heterologous and homologous tetanus antitoxin following passive immunization in humans Smolens *et al.* (1961) calculated the half-life of horse tetanus globulin in man to be only 7 to 14 days, whereas the half-life of homologous (human) tetanus globulin was about 4 weeks.

The difficulties of obtaining a human antitoxin to replace animal products for the treatment of botulism are, however, of a greater magnitude than those encountered in the collection of tetanus antitoxins. These difficulties have been adequately discussed elsewhere (Habermann and Bernáth, 1975).

In this report the efficacy of a commercially available trivalent heterologous (horse) antitoxin and three monovalent homologous (guinea pig) antitoxins are evaluated for the prophylaxis and treatment of botulism in guinea pigs. The half-life for the same heterologous antitoxin was determined in a human patient intoxicated with Type A toxin. Also, the anamnestic response of the donors of human botulism immune plasma to a booster dose of pentavalent toxoid is presented. Furthermore, the relationship of clinical signs of botulism, time of passive immunization or treatment with Botulism Immune Plasma (Human) (Lewis and Metzger, 1978) and survival are examined in guinea pigs.

MATERIALS AND METHODS

Female Hartley guinea pigs, 200 to 300 g body weight, were used in each study described.

The horse-derived antitoxin was produced by Connaught Medical Research Laboratories, Toronto, Canada, and labeled as Botulism Antitoxin Trivalent (Equine) Types A, B, and E. Monovalent antitoxins, A, B and E, were raised in guinea pigs by repeated intramuscular inoculations with 0.6 per cent formaldehyde toxoids. All antitoxin dilutions were prepared in a standard phosphate gelatin buffer (0.2 per cent gelatin in phosphate buffered saline at pH 6.2).

International units (IU) of antitoxin contained in sera examined and in each dilution of antitoxin used were determined by the standard mouse serum neutralization test using the standard Types A, B and E antitoxins provided by Statens Serum Institute, Copenhagen, Denmark.

Types A, B and E crude toxins were produced in static cultures and concentrated by sequential steps of acid precipitation, extraction, and ammonium sulfate precipitation, then stored frozen in phosphate gelatin buffer.

STUDY DESIGN AND RESULTS

Heterologous vs. Homologous Antitoxin in Guinea Pigs

The efficacy of heterologous (horse) antitoxin as compared to homologous (guinea pig) antitoxin was examined in guinea pigs (Table 1). Eighteen groups (4 animals per group) of guinea pigs were injected intramuscularly with one of the three monovalent homologous antitoxins, or with the trivalent heterologous antitoxin. Homologous and heterologous antitoxins were diluted to contain equivalent international units. Guinea pigs were challenged subcutaneously with buffered crude toxin at 18 hr before the treatment with either homologous or heterologous antitoxin, at 24 hr after, or at 18 days, after treatment with antitoxin.

Guinea pigs treated with homologous or heterologous antitoxin and challenged with Types A, B or E toxin at 18 hr before or 24 hr after treatment demonstrated 0 to 100 per cent survival rates depending on time, type and species of antitoxin administered (Table 1). When guinea pigs were challenged with Types A, B or E toxin 18 days after treatment with either homologous or heterologous antitoxin, only those treated with homologous antitoxin survived. Thus, equated doses of the homologous antitoxin were shown to be as efficacious as the heterologous equine antitoxin when administered within 18 hr before or at 24 after exposure to toxin. However, the homologous antitoxins persisted at or above protective levels much longer than did the horse-derived antitoxin.

TABLE 1 Efficacy of Homologous (Guinea Pig) and Heterologous (Horse) Antitoxin for the Prophylaxis and Treatment of Botulism in Guinea Pigs

Antitoxin Treatment	International Units	% Survival Time of Toxin Challenge 18 hr Before	 24 hr After	 18 days After	Toxin dose Guinea Pig Intraperitoneal LD50
Type A					
Homologous	0.6	50	100	100	4.5
Heterologous	0.6	75	100	0	4.5
Type B					
Homologous	0.6	0	100	100	6.3
Heterologous	0.6	25	100	0	6.3
Type E					
Homologous	0.5	75	100	100	5.0
Heterologous	0.5	75	100	0	5.0

Heterologous Antitoxin in a Human

The decay rate of trivalent heterologous (horse) antitoxin was determined in a human by examination of sera collected from a patient who was treated for food-borne, Type A intoxication (Fig. 1). The decay rates for Types A, B and E antitoxin activity were similar and reflected a half-life of 5 to 7 days for the heterologous (horse) antitoxin.

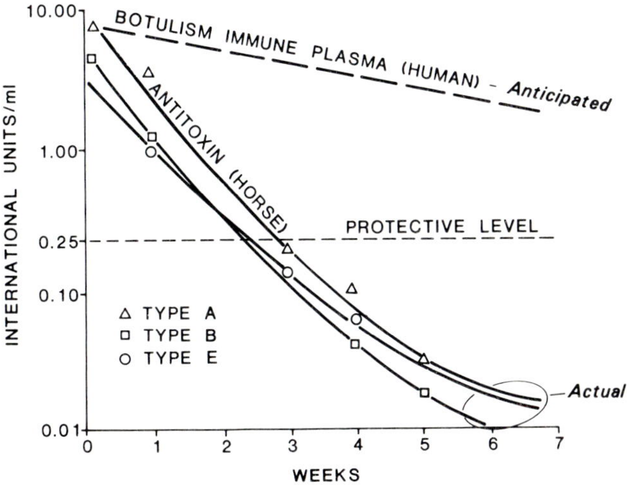

Fig. 1. Actual decay rate of heterologous (horse) trivalent antitoxin and anticipated decay rate of Botulism Immune Plasma (Human) in a patient with botulism

A protective level of 0.25 unit would be maintained for only 3 weeks with equine antitoxin while it would be anticipated that a comparable dose of homologous antitoxin would afford the same level for 22 weeks (Fig. 1).

The prophylactic use of homologous rather than heterologous antitoxin might well be crucial to recovery in an untimely exposure to preformed botulinal toxin or where the persistence of antitoxin is required for the neutralization of continued production of toxin from the intestine or from a contaminated wound.

Acquisition of a Homologous (Human) Antitoxin

It has long been recognized that a homologous, specifically-immune serum, plasma or globulin would be a valuable asset in the therapy of human botulism. A homologous (human) botulism antitoxin program was initiated utilizing a group of 24 volunteers who had been previously immunized with Botulinum Toxoid Adsorbed Pentavalent (ABCDE). Upon entering the program a booster dose of 0.5 ml was administered. Each individual had previously received 7 to 11 immunizations with the same toxoid but none had received the toxoid for 7 to 8 years prior to the booster re-immunization. The geometric mean of the group serum titers to Type A toxin was 0.82 IU/ml, at the time of boosting and 8.98 IU/ml for sera collected 28 days later (Table 2). The prebooster group geometric mean Type B titer was 0.06 IU/ml while the 28-day postbooster titer was 0.52 IU/ml. The anamnestic response to Type E was even greater. The approximate 10-fold increase in neutralizing antibodies in response to a single booster after a 7 to 8 year lapse in immunization is highly significant ($p < 0.001$), and represents an excellent anamnestic response.

After re-immunization a total of 500 liters of Botulism Immune Plasma (Human) was collected by plasmapheresis and stored as single donor units of fresh, frozen plasma.

TABLE 2 Anamnestic Response to a Single Booster Dose of Botulinum Toxoid in 24 Donors of Botulism Immune Plasma (Human)

Type	Geometric Mean Titer (IU/ml)		p
	Before (Day 0)	After (Day 28)	
A	0.82	8.98	< 0.001
B	0.06	0.52	< 0.001
E	0.16	2.30	< 0.001

Efficacy of Botulism Immune Plasma (Human) in Guinea Pigs

Guinea pigs were utilized to determine the efficacy of Botulism Immune Plasma (Human) for the prophylaxis and treatment of Type A botulism. The relationship of the time of antitoxin (plasma) administration, appearance of clinical signs of toxemia, detection of serum toxemia, and survival were evaluated (Table 3).

Guinea pigs were inoculated intramuscularly with 10 IU of the immune plasma 4 hr before or 4, 8, 12 and 34 to 44 hr after the oral administration of 4 guinea pig oral LD_{50} ($GPOLD_{50}$) of buffered crude Type A toxin.

Circulating toxin could be detected in the serum of guinea pigs 4 hr after oral ingestion. However, clinical signs of botulism were not evident until 12 to 24 hr later. When Botulism Immune Plasma (Human) was administered intramuscularly 4 hr before or 4 or 8 hr after oral toxin, survival was 100 per cent and clinical signs did not develop. Plasma administered at 12 hr effected a 66 per cent survival rate and at 34 to 44 hr, when clinical signs were very prominent, a 45 per cent survival rate. All untreated guinea pigs died within 4 days. However, the time to death for many of those which were treated at 34 to 44 hr, but eventually died, was extended to as long as 10 days after exposure to toxin. These toxemic guinea pigs did not receive any supportive care, as a hospitalized human patient would. The extended

TABLE 3 Efficacy of Botulism Immune Plasma (Human) for the Prophylaxis and Treatment of Botulism in Guinea Pigs

Application*	Time (hr)**	Clinical Signs of Toxemia	Toxin Detected in Serum	% Survival
Prophylaxis	-4	None	No	100
	4	None	Yes	100
	8	None	Yes	100
Treatment	12	Slight in some	Yes	67
	34 to 44	Present	Yes	45
None	24	Present	Yes	0
	34	Present	Yes	0

*10 IU of botulism immune plasma per guinea pig, administered intramuscularly.
**4 Guinea pig oral LD_{50} of Type A toxin per guinea pig, administered orally at 0 hr.

survival of toxemic guinea pigs, treated with antitoxin at a time when clinical signs were present, may well be correlated with the survival of intoxicated humans treated with Botulism Immune Plasma (Human).

DISCUSSION

In the present work, it was revealed that circulating botulinum neurotoxin could be detected well before clinical signs of botulism appeared and that passive immunization with Botulism Immune Plasma (Human), guinea pig antiserum, or equine antitoxin is effective in the prophylaxis and treatment of botulism in guinea pigs.

The effective half-life of heterologous (equine) antitoxin was determined to be 5 to 7 days in man. Habermann and Bernáth (1975) reported on the preparation of a small quantity (serum from 500 ml of blood) of human antibodies to botulinal toxins A, B and E by repeated injections of pentavalent toxoid in a healthy volunteer. They demonstrated the efficacy of their human antitoxin in mice and reported its ability to retard the progress of intoxication and improve survival rates even when antitoxin was given 8 hr after poisoning. However, in man, due to the scarcity of this valuable human antiserum, it was suggested that therapy should be started with high-titer heterologous antitoxin and later continue with the human antiserum.

The feasibility of clinical application of homologous antibotulin plasma and its medical value in 16 patients were first reported by Piven' et al. (1975). Subsequently the treatment of 4 children with antibotulinal homologous plasma was described and compared to children treated with heterologous (horse) antitoxin. In this same study Fekliosova et al. (1977) reported that serum sickness, as a complication of serum therapy, developed in 1/3 of the cases treated with a heterologous (horse) product. Because of the rarity of homologous antitoxin, Sinel'nikov et al. (1978) suggested that a purified antibotulinal serum from a second heterologous species (cattle) be manufactured and used to assure a lesser degree of reactogenicity to prophylactic and therapeutic preparations.

Evidence concerning the exact amount of circulating heterologous or homologous antitoxin needed to neutralize experimental botulinum toxin poisoning is incomplete. Results from animal experimentation suggest that the success of treatment depends, as it does in other comparable conditions, largely on the time interval elapsing between the onset of symptoms and the peak of circulating administered antitoxin is reached.

Although the efficacy of Botulism Immune Plasma (Human) has not been substantiated in human botulism, the 500 liters of this human immune product we have collected should offer two advantages over heterologous antitoxins: (1) lack of a foreign protein reaction and (2) a prolonged level of effective homologous antibody. Antitoxin immunoglobulins of human origin, which could persist for several weeks after administration would be highly desirable, particularly for the treatment of infant botulism (Arnon *et al.*, 1978).

ACKNOWLEDGEMENTS

The volunteers were civilian United States Government employees. These tests were governed by the principles, policies, and rules for medical volunteers as established by Army Regulation 70-25 and the Declaration of Helsinki. The study was conducted as part of a long-term program for the investigation of mechanisms of vaccine efficacy and host responses to infectious diseases.

In conducting the research described in this report, the investigators adhered to the "Guide for the Care and Use of Laboratory Animals," as promulgated by the Committee on Care and Use of Laboratory Animals of the Institute of Laboratory Animal Resources, National Research Council. The facilities are fully accredited by the American Association for Accreditation of Laboratory Animal Care. The views of the authors do not purport to reflect the positions of the Department of the Army or the Department of Defense.

We are very grateful for the outstanding technical support provided by Robert M. Wood.

REFERENCES

Arnon, S. S., T. F. Midura, K. Damus, R. M. Wood, and J. Chin (1978). Intestinal infection and toxin production by *Clostridium botulinum* as one cause of sudden infant death syndrome. *Lancet, I*, 1273-1277.

Cooper, M. S. (1964). In K. H. Lewis and K. Cassel, Jr. (Ed.), *Botulism*. U.S. Public Health Service, Cincinnati, Ohio. pp. 146-164.

Fekliosova, L. V., E. S. Safonova, S. G. Pak, E. N. Levina, and V. S. Vinogradov (1977). Characteristics of botulism (serotype A) in children. *Sov. Med., 40(5)*, 70-72.

Habermann, E., and S. Bernáth (1975). Preparation, measurement and possible use of human antitoxin against *C. botulinum* A, B, and E toxins. *Med. Microbiol. Immunol.*, *161*, 203-210.

Lewis, G. E., Jr., and J. F. Metzger (1978). Botulism Immune Plasma (Human). *Lancet, II*, 634-635.

Merson, M. H., J. M. Hughes, V. R. Dowell, A. Taylor, W. H. Barker, and E. J. Gangarosa (1974). Current trends in botulism in the United States. *J. Am. Med. Assoc., 229*, 1305-1308.

Piven', I. N., T. V. Golosova, and A. V. Sidorova (1975). Therapeutic efficacy of homologous antibotulism plasma. *Probl. Gematol. Pereliv. Krovi, 20(11)*, 46-49.

Sinel'nikov, G. Ye., S. M. Preger, and N. Kh. Muzafarova (1978). Anaphylactogenic, antigenic and avid properties of antibotulin serum from the blood of various species of animals. *Zh. Mikrobiol. Epidemiol. Immunobiol., 55(1)*, 123-127.

Smolens, J., A. B. Vogt, M. N. Crawford, and J. Stokes, Jr. (1961). The persistence in the human circulation of horse and human tetanus antitoxins. *J. Pediatr., 59*, 899-902.

EFFECT OF TETANUS TOXIN ON THE EXCITATORY TRANSMISSION OF THE MOTONEURONE AND OTHER SYNAPSES IN THE MOTOR SYSTEM

K. Takano*, K. Kanda, F. Kirchner*, H. Kretzschmar*, M. Mizote** and P. Terhaar***

**Department of Physiology, University of Göttingen, Humboldtallee 7, D-3400 Göttingen, Federal Republic of Germany*
***Department of Physiology, Chiba University, Chiba, Japan*

ABSTRACT

The monosynaptic reflex was partially or totally blocked by tetanus toxin at relatively low doses, when toxin was injected into the muscle. Depression of the IPSP was followed by that of the EPSP. Tetanus toxin blocks the endplate of the phasic muscle more strongly than that of the tonic muscle. Cholinergic transmission of the Renshaw cell is left intact. There is no selective blocking of inhibitory synapses by tetanus toxin in the strict sense.

KEYWORDS

Tetanus toxin; local tetanus; monosynaptic reflex; stretch reflex; motoneurone; EPSP and IPSP; neuromuscular transmission, fast and slow muscle; Renshaw cell.

MONOSYNAPTIC REFLEX

Since the classical study of Brooks, Curtis and Eccles (1957), it is generally accepted that tetanus toxin blocks the inhibitory synapses on the spinal motoneurone without affecting the excitatory transmission, because (they wrote) the monosynaptic reflex is not affected by tetanus toxin. Sverdlov (1960) reported a depression of the monosynaptic reflex; however, this study received little attention or was interpreted incorrectly, (e.g. Zacks and Sheff, 1970; Laurence and Webster, 1963). Brooks, Curtis and Eccles (1957) tested the monosynaptic reflex in the early period after the injection of high doses of tetanus toxin into the sciatic nerve or into the spinal cord of the cat. They did not test the monosynaptic reflex in the later stage of tetanus intoxication.

In our study (including Terhaar and others, 1977) tetanus toxin (T9, Behringwerke) at various doses (1-2000 mouse MLD/kg) was injected into the left gastrocnemius muscle of the cat. The input-output relation of the motoneurone was investigated at various stimulus strength and the reflex amplitude was plotted. In the early period (e.g. 50 h after toxin injection, 500 mouse MLD/kg) the monosynaptic reflex as well as the phasic stretch reflex in response to a short rapid stretch of the muscle were enhanced. But in cats a depression of the monosynaptic reflex could be found 7 days after the injection at the dose of only 1 mouse MLD/kg.

Analyzing such input-output relations of the monosynaptic as well as of the stretch reflex, it could be concluded that the motoneurone could be excited with a smaller amount of afferent input in the early period, whereas in the later period the motoneurone needed greater input to fire. The monosynaptic reflex was highly depressed or totally blocked in the later period also in animals which received low doses of toxin intramuscularly. The general tendency was that in the early period the stretch reflex was more activated than the monosynaptic reflex. This suggests the higher sensitivity of the muscle spindle and supports our suggestion that the gamma-motor-system is activated and so mediates high motor activity in the early period of local tetanus (e.g. Takano and Kano, 1973). There is also some possibility that the spontaneous inhibitory inflow into the motoneurone decreases and therefore the motoneurone is more sensitive to the excitatory input in the early period.

IPSP AND EPSP

Gushchin, Kozhechkin and Sverdlov (1969) observed abolition of the inhibitory postsynaptic potential (IPSP) of the motoneurone recorded intracellularly in tetanus intoxication. Since excitatory transmission in the endplate (e.g. Kryzhanovsky, 1967) or in the terminals of the Sphincter pupille (e.g. Ambache, Morgan and Wright, 1948) can be blocked by tetanus toxin, the excitatory synapse of the motoneurone might be also blocked. When the monosynaptic reflex is reduced in the later period of tetanus intoxication it is possible that the excitatory postsynaptic potential (EPSP) is depressed or blocked by tetanus toxin. Tetanus toxin at the dose of 100 mouse MLD/kg was injected into the gastrocnemius muscle of the left hind leg of the cat. The postsynaptic potential of the motoneurone to the gastrocnemius in response to the stimulus of the group Ia nerve fibres was recorded, using an intracellular micropipette electrode (for the method see e.g. Eccles, 1953). Within 3 days after the injection of toxin, IPSPs were still detectable but their amplitudes were minimal. Fig. 1 shows the number of gastrocnemius motoneurones (ordinate) and the postsynaptic hyperpolarisation (IPSP) in response to the antagonistic deep peroneal nerve stimulation. Control (a); 30-48 h (b) and 55-72 h (c) after tetanus toxin (100 mouse MLD/kg) injection into the gastrocnemius muscle of the cat.

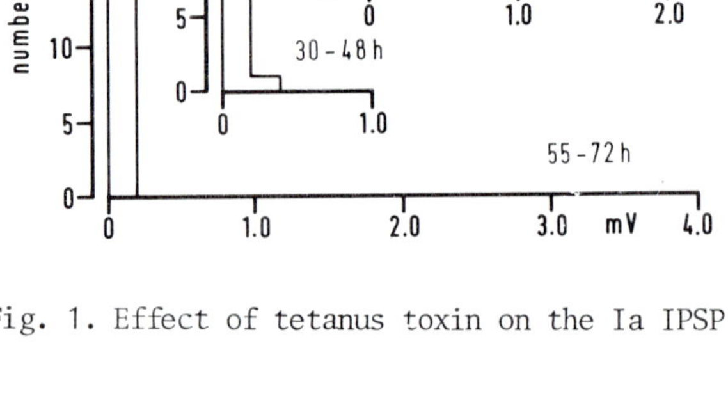

Fig. 1. Effect of tetanus toxin on the Ia IPSP

The EPSP was also greatly depressed or diminished during the five days as shown in Fig. 2 by the number of gastrocnemius motoneurones with EPSPs in response to stimulation of the Ia afferent fibres.

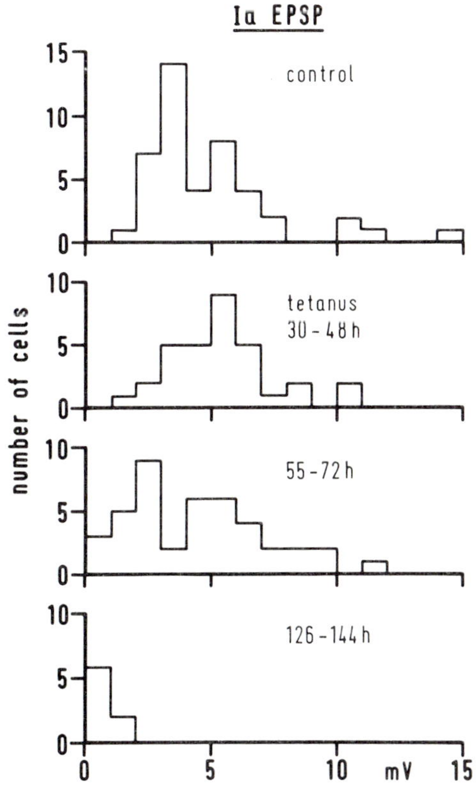

Fig. 2. Effect of tetanus toxin on the Ia EPSP

From the experiment of the monosynaptic reflex and of the EPSP it was clearly shown that tetanus toxin at rather low doses blocks not only inhibitory synapses but also excitatory synapses on the motoneurone.

Sherrington (1906) wrote that tetanus toxin converts inhibition into excitation in the spinal reflex pathway. This comment is correct, if we observe the reflex as an integrated action (see Takano and Henatsch, 1973; Fig. 5). This conversion of inhibition into excitation could be observed, when we stimulated the sural nerve. In response to sural nerve stimulation in nonintoxicated animals about 2/3 of PSPs were IPSPs and 1/3 were of the mixed type (EPSP and IPSP), while only 2 cells of 33 showed predominantly depolarization. Two days after tetanus intoxication almost all cells showed only depolarizing PSPs while some cells showed mixed type but none of them showed hyperpolarization (Fig. 3). The duration of the afterhyperpolarization and input resistance of motoneurone showed no or little, if any, change throughout the investigated period.

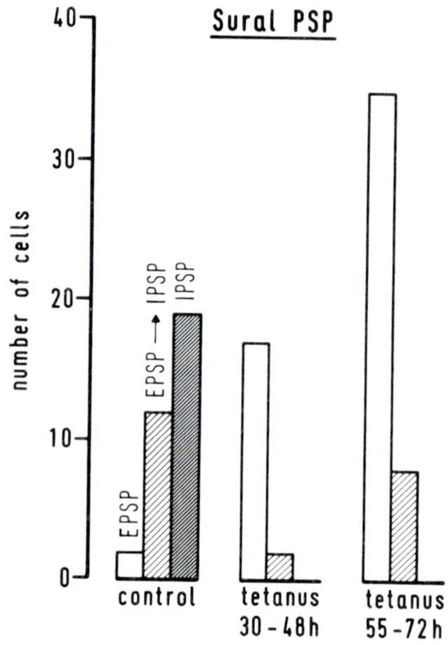

Fig. 3. Change in PSP of the intoxicated gastrocnemius motoneurone in response to stimulation of the sural nerve at stimulus strength five times that of threshold. Those cells indicated "EPSP" or "IPSP" showed predominantly EPSPs or IPSPs respectively, the cells indicated "EPSP → IPSP" showed first depolarization followed by hyperpolarization.

Since it might be possible that tetanus toxin acts on membranes, various authors studied the effect of it on the conduction velocity of the nerves in which tetanus toxin is transported intracellularly (e.g. Price and coworkers, 1975). Westhues (1964) found no change in the conduction velocity of myelinated as well as non-myelinated fibres bathed in Locke solution with tetanus toxin for 4 h. Wiegand, Hilbig and Wellhöner (1977) reported no change of latency between stimulation of the gastrocnemius nerve and responses of the dorsal root until 12 h after toxin injection into the gastrocnemius muscle of the cat. There was also no change in the latency of the muscle action potential in response to nerve stimulation 58 h after the toxin injection into the muscle (Takano, 1976). The conduction velocity of the single alpha- motor fibre was measured during the identification of the motoneurone. We found that there is no change in the conduction velocity in the individual motor fibres up to 140 h after toxin injection (Fig. 4).

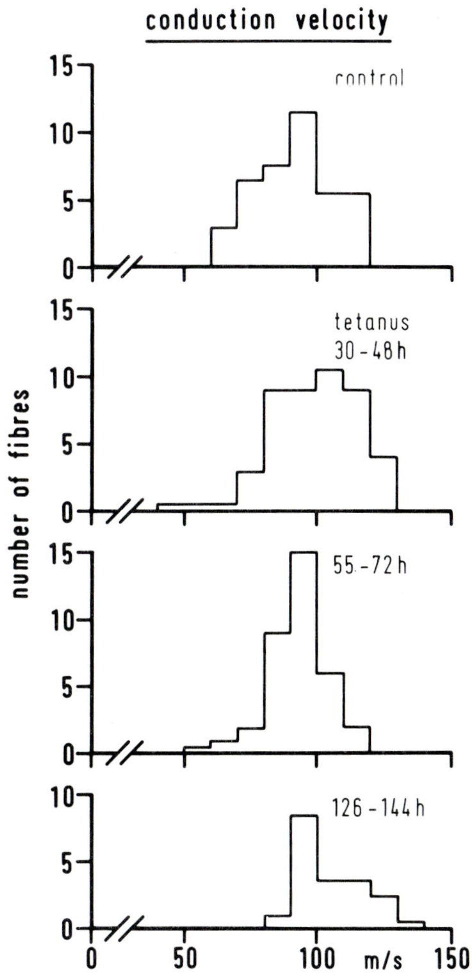

Fig. 4. Conduction velocity of the alpha-motor-nerve fibres to the gastrocnemius muscle of control and after tetanus intoxication.

NEUROMUSCULAR TRANSMISSION

Duchen and Tonge (1973) concluded that the neuromuscular transmission of the slow muscles is more sensitive to tetanus toxin than that of the fast muscles in the mouse. However, we observed the opposite effects in the cat (Takano, 1978). We resolved the discrepancy by injecting small volumes of toxin into the muscle of the rat. Fig. 5 shows the dose-effect-relation in the tibialis anterior (●), gastrocnemius (O) and soleus (▲) muscles of the hind leg. The effect (ordinate) shows reduction of the amplitude of the electromyogram following nerve stimulation. 100% means a total blockage of the neuromuscular transmission. The neuromuscular transmission of the fast tibialis anterior was about 4 times more sensitive than that of the slow soleus. The gastrocnemius and two forelimb muscles (not shown here), the extensor carpi radialis and the flexor carpi ulnaris, showed medium sensitivity. In all five muscles the contraction time was measured and correlated with their blocking dose. The faster the muscle, the more sensitive is the neuromuscular transmission to the action of tetanus toxin. The fibres of the muscle were stained and the numbers of red, intermediate and white fibres were counted. The percentage of white fibres in the muscle was negatively correlated with the minimal blocking dose needed for total blocking of neuromuscular transmission. For further information see Kretzschmar, Kirchner and Takano (1980).

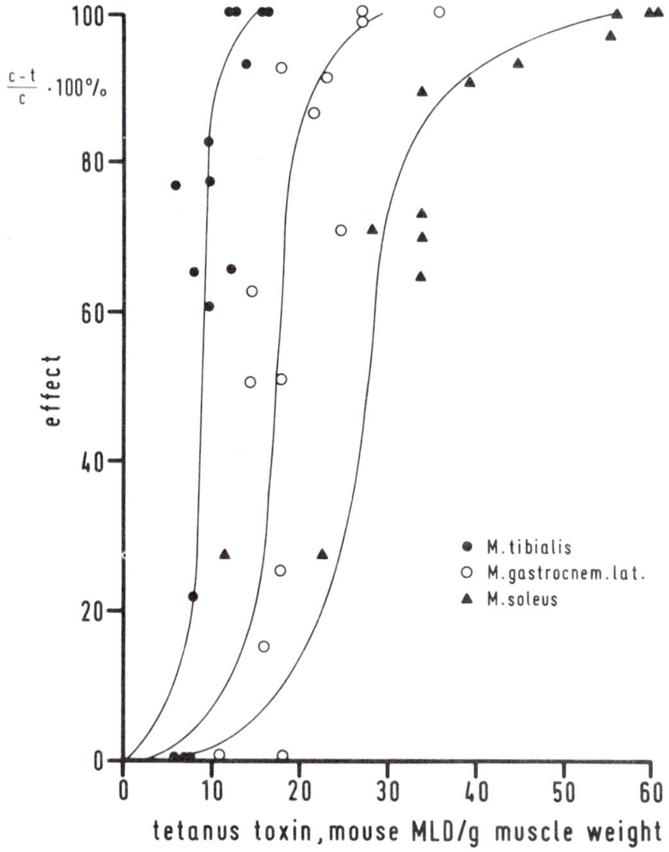

Fig. 5. Tetanus toxin dose-effect-relation of three hind leg muscles of the rat.

CHOLINERGIC SYNAPSE ON THE RENSHAW CELL.

The Renshaw cell is excited by the impulses of the collateral of the motor axon. The transmission to the Renshaw cell is cholinergic. This transmission was not affected by toxin for 18 h, when toxin was injected into the sciatic nerve (Brooks, Curtis and Eccles, 1958). Curtis and de Groat (1968) injected toxin close to the cell and found no effect on the cholinergic transmission in several hours. Curtis (1971) stated: "It is possible that sufficient time was not allowed in these investigations for tetanus toxin to affect cholinergic transmission, ...". We could always bring the Renshaw cell to fire by stimulating the motor nerve also long after toxin injection into muscle (44 h, after the application of lethal doses, Benecke and coworkers, 1978; 24 days, sublethal doses, Kirchner and Takano, 1977). The cholinergic synapse on the Renshaw cell seems not to be influenced at least in clinical tetanus and also in experimental local tetanus, when toxin is injected into the muscle. We do not rule out the possibility that this synapse can be blocked at a higher local toxin concentration.

ACKNOWLEDGEMENT

This study was supported by the Deutsche Forschungsgemeinschaft (SFB 33). Tetanus toxin was kindly supplied by Behringwerke AG (Marburg). Technical assistance of Ms. G. Federkeil and Ms. G. Thiele are greatfully acknowledged. English text was checked by Mr. D. Shefcyk.

REFERENCES

Ambache, N., R.S. Morgan and G.P. Wright (1948). The action of tetanus toxin on the rabbit's iris. J. Physiol. (Lond.) 107, 45-53.

Benecke, R., K. Takano, J. Schmidt and H.-D. Henatsch (1977). Tetanus toxin induced actions on spinal Renshaw cells and Ia-inhibitory interneurones during development of local tetanus in the cat. Exp. Brain Res. 27, 272-286.

Brooks, V.B., D.R. Curtis and J.C. Eccles (1957). The action of tetanus toxin on the inhibition of motoneurones. J. Physiol. (Lond.) 135, 655-672.

Curtis, D.R, (1971). Tetanus toxin as a neuropharmacological tool. In L.L. Simpson (Ed.), Neuropoisons - Their Pathophysiological Actions, Vol. 1. Poisons of animal origin. Plenum Press, London, pp. 263-281.

Curtis, D.R. and W.C. de Groat (1968). Tetanus toxin and spinal inhibition. Brain Res. 10, 208-212.

Duchen, L.W. and D.A. Tonge (1973). The effect of tetanus toxin on neuromuscular transmission and on the morphology of motor end-plates in slow and fast skeletal muscle of the mouse. J. Physiol. (Lond.) 228, 157-172.

Eccles, J.C. (1953). The Neurophysiological Basis of Mind. The Principles of Neurophysiology. Clarendon Press, Oxford.

Gushchin, I.S., S.N. Kozhechkin and Y.S. Sverdlov (1970). Hyperpolarizing action of glycine on motoneurones blocked by tetanus toxin. Byull. eksp. Biol. Med. 70, 29-32.

Kirchner, F. and Takano, K. (1977). The activity of the Renshaw cell in the later period of local tetanus. In Proc. IUPS 13, p. 388.

Kretzschmar, H., F. Kirchner and K. Takano (1980). Relations between the effect of tetanus toxin on the neuromuscular transmission and histological functional properties of various muscles of the rat. Exp. Brain Res. (in the press).

Kryzhanovsky, G.N. (1967). The neural pathway of toxin: its transport to the central nervous system and the state of the spinal reflex apparatus in tetanus intoxication. In L. Eckmann (Ed.) Principles of Tetanus, H. Huber, Bern, pp. 155-168.

Laurence, D.R. and R.A. Webster (1963). Pathologic physiology, pharmacology and therapeutics of tetanus. Clin. Pharmacol. Therap. 4, 36-72.

Price, D.L., J. Griffin, A. Young, K. Peck and A. Stocks (1975). Tetanus toxin: Direct evidence for retrograde intraaxonal transport. Science 188, 945-947.

Sherrington, C.S. (1906). The Integrative Action of the Nervous System, Yale University Press, New Haven.

Sverdlov, Y.S. (1960). The spinal cord reflex activity under local tetanus (electrophysiological study). J. Physiol. USSR 46, 941-947.

Takano, K. (1976). The effect of tetanus toxin on the extensor and flexor muscles of the hind leg of the cat. In A. Ohsaka, K. Hayashi and Y. Sawai (Eds.), Animal, Plant and Microbial Toxins, Vol. 2, Plenum Publ. London, pp. 363-378.

Takano, K. and H.-D. Henatsch (1973). Tension-extension diagram of the tetanus intoxicated muscle of the cat. Naunyn-Schmiedeberg's Arch. Pharmacol. 276, 421-436.

Takano, K. and M. Kano (1973). Gamma-bias of the muscle poisoned by tetanus toxin. Naunyn-Schmiedeberg's Arch. Pharmacol. 276, 413-420.

Terhaar, P., B. Tiebert, F. Kirchner and K. Takano (1977). Monosynaptic reflex during local tetanus. Pflügers Arch. 368, R 35.

Westhues, M. (1964). Untersuchungen an marklosen Nervenfasern über den Wirkungsort von Botulinus- und Tetanustoxin. Naunyn-Schmiedeberg's Arch. Pharmacol. 246, 309-315.

Wiegand, H., G. Hilbig and H.H. Wellhöner (1977). Early local tetanus: Does tetanus toxin change the stimulus evoked discharge in afferents from the injected muscle? Naunyn-Schmiedeberg's Arch. Pharmacol. 298, 189-191.

Zacks, I and M.F. Sheff (1970). Tetanism: Pathobiological aspects of the action of tetanal toxin in the nervous system and skeletal muscle. Neurosci. Res. 3, 209-287.

NEW TRENDS IN THE STUDY OF THE PATHOGENESIS OF TETANUS SYMPTOMS IN THE MOTOR SYSTEM

K. Takano, F. Kirchner, H. Kretzschmar, P. Terhaar and B. Tiebert

Department of Physiology, University of Göttingen, Humboldtallee 7, D-3400 Göttingen, Federal Republic of Germany

ABSTRACT

This communication aims to clarify the cause of some of the controversial observations in the neurophysiological experiments on tetanus and to point out future trends. It is concluded: The hypothesis that the hyperactivity of the motor system in tetanus is caused by disinhibition, must be critically examined.

KEYWORDS

Local tetanus; generalized tetanus; presynaptic inhibition; polysynaptic reflex; proprioceptive reflex; tremor; EEG; electrospinogram.

PRESYNAPTIC INHIBITION

When a primary afferent fibre is depolarized through axo-axonal synapses the amplitude of its spike is decreased causing a decrease of transmitter release from its presynaptic terminal. Thus the EPSP on the motoneurone is depressed. This is known as presynaptic inhibition. The electrotonic spread of the primary afferent depolarization can be recorded on the surface of the dorsal root as the "dorsal root potential". Presynaptic inhibition is characterized by its appearance and prolonged duration. Sverdlov and Alekseeva (1965) reported that presynaptic inhibition diminished in local tetanus following intramuscular toxin injection, but the dorsal root potential was not changed. Kano and Ischikawa (1972) demonstrated a blocking effect of tetanus toxin on the inhibitory synapses of the crayfish. The transmitter of this synapse and that of the axo-axonal synapse of the primary afferent fibres of the mammalian spinal cord is supposed to be GABA. Curtis and his coworkers (1973) found neither dorsal root potential nor presynaptic inhibition when they injected a high dose of tetanus toxin into the spinal cord. However, Kryzhanovsky and Lutsenko (1969) found an increase of dorsal root potential when they injected toxin intramuscularly.

In our study (Tiebert and others, 1977), we could observe delayed prolonged inhibition in almost all experiments provided that the monosynaptic reflex was present (see Takano and others, in this book). We injected tetanus toxin into the gastrocnemius muscle at high doses and the experiment was performed when local tetanus was well developed. The test stimulus was given to the nerves to the gastrocnemius after a conditioning stimulus on the deep peroneal nerve. The time course of the delayed inhibition was lengthened sometimes to as long as 3 sec after the conditioning inhibitory stimulus. The local concentration of toxin in the experiment of Curtis and his coworkers must have been far higher than that in the experiment with intramuscular toxin injection. The toxin concentration in the spinal segment was also very high in the above mentioned experiments (including ours with intramuscular injection) when we compare it with that of clinical tetanus. Thus it is suggested that the presynaptic inhibition is not blocked in clinical tetanus.

GENERALIZED TETANUS

As mentioned above, the local concentration in experimental local tetanus might be too high compared to that in clinical tetanus. In clinical tetanus the usual manifestation of the disease is generalized tetanus. In our study, tetanus toxin at high lethal doses was injected intravenously. The acute experiments were performed after the maximal symptoms of convulsion and tremor had developed. The animal was anaesthetized shortly before the time in which the animal would otherwise die. The spontaneous high electromyographic (EMG) activity of the gastrocnemius muscle of the cat could be increased by passive stretching of the muscle to a certain length, but with additional stretching the activity was depressed showing the action of autogenic Group Ib inhibition on the stretch reflex. The antagonistic peroneal nerve was stimulated with single electrical stimuli of various strengths. This produced a flexor muscle twitch and thereby stretched the extensor muscle. The EMG of the stretch reflex in the gastrocnemius muscle (extensor) could be depressed partly or totally when the stimulus strength was respectively 3 or 4 times the threshold. The amplitude of flexor contraction did not change and therefore there was no change of muscle stretching. The muscle stretch was preceded at various intervals by conditioning inhibitory stimuli. The postsynaptic as well as delayed presynaptic inhibition was pronounced in the severe case of tetanus. Mutual inhibition between Renshaw cells may be mediated by glycine, and was blocked in the later stage of local tetanus (Kirchner and Takano, 1977). The mutual inhibition of Renshaw cells could always be observed during severe generalized tetanus in rabbits.

In generalized tetanus of rabbits, rhythmic EEG activity of the cerebellum could be observed (Huck, Gogolák and Stumpf, 1976). A rhythmic activity synchronized to that of the cerebellum could be observed also in the electrospinogram. After transection of the spinal cord this rhythm disappeared only distally from the transection. In the extracellular recording in immobilized animals, a very high number of alpha- and gamma-motoneurones and Renshaw cells innervating or belonging to the hind limb flexor and extensor muscles showed rhythmic activity correlated to the cerebellar rhythm. The rhythmic activity is of central origin and is transmitted to alpha- and gamma-motoneurones. Rhythmic activity in Renshaw cells might reflect motoneuronal activity or also be of supraspinal origin (Huck, Kirchner and Takano, 1977a, 1977b). Thus under our experimental conditions the hyperactivity of the spinal motor system of generalized tetanus was not caused by disinhibition of the spinal alpha motoneurone but by activation of the spinal cord modulated by the supraspinal structures.

GAMMA-MOTOR-SYSTEM

Without doubt there is a hyperactivity of spinal reflexes in clinical tetanus. There are direct and indirect ways of activating the muscle. The motoneurones innervating the muscle can be directly activated. The second way of activation is via gamma-motoneurones. When the gamma-motoneurone is activated the intrafusal muscle fibre in the muscle spindle contracts and sends more impulses through the primary fibre of the muscle spindle to the motoneurone which consequently fires more strongly.

The hyperactivity of the gamma-motor-system in tetanus was suggested by Rushworth (1960) and Erzina (1961), but questioned by Andrew and Barr (1958). Kano and Takano (1969) and Takano and Kano (1973) have presented experimental evidence showing that the gamma-motor-system plays an important role at least in the early period of local tetanus. They measured the change of gamma-bias (Eldred, Granit and Merton, 1953), and concluded that rough pathological augmentation of the bias was more than 10 mm in the triceps surae muscle of the cat, which is beyond the physiological range (Takano and Kano, 1973). Further Takano and Henatsch (1973) observed a parallel shift of the tension-extension curve to the left during the development of tetanus symptoms. The curve could be shifted back parallel to the right with a selective blocking of the gamma motor fibres by procaine. Under experimental conditions (10^4 mouse MLD/kg , intracellularly injected), the tetanus symptom could not be observed in the muscle lacking the gamma-motor-system (Takano and Kano, 1973; Takano, 1976). In a preliminary study in our laboratory, the muscle spindle was activated by frequency modulated vibration (for the method see Mizote, 1976), and we found evidence for a strong activation of the nuclear bag fibres in the muscle spindle in the early period of local tetanus. In the later period the Ia fibre discharge lost its dynamic pattern showing a rigid state of the nuclear bag fibres (contracture?). On the other hand Webster (1967) reported that he found no hyperactive gamma-efferents in rabbits with local tetanus. He used intracollicular decerebrate animals, which have elevated gamma-bias. Therefore the effects of tetanus toxin might be at least partly covered by decerebration. One should take into account that the muscle spindle does not fire when the extrafusal muscle is shortened by contraction. Further one should not take tension as the parameter of muscle stretch, since the stiffness of the muscle is far greater in the intoxicated muscle than the control one, due to physiological (active tension) and physical (passive tension) change of the muscle (Takano and Henatsch, 1973; Takano, 1976). Such factors should be taken into consideration in the experiments with the gamma-system, otherwise the results are not relevant.

Diazepam is extensively used by clinicians in the treatment of tetanus. Brausch and others (1973) and Takano and Student (1978) have shown that diazepam acts far more strongly on the gamma-motor-system than on the alpha-system. This is an indirect support of our hypothesis concerning the role of the gamma-system in tetanus intoxication. There are, however, some clinical studies which report that in severe cases of tetanus, diazepam is not effective. In the severe case of tetanus the alpha-motoneurone is also directly hyperactivated and the reduction of Ia-impulses (therefore, of gamma activity) cannot reduce the elevated hypersensitivity of the motoneurone. In such cases diazepam has no effect on the motor activity and the additional depressant drugs (e.g. barbiturate acting also in the alpha-system) must be used. In modern experimental tetanus with high doses of toxin, local tetanus can still be observed in a completely de-afferentated limb. This fact does not mean that the gamma-motor-system is not affected by toxin. The motoneurone is so sensitive (regardless of the presence or absence of disinhibition) that any tiny excitable input causes the firing of the motoneurone and the Ia-input is not necessary to excite the alpha-motoneurone. In old studies such as Liljestrand and Magnus (1919) with lower doses of toxin, we can find a more clinically relevant experiment supporting the gamma-hypothesis.

Tetanus toxin has a multimodal effect, changing its features according to the dose used and the form of application. A gross tentative speculation of the effect of tetanus toxin on various components of the motor system at different doses is shown in Fig. 1. For example, in generalized tetanus at just lethal dose (1 MLD), the higher central nervous system is also activated. The alteration of the alpha

TENTATIVE SCHEMA OF PATHOLOGICAL CHANGE OF VARIOUS COMPONENTS OF THE MOTOR SYSTEM IN TETANUS

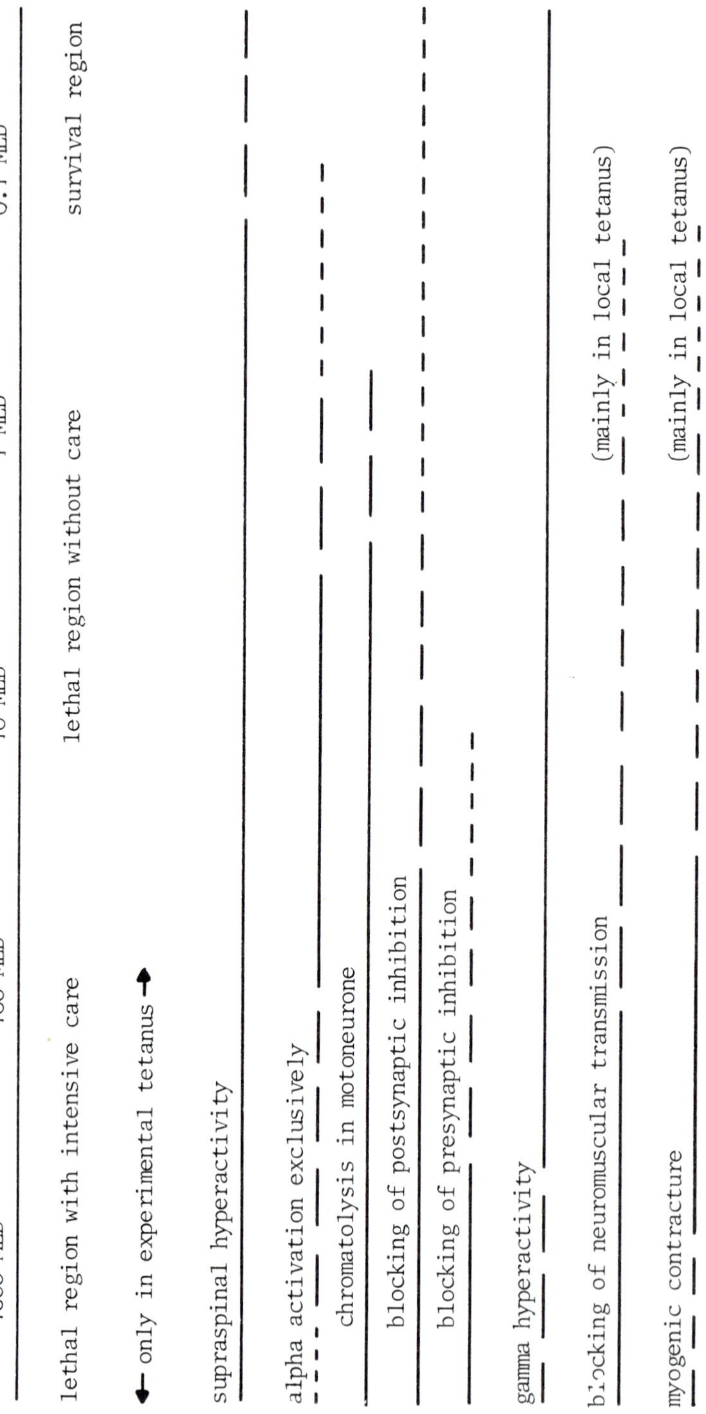

Fig. 1.

motoneurone might be slight (long interrupted line), the postsynaptic inhibition might be almost intact (short interrupted line), and the presynaptic inhibition might not be affected. Blocking of the endplate does not occur as long as there is no local tetanus. Myogenic contracture might exist in the extensor muscle, when a very high muscle activity develops.

ACKNOWLEDGEMENT

This study was supported by the Deutsche Forschungsgemeinschaft (SFB 33). Tetanus toxin was kindly supplied by Behringwerke AG (Marburg). Technical assistance of Ms. G. Federkeil and Ms. G. Thiele are greatfully acknowledged. The discussion of Dr. Fedenic during the Symposium in Uppsala was greatly appreciated.

REFERENCES

Andrew, B.L. and M.N. Barr (1958). Anaesthesia and local tetanus intoxication. J. Physiol. (Lond.) 141, 40-41.

Brausch, U., H.-D. Henatsch, C. Student and K. Takano (1973). Effect of Diazepam on the development of stretch reflex tension. In S. Garattini, E. Mussini and L.O. Randal (Eds.), The Benzodiazepines, Raven Press, New York. pp 531-543.

Curtis, D.R., D. Felix, C.J.A. Game and R.M. McCulloch (1973). Tetanus toxin and the synaptic release of GABA. Brain Res. 51, 358-362.

Eldred, E.R., R. Granit and P.A. Merton (1953). Supraspinal control of the muscle spindles and its significance. J. Physiol. (Lond.) 122, 498-523.

Erzina, G.A. (1961). Effects of the gamma-neurone system on the electrical activity of muscle spindles during local tetanus in the cat. Sechenow J. Physiol. (Eng.) 47, 30-33.

Huck, S., G. Gogolák and Ch. Stumpf (1976). Rhythmic cerebellar and cortical electric activity in tetanus intoxicated rabbits. Experientia 32, 200-201.

Huck, S., F. Kirchner and K. Takano (1977a). Tetanus intoxication in rabbits: Propagation of a supraspinal rhythm into the spinal cord. Pflügers Arch. 368, R 36.

Huck, S., F. Kirchner and K. Takano (1977b). Correlation between tetanus toxin induced rhythm of the cerebellum and the spinal motor output in rabbits. In "Joint Meeting of German and Italian Pharmacologists", Venecia, October 4-6, p.382.

Kano, M. and K. Ishikawa (1972). Effect of tetanus toxin on the inhibitory neuromuscular junction of crayfish muscle. Exp. Neurology. 37, 550-561.

Kano, M. and K. Takano (1969) Gamma activity of rigid cat caused by tetanus toxin. Japan J. Physiol. 19, 1-10.

Kirchner, F. and K. Takano (1977). The activity of the Renshaw cell in the later period of local tetanus. In Proc. IUPS 13, p. 388.

Kryzhanovsky, G.N. and V.K. Lutsenko (1969). Dorsal root potential of the spinal cord in rats with convulsions due to ascending tetanus. Byull. eksp. Biol. Med. 67, 16-19.

Liljestrand, G. and R. Magnus (1919). Über die Wirkung des Novokains auf den normalen und den tetanusstarren Skelettmuskel und über die Entstehung der lokalen Muskelstarre beim Wundstarrkrampf. Pflügers Arch. 176, 168-208.

Mizote, M. (1976). Effect of FM vibration on muscle spindles in the cat. In S. Homma (Ed.) Progress in Brain Res. Vol.44, Understanding the stretch reflex, Elsevier, Amsterdam, p. 133-140.

Rushworth, G. (1960) Spasticity and rigidity: An experimental study and review. J. Neurol. Neurosurg. Psychiatr. 23, 99-118.

Sverdlov, Y.S. (1960). The spinal cord reflex activity under local tetanus (electrophysiological study). J. Physiol. USSR 46, 941-947.

Sverdlov, Y.S. and V.I. Alekseeva (1965). Effect of tetanus toxin on presynaptic inhibition in the spinal cord. J. Physiol. USSR 51, 1441-1452.

Takano, K. (1976). The effect of tetanus toxin on the extensor and flexor muscles of the hind leg of the cat. In A. Ohsaka, K. Hayashi and Y. Sawai (Eds.), Animal, Plant and Microbial Toxins, Vol. 2, Plenum Publ. London, pp. 363-378.

Takano, K. and H.-D. Henatsch (1973). Tension-extension of the tetanus intoxicated muscle of the cat. Naunyn-Schmiedeberg's Arch. Pharmacol. 276, 421-436.

Takano, K. and M. Kano (1973). Gamma-bias of the muscle poisoned by tetanus toxin. Naunyn-Schmiedeberg's Arch. Pharmacol. 276, 413-420.

Takano, K. and J.C. Student (1978). Effect of diazepam on the gamma motor system indicated by the responses of the muscle spindle of the triceps surae muscle of the decerebrate cat to the muscle stretch. Naunyn-Schmiedeberg's Arch. Pharmacol. 302, 91-101.

Tiebert, B., P. Terhaar, F. Kirchner and K. Takano (1977). Presynaptic inhibition during local tetanus. Pflügers Arch. 368, R 36.

Webster, R.A. (1967). The effect of tetanus toxin on motor nerve activity in the rabbit. Int. J. Neuropharmacol. 6, 207-215.

Novel Toxins and Toxic Effects

STRUCTURE-ACTIVITY STUDIES ON BEE VENOM POLYPEPTIDES

B. E. C. Banks*, C. Dempsey and A. J. Garman****

**Department of Physiology*
***Department of Chemistry, University College London, Gower Street, London WC1E 6BT, UK*

ABSTRACT

Peptide 401, a twenty-two residue peptide from bee venom that has mast-cell degranulating and anti-inflammatory activity, has been modified selectively for structure-activity studies. The reductively alkylated derivative is active as a degranulator of rat peritoneal mast cells, but is devoid of anti-inflammatory activity and it therefore seems unlikely that the peptide acts simply as a counter-irritant. The peptide has been found to be effective against skin-blueing in the guinea pig but does not release histamine from guinea pig mesenteric mast cells.

KEYWORDS

Apamin; peptide 401; mast-cell degranulation; anti-inflammatory agent.

INTRODUCTION

The two most important minor polypeptide constituents of the venom of the common European honey bee, Apis mellifera, are the centrally-acting eighteen-residue neurotoxin called apamin (Habermann & Reiz, 1965), and the twenty-two residue components called by Habermann (Breithaupt & Habermann, 1968) mast-cell degranulating peptide and by Vernon (Vernon and others, 1969) peptide 401. The structures of these two peptides given in Fig. 1 are superficially similar in that both contain two disulphide bridges with the same number of residues between the relevant half-cystines, both are basic and both have the C-terminal residue amidated (Shipolini & others, 1967; von Haux, 1969; Gauldie & others, 1978). Neither contains an aromatic amino acid residue. However, the biological effects of the two peptides are quite dissimilar. Apamin crosses the blood-brain barrier to act centrally by whatever route of administration, whereas peptide 401 only shows central nervous activity when injected directly into the cerebral ventricles. The symptoms of central intoxication are different in the two cases (Habermann, 1977). In addition, apamin has recently been found to have peripheral effects, in particular as a blocker of the inhibitory innervation of the smooth muscle of the gut (Vladimirova & Shuba, 1978; Banks and others, 1979). Peptide 401, on the other hand, has paradoxical activities. As a degranulator of rat peritoneal mast cells, the peptide produces an inflammatory response at the site of injection in rats due to release of histamine and 5-hydroxytryptamine, whereas it is as potent as an anti-inflammatory agent in rat models of both acute and chronic inflammation as any therapeutic agent presently available (Billingham & others, 1973; Hanson, Morley & Sorria-Herrera, 1974). We have sought to dissociate the various activities of the two peptides by selective chemical modification of side-chain residues.

A preliminary account of some of the results has been published, (Banks, Garman & Habermann, 1978). Only results relating to Peptide 401 will be given here.

MATERIALS AND METHODS

Chromatography. Peptide 401 and apamin were isolated from freeze dried bee venom, purchased from Bulgarcoop; Sofia, Bulgaria, essentially by the methods described by Gauldie and others, 1976, except that the ion exchange chromatography was on CM Sephadex C-25 rather than on SP-Sephadex C25. The eluant was ammonium formate buffer, pH4.7, 0.1*M* with linear salt gradients of 1.2 to 1.6 *M* in the case of Peptide 401 and 0.5 to 0.8 *M* for apamin. The relevant fractions were repeatedly chromatographed, (at least three times), before all traces of contaminating melittin were removed. The purity of peptides was checked by thin layer chromatography.

Chemical Modifications.

Acetamidation of disulphides. Peptide 401 was reduced with dithioerythritol and treated with iodo acetamide under nitrogen.

Modification of histidines was carried out by the method of Gleisner & Liener (1973) giving a di-acetonylated derivative.

Modification of arginines by reaction with 2,4-pentanedione was by the method of Gilbert & O'Leary (1975).

Modification of lysines by reaction with O-methyl isourea to form homoarginine was the method of Chervenka & Wilcox (1957). Formylation was carried out both by the methods of Sheehan & Yang (1958) and of Okawa & Hase (1963) and reductive alkylation by the method of Means & Feaney (1968).

Histamine release from mast cells. Degranulation of rat peritoneal mast cells or guinea pig mesenteric mast cells was determined as described by Atkinson, Ennis & Pearce (1979).

Rat paw oedema test. Inhibition of carrageenan induced oedema in rat hand paw was assessed by plenthysmography, (Billingham, Robinson & Robson 1969).

Neurotoxicity was assessed by Prof. E. Habermann using intracerobroventricular injection in mice.

RESULTS

The mast cell degranulating, anti-inflammatory and central nervous activities of Peptide 401 and the chemically modified variants of the peptide are given in Table 1.

The dose-response curve from which the histamine release caused by Peptide 401 is estimated, is illustrated in Fig. 2. and, for comparison, the degranulation caused by D-4-18 a polypeptide isolated from the venom of *Dendroaspis viridis* is included. The sequences of the largest loop of Peptide 401 and a fragment of the snake peptide are given in Fig. 3. Also included in Fig.2. is the effect of Peptide 401 on guinea pig mesenteric mast cells.

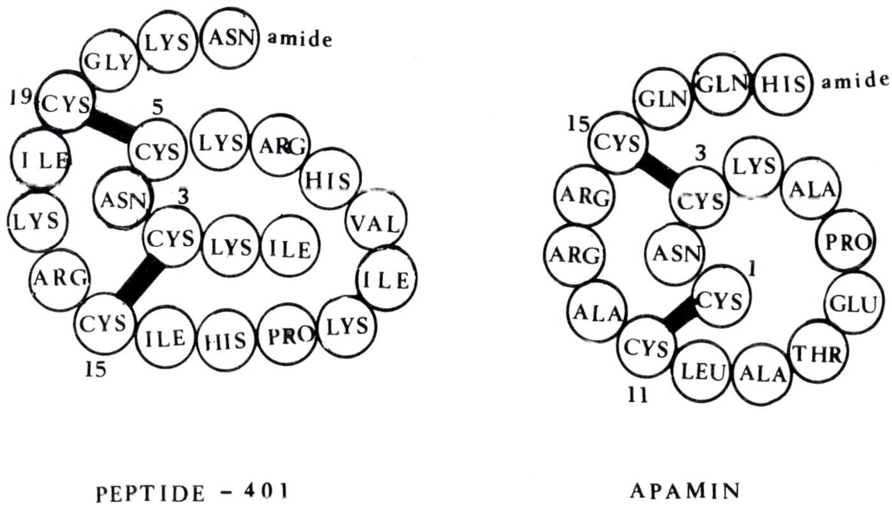

Fig.1. Amino acid sequences & disulphide bridge positions.

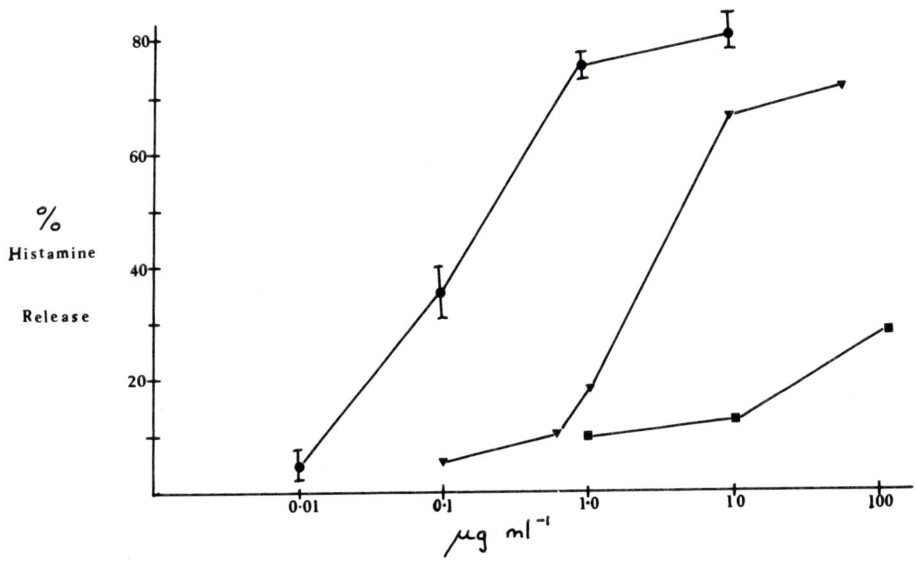

Fig.2. Histamine release from mastcells ● and ▼ rat peritoneal,■guinea pig mesenteric, ● & ■ Peptide 401, ▼ Dendroaspis viridis peptide.

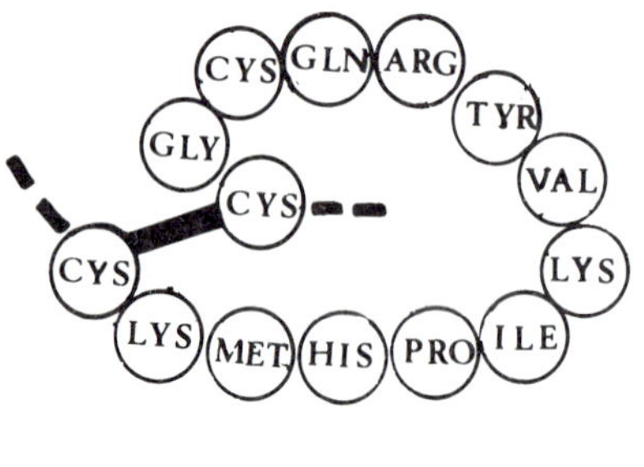

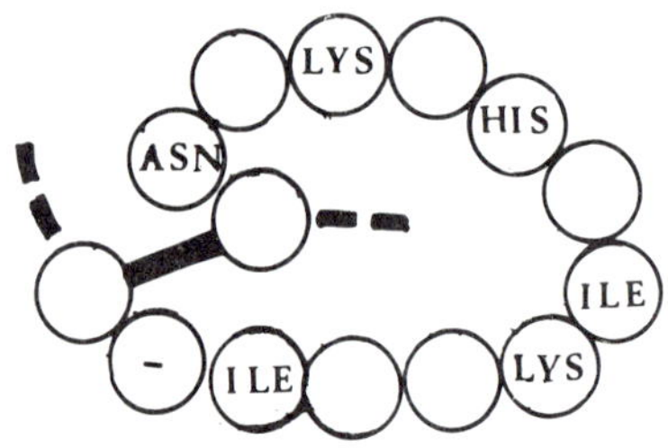

Fig.3. Homologous sequences in Peptide 401 & the Dendroaspis viridis peptide.

TABLE 1.

RESIDUE	MODIFICATION	MCD[a]	AI[b]	CNS[c]
	Native	1	1	1
Cys-Cys	Acetamidation	<0.003	<0.1	<0.015
Histidine (2)	Acetonylation	0.3	0.8	0.08
Arginine (2)	2,4 Pentanedione	0.05	<0.1	<0.015
Lysine (5)	guanidination	1.1	1.4	0.05
Lysine (1)	formylation (positions 2,17 or 21)	1	1	2
Lysines (5+N term)	formylation d.	0.03	?	0.04
Lysines (5+N term)	formylation e.	0.03	<0.1	-
Lysines (5+N term)	reductive alkylation	0.8	<0.1	-

a. Mast cell degranulating activity.
b. Anti-inflammatory activity in rat paw oedema test.
c. Central nervous activity on intraventicular injection.
d. Formylation by formic acid and acetic anhydride.
e. Formylation by reaction with p-nitrophnenylformate.

DISCUSSION

The presence in bee venom to the extent of ca.40% of melittin, the 26 residue detergent, makes the isolation of minor components a time consuming process. Up to three passages through an ion exchange column may be necessary to remove the last traces of melittin from samples of apamin or Peptide 401. Melittin has a lytic effect against all cells while other peptides have marked and varied biological effects at low concentrations so the isolation of pure peptides is an important prerequisite to any study of structure-activity relations.

In the original paper on the anti-inflammatory effects of Peptide 401, (Billingham & others, 1973), it was reported that the anti-inflammatory activity in the rat paw oedema test was unimpaired by pretreatment of the rats with mepyramine and methysergide at levels sufficient to protect the animals against the effects of histamine and 5-hydroxytryptamine respectively. It was concluded that the anti-inflammatory activity might well be independent of the mast cell degranulating activity and it was therefore decided to try to dissociate the two effects by selective chemical modification of amino acid side chains. Such a study depends heavily on the extent to which the chemical variants are purified and characterised for it is impossible to interpret results obtained with ill-characterised mixtures that may well contain unmodified peptides as contaminants. In the present work, all modified peptides have been separated by column chromatography shown to give single spots on TLC and subjected to amino acid analysis to check on the extent of modification of individual residues.

From the results in the table, it appears that the disulphide bridges are essential for all three activities of Peptide 401 and it is therefore unlikely that any smaller linear sequence of residues from the peptide will show any of the biological effects of the whole molecule. This finding also means that it is not possible to place any simple interpretation on the results of side chain modification in the sense of associating particular residues with an "active site", since a change in the three dimensional shape of the molecule may be sufficient to abolish activity. A case in point is the change in the arginine side chains since the 2,4-pentanedione derivative will be considerably bulkier than the unmodified residue. The evidence for arginine involvement in the central effects of apamin based on the use of synthetic analogues (Granier & others, 1978), is more convincing than the present evidence that arginines are needed for all the activities of Peptide 401. The effect of modifying the two histidine residues is interesting since there is here some evidence for partial dissociating of the three activities. The central nervous activity is very much reduced while the mast cell degranulating activity is more affected than is the anti-inflammatory activity. Guanidination of lysines again reduced the central activity without, in this case, significantly altering either of the other activities. The monoformyl derivative of Peptide 401 is a naturally occurring variant (Doonan & others, 1978) in which the formyl group is found on any one of three of the five lysines. It is fully active. Complete formylation of the molecule has been carried out by two methods, the first of which(formic acid and acetic anhydride) gave, on one occasion, a mixture of the penta and hexaformyl derivatives that retained some 30% of the anti-inflammatory activity while both mast cell degranulating and central nervous effects were very low. The hexaformyl derivative prepared by reaction with p-nitrophenyl formate was, on the other hand, inactive as an anti-inflammatory agent as well as against mast cells. The discrepancy between these results has yet to be resolved. Almost complete dissociation of anti-inflammatory and mast cell degranulating effects has been achieved by reductive methylation. It is unfortunate that it is the undesirable activity that has been retained while the desirable property is lost.

In the course of structure determination on a non-neurotoxic peptide isolated from the venom of *Dendroaspis viridis*, a degree of homology was observed between a sequence close to the C-terminus and the sequence of the larger loop of Peptide 401 (R.A. Shipolini, private communication). The peptide was found to be only one tenth as potent on a weight basis as 401 in degranulating mast cells but on a molar basis there was only a three fold difference. It seems possible that the degranulating effect may be associated with the larger loop of Peptide 401.

The principal objective in the present study was dissociation of the two paradoxical activities of Peptide 401 since there is no intrinsic reason why the two opposing effects should be associated with the same structural features of the molecule. As a secondary objective, it was hoped to find a method of labelling the molecule without change in activity since the anti-inflammatory effects are only observed after a delay of a half to one hour and the fate of the peptide in this period is of considerable interest. The first objective has been achieved in the hexadimethyl derivative but since the compound is inactive in the rat paw oedema test it cannot be used for tracer studies. The existence of a derivative with unimpaired mast cell degranulating activity but no anti-inflammatory effects lends support to the view that Peptide 401 is not simply acting as a counter irritant.

Further evidence against the counter-irritation hypothesis comes from experiments in guinea pigs in which the peptide was mistakenly reported not to be anti-inflammatory (Hanson and others, 1974). In fact it is as active against skin blueing in guinea pigs as it is in rats but, on the other hand, it does not degranulate mast cells prepared from guinea pig mesentery, at least in the presence of physiological concentrations of calcium ions. The two activities of the peptide are therefore dissociated in guinea pigs.

Peptide 401 is a useful tool for the investigation of a number of pharmacological effects including mechanisms of mast cell degranulation and inflammation and the properties of the blood-brain barrier. Dansylation of the peptide gives a fluorescent derivative that has been used to show that the peptide binds first to the cell membrane of mast cells in a mixed cell population and then, as degranulation occurs, to the granule membranes.

ACKNOWLEDGEMENT

Professor C.A. Vernon is thanked for valuable discussion. An SRC studentship (AJG) and a CASE award with Roche Products Ltd. (CD) are gratefully acknowledged. We wish to thank Dr. F.L. Pearce, Dr. M. Ennis and Mr. J. White for carrying out some of the mast cell degranulating experiments and Miss J. Yarney for some anti-inflammatory testing.

REFERENCES

Atkinson, G., M. Ennis, and F. L. Pearce (1979). The effect of alkaline earth cations on the release of histamine from rat peritoneal mast cells treated with compound 48/80 and peptide 401. Br. J. Pharmac., 65, 395-402.

Banks, B. E. C., C. Brown, G. M. Burgess, G. Burnstock, M. Claret, T. Cocks, D. H. Jenkinson, and H. Parsons (1979). Some peripheral activities of apamin. Toxicon, 17, Suppl. 1, 4.

Banks. B. E. C., A. J. Garman, and E. Habermann (1978). Structure-activity studies on apamin and mast-cell degranulating peptide (MCDP)-401. J. Physiol., 284, 160-161p.

Billingham, M. E. J., J. Morley, J. M. Hanson, R. A. Shipolini, and C. A. Vernon (1973). An anti-inflammatory peptide from bee venom. Nature, 245, 163-164.

Billingham, M. E. J., B. V. Robinson, and J. M. Robson (1969). Partial purification of the anti-inflammatory factor(s) in inflammatory exudates. Br. J. Pharmac., 35, 543-557.

Breithaupt, H., and E. Habermann (1968). Mastzelldegranulierendes Peptid (MCD-Peptid) aus Bienengift: Isolierung, biochemische und pharmakologische Eigenschaften. Naunyn-Schmiedebergs Arch. Pharmak. u. Path., 261, 252-270.

Chervenka, C. H., and P. E. Wilcox (1957). Chemical derivatives of chymotrypsinogen. II: Reaction with O-methylisourea. J. Biol. Chem., 222, 635-647.

Doonan, J., A. J. Garman, J. M. Hanson, A. G. Loudon, and C. A. Vernon (1978). Identification by mass-spectrometry of Nε-formyllysine residues in a peptide from bee venom. J. Chem. Soc. Perkin Trans. 1., 1157-1160.

Gauldie, J., J. M. Hanson, F. D. Rumjanek, R. A. Shipolini, and C. A. Vernon (1976). The peptide components of bee venom. Eur. J. Biochem., 61, 369-376.

Gauldie, J., J. M. Hanson, R. A. Shipolini, and C. A. Vernon (1978). The structures of some peptides from bee venom. Eur. J. Biochem., 83, 405-410.

Gilbert, H. F., and M. H. O'Leary (1975). Modification of arginine and lysine in proteins with 2,4-pentanedione. Biochemistry, 14, 5194-5198.

Gleisner, J. M., and I. E. Liener (1973). Chemical modification of the histidine residue located at the active site of ficin. Biochim. Biophys. Acta, 317, 482-491.

Granier, C., E. Pedroso Muller, and J. van Rietschoten (1978). Use of synthetic analogs for a study on the structure-activity relationships of apamin. Eur. J. Biochem., 82, 293-299.

Habermann, E. (1977). Neurotoxicity of apamin and MCD peptide upon central application. Naunyn-Schmiedeberg's Arch. Pharmacol., 300, 189-191.

Habermann, E., and K. G. Reiz (1965). Ein neues Verfaren zur Gewinnung der Komponenten von Bienengift, insbesondere des zentral wirksamen Peptids Apamin. Biochem. Z., 341, 451-466.

Hanson, J. M., J. Morley, and C. Soria-Herrera (1974). Anti-inflammatory property of 401 (MCD-peptide), a peptide from the venom of the bee (Apis mellifera). Br. J. Pharmac., 50, 383-392.

Means, G. E. and R. E. Feaney (1968). Reductive alkylation of amino groups in proteins. Biochemistry, 7, 2192-2201.

Okawa, K., and S. Hase (1963). The synthesis of N_ω-formyl basic amino acids. Bull. Chem. Soc. Japan, 36, 754.

Sheehan, J. C., and D. D. H. Yang (1958). The use of N-formylamino acids in peptide synthesis. J. Am. Chem. Soc., 80, 1154-1158.

Shipolini, R. A., A. F. Bradbury, G. L. Callewaert, and C. A. Vernon(1967). The amino acid sequence of apamin. Chem. Commun., 679-680.

Vernon, C. A., J. M. Hanson, and R. W. Brimblecombe (1969). British Patent No. 1314823.

Vladimirova, I. A., and M. F. Shuba (1978). Strychnine, hydrastine, and apamin effect on synaptic transmission in smooth muscle cells. Neurofiziologiya, 10, 295-299.

Von Haux, P. (1969). Die Aminosaurensequenz von MCD-Peptid, einem spezifisch Mastzellen-degranulierenden Peptid aus Bienengift. Hoppe-Seyler's Z. Physiol. Chem.,350, 536-546.

ISOLATION, PURIFICATION AND SOME PROPERTIES OF SUBERITINE, THE TOXIC PROTEIN FROM THE MARINE SPONGE, *SUBERITES DOMUNCULA*

L. Cariello*, L. Zanetti* and W. Rathmayer**

**Stazione Zoologica, Villa Comunale, Napoli, Italy*
***Fachbereich Biologie Universität, Konstanz, Federal Republic of Germany*

ABSTRACT

In this work suberitine, a neurotoxic protein from marine sponge, *Suberites domuncula*, has been purified by fractional precipitation with ethanol and by gel chromatography. The purified protein is homogeneous in electrophoresis and in analytical ultracentrifuge. The molecular weight is 28000; the lethal dose for the crab, *Carcinus maenas* is 0.8 µg per 10 g. The neurotoxin shows ATPase and haemolytic properties. The neurotoxic activity was studied on the giant axon of the crayfish, *Astacus leptodactylus*.

KEYWORDS

Suberitine, *Suberites domuncula*, neurotoxin.

INTRODUCTION

The work of Richet (1960a) exaustively describing the symtoms following the injection of watery extracts of the marine sponge, *Suberites domuncula* into laboratory animals is well known. He called this toxin suberitine (Richet, 1906b and Lassabliere, 1906). However, as yet the nature and the toxic properties of suberitine are completely unknown. In this work we describe the isolation and characterization of this toxin

MATERIALS AND METHODS

Living samples of *S. domuncula* were squeezed twice with a bench press; the juice was centrifuge in the cold at 27.000 x g for 1 hr. About 800 ml of juice is obtained from 1.7 Kg of material. The sediment was resuspended in the minimum amount of sea water and centrifuged as before. To the combined original juice and sea water supernatants cold ethanol was added (4:1 vol/vol) and the large precipitate was removed by centrifugation. The sediment was extracted with a minimum amount of sodium acetate 0.15 M pH 7.6. This suspension was centrifuged and the precipitate reextracted with the same buffer. This procedure was repeated until the supernatant showed no lethal activity. The combined supernatants (about 400 ml) were concentrated to a small volume (about 200 ml) by ultrafiltration with a UM2 Diaflo membrane.

Figure 1 shows the steps of the isolation and purification of suberitine.

The toxic activity was estimated from the minimum amount of the protein wich causes paralysis within 1 min when injected into crabs, *Carcinus maenas* weighing ten grams. Elctrophoretic techniques were performed according to Weber and Osborn (1969).

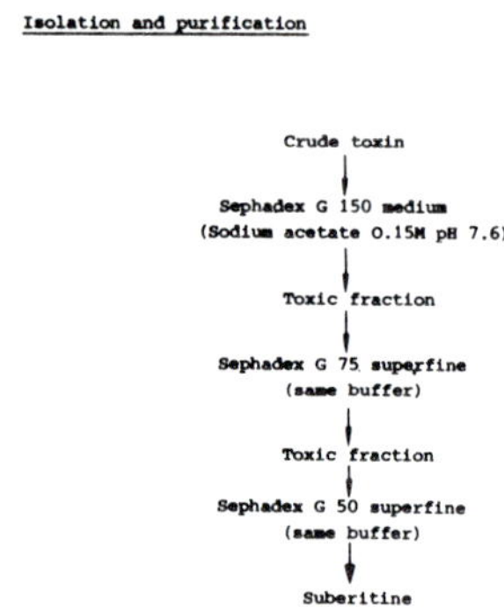

Fig. 1. Steps of suberitine purification.

RESULTS AND DISCUSSION

A column of G-150 Sephadex, medium grade was used to fractionate the crude toxin. The results are shown in Fig. 2.

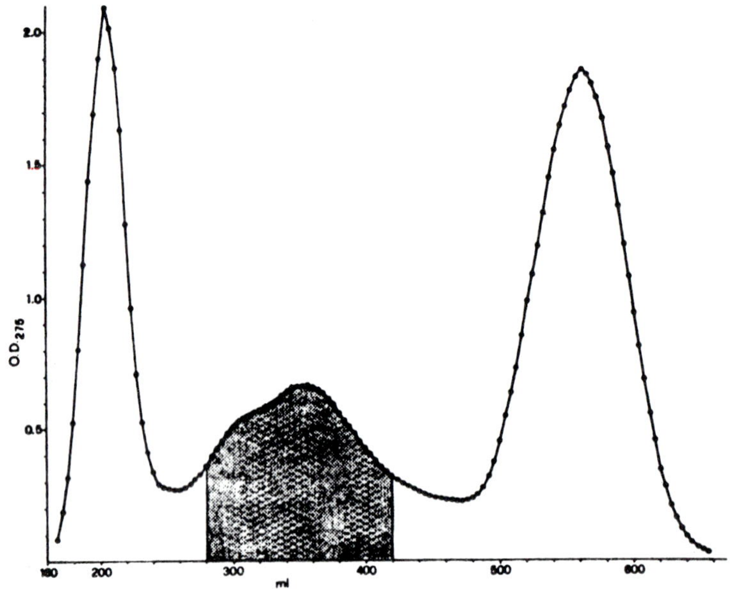

Fig. 2. First fractionation of the crude extract of *Suberites domuncula*. The hatched area indicates the toxic fractions. The samples contained 128 mg of protein.

The toxic fraction was further purified on a Sephadex G-75 superfine and on Sephadex

G-50 superfine columns (Fig. 3 and 4). The homogeneity was examined by SDS-poly-

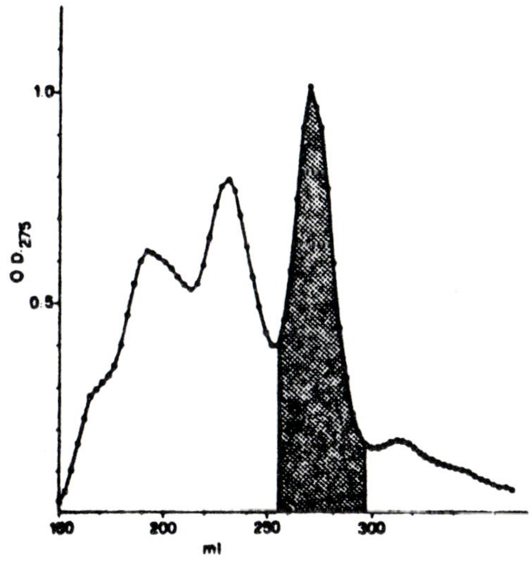

Fig. 3. Further purification of suberitine on Sephadex G-75 superfine. All of the toxicity was contained in the third peak (hatched area). The sample contained 91 mg of protein.

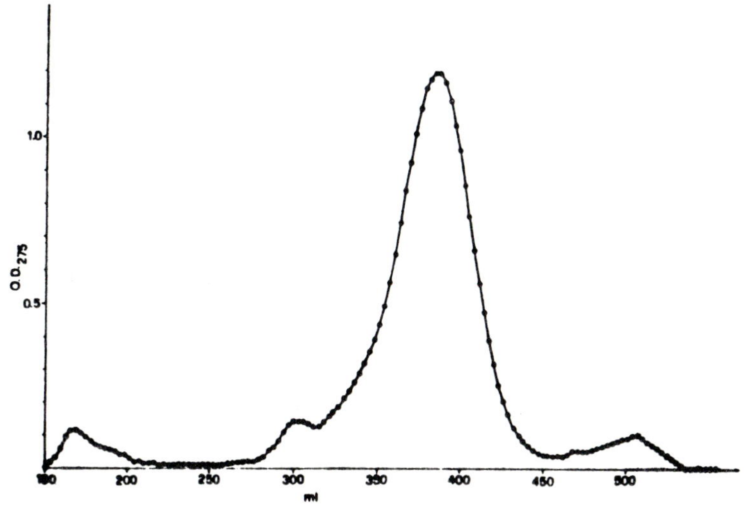

Fig. 4. Purification of suberitine on Sephadex g-50 superfine. The sample contained 53 mg of protein.

acrylamide gel electrophoresis (Fig. 5). The molecular weight of suberitine was estimated from its mobility in SDS-polyacrylamide gel electrophoresis (Fig. 6)

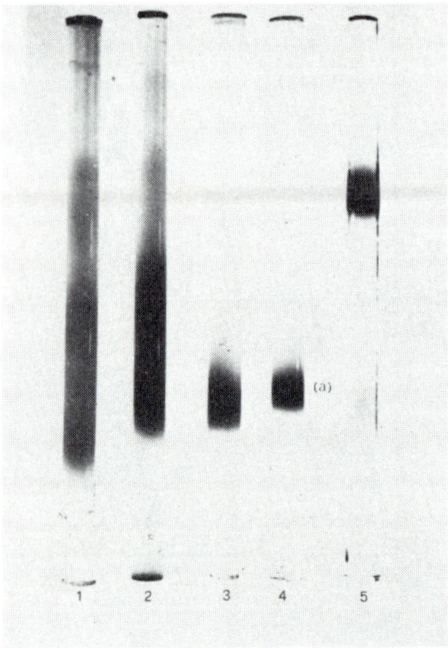

Fig. 5. Evidence of purification by electrophoresis. 1 - Crude extract. 2 and 3 - The fraction obtained from the first and second fractionation respectively. 4 - Purified suberitine. 5- Purified suberitine without treatment with urea and β-mercaptoethanol.

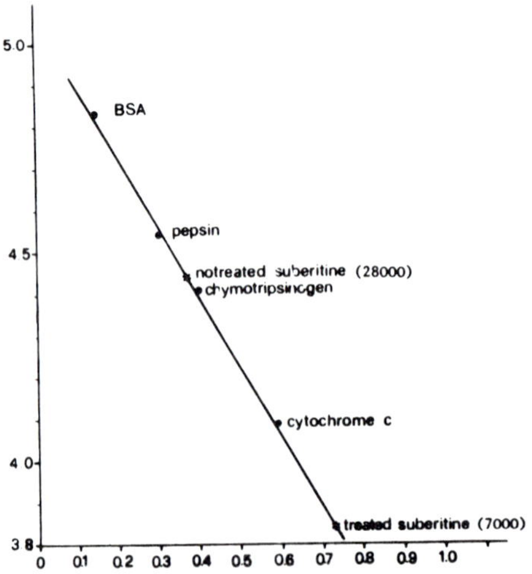

Fig. 6. Determination of the molecular weight of suberitine before and after treatment with 4M urea or 2% β-mercaptoethanol.

and by analytical ultracentrifuge (Fig. 7). It can be noted that when the toxin was treated with 4M urea and/or β-mercaptoethanol and then submitted to electrophoresis, the resulting molecular weight was about 7000, while the untreated protein shows a molecular weight of about 28000.
The values calculated for S and D are 2.32 and 8.29 respectively.

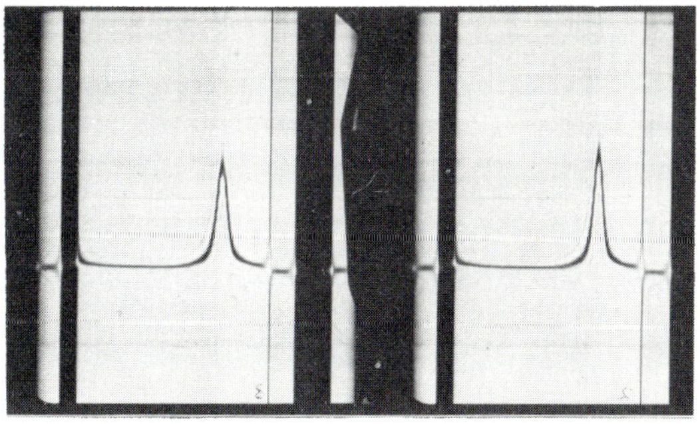

Fig. 7. Sedimentation of suberitine.

We studied some properties of suberitine and found haemolytic activity against human erythrocytes and some ATPase activity. We also studied the neurotoxic activity: suberitine at concentrations of 4.4 ng/ml gradually blocked the action potentials elicited by indirect stimulation within 7 to 40 min (Fig. 8).

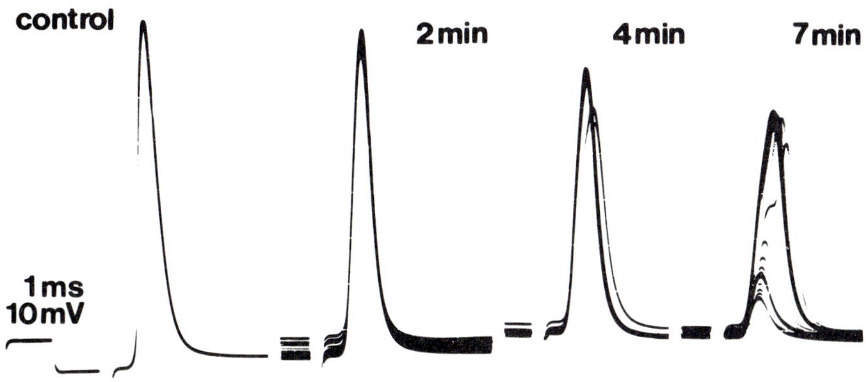

THE BLOCKING EFFECT OF SUBERITES TOXIN ON ACTION POTENTIALS IN THE LATERAL GIANT AXON OF THE CRAYFISH ASTACUS LEPTODACTYLUS

THE RECORDS, TAKEN 2, 4 AND 7 MIN AFTER APPLICATION OF 4.4 ng/ml SUBERITINE, REPRESENT CONTINOUS REGISTRATION OF SUPERIMPOSED SWEEPS AT 0.5 Hz STIMULATION. THE TOXIN, BESIDES BLOCKING THE ACTION POTENTIAL, DEPOLARIZED THE MEMBRANE POTENTIAL FROM INITIALLY -73 mV TO -63 mV. THE EFFECTS WERE IRREVERSIBLE WITHIN SEVERAL HOURS OF WASHING THE PREPARATION WITH TOXIN-FREE SOLUTION.

At ten times higher concentrations the block developed quickly within few min. The decrease in amplitude was always accompanied by a decrease in the rate of rise of the action potential. The block was sometimes preceeded by a depolarization of 2 to 15 mV. Block of action potentials may be one explanation for the flaccid paralysis observed in crabs upon direct injection of suberitine into the haemolymph. The effect of suberitine on the axon were irreversible within several hours of washing. The mechanism of the block will be studied in further experiments.

REFERENCES

Lassabliere, M.P. (1906). C.R. Sèance Soc. Biol., 61, 600.
Richet, C. (1906a). C. R. Sèance Soc. Biol., 61, 598.

Richet, C. (1906b). *C. R. Sèance Soc. Biol., 61*, 686.
Weber, K. and M. Osborn (1969). *J. Biol. Chem., 244*, 4406-4411.

TOXINS SELECTIVE TO INSECTS DERIVED FROM SCORPION VENOMS

E. Zlotkin*, Z. Teitelbaum, D. Lester* and P. Lazarovici***

**Department of Zoology, The Hebrew University of Jerusalem, Jerusalem, Israel*
***Department of Radiochemistry, Nuclear Research Center, Negev, Israel*

ABSTRACT

1. Scorpion venoms contain different groups of neurotoxic polypeptides specifically affecting different groups of animals; 2. Six insect toxins were isolated from the venoms of four different scorpion species and compared, on the level of their amino acid composition, to the so-called mammal and crustacean toxins derived from the same venoms; 3. On the basis of their symptoms of paralysis the above insect toxins were classified as excitatory and depressory toxins; 4. The unique and selective affinity of the Androctonus - insect toxins to insect neuronal tissue enables their employment as pharmacological tools in the study of insect neurobiology.

KEYWORDS

Scorpion venom, insect toxins, crustacean toxins, mammal toxins, column chromatography, selective action, specificity, amino acid composition, Androctonus australis Hector, Androctonus mauretanicus mauretanicus, Buthotus judaicus, Scorpio maurus palmatus.

SCORPION ENVENOMATION

Like in many other topics in the field of toxinology, the study of the chemistry and pharmacology of scorpion venoms was mainly motivated by medical aspects, thus employing vertebrates and mainly mammals as experimental animals. The capacity of a scorpion sting to kill a human being is astonishing when taking into consideration the relatively small amount of active substance injected (Yahel-Niv and Zlotkin, 1979), which is about three orders of magnitude less than that released, for example, by a bite of an average viperid or elapid snake. On the background of the accumulated and recently reviewed (Zlotkin and others, 1978a) pharmacologic information, it may be concluded that the different cardio-vascular, muscular and respiratory manifestations associated with the pathology of scorpion envenomation, are a consequence of a general sympathetic and parasympathetic discharge due to the peripheral axonal excitatory effect of scorpion venoms.

In nature, however, the rendezvous between scorpions and humans is coincidental. The stinging activity of scorpions, in the field, is mainly directed to arthropods and especially soft-bodied insects which serve as their prey food. The symptoms of scorpion envenomation in arthropods as previously demonstrated in locusts, terrestrial crustaceans and blowfly larvae (Zlotkin and others, 1978b) clearly indicate a stimulatory effect on the skeletal musculature. Employing crustacean and insect neuromuscular preparations and the crude venoms of Centruroides and Leiurus scorpions it has been shown (Parnas and Russell, 1967; Parnas and others, 1970) that the above typical spastic-excitatory paralysis is actually due to a peripheral presynaptic action. This was expressed in the increase of quantal content and in the spontaneous contraction of the muscle which was correlated to the repetitive firing of the motor nerve. Both the axonal excitation and conduction block were assumed to result from the axonal membrane depolarization.

As predators scorpions possess slow mobility and undeveloped vision and smell senses emphasizing the necessity of a device for paralyzing the prey at the earliest moment of contact. This function is carried out by their venom apparatus. In spite of the general resemblance in the paralytic action of scorpion venoms on vertebrate (Katz and Edwards, 1972; Brazil and others, 1973) and arthropod neuromuscular systems, as it will be shown below, these effects are due to separate and special groups of neurotoxic polypeptides present in the crude venoms.

INSECT TOXINS

By the aid of the assay of the contraction paralysis of blowfly larvae it has been found that there was no correlation between larvae paralysis and mice lethal potencies of sixteen different Buthidae scorpion venoms (Zlotkin and others, 1971a), hinting at the possibility that the two toxic activities may result from different factors. This assumption was strongly supported by the finding that the potent toxins I and II derived from the venom of A. australis, which are strongly lethal to mammals and were previously isolated and purified according to the biological criterion of mice lethality (Miranda and others, 1964 a, b; Rochat and others, 1967; Miranda and others, 1970), were completely inactive to blowfly larvae. The final proof of the diversity between factors affecting mammals and those paralyzing insects in scorpion venoms, was obtained by starch gel electrophoretical separation of the venom of A. australis (Zlotkin and others, 1971b) and six other Buthinae venoms (Zlotkin and others, 1972a). It has been shown that three of the above venoms contain more than one fraction paralytic and lethal to fly larvae.

Insect toxins derived from the venom of Androctonus scorpions. With the aid of the above fly larvae contraction paralysis assay coupled with a series of steps of fractionation of the Androctonus australis Hector venom, the first insect toxin was obtained (Zlotkin and others, 1971c). The final product, 267-fold purified and with a yield of 95% toxicity, is a single chained protein composed of 67 amino acids (Table 1) and crosslinked by four disulfide bridges. In constrast to the crude venom of A. a. Hector, the insect and the so-called mammal toxins derived from the same venom were unable to affect an isopod (terrestrial crustacean) or a scorpion (arachnid) (Zlotkin and others, 1972b). This led to the isolation and purification of the so-called crustacean toxin from the same venom - which was also a low molecular weight (69 amino acids) basic polypeptide (Zlotkin and others, 1975 and Table 1). For comparative purposes an additional insect toxin was isolated from the venom of a related species of scorpion, that of Androctonus mauretanicus mauretanicus (Zlotkin and others, 1979). The purified toxin is about 330 times more toxic than the crude venom in its larvae contraction paralysis activity, and is composed of 67 amino acids with an estimated molecular weight of 8129 (Table 1). The present insect toxin strongly resembles the toxin purified from the venom of the scorpion A. a. Hector in terms of its toxicity, amino acid composition, molecular weight and selective binding affinity to insect nervous tissue (see next section). Like A. a. Hector venom, the crude venom of A. m. mauretanicus also possesses toxins specifically affecting crustaceans and mammals (Table 1).

Insect toxins derived from the venom of a Buthotus scorpion. On the background of the strong resemblance between the two previous insect toxins derived from scorpions belonging to the genus Androctonus (Buthinae) and the chemical and pharmacological diversity among the abundant scorpion venom mammal toxins (Zlotkin and others, 1978a) it has been decided to examine several additional insect toxins derived from taxonomically different groups of scorpions. The venom of the Israeli black scorpion Buthotus judaicus (Buthinae) apart from belonging to a different genus of a scorpion and being relatively limited in its geographical distribution (Levy - personal communication), is characterized by a very low toxicity to mammals (about 1.2 mg/mouse - Lester, unpublished) and the induction of excitatory and depressory symptoms in arthropods. Using paralysis and lethality assays on fly larvae, locusts and isopods coupled with gel filtration and different combinations of ion exchange column chromatographies (Fig. 1) two different insect toxins have been isolated and purified from the venom of B. judaicus. The first toxin (TxI, mw 8737, pHi 8.24 with about 60% of the yield of toxicity to fly larvae and 40-fold of increase in specific activity) induces an immediate contraction-paralysis of fly larvae. The second, insect toxin (TxII, mw 8987, pHi 8.3, possessing about 40% of the crude venom's toxicity to fly larvae and about 40-fold of increase in its specific toxicity) causes a gradual slow, flaccid paralysis of fly larvae. As indicated in Table 1, the two toxins differ in their amino acid composition.

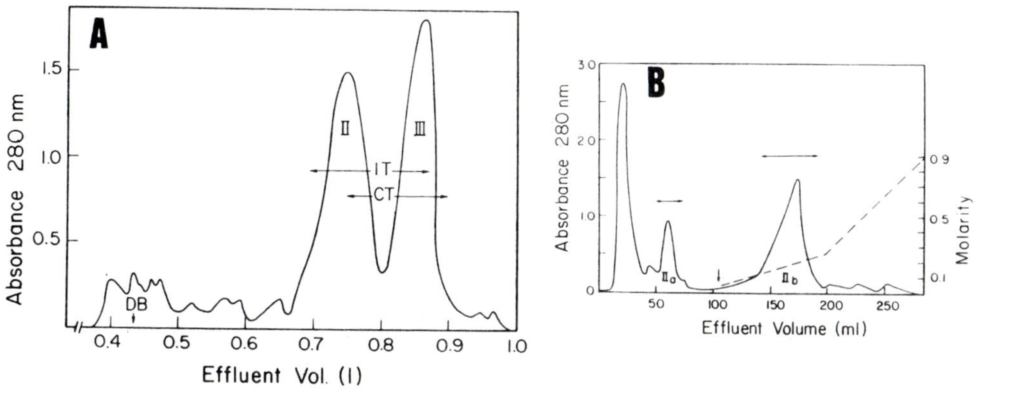

Fig. 1. The initial steps in the purification of the two insect toxins derived from the venom of the scorpion Buthotus judaicus. (A) Gel filtration on Sephadex G-50 fine (Pharmacia) of 200 mg Lowry protein of the water extract of the crude venom of B. judaicus. Two columns, 202x1.94cm in series. Ammonium acetate buffer 0.1M pH 8.5. Flow rate 15ml/hr. The vertical arrow indicates elution volume of Dextran Blue (DB=void volume). IT corresponds to the region of separation where toxicity was found for fly larvae (according to the contraction paralysis assay) and locusts (according to paralysis or excitation). CT represents the region of crustacean toxicity (according to paralysis of isopods). Fraction II, which contained about 70 percent of the toxicity to fly larvae and locusts, was employed for further purification. (B) Cation-exchange chromatography on CM-Cellulose CM 52 (Whatman) of 30 mg of Sephadex G-50 FII, using ammonium acetate buffer. Column: 1.5 x 8.0 cm. 1 ml of Sephadex G-100 was placed on the filter. Equilibrium conditions; buffer 0.05M pH 6.9. Free flow rate 75ml/hr. First gradient: 0.05-0.25M pH 6.9 buffer. 2nd gradient: 0.25-1.0M pH 6.9 buffer. Gradients flow rate 5ml/hr. Fraction IIa represents the immediate insect paralytic factor (as assayed on locusts) which was finally purified by two additional steps of chromatography: DEAE-Cellulose and CM-Sephadex columns, Fraction IIB represents the slow paralytic factor to fly lar-

vae and to locusts which was finally purified by two additional column chromatographical applications both with CM-Cellulose columns.

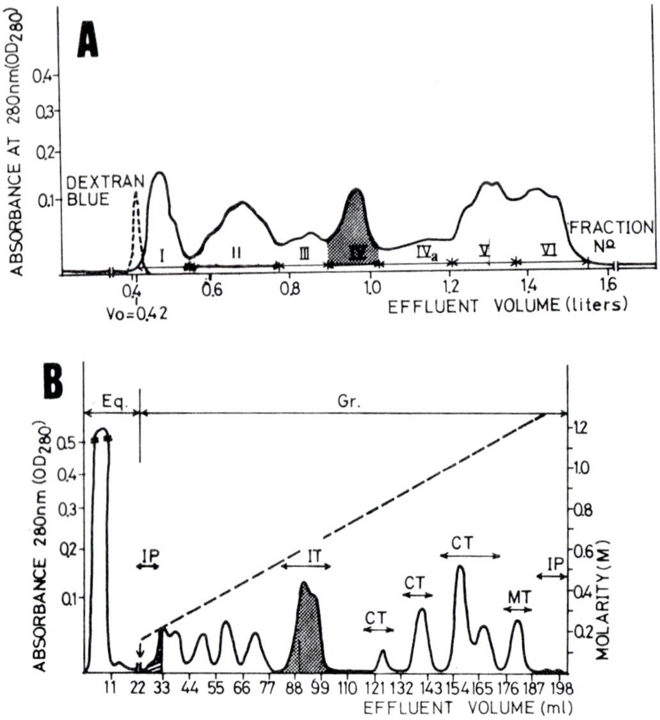

Fig. 2. The different pharmacologically active fractions isolated from the venom of the scorpion Scorpio maurus palmatus (Scorpionidae). (A) Sephadex G-50 column chromatography. 680 OD units of water extract were charged on two columns of ^{280} 198x1.7cm connected in series and eluted by ammonium acetate 0.1M pH 8.5 buffer. Flow rate of 15ml/hr was applied and fractions of 10ml were collected. Absorbance at 280nm was automatically recorded (Full line). Fractions collected are indicated by horizontal double headed arrows. Fractions I, to IV contain: high molecular enzymes such as hyaluronidase and phosphatase (I), phospholipases (II), direct lytic factors (III) and neurotoxic polypeptides (IV). Fractions IVa-VI are non-proteic substances. (B) CM-Sephadex C-25 cation-exchange chromatography of the Sephadex G-50 toxic fraction IV. Column: 20x1cm; buffer; ammonium acetate. At equilibrium conditions (Eq): 0.1M, pH 8.5. Linear gradient of molarity up to 2.0M, pH 8.5. Flow rate of 4ml/hr was applied and fractions of 1.25ml were collected. 49 OD units were charged on the column. Full line, absorbance^{280}at 280nm; dotted line, linear gradient of buffer concentration. IP = Insect immediate and reversible paralysis. IT - insect toxicity, CT - crustacean toxicity, MT - mammal toxicity. The insect toxic (IT) fraction was further treated on a column of CM-Sephadex C-25 resulting in the purification of the two insect toxins (Table 1).

TABLE 1 The Amino Acid Composition of Different Toxins Derived from the Venoms of Several Scorpion Species

	Insect Toxins						Crustacean Toxins				Mammal Toxins						
	(a	(b	(c	(c	(d	(d	(e	(d	(d	(d	(f	(f	(f	(g	(g	(c	(d
Amino acid	Aa	Am	BI	BII	SI	SII	Aa	SI	SII	SIII	AaI	AaII	AaIII	AmI	AmII	B	S
Aspartic acid	11	11	8	7	2	3	6	2	3	2	9	8	8	9	10	10	2
Threonine	4	3	3	4	0	4	4	3	2	2	2	3	0	1	1	3	2
Serine	6	5	3	4	1	2	4	3	3	3	6	2	6	4	3	3	2
Glutamic acid	3	3	4	4	3	1	10	1	1	1	0	4	0	4	4	2	2
Proline	1	1	4	0	3	2	2	1	2	1	6	3	6	3	3	3	2
Glycine	4	4	7	10	2	2	4	4	3	3	6	7	6	6	7	7	3
Alanine	3	3	4	4	1	2	2	2	2	2	1	3	3	3	3	6	2
Half-cystine	8	8	6	6	4	6	10	8	8	8	8	8	8	8	8	6	8
Valine	3	4	3	4	2	2	4	1	1	1	5	4	6	1	1	2	1
Methionine	0	1	0	0	0	0	0	0	0	0	0	0	0	0	0	0	1
Isoleucine	2–3	3	4	2–3	1	3	2	1	1	1	2	1	3	3	3	4	0
Leucine	5–6	4	2	2	2	1	2	0	0	0	4	2	4	3	3	3	0
Tyrosine	5	6	5	3	1	2	4	1	2	1	3	7	3	5	6	4	1
Phenylalanine	1	1	1	2	0	0	0	0	0	0	1	1	1	2	2	0	0
Lysine	7	7	8	5	4	3	4	4	5	4	6	5	6	5	6	3	5
Histidine	1	1	1	1	0	0	0	0	0	0	1	2	2	0	0	0	0
Arginine	1	1	1	2	2	3	9	2	1	2	2	3	1	2	3	3	1
Tryptophan (h	1	1	3	8	0	0	2	0	0	0	1	1	1	2	2	3–4	0
Total	67	67	**67**	68–69	28	36	69	33	34	31	63	64	64	61	65	62–63	32

Legend and remarks: Aa –*Androctonus australis Hector*. Am – *Androctonus mauretanicus mauretanicus*. B – *Buthotus judaicus*. S – *Scorpio maurus palmatus*. a) Zlotkin and others, 1971c. b) Zlotkin and others, 1979. c) Lester – unpublished. d) Lazarovici – unpublished. e) Zlotkin and others, 1975. f) Miranda and others, 1970. g) Zlotkin and others, 1978a. h) Spectophotometrically determined.

Insect toxins derived from the venom of Scorpio marus palmatus (Scorpionidae). This scorpion belongs to a different family, that of Scorpionidae, and its venom possesses several unique properties:
1. Very low toxicity to mammals (LD_{50} of about 2.5 mg/20mg mouse - Lazarovici, unpublished) in contrast to its relatively strong toxicity to arthropods. 2. In contrast to buthid scorpion venoms (Zlotkin and others, 1971a), it induces a gradual slow flaccid paralysis of blowfly larvae instead of the common immediate contraction paralysis. 3. In contrast to a well-known buthid venoms, this venom possesses (in addition to neurotoxic polypeptides) toxic phospholipases and direct lytic factors (Fig. 2A). The employment of different techniques of column chromatography coupled with different bioassays, based on paralysis and lethality of several insect species (including blowfly larvae), isopods (crustaceans), and mice, enabled the isolation of several fractions possessing specific toxicities to insects, crustaceans and mammals (Fig. 2B). An additional step of fractionation on a column of CM-Sephadex C-25 of the insect toxin fraction obtained in the previous step (IT Fig. 2B) enabled the purification of two insect toxins. Both are low molecular weight (3232 and 3963 daltons) basic polypeptides characterized by a relative abundance of half cystines and lysines and the absence of several common amino acids in their compositions (Table 1). Table 1 presents the amino acid compositions of the different insect toxins. For comparative purposes the so-called crustacean and mammal toxins derived from the respective venoms were also added.

ACTION AND SPECIFICITY

The vast majority of information concerning the pharmacology and action of insect toxins has been obtained with the toxin derived from the venom of A. a. Hector, which was the first to be isolated (Zlotkin and others, 1971c). Preliminary studies and observations (Zlotkin and others, 1971b; D'Ajello and others, 1972; Pansa and others, 1973) have indicated that its specificity or selectivity is based on a specific affinity to the insect neural system and that its paralytic effects are due to peripheral action on the level of the neuromuscular junctions. On the background of these considerations the action of the insect, crustacean and mammal I and II toxins all derived from the venom of A. a. Hector were investigated in a series of neuromuscular preparations: those of a mammal (Tintpulver and others, 1976), crustacean (Rathmayer and others, 1977), arachnid (Ruhland and others, 1977) and insect (Walther and others, 1976, Fig. 3). It was concluded that the muscular stimulatory effects of the different toxins on the different preparations were basically due to an excitatory presynaptic action on the motor axons. The crustacean and the mammal toxins have demonstrated a relative specificity to the corresponding neuromuscular preparations. The insect toxin, however, was the most potent and active only on the insect nerve muscle preparation (Rathmayer and others, 1978). The axonal effect of the insect toxin was mainly expressed by the induction of repetitive firing (Fig. 3) without affecting the time-course of the action potentials (Walther and others, 1976). The selective affinity of the A. a. Hector insect toxin to insect nervous tissue was further established in a series of binding experiments with the radioiodinated insect toxin to different tissue preparations of a locust. A clear, specific binding of a high affinity was obtained only between the toxin and the nervous tissue extracts. Assays with a similar nervous tissue preparation derived from the crustacean (crayfish) resulted in low and nonspecific binding of the toxin (Table 2, Teitelbaum and others, 1979).

The question we encounter is how may the above information concerning the mode of action of the A. a. Hector insect toxin, be also applied to the additional insect toxins derived from the different scorpion venoms (Table 1). It may be safely concluded that the A.m. mauretanicus insect toxin, which strongly resembles the previous one by its composition, specific toxicity and its binding and competitive displacement properties (Zlotkin and others, 1979), is pharmacologically identical.

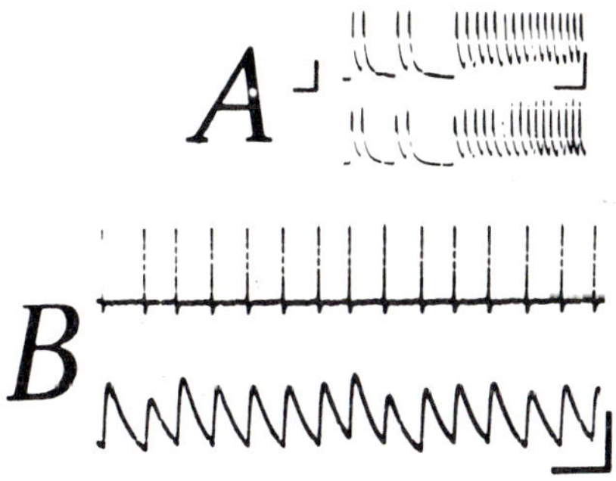

Fig. 3. A. Neuromuscular effect of the A. a. Hector - Insect Toxin on the locust hind leg extensor tibiae nerve muscle preparation. A. start of two trains of slow ejps synchronously recorded from two distant locations on the muscle 50 min after application of 0.15 μg/ml of insect toxin. Calibration: 10 mV, 100 msec. B. Spontaneous neuromuscular activity caused by insect toxin. Synchronous recording from the "slow" motor axon (upper trace) and a fibre in the main part of the extensor tibiae muscle (lower trace) 65 min after application of approximately 0.5 μg/ml of toxin. Calibration: 50 msec; upper 0.5 mV lower 10 mV.. These data (A,B) clearly indicate a presynaptic excitatory action. (Taken from Walther and others, 1976).

TABLE 2 Specific Binding of $|^{125}|$-IT to Locust and Crayfish Nervous Tissue and Non-innervated Locust Tissues*

Preparation	Unlabelled IT† (μg)	$\vert^{125}\vert$-IT bound (ng/mg protein)	Specifically bound $\vert^{125}\vert$-IT** (ng/mg protein)
Locust nervous tissue	0	0.47 ± 0.013	0.20 ± 0.023
	20	0.27 ± 0.010	
Locust Malpighian tubules	0	0.32 ± 0.020	0.03 ± 0.035
	20	0.29 ± 0.015	
Locust fat body	0	0.49 ± 0.010	0.00 ± 0.026
	20	0.49 ± 0.016	
Crayfish nervous tissue	0	0.12 ± 0.007	0.01 ± 0.012
	20	0.11 ± 0.005	

* For each tissue preparation four to six determinations were performed. The results are expressed as the mean ± S.D.

† Doses of unlabelled IT present in the incubation mixture. The binding obtained in absence of unlabelled IT represents total binding while that obtained in the presence of 20 μg represents non-specific binding.

** Calculated as the difference between total and non-specific bindings measured for each tissue preparation.

To the same category we may, possibly, associate also the B. judaicus - insect toxin I which in spite of the clear difference in its composition (Table 1), it mimics the previous two toxins in the induction of the typical immediate contraction paralysis. The B. judaicus - insect toxin II and S. m. palmatus toxins I and II - belong to different categories. They do not induce the immediate spastic paralysis but rather a slow and flaccid paralysis as demonstrated on fly larvae and locusts. Their mode of action deserves further study. It has to be determined whether their neurotoxic action is central or peripheral and if peripheral is it pre- or postsynaptic. The two insect toxins of S. m. palmatus, in contrast to those derived from buthid scorpion venoms, demonstrate an evident degree of cooperativity (Fig. 4) which deserves further clarification. Separately, the two insect toxins yielded only about 1.5 percent of the total crude venoms' toxicity each. Their combination, however, resulted in an evident degree of recovery (of about 25%) of the crude venoms' toxicity (Fig. 4). An additional feature of the S. m. palmatus insect toxins when compared to those derived from buthid scorpion venom is their toxicity to isopods (about 30 to 100 times less toxic than to insects).

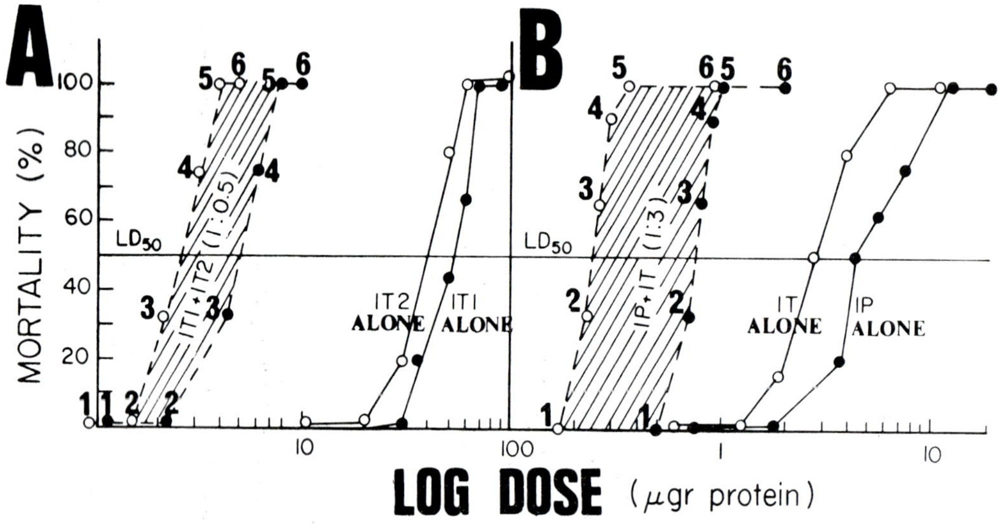

Fig. 4. Cooperative interactions between the insect toxic components derived from the venom of the scorpion S. m. palmatus. A. synergic interaction in lethality to locusts (Locusta migratoria) between the two insect toxins: ITI (●—●) and ITII (○—○) when applied separately and in combination (molar ratio of 1:0.5). B. synergic interactions in lethality to flies (Sarcophaga falculata) between the insect toxic fraction (IT-Fig. 2B○—○) and the insect paralytic fraction (IP-Fig. 2B●—●) when applied separately and in combination (in ratio of 1:3).

CONCLUDING REMARKS

1. Scorpion venoms contain discrete groups of neurotoxic polypeptides specifically affecting different groups of animals. The insect and arthropod active toxins are essential tools, for scorpions' survival and food obtaining.
2. The six insect toxins presented can be classified into two categories: (a) excitatory toxins - inducing the typical immediate contraction paralysis of blowfly larvae. This may include the toxins derived from the A. a. Hector and A. m. mauretanicus scorpions and toxin I from B. judaicus. (b) depressory toxins - inducing

a delayed flaccid paralysis of blowfly larvae. To this category we may associate the toxin II of *B. judaicus* and the two toxins derived from the venom of *S. m. palmatus*. This is, however, a very rough classification which cannot replace essential neurophysiological-pharmacological studies. The phenomenon of cooperativity, as was clearly demonstrated with the insect toxic components of the venom of *S. m. palmatus*, contributes an additional interesting dimension.

3. In spite of the temptation to associate the apparent resemblance and consistency in the chemical compositions of the two *Androctonus* insect toxins with their unique and selective mode of action, such conclusions should be carefully considered. When comparing the compositions of the different groups of toxins presented in Table 1, it appears that the resemblance in the amino acid compositions is basically associated with the biological source of the substances rather than with their specificities. This element is strongly emphasized when considering, for example, the amino acid composition of the mammal toxin of *S. m. palmatus* venom, which clearly resembles the different arthropod toxins derived from the same venom and differs from the mammal toxins derived from the venom of the other three scorpions species.

4. The fact that different neurotoxic polypeptides are able to discriminate between phylogenetically and taxonomically related groups of arthropods such as insects and crustaceans is curious. According to common knowledge the above two groups of organisms share identical nervous systems from an anatomical, physiological, pharmacological and chemical point of view. This concept has to be revised and reconsidered. The presence of toxins such as the *Androctonus* insect toxins possessing a selective affinity for insect neuronal tissue may indicate a structural and functional uniqueness of these tissues. These substances may serve as important pharmacological tools in the study of insect neurobiology.

ACKNOWLEDGEMENT

The authors would like to express their gratitude to the US-Israel Binational Science Foundation (BSF) for support of the studies presented.

REFERENCES

Brazil, O. V., A. C. Neder, and A. C. Corrado (1973). *Pharmac. Res. Comm., 5,* 137-150.

D'Ajello, V., E. Zlotkin, F. Miranda, S. Lissitzky, and S. Bettini (1972). *Toxicon, 10,* 399-404.

Katz, N. L. and C. Edwards (1972). *Toxicon, 10,* 133-137.

Miranda, F., H. Rochat, and S. Lissitzky (1964a). *Toxicon, 2,* 51-69.

Miranda, F., H. Rochat, and S. Lissitzky (1964b). *Toxicon, 2,* 113-121.

Miranda, F., C. Kopeyan, C. Rochat, H. Rochat, and S. Lissitzky (1979). *Eur. J. Biochem., 16,* 514-523.

Pansa, M. C., G. Migliori-Natalizi, and S. Bettini (1973). *Toxicon, 11,* 361-368.

Parnas, I., D. Avgar, and A. Shulov (1979). *Toxicon, 8,* 67-79.

Parnas, I., and F. E. Russell (1967) In: F. E. Russell and P. R. Saunders (eds.) *Animal Toxins,* Pergamon Press, Oxford, pp. 401-415.

Rathmayer, W., C. Walther, and E. Zlotkin (1977). *Comp. Biochem. Physiol., 56c,* 35-39.

Rathmayer, W., M. Ruhland, M. Tintpulver, C. Walther, and E. Zlotkin (1978). In: P. Rosenberg (ed.). *Toxins: Animal, Plant and Microbial,* Pergamon Press, pp. 629-637.

Rochat, C., H. Rochat, F. Miranda, and S. Lissitzky (1967). *Biochemistry, 6,* 578-585.

Ruhland, M., E. Zlotkin, and W. Rathmayer (1977). *Toxicon, 15,* 157-160.

Teitelbaum, z., P. Lazarovici, and E. Zlotkin (1979). Insect Biochem., 9, 343-346.
Tintpulver, M., T. Zerachia, and E. Zlotkin (1976). Toxicon, 14, 371-377.
Walther, C., E. Zlotkin, and W. Rathmayer (1976). J. Insect Physiol., 22, 1187-1194.
Yahel-Niv, A., P. Lazarovici, and E. Zlotkin (1979). Toxicon, 17, 435-446.
Zlotkin, E., G. Fraenkel, F. Miranda, and S. Lissitzky (1971a). Toxicon, 9, 1-8.
Zlotkin, E., F. Miranda, C. Kupeyan, and S. Lissitzky (1971b). Toxicon, 9, 9-13.
Zlotkin, E., H. Rochat, C. Kupeyan, F. Miranda, and S. Lissitzky (1971c). Biochemie (Paris), 53, 1073-1078.
Zlotkin, E., F. Miranda and S. Lissitzky (1972a). Toxicon, 10, 207-210.
Zlotkin, E., F. Miranda and S. Lissitzky (1972b). Toxicon, 10, 211-216.
Zlotkin, E., G. Martinez and H. Rochat and F. Miranda (1975). Insect Biochem., 5, 243-250.
Zlotkin, E., F. Miranda and H. Rochat (1978a). In: Bettini, S. (ed.), Arthropod Venoms, Springer, pp. 317-369.
Zlotkin, E., W. Rathmayer and S. Lissitzky (1978b). In: Shankland, D.L., Hollingworth, R.M. and T. Smyth (eds.), Pesticides and Venom Neurotoxicity, Plenum Press, pp. 227-246.
Zlotkin, E., Z. Teitelbaum, H. Rochat and F. Miranda (1979). Insect Biochem., 9, 347-354.

TOXIC EFFECTS OF CYCASIN, THE GLYCOSIDE OF CYCAD PLANT, UPON SEVERAL BIOLOGY SPECIES

A. Kobayashi, K. Tadera and F. Yagi

Lab. of Biochem. and Nutr. Chem., Faculty of Agriculture, Kagoshima University, Kagoshima, Japan

ABSTRACT

Toxic effects of cycasin, a carcinogen present in cycad plant, were examined on biology species other than animals for the purpose of looking for a general as well as a possible common toxicological scope.

Cycasin developed generally not only retardation of growth but reduction in the characteristic products of each microorganism. The production of kojic acid by *Aspergillus oryzae* K was exceptionally accelerated. Spore-formation was specifically inhibited in fungi. Germination and growth of various cereal seeds were interfered by cycasin. Respiration of the treated seedlings was low, and necrosis and death occurred. The activity of α-amylase and the content of gibberellin were low. An emergence-mechanism of cycasin-toxicity was proposed; cycasin is hydrolyzed by β-glucosidase, and the liberated aglycone might be oxidized by alcohol dehydrogenase to give the aldehyde-form of the aglycone, which would interfere the formation of gibberellin in the embryo parts and/or the *de novo* synthesis of α-amylase. Larvae of cabbage army worm and silk worm melaninized themselves heavily, pupated incompletely and died. As a whole the respiratory or red-ox system was disturbed by the aglycone of cycasin.

KEYWORDS

Cycasin; methylazoxymethanol; kojic acid; α-amylase; gibberellin; alcohol dehydrogenase; β-glucosidase; toxicity of cycasin.

INTRODUCTION

The seeds of cycad plants were formerly used as foods, especially in famine years, while inadequate removal of the toxin brought about human poisoning. Ingestion of the leaves caused paralysis in grazing livestocks. The toxic principle of Japanese cycad, *Cycas revoluta* Thunb., was isolated and elucidated in our laboratory (Nishida, Kobayashi and Nagahama, 1955) as cycasin, methylazoxymethyl-β-D-glucoside. During the pursuit of a presumed relationship between the utilization of cycad and a high incidence of amyotrophic lateral sclerosis in the Chamorro population of Guam, the seeds were found to be carcinogenic for experimental animals (Laqueur and co-workers, 1963). Many papers were published thereafter on carcinogenic action, neurotoxicity or micrencephaly due to cycasin or its aglycone (6th International Cycad Conference, 1972).

In this study, toxic effects of cycasin were examined on biology species other than animals, namely microorganisms, plants and insects for the purpose of looking for a general, and a possible, common toxicological scope.

MATERIALS AND METHODS

Cycasin was isolated from the seeds of Japanese cycad. Microorganisms were supplied from the type-cultures maintained in Laboratory of Applied Microbiology in this Faculty, and partly in Faculty of Agriculture, Kyoto University. *Aspergillus oryzae* K was from Kawachi Co., Kagoshima. The seeds of rice plant, Ariake, were those harvested in this University Farm. Other seeds were of commercial sources.

Gibberellin A_3 was from Kanto Chemical Co., crystalline α-amylase of *Bacillus subtilis* was from Seikagaku Kogyo Co., NAD from Kyowa Hakko Co., and yeast alcohol dehydrogenase from Boehringer Mannheim Co.

Oxygen-uptake was measured with a Warburg manometer or an O_2 Uptester of Taiyo Co. The enzyme activities were determined as follows; α-amylase by blue-value method (Akabori, Ikenaka and Hagihara, 1956), catalase by Hennick's method (Tamari and Kaji, 1952), peroxidase by guaiacol method (Kondo and Morita, 1951), β-glucosidase from the amount of *o*-nitrophenol liberated from *o*-nitrophenyl-β-D-glucoside as the substrate (Miwa and Suzuki, 1956), and alcohol dehydrogenase from the absorption at 340 nm of NADH produced (Hatanaka and Sekiya, 1976). Protein was determined by the modified Lowry's method (Hartree, 1972).

RESULTS AND DISCUSSION

MICROORGANISMS

Effects on Various Microorganisms

Cycasin added to the culture medium generally developed the retardation of growth as well as the reduction in the characteristic products of each organism. The following bacteria were examined for their growth; *Bacillus subtilis* IFO 3007, *Bacillus cereus* IFO 3001, *Escherichia coli* IAM 1016, *Leuconostoc mesenteroides* B07 and *Streptomyces griseus* IAM 0084. They showed a fairly good tolerance to the added cycasin in 0.01 or 0.1% concentration, while they were affected with 1% cycasin. *E. coli* was exceptional, since its growth was accerelated by the added cycasin. One yeast, *Saccharomyces cerevisiae* IAM 4702, and a microalgae, *Chlorella vulgaris* IAM C-30, also showed a similar intoxication. In the latter, when grown on glucose as its carbon-source, it lost chlorophyll in the later period of culture, while the added cycasin brought a delay in decoloration. Fungi were intoxicated more clearly and their spore-formation was inhibited. The examined strains were *Penicillium chrysogenum* IFO 4626, *Aspergillus niger* Sz-2, *Aspergillus kawachii* IFO 4308 and *Aspergillus oryzae* K.

The production of lactic acid by *L. mesenteroides* or citric and gluconic acids by *Asp. niger* was low in the cycasin-added medium. An attempted observation of the increased production of riboflavin by *Eremothecium ashbyii* IFO 0952 and streptomycin by *St. griseus* FKU 3021 were in the negative results.

Kojic Acid and Its Related Substances Produced by *Asp. oryzae* K

Kojic acid, determined by Yabuta (1912, 1924) to be 5-hydroxy-2-hydroxymethyl-γ-pyrone, is known as a usual product of *Aspergillus*. Its production by *Asp. oryzae* K was exceptionally increased by the added cycasin; a maximum, 15 mg/ml on the 9th day of culture in the medium containing 0.2% cycasin. A maximum value in the medium without cycasin was 1 mg/ml. About one half of the added cycasin had been consumed by the fungus at the end of the 1st week, and almost all the cycasin in the 2nd week. In the later period of culture, 2nd to 4th week, several products with the same yellow fluorescence as kojic acid were observed on paper chromatograms under an ultraviolet lamp. Two major ones, referred as compounds 1 and 2, were isolated. A maximum accumulation of the compound 1 in the medium containing 0.2% cycasin was about 5 mg/ml on the 15th day. The structure of those was studied by infrared, nuclear magnetic resonance and mass spectrometries. Their acetyl derivatives prepared in the usual way were also analyzed. The compound 1 was concluded to be a dimer of kojic acid, 2,2'-dihydroxymethyl-6,6'-dikojyl-methane. The methylene group bridging two kojic acid moieties was assumed to have been derived from formaldehyde, which is one of the degradation products of the aglycone of cycasin. Ichimoto, Fujii and Tatsumi (1965) showed in the organic reaction of kojic acid with formaldehyde that 6-hydroxymethyl kojic acid was produced as a main product and that the dimer as a by-product. In our reaction of kojic acid with an enzymatic hydrolyzate of cycasin, the former was little produced, while the latter, the dimer, was obtained as the major product. The compound 2 was assumed to be a tetramer of kojic acid.

In a separate preliminary experiment, an enhanced oxygen-uptake was observed in the fungus which was on the stage of producing kojic acid. This acid is known to be synthesized by a direct oxidation of glucose (Arnstein and Bentley, 1953). A possible relationship between the respiration of the fungus and the kojic acid production is suggested.

PLANTS

Effects on Various Plant Seedlings

Several sorts of seeds of *Gramineae, Cruciferae* or *Leguminosae* were sown on cotton layers containing solutions of cycasin of various concentrations. Fig. 1 shows the seedlings of chinese cabbage, rice plant and soybean grown on cycasin-beds.

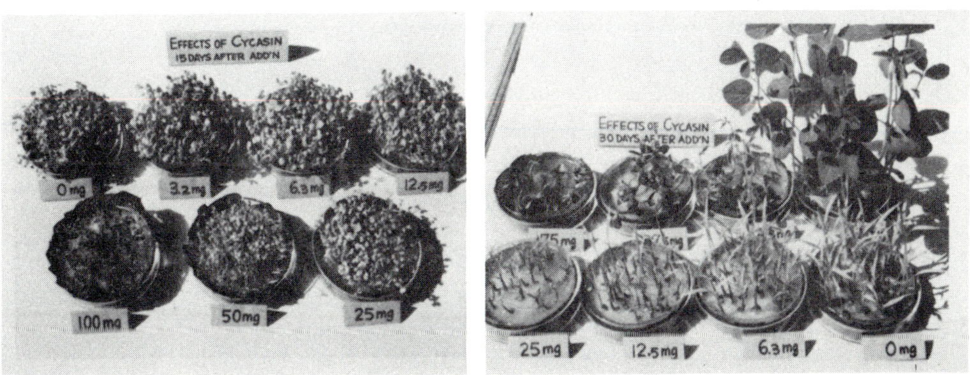

Fig. 1. Effects of cycasin on some plant seedlings.

The affected shoots and roots of the seedlings showed wilting, chlorosis and necrosis, as compared with those grown on water. Rice plant was most affected and did not germinate in a higher concentration of cycasin. Soybean seemed to be more tolerant.

The oxygen-uptake and the activities of catalase and peroxidase were measured on shoots or roots of rice, corn, soybean and kidney bean. In these experiments, the seeds were germinated on water for 13-20 days to get healthy seedlings grown to some extent and then they were transplanted for a few days to beds of 5-10 mM cycasin solution (the cycasin group) or water (the control group). The respiration was suppressed as a whole by cycasin, but both enzyme activities in the cycasin group were rather higher than those in the control group.

Rice Plant Seedlings

The rice plant was chosen as the most sensitive one to the effects due to cycasin. The seedlings grown for 10 days on 10 mM cycasin-bed were compared, every day, with those grown on water-bed. The fresh weight of the shoots and roots of the cycasin group was about half of that of the control group after 10 days. Oxygen-uptake became different between the two groups after 4 days, and showed 4 times in the control group of that in the cycasin group on the 7th day. The differences in the shoot-length and the activity of α-amylase also began to be clear on the 6th day; on the 10th day in the control group the shoot-length showed twice and the activity of α-amylase 2.4 times as long and as good as that in the cycasin group.

The biosynthesis of α-amylase in the germinating cereal seeds is, as well known (Yomo, 1960; Paleg, 1960; Varner and Chandra, 1964), closely related to the function of gibberellin (GA), one of the growth hormones for plants. Fig. 2 shows the effect of GA on the cycasin-treated rice seedlings. The group (a) is the control seeds grown on water during the whole experimental period of 9 days. Samples on

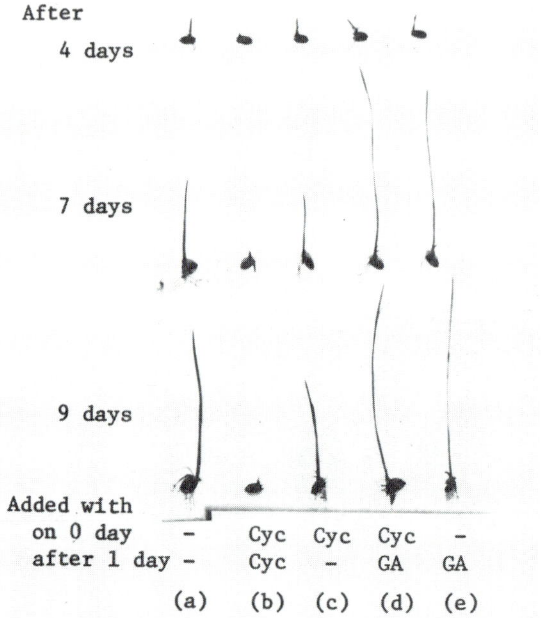

Fig. 2. Recovery of the ill-effect of cycasin by gibberellin.

the 4th, 7th and 9th days are shown. The group (b) grown on 10 mM cycasin for 9 days gave the worst result of no-germination. The group (c) was seeded on cycasin-bed and then transferred to water-bed on the 2nd day. Slightly better growth was observed. The group (d) was seeded on cycasin-bed and then grown on 0.3 mM GA_3-bed from the 2nd to the 9th day. A good recovery from the ill-effect of cycasin was attained. The group (e) was seeded on water-bed and transferred to GA_3-bed.

These sampled seedlings were assayed, respectively. The fresh weight of the part of paddy on the 9th day in the groups (a) to (e) was in a ratio of 1.00 : 2.00 : 1.50 : 1.31 : 1.34. The group (b) grown on cycasin through the whole period did not show so much decrease in weight. It means that the reserved carbohydrate in the endosperm was not consumed, and remained as it was at the initial stage. The ratio in the shoot-length on the 9th day was 1.00 : 0.07 : 0.31 : 0.57 : 1.64. The activity of α-amylase was in a ratio of 1.00 : 0.17 : 0.30 : 0.61 : 1.06. The treatment with cycasin clearly suppressed the development of α-amylase.

In the separate *in vitro* experiments, it was confirmed that the aglycone of cycasin did not inhibit at all the activities of hydrolytic enzymes themselves. The examined enzyme preparations were a commercial crystalline α-amylase from *B. subtilis*, and α-amylase and β-glucosidase in crude preparations obtained from the healthy rice seedlings grown on water.

Enzymatic Studies: Mechanism of the Toxification Due to Cycasin

The above mentioned experiments cleared that the toxicity of cycasin for germinating rice-seedlings was found in the suppression of the biosynthesis of α-amylase, and that this suppression was recovered by GA. An assay system with half-cut barley seeds, which is usually applied for the determination of GA (Jones and Varner, 1967), was used in order to study the effect of cycasin on the biosynthesis of α-amylase. The seeds of barley were cut in half, and the embryoless part of these containing no GA were put on a layer of quartz-sand containing water, or 10 mM solution of cycasin or pyrazole at room temperature for 3 days. Pyrazole will be described in the later experiment. The seeds were then transferred into acetate buffer, pH 4.8, containing 1×10^{-3} to 10 μg/ml of GA_3, calcium chloride and chloramphenicol, and were shaken at 25° for 24 hr. They were homogenized with the buffer, and the centrifuged supernatant was assayed for the α-amylase activity. The activity increased from 3×10^3 to 13×10^3 units in the control group with an increased amount of GA_3 added. The activity in the cycasin group was always lower than in the control group. More GA was clearly needed for the biosynthesis of α-amylase in the barley seeds treated with cycasin. The content of GA in the rice seedlings grown for 2 days on water or 10 mM cycasin was assayed by the use of the same assay system. GA found in 10 seedlings treated with cycasin was practically zero, as compared with the amount of GA in the control group, 0.04 μg.

Grab and Zedeck (1977) have recently reported that NAD-dependent alcohol dehydrogenase (ADH) is concerned with the carcinogenesis in the rats due to the aglycone of cycasin. They also examined the effect of pyrazole, a specific inhibitor for ADH. After the embryoless half seeds of barley was treated with water, 10 mM pyrazole, 10 mM cycasin, or with pyrazole and cycasin, they were incubated with acetate buffer containing 1 μg/ml of GA_3, and the activity of α-amylase was assayed as shown in the above experiment. The activities found in 10 half seeds were 11.85, 11.79, 8.91 and 12.06×10^3 units, respectively. Pyrazole did not affect the α-amylase formation, while the ill-effect of cycasin was recovered by pyrazole. This shows that ADH has some role in this case, too.

Cycasin added to the germinating seeds should first be hydrolyzed by β-glucosidase to liberate its aglycone, methylazoxymethanol (MAM), which would be a substrate of

ADH. These two enzyme activities were determined for a few plant seeds as shown in Table 1. The activities were especially high in the embryo of rice plant, and higher activities were parallel with the lower tolerance of the plants observed in the *in vivo* experiments. Kidney bean was the most resistant species. The total activities of ADH in embryo and endosperm of 10 rice seeds were 318.3 and 141.8, respectively, expressed in nmole of reduced NADH per min. β-Glucosidase activity in the same sample was 14.90 and 3.18 nmoles of liberated *o*-nitrophenol per min. Thus, the toxicity of cycasin can be closely correlated with these two enzymes.

TABLE I Activities of Alcohol Dehydrogenase and β-Glucosidase in Some Plant Seeds

Seeds	Alcohol dehydrogenase		β-Glucosidase	
	1	3	2	3
Rice	218.3	2.10	8.58	0.08
embryo	339.5	24.50	15.89	1.14
endosperm	121.2	0.69	2.72	0.02
Barley	66.9	1.25	127.00	3.02
Radish	9.2	1.45	1.90	0.02
Kidney bean	0.4	0.10	0.61	0.08

1. nmole NADH/min, mg protein
2. nmole *o*-nitophenol/min, mg protein
3. converted to mg basis of seeds

In the two preceding experiments, the dehydrogenase activity was determined for ethanol as its substrate. Whether the aglycone of cycasin, MAM, could become virtually a substrate of this enzyme or not should be ascertained. A commercial yeast ADH and an extract of rice bran were used as the enzyme preparations. The observed specific activities of yeast ADH to ethanol, methanol and MAM in 10 mM concentration were 38.600, 0.120 and 0.087 μmoles NADH/min, mg protein. The values for rice bran were 0.294, 0.003 and 0.002. Although the activity was low toward methanol and MAM, as compared with ethanol, these two enzyme preparations did catalyze the dehydrogenation of MAM. The liberated aglycone of cycasin, MAM, spontaneously degrades to give methanol (Kobayashi and Matsumoto, 1965), which would become the substrate for the dehydrogenase to yield formaldehyde. Grab and Zedeck (1977) found this aldehyde in the similar system with a rat liver preparation. This possibility was examined with a reaction system of 0.5 mM MAM, 0.756 mg/ml of yeast ADH in 10 mM pyrophosphate buffer, pH 8.5, at 25° for 60 min in the presence or absence of 0.6 mM NAD. The amount of NADH produced in the NAD-present system was 47.1 nmoles/ml. The decreased amount of MAM was 17.8 in the absence of NAD, and 55.6 in the presence of NAD, and the difference of them was 37.8 nmoles/ml. For formaldehyde, 17.2, 11.8 and -5.4 nmoles/ml were obtained, respectively. These results showed that the yeast ADH consumed MAM as its substrate in this experiment, too. The production of formaldehyde, however, was not observed, which is different from the case of an animal enzyme.

A proposed mechanism of emergence of cycasin-toxicity in germinating cereal seeds is illustrated in Fig. 3.

INSECTS

Larvae of silk worm, *Bombyx mori*, ingested the mulberry leaves sprayed with dilute solution of cycasin, were intoxicated, melaninized themselves heavily and died. Cabbage army worm, *Mamestra brassicae* L., were maintained on an artificial feed.

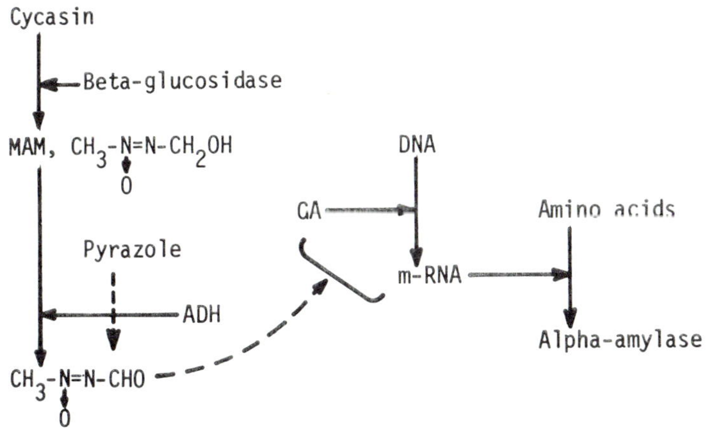

Fig. 3. A proposed mechanism of emergence of cycasin-toxicity in germinating cereal seeds.

They were given the feed containing cycasin at the 6th age of larvae. The actual amount of cycasin ingested by these two kinds of worms was not ascertained exactly. The larvae of cabbage army worms fed with 0.5 - 4 mg% cycasin-feed also melaninized themselves, pupated incompletely and died. Their pupation-ratio was 90 - 70%, and the weight of pupa fed with 4 mg% cycasin remained in 76% of the control.

The experiments are still on a preliminary stage, but these melaninized worms, being of interest to us, might have something in common with the necrosis observed in the intoxicated plants.

ACKNOWLEDGMENT

This study was partly supported by the Grant of Ministry of Education, Japan, No. 356064 in 1978, to which we are grateful. We also express our gratitudes to the students, Messrs. H. Terazono, S. Minemoto, H. Nakamura and Y. Onoyama, who engaged in each division of this work, and to the suppliers of the type-cultures of microorganisms.

REFERENCES

Akabori, S., T. Ikenaka, and B. Hagihara (1956). α-Amylase. In S. Akabori (Ed.), *Koso Kenkyu-ho (Methods in Enzymology)*, Vol. 2. Asakura, Tokyo. pp. 108-110.

Arnstein, H. R. V., and R. Bentley (1953). The biosynthesis of kojic acid (1). *Biochem. J.*, 54, 493-508.

Grab, D. J., and M. S. Zedeck (1977). Organ-specific effects of the carcinogen methylazoxymethanol related to metabolism of nicotinamide adenine dinucleotide-dependent dehydrogenases. *Cancer Res.*, 37, 4182-4189.

Hartree, E. F. (1972). Determination of protein: a modification of the Lowry method that gives a linear photometric response. *Anal. Biochem.*, 48, 422-427.

Hatanaka, A., and J. Sekiya (1976). Alcohol dehydrogenase from tea seeds. In *Tanpaku-shitsu, Kakusan, Koso (Protein, Nucleic acid and Enzyme).* 76:2, Kyoritsu, Tokyo. pp. 255-260.

Ichimoto, I., K. Fujii, and C. Tatsumi (1965). Studies on kojic acid and its re-

lated γ-pyrone compounds (14). *Agr. Biol. Chem.*, 29, 325-330.
Jones, R. L., and J. E. Varner (1967). The bioassay of gibberellin. *Planta*, 72, 155-161.
Kobayashi, A., and H. Matsumoto (1965). Studies on methylazoxymethanol, the aglycone of cycasin. Isolation, biological and chemical properties. *Arch. Biochem. Biophys.*, 110, 373-380.
Kondo, K., and Y. Morita (1951). Studies on phyto-peroxidase (1). *Bull. Res. Inst. Food Sci. Kyoto University*, 4, 12-23.
Laqueur, G. L., O. Mickelsen, M. G. Whiting, and L. T. Kurland (1963). Carcinogenic properties of nuts from *Cycas circinalis* L. indigenous to Guam. *J. Natl. Cancer Inst.*, 31, 919-951.
Miwa, T., and H. Suzuki (1956). Glycosidase. In Nippon Kagaku-kai (Japan Chem. Soc.) (Ed.), *Jikken Kagaku Koza (Handbook of Experimental Chemistry)*, Vol. 24. Maruzen, Tokyo. pp. 305-307.
Nishida, K., A. Kobayashi, and T. Nagahama (1955). Studies on cycasin, a new toxic glycoside of *Cycas revoluta* Thunb. (1). *Bull. Agr. Chem. Soc. Japan*, 19, 77-83.
Paleg, L. G. (1960). Physiological effects of gibberellic acid (2). *Plant Physiol.*, 35, 902-906.
Sixth International Cycad Conference (1972). *Fed. Proc.*, 31, 1465-1546.
Tamari, K., and J. Kaji (1952). Injurious action of fusarinic acid on plant growth (1). *Nippon Nogeikagaku Kaishi (J. Agr. Chem. Soc. Japan)*, 26, 223-227.
Varner, J. E., and G. R. Chandra (1964). Hormonal control of enzyme synthesis in barley endosperm. *Proc. Natl. Acad. Sci. U. S.*, 52, 100-106.
Yabuta, T. (1912). On kojic acid, a new organic acid formed by *Aspergillus oryzae*. *Mem. Coll. Agr. Tokyo*, 5, 51-58.
Yabuta, T. (1924). The constitution of kojic acid, a γ-pyrone derivative formed by *Aspergillus oryzae* from carbohydrates. *J. Chem. Soc.*, 125, 575-587.
Yomo, H. (1960). Studies on the amylase activating substance (5). *Hakko Kyokaishi (J. Ferm. Soc. Japan)*, 18, 603-606.

ENZYMATIC HYDROLYSIS OF AMYGDALIN BY FECAL SAMPLES AND SOME FOODS

B. Stavric and R. Klassen

Toxicology Research Division, Food Directorate, Health Protection Branch, Health and Welfare Canada, Ottawa, Ont. K1A 0L2, Canada

ABSTRACT

Toxic effects and deaths in humans due to consumption of nuts or other foods containing amygdalin have been reported by many investigators. The toxicity is due to the release of HCN in gut, upon hydrolysis of amygdalin. Meanwhile, similar toxic effects have not been observed in experimental animals. We investigated the effect of intestinal and fecal flora from various species on hydrolytic breakdown of amygdalin. A recently developed gas liquid chromatographic method for quantitation of amygdalin by measuring underivatized benzaldehyde extracted from the anaerobically conducted enzymatic hydrolysis with emulsin, was employed. Samples of feces of mouse, rat, hamster, guinea pig, monkey and man were analyzed for their ability to hydrolyze amygdalin. A great variation was found in the relative potency to hydrolyze amygdalin among different individuals of the same species, but even greater variations were found between different species. These preliminary data suggest that man may be more susceptible to amygdalin poisoning than other tested species. It was also found that some foods possess enzyme(s) which can hydrolyze amygdalin. These data suggest that severe toxic effects could be expected if individuals taking amygdalin (in foods or as tablets) are simultaneously consuming diets containing emulsin or other similar enzymes.

KEYWORDS

Amygdalin; hydrolysis of cyanogenetic glycoside; β-glucosidase in foods; release of hydrogen cyanide; toxicity of amygdalin.

INTRODUCTION

Amygdalin [D-mandelonitrile-β-D-glucosido-6-β-D-glucoside] is a naturally occurring cyanogenetic glycoside, which appears in variable quantities in almonds and other stone fruit kernels like apricot, cherry, prune, plum, peach (Dorr and Paxinos, 1978; Montgomery, 1969). Reports are accumulating describing fatal or toxic effects in some people consuming foods or tablets containing amygdalin (Braico and co-workers, 1979; Humbert, Tress and Braico, 1977; Rubino and Davidoff, 1979; Sadoff, Fuchs and Hollander, 1978; Sayre and Kaymakcalan, 1964; Smith and co-workers, 1977; Townsend and Boni, 1975). An apparent discrepancy between animal and human data and the recent interest and availability of amygdalin

(C.H., 1977; Culliton and Waterfall, 1979; Jukes, 1976), prompted us: (i) to investigate the difference in intestinal content and/or fecal flora from various species in hydrolyzing amygdalin to form toxic hydrocyanic acid (HCN) (Dorr and Paxinos, 1978), and (ii) to determine the presence and ability of enzyme(s) in some fruit pits capable of hydrolyzing amygdalin.

The enzymes which hydrolyze amygdalin are β-glucosidases (amygdalaze, emulsin) and probably in weaker capacity some digestive enzymes. The rate of hydrolysis of amygdalin to form equimolar amounts of toxic HCN and non-toxic benzaldehyde depends on the concentration of the enzyme(s) (Dorr and Paxinos, 1978).

Since the liberation of HCN from its glycoside precursors is an enzymatic reaction, heat treatment would be expected to render plants containing glucosidases relatively non-toxic (Herbert, 1979). Nevertheless, serious outbreaks of cyanide poisoning from cooked lima beans have been known to occur in various parts of the world (Montgomery, 1969). Some experiments with lima beans raised the possibility that the body itself may contain enzymes capable of releasing HCN from cyanogenetic glycosides. It was also reported, that very little HCN was released from cooked lima beans exposed to human gastric juices, although fecal extract and *Escherichia coli* did release significant amounts of HCN (Winkler, 1958). It is conceivable, therefore, that the toxic effects of cyanogenetic glycosides in humans may arise from the absorption of HCN in the colon through the action of the enzymes obtained with food or from bacterial origin. The body itself may also contain enzymes capable of releasing HCN (Liener, 1966).

The rate of hydrolysis of amygdalin is very important, because HCN once formed, is rapidly absorbed from the gastrointestinal tract. If the rate of formation of HCN is greater than the detoxification rate (by forming thiocyanate), toxic or fatal concentration of HCN in blood (0.5-1.0 mg HCN/kg b.w.; Herbert, 1979) could easily occur.

In this report the relative enzymatic activity in hydrolyzing amygdalin of fecal samples from various species or of fruit kernels is described. This procedure utilizes the measurement of benzaldehyde formed when amygdalin is added to the test samples (feces, intestinal content, fruit pits, food component) and incubated anaerobically.

MATERIALS AND METHODS

Samples

Fresh fecal samples (approx. 1-2 g) were obtained from healthy laboratory animals, fed normal diets. When necessary (mouse), feces of a few animals were pooled for a test. Fecal samples from children (3-6 years) or adult healthy volunteers (35-55 years) were obtained from people consuming normal diets, and analysed not later than 3 hours after the collections. Fruits and/or pit kernels were obtained from local food markets.

Standard solution: 1% amygdalin (Aldrich Chem. Co. purity unspecified) in H_2O.
Internal standard: o-toluidine (Eastman Kodak, Co.) (100 μl/200 ml ethyl acetate).

Methods

The amount of benzaldehyde formed after hydrolysis of amygdalin was measured by gas liquid chromatography (GLC). A preliminary report of this method was presented [column : 3% DEGS on Gas Chrom Q; isothermal, temp. column 100°C;

ret. times : amygdalin 2.42 min; int. standard (o-toluidine) 8.07 min] (Klassen and Stavric, 1977)[1].

Fecal samples. Fresh samples (1-2 g) were homogenized in 0.9% saline (1 g/5 ml) and centrifuged. The supernate served as a stock solution for three (i, ii, iii) 1 ml aliquots. (i) A first 1 ml aliquot was injected into a 10 ml vacutainer-tube in which 1 ml amygdalin standard solution was already injected. The mixture was anaerobically incubated at 37°C for 2 h and then mixed with 3 ml of ethyl acetate internal standard. After separation, an aliquot (3 µl) of the ethyl acetate was injected into the GLC. - (ii) A second 1 ml of the supernate was injected into a vacutainer containing only 1 ml water (blank), and the procedure followed as described in (i). - (iii) A third 1 ml aliquot was freeze-dried to obtain the weight of the dry feces used in the test.

Fruit kernel. Fruit kernels (or other food samples) (approx. 2-3 g) were homogenized in water (1 g/10 ml), centrifuged and the two 1 ml aliquots of the supernate were used for the test of enzymatic activity (i) and as a blank (ii). Incubation time for the determination was 16h at 37°C.

By taking in consideration the weight of sample used in the tests (for fecal samples the freeze dried weight), dilutions, the aliquot injected into GLC and the peak heights obtained for benzaldehyde of the sample (and of the blank as well), it was possible to determine the potency of hydrolyzing enzymes in fecal samples or in kernels. For the calculation of the relative enzymatic activity of the fecal sample, the following formula was used:

$$\text{relative enzymatic activity} = \frac{\%\ \text{converted (sample)} \div \text{wt. freeze dried feces sample}}{\%\ \text{converted (mouse)} \div \text{wt. freeze dried feces mouse}}$$

RESULTS AND DISCUSSION

Our preliminary results (Klassen and Stavric, 1977) demonstrated that identical hydrolytic breakdown products, HCN and benzaldehyde, were obtained when amygdalin was treated either with commercial β-glucosidase, or with water extract from the peach kernel homogenate or from the fecal extract.

Table 1 summarizes the results concerning the enzymatic potency of enzymes in various fecal samples to hydrolyze amygdalin. Only 0.7% (averages of several tests) of amygdalin added to mouse feces was hydrolyzed after 2 hours of incubation, while the obtained values for other species were: guinea pig 2.2%; monkey 2.7%; rat 3.4%; hamster 13%. Under the same experimental conditions, feces from healthy humans hydrolyzed 29% of amygdalin, with some individuals hydrolyzing as much as 45% of the added amygdalin. When the enzymatic activity of 1 mg of dry mouse feces is taken as 1, the average relative enzymatic activity of 1 mg dry human feces was 46 times greater than that observed for the mouse.

---

[1]More information about the methodology (optimum conditions, confirmation, recovery) and use of this method in the quantitation of amygdalin in various foods will be published elsewhere (Klassen and Stavric, 1977).

TABLE 1 Potency of Fecal Samples to Hydrolyze Amygdalin

Species	% amygdalin converted*	Weight of freeze-dried feces (mg)	Relative enzymatic activity per 1 mg dry feces**
mouse	0.74	30.5	1.0
guinea pig	2.16	22.6	4.0
monkey	2.72	25.5	3.3
hamster	13.0	16.4	33.0
rat	3.4		6.4
individual:	3.7	18.0	8.6
	0.7	25.0	1.2
	6.0	25.0	10.0
	3.2	22.4	6.0
human (child)	30.6	28.7	44.4
human (adult)	27.6		48.0
individual:	7.45	17.4	17.8
	45.2	28.3	66.6
	30.1	21.9	58.4
	27.8	28.5	48.5

* average of 4-10 individual tests

** enzymatic activity of 1 mg dry mouse feces = 1

Our results indicate some variations in potential toxicity of ingested amygdalin between individual members of the same species, but a greater variation exists between different species (Table 1). The observed variations in relative enzymatic activity for the same individual is probably dependent on the ingested food, which may possess more or less of the glucosidase-type enzymes, or colonic bacteria capable of hydrolyzing cyanogenetic glycosides.

Table 2 summarizes the results on the relative activity of enzymes capable of hydrolyzing amygdalin. For comparative purposes the enzymatic activity of different fruits was compared to the activity of 0.1 g of peach kernel taken as 1.00. Our results indicate that although certain kernels do not contain amygdalin, they still possess a strong enzymatic capacity to hydrolyze amygdalin.

Recently, experimental evidence was presented (Schmidt and co-workers, 1978) for the significance of a mixed diet to obtain toxic effects of amygdalin in dogs. Toxicity and deaths occurred to dogs when "laetrile" was digested together with a sweet almond extract prepared just prior to administration. In a series of preliminary experiments with rats (Wistar, females, 225-240 g) we tried to create a condition for potential toxicity by feeding rats a diet containing β-glucosidase (50% ground rat chow + 50% ground sweet almonds). A three to four fold increase in the enzymatic potency of rat feces to hydrolyze amygdalin was obtained after 1-2 days on this diet. These rats were then dosed via gastric tube with 20 mg amygdalin (app. 5.0 mg HCN/kg b.w.). No toxic effects were observed.

Toxic effects and deaths were observed in the next series of tests, when variable amounts of amygdalin were given by gastric tube simultaneously with an optimized concentration of the enzyme preparation (EP). Out of 4 rats given 20 mg amygdalin

TABLE 2 The Relative Potency of Enzymes from Different Foods to Hydrolyze Amygdalin.

Kernel	Enzymatic potency*
peach	1.00
brazil nut	0.76**
walnut	0.02**
almond (sweet)	0.99**
flbert	0.04
lima beans	0.25
red walnut	0.02**
prune	0.46
nectarine	0.71**
apple seeds	0.98
apricot	0.96

* 0.1 g of the peach kernel will hydrolyze approximately 7 mg of amygdalin in 16 h. This unit was used as 1.00 in calculating the relative potency of other tested foods.

** Preliminary evidence indicates that no detectable amounts of amygdalin were present in tested samples.

+ EP (≡5.0 mg HCN/kg b.w.) no deaths occurred, although one rat was in poor condition for almost 1 hour after the dosing. After recovery period of a few days the same group of rats were treated with the dose of 25 mg amygdalin + EP (≡6.5 mg HCN/kg b.w.). One rat died shortly after the dosing, and two were severely affected but recovered. Subsequently, after a few days the remaining 3 rats were treated with a dose of 30 mg amygdalin + EP (≡7.5 mg HCN/kg b.w.) and two of them died. The third one, although comatose for more than 1 hour survived and completely recovered. A dose of 35 mg amygdalin + EP (≡8.7 mg HCN/kg b.w.) was required to kill this rat. The clinical signs and the subsequent deaths of the HCN poisoned rats, as well as the doses of HCN required for toxic manifestations, were in agreement with the recently reported cyanide toxicity in rats dosed with potassium cyanide (Egekeze and Oehme, 1979).

These results suggest a variation in lethal dose for rats exposed to HCN gastrically developed from amygdalin. The observed minimal lethal dose of LD_{25} = 6.5 mg HCN/kg b.w. is much higher than the lethal dose reported for human (0.5-1.0 mg/kg b.w.). This, as well as the fast recovery of the intoxicated rats indicates a faster detoxification mechanism for HCN in rats than in humans, where the comatose state tends to last up to several days (Braico and co-workers, 1979; Herbert, 1979; Humbert, Tress and Braico, 1977). These findings, coupled with the relative lack of an appropriate enzymes(s) to hydrolyse amygdalin in the rat, indicate that the rat is not an appropriate animal model for feeding studies with amygdalin.

SUMMARY

Our results so far suggest that the efficacy of human fecal enzymes to hydrolyze amygdalin significantly exceeds the potency of enzymes in all tested animals. It seems that most of the animals do not possess enough of these enzymes for a fast hydrolysis of amygdalin, therefore, these animals can consume large amounts of amygdalin without apparent toxic effects. Our data suggest that man may be more susceptible than other species to amygdalin poisoning, because of the possibility for faster hydrolysis of amygdalin in human gut to form toxic HCN. Toxic effects could be enhanced if individuals taking amygdalin (in foods or as tablets) are simultaneously consuming diets containing emulsin.

REFERENCES

A.J.L. (1959). Quarterly report to the editor on topics of current interest (hydrogen cyanide and amygdalin). Association of the Food and Drug Officials of the United States 23, 55-58.

Braico, K.T., J.R. Humbert, K.L. Terplan and J.M. Lehatay (1979). Laetrile intoxication. New Engl. J. Med. 300, 238-240.

-C.H. (Editorial) (1977). Science 196, 854.

Culliton, B.J. and W.K. Waterfall (1979). Apricot pits and cancer. Brit. Med. J. 1, 802-803.

Dorr, R.T. and J. Paxinos (1978). The current status of laetrile. Ann. Interm. Med. 89, 389-397.

Egekeze, J.O. and F.W. Oehme (1979). Blood and liver cyanide concentrations in rats poisoned with oral doses of potassium cyanide. Toxicology Letters 3, 243-247.

Herbert, V. (1979). Laetrile: the cult of cyanide promoting poison for profit. Amer. J. Clin. Nutr. 32, 1121-1158.

Humbert, J.R., J.M. Tress and K.T. Braico (1977). Fatal cyanide poisoning: accidental ingestion of amygdalin. J. Amer. Med. Ass. 238, 482.

Jukes, T.H. (1976). Laetrile for cancer. J. Amer. Med. Ass. 236, 1284-1286.

Klassen, R. and B. Stavric (1977). Hydrolysis of amygdalin: potency of intestinal/fecal flora of various species. 191st Ann. Meeting Assoc. Offic. Anal. Chemists, Washington, D.C. October 17-20, abstract 52. Manuscript will be submitted for publication to the Journal of the Ass. Off. Anal. Chem. (1979).

Liener, I.E. (1966). Cyanogenetic Glycosides. In Toxicants Occurring Naturally in Foods, NAS/NRC, Washington, pp. 58-61.

Montgomery, R.D. (1969). Cyanogens. In I.E. Liener (Ed.) Toxic Constituents of Plant Foodstuffs, Academic Press, New York, pp. 143-157.

Rubino, M.J. and F. Davidoff (1979). Cyanide poisoning from apricot seeds. J. Amer. Med. Ass. 241, 359.

Sadoff, L., K. Fuchs and J. Hollander (1978). Rapid death associated with Laetrile ingestion. J. Amer. Med. Ass. 239, 1532.

Sayre, J.W. and S. Kaymakcalan (1964). Cyanide poisoning from apricot seeds among children in Turkey. New Engl. J. Med. 270, 1113-1115.

Schmidt, E.S., G.W. Newton, S.M. Sanders, J.P. Lewis and E.E. Conn (1978). Laetrile toxicity studies in dogs. J. Amer. Med. Ass. 239, 943-947.

Smith, F.P., T.P. Butler, S. Cohan and P.S. Schein (1977). Laetrile toxicity: A report of two cases. J. Amer. Med. Ass. 238, 1361.

Townsend, W.A. and B. Boni (1975). Cyanide poisoning from ingestion of apricot kernels. Morbidity and Mortality Weekly Report Dec. 13, 427.

Winkler, W.O. (1958). Study of methods for glucosidae HCN in lima beans. J. Assoc. Offic. Agr. Chem. 41, 282-287.

Mycotoxins

TOXICOLOGICAL EVALUATION OF TRICHOTHECENE MYCOTOXINS

Y. Ueno

Department of Toxicology and Microbial Chemistry, Faculty of Pharmaceutical Sciences, Tokyo University of Science, Ichigaya, Shinjuku-ku, Tokyo, Japan

ABSTRACT

Among 40 kinds of trichothecenes, nivalenol and deoxynivalenol of *Fusarium graminearum* are the dominant pollutants of cereal grains. Pharmacological mechanisms of vomiting and skin toxicity, immunological disorders, metabolism in animal tissues and epoxide-specific detection method were summerized.

KEYWORDS

Trichothecenes; nivalenol; deoxynivalenol; T-2 toxin; *Fusarium spp.*; vomiting; central depressants; mast cells; delayed hypersensitivity; blue-spot test.

INTRODUCTION

The first trichothecene compound, trichothecin, was isolated as an antifungal metabolite of *Trichothecium roseum* (Freeman *et al.*, 1959). Mycotoxicologically important finding was carried out by Bamburg *et al.* (1968), who reported T-2 toxin as a causative toxicant of the moldy corn toxicosis in the U.S.A. Red-mold diseases prevailed in barley and wheat in Japan, and the uptake of these moldy cereals caused vomiting, diarrhea and hemorrhage. Rabbit reticulocyte bioassay (Ueno *et al.*, 1969a) and pathological observation revealed nivalenol (Tatsuno *et al.*,1969), fusarenon-X (Ueno *et al.*, 1969b) and others. Yoshizawa *et al.* (1973) discovered deoxynivalenol, which was identical with vomitoxin (Vesonder *et al.*,1973).
Alimentary toxic alukia (ATA) has been recorded in Russia since the 19th century. The characteristic symptoms of the disease were fever, hemorrhage, necrotic angina, leukopenia and exhaustion of bone marrow. In view of sudden outbreaks and a high mortality (up to 60 %), ATA was first considered to be an epidemic disease of infectious origin, but recent research has led to the conclusion that the trichothecenes produced by *F.sporotrichioides* and F.poae are responsible for the outbreak of this endemic food-borne disease (Ueno, 1977a).
In early 1931, a fatal disease of unknown origin prevailed in Ukranian horses. Russian workers found that the disease was associated with fungi-contaminated feed and hay, and they classified it as a mycotoxicosis. This disease could be designated as stachybotryotoxicosis, since the toxic agents of unknown structure are elaborated by certain strains of the fungus *Stachybotrys alternans* (*S.atra*). FDA group presented indirect evidence that the toxic agents responsible for stachybotryotoxicosis are satratoxins, a macrocyclic 12, 13-epoxytrichothecene

(Eppley *et al.*, 1977).
These epidemiological and mycotoxicological surveys have thus revealed that "red-mold disease" in Japan, "moldy corn toxicosis" in the U.S.A., "ATA" in Russia and central Europe, and "stachybotryotoxicosis" in Russia and Hungary are caused by common toxicants, "trichothecene mycotoxins" (Ueno, 1977a and 1977b).
A comprehensive review by Bamburg *et al.*(1971) covered the literature available through the first half of 1970s. At that time, 22 naturally occurring members of trichothecenes had been discovered. During the past nine years, the development of improved analytical and bioassay screening methods provided rapid progress in detection of new trichothecenes. At the present time, more than 40 kinds of naturally occurring trichothecenes have been elucided, and the author proposed the classification system for trichothecenes into four groups according to their structural and fungal characteristics as follows: type-A (T-2 toxin, HT-2 toxin, diacetoxyscirpenol etc.); type-B (nivalenol, deoxynivalenol etc.); type-C (crotocin etc.); and type-D (verrucarins and other macrocycles) (Ueno, 1977a, 1977b, 1978).
In this Symposium, the author aimed to summerize the recent progress on the mycology of trichothecene-producing *Fusarium spp.*, natural occurrence of trichothecenes in cereal grains in Japan, toxicological and pharmacological characteristics of trichothecenes, and the fate and metabolism of some of trichothecenes in animals. An improved method, so-called "blue-spot test", was also established and its application for screening of trichothecene-producing fungi and detection in animal excreta was reported.

TRICHOTHECENE-PRODUCING *FUSARIUM* SPECIES

In a preceding paper (Ueno *et al.*, 1973), the author has reported the trichothecene-producing *Fusarium spp.* in domestic and imported cereal grains. The dominant species are *F.tricinctum, F.sporotrichioides and F.poae* for the type-A toxins (T-2 toxin etc.), and *F.nivale, F.oxysporum* for the type-B toxins (nivalenol etc.). In general, the type-A trichothecene producers are not able to produce the type-B toxins. For example, *F.tricinctum* produces T-2 toxin and related compounds, and *F.nivale* produces the C-8 keto trichothecenes such as nivalenol. Exceptionally, *F.lateritium* and *F.semitectum* are capable of producing both the type-A and B trichothecenes. *F.roseum* is known to produce various kinds of the type-A and B toxins. Taxonomically, this fungus is subdivided by "forma specialis" into *F.roseum "culmorum", "avenaceum", scirpi", gibbosum" and "graminearum"*. *F.roseum "gibbosum"* produces monoacetoxyscirpenol (type-A) and *F.roseum "graminearum"* produces nivalenol and deoxynivalenol.

TABLE 1 Trichothecene Producibility of *Fusarium* Species

Species	Trichothecenes					
	Type-A			Type-B		
	T-2	NS	DAS	NIV	FX	DEN
F.tricinctum	+	+	+			
F.sporotrichioides	+	+	+			
F.poae	+	+	+			
F.acuminatum	+	+				
F.graminearum				+	+	+
F.nivale				+	+	
F.lateritium		+	+	+		
F.equiseti		+	+	+	+	
F.semitectum		+	+	+	+	

F.nivale Fn 2B is the first isolated producer of nivalenol and its acetylated fusarenon-X. This species was isolated by Tsunoda *et al.* (1968) from moldy wheat at Kumamoto district in Japan when a massive outbreak of Akakabi (red-mold) disease occurred. For identification of this fungus, he compared the mycological charactors with those of *F.nivale* NRRL 3249, which now recognized as an abnormal strain of *F.tricinctum*. Recent surveys by Yoshizawa & Morooka (1977) demonstrated that *F.roseum "graminearum"* is responsible for the production of nivalenol and its derivatives. As for *F.solani* M-1-1, which was isolated by Tsunoda from dried bean-hulls in relation to "bean-hulls poisoning of horses", the author have demonstrated several type-A trichothecenes such as T-2 toxin, neosolaniol and related compounds (Ueno *et al.*, 1972). According to Ichinoe (1978), however, this fungus should be classified as *F.sporotrichioides*.
An interesting finding was the geographic distribution of trichothecene-producing *Fusarium* species. As cited in a preceding paper (Ueno *et al.*, 1973), the type-A trichothecene producers such as *F.sporotrichioides* and *F.poae* are distributed in the northern district of Japan and the type-B trichothecene producers such as *F.graminearum* are frequently detected in the southern part of Japan. This finding was recently confirmed by the extensive survey of Ichinoe (1978) and Yoshizawa (1978). These mycological investigations support an assumption that the red-mold diseases prevailed in Kyushu, Shikoku and other southern part of Japan were originated by the toxic metabolites of *F.graminearum*, nivalenol and deoxynivalenol.

NATURAL OCCURRENCE OF TRICHOTHECENES

Publications on the occurrence of trichothecenes in foodstuffs have been scarce because of the lack of detection methods as well as due to the complexity of the trichothecene family. The trichothecene mycotoxins consist of about 40 kinds of derivatives, however, the mycotoxins detected in natural environment are limited to a relatively small number of toxins such as T-2 toxin, diacetoxyscirpenol, nivalenol and deoxynivalenol, as summarized in TABLE 2.

TABLE 2 Natural Occurrence of Trichothecenes

Trichothecenes	Source	Country	Yield (mg/kg)	Content (ppm)	Ref.
T-2 toxin	Corn	U.S.A.	2		Hsu *et al.*(1972)
	Barley	Canada		25	Greenway & Puls (1976)
	Mixed feed	U.S.A.		0.075	Mirocha *et al.*(1976)
Deoxynivalenol	Corn	U.S.A.	3		Vesonder *et al.*(1973)
	Corn	U.S.A.	8		Ishii *et al.*(1975)
	Corn	U.S.A.		8	Yoshizawa *et al.*(1977)
	Barley	Japan		5	ibid.
	Corn	France		0.1-0.6	Jemmali *et al.*(1978)
	Mixed feed	U.S.A.		1	Mirocha *et al.*(1976)
	Maize kernel	U.S.A.		0.1	ibid.
	Corn	U.S.A.		0.5-10	Vesonder *et al.*(1978)
Nivalenol	Corn	France		1-4	Jemmali *et al.*(1978)
	Barley	Japan		0.1-22.9	Yoshizawa *et al.*(1978)
Diacetoxyscirpenol	Mixed feed	U.S.A.		0.4-0.5	Mirocha *et al.*(1976)
	Seed	India		not cited	Ghosal *et al.*(1977)

During the past two years (1977-1978), the red-mold disease research term carried out extensive survey on the natural occurrence of trichothecenes in domestic barley and wheat. The results (unpublished) revealed that over a half of samples tested was contaminated by nivalenol (0.02-9.47 ppm) and deoxynivalenol (0.04-3.0

ppm). Furthermore, according to Kamimura *et al.* (1978), about 50% of nivalenol and deoxynivalenol added to flour remained after food processings such as baking (210°C), frying (140°C) or boiling. These evidences strongly suggest that the barley and wheat harvested in the southern part of Japan are polluted by the trichothecene mycotoxins, especially nivalenol and deoxynivalenol of *F.graminearum*, and once contaminated in natural environment, these toxins are hard to remove by ordinary food processing.

PHARMACOLOGY OF TRICHOTHECENES

All the trichothecene mycotoxins are highly toxic to experimental animals such as mice, rats, cats, guinea-pigs, dogs and avians. Characteristic symptoms are, in general, vomiting, diarrhea, hyperemia of the intestinal tract, leukocytosis and leukopenia. Pathologically, the actively-dividing cells of the gastro-intestinal tract, thymus, bone marrow, lymph node, testis and ovary were affected (Saito & Tatsuno, 1971; Ueno *et al.*, 1971). Recently, Matsuoka and the author (Matsuoka *et al.* 1979) have examined the general pharmacological effect of fusarenon-X to mice, rats and dogs. In mice i.p. injected with fusarenon-X, a slight ataxic gait and a fall of the body temperature were observed. In rats, an elevation of blood pressure and a depression of respiratory rate were evident in the early stage of intoxication. In isolated organs such as fundus, vas deferens, tracheal muscle and ileum of rats and guinea-pigs, none of responses were affected by the mycotoxin. These results suggest that fusarenon-X has no significant effect on the muscle cell membrane or on the nerve elements of these isolated organs.
Interesting finding was that the i.v. injected fusarenon-X caused a partial inhibition of intestinal peristalsis 30 min after the injection and a complete inhibition after 40 min. This inhibition was antagonized by pilocarpine. These evidences suggest that the trichothecene may induce desquamation of intestinal epithelium cells and thereby cause leaking of body fluids leading to the enhancement of the propulsion of intestinal contents. These pharmacological effects are presumed to be one of the reason of heavey diarrhea in animals administered with the trichothecenes.
Vomiting is one of the most significant symptoms in cats, dogs, swines, ducklings, and sometimes in man, when the purified toxins or damaged cereals were consumed, and by employing ducklings as a bioassay tool the author isolated deoxynivalenol from corn polluted by *Fusarium* species (Ishii *et al.*, 1975). TABLE 3 summarizes the data on vomiting effect of trichothecenes.

TABLE 3 Vomiting Doses of Trichothecenes

Trichothecenes	Vomiting Doses (mg/kg, s.c.)			
	Duckling[a)]	Cat	Dog	Swine
T-2 toxin	0.1	0.1[b)]		
HT-2 toxin	0.1			
Diacetoxyscirpenol	0.2			
Neosolaniol	0.1			
Nivalenol	1.0			
Fusarenon-X	0.4	1[c)]	0.3 (i.v.)[d)]	
Diacetylnivalenol	0.4			
Deoxynivalenol (Vomitoxin)	10.0[e)]	0.1	0.1	0.05 (i.p.)[f)]
Acetyldeoxynivalenol	10.0		0.2	

a) Ueno *et al.* (1974); b) Sato *et al.* (1975); c) Ueno *et al.* (1971); d) Matsuoka *et al.* (1979); e) Yoshizawa *et al.* (1977); f) Vesonder *et al.* (1973).

As for the vomiting mechanism, Matsuoka *et al.* (1979) investigated the effect of central depressants. Intravenously administered fusarenon-X of 0.3 mg/kg induced emesis in dogs. Vomiting appeared 5 to 15 min after the administration and occured repeatedly at intervals of 30 to 40 min for 1 to 3 hr. This vomiting action of fusarenon-X was antagonized by an injection of 0.5 mg/kg of metoclopramide·HCl or 1.0 mg of chloropromazine·HCl 1 hr before the administration of fusarenon-X. This suppressive effect of central depressants strongly suggest the possible action of fusarenon-X to stimulate the chemoreceptor trigger zone (CTZ) in medulla oblongata.

Skin toxicity is another characteristic effect to animals, and this biological action of trichothecenes was applied for screening of trichothecene-producing fungi for a long time without any scientific basis. In a preceding paper (Ueno *et al.*, 1970), the author compared the skin toxicity of several trichothecene mycotoxins in mice, rats, rabbits and guinea-pigs. The data revealed that the toxicity of trichothecenes differs markedly depending on their chemical structure, and guinea-pigs are most sensitive among the animals tested. Recent experiments indicate that as little as 0.005 µg of T-2 toxin is enough to induce skin reddening in gunea-pigs. In general, the type-A and D toxins, such as T-2 toxin and verrucarin A, respectively, are highly toxic and the type-B toxins such as nivalenol and deoxynivalenol are less toxic than the formers in this respect. A noticeable finding was the rapid appearance of skin toxicity when crotocin and trichothecin, both possessing an isocrotonyl residue at C-4, were applied to skin tissue (Shimada and Ueno, unpublished).

The mechanism of the skin toxicity is not fully clarified at the present time. In order to elucidate the effect of trichothecene on vascular permeability, the back skin of rabbit was painted by fusarenon-X for varied intervals, and pontamine sky blue was i.v. injected 1 hr before sacrifice. The amount of dye deposited in the toxin-painted skin tissue was used as a parameter of increment of vascular permeability. As shown in Fig. 1, fusarenon-X caused a biphasic increment of vascular permeability 5 and 24 hr after the painting (Shimada & Ueno, unpub). A similar biphasic response was observed in foot pad swelling when the toxin was administered into rat hind paw (Matsuoka *et al.*, 1979).

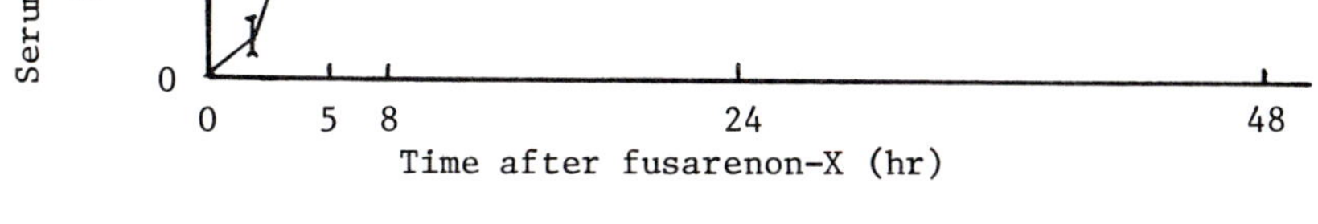

Fig. 1. Effect of fusarenon-X to vascular permeability (10 µg of fusarenon-X, s.c.).

Since the preliminary experiment revealed the disruption of mast cells by a low concentration of fusarenon-X or T-2 toxin, the first increment in permeability is presumed by mediated by chemical mediator(s). As for the second phase, the toxin cause the increment of permeability by acting directly on capillary vessel, since the trichothecene mycotoxins possess a potent cytotoxicity to animal cells. It is very important finding that the macrocyclic trichothecenes such as verrucarin A are characterized by edematous damages of skin tissues and the type-B toxins are characterized by skin reddening. Since the cytotoxicity of varrucarin A is around 100 times higher than that of fusarenon-X, the inflammatory properties of the macrocyclic trichothecenes are well correlated with their potent cytotoxicity.

IMMUNOTOXICITY OF TRICHOTHECENES

It is well established that the trichothecene mycotoxins have a characteristic biological activity to cause marked damages to the proliferating cells of the hematopoietic tissues in the bone marrow, spleen, thymus and lymph nodes. Treatment of the mouse with high doses of these toxins brings about a rapid decrease in the weight of thymus and spleen (Sato *et al.*, 1978). This suggests that these toxins may cause immunological deficiencies in animals.

According to Rosenstein *et al.* (1979), T-2 toxin and diacetoxyscirpenol caused a significant reduction in thymus weight and inhibited immunological responsiveness to sheep red blood cells (SRBC) in the mouse. This suppressive effect of trichothecenes may partly be explained by the ability of these toxins to inhibit protein synthesis in eukaryotic cells(Ueno *et al.*, 1975).

Another interesting approach was made by Masuko *et al.* (1977) and Otokawa *et al.* (1979), who observed the effect of T-2 toxin on delayed hypersensitivity (DH) in mice. Female mice were sensitized by s.c. injection of SRBC, and the mycotoxin was i.p. injected within several days before, at the time of, or several days after sensitization, and DH response was observed as footpad swelling, as shown in TABLE 4.

TABLE 4 Effect of Time of T-2 Toxin on Footpad Response and Antibody Formation

Treatment	Day	Footpad swelling ar 24 hr (1/10 mm) Day 7	enhancement	Hemagglutinin titer ($\log_2$) Day 8	enhancement
None		5.79 ± 0.47	-	4.0 ± 0.2	-
Olive oil	3	5.74 ± 0.50	no	3.8 ± 0.2	no
	-3	6.21 + 0.74	no	4.3 ± 0.3	no
	-2	6.27 ± 0.96	no	4.3 ± 0.2	no
T-2 toxin	0	5.34 ± 0.50	no	5.0 ± 0.2	no
	2	11.38 ± 1.06	yes	4.5 ± 0.2	no
	3	8.43 ± 0.74	yes	4.0 ± 0.4	no
Cyclophosphamide	-3	15.04 ± 1.13	yes	1.8 ± 0.6	suppress

The mice treated with the toxin before the sensitization exhibited no appreciable effect on the DH response. However, when the toxin was administered 2-3 days after the sensitization, marked enhancement of the DH response was observed on day 7. A similar data was obtained on day 14 (data not presented). Cyclophosphamide also caused enhancement but the effective timing of drug administration was 3 days before the sensitization. As for the antibody formation, T-2 toxin exhibited no significant effect, whereas cyclophosphamide induced marked suppression, as expected.

It is well established that the DH response as well as antibody formation are controled by suppressor T-cells, and cyclophosphamide attacks the precursor of suppressor cells, causing the enhancement when administered several days before sensitization. However, in the case of T-2 toxin, the DH response was enhanced only when the drug was injected several days after sensitization, and no effect was observed for the formation of antibody. These data strongly suggest that the trichothecenes selectively interfere with the function of suppressor T-cells. Detailed analysis of the mechanism of action of T-2 toxin on DH response revealed that, in mice i.v. injected with tolerance SRBC the cell population of the spleen was increased and that of the thymus decreased, whereas T-2 toxin treatment 2 days after the i.v. injection caused only the marked decline of the cell population in the thymus. This fact may indicate that T-2 toxin inhibits a transfer of T-cells of the thymus into the spleen. The ratio of θ -bearing cells was increased in the spleen after the i.v. injection of SRBC. However, such increase was not observed after T-2 toxin. Furthermore, Ig-bearing cells (B-cells) were not changed after the i.v. injection and the T-2 toxin treatment after the i.v. injection. These data indicate that T-2 toxin seems to interfere with generation of suppressor cells for the DH response.

METABOLISM OF TRICHOTHECENES

In some preceding papers (Ohta *et al.*, 1977, 1978), the author have reported that the C-4 acetyl residue of T-2 toxin, fusarenon-X and other trichothecenes was selectively hydrolyzed by microsomal carboxyesterase, and that the resulting HT-2 toxin and nivalenol are the end product of this *in vitro* system. ^{3}H-labeled T-2 toxin was also eliminated into feces and urine after the biotransformation into deacetylated metabolites (Matsumoto *et al.*, 1978).
With an aim to demonstrate whether HT-2 toxin is a metabolite in *in vivo* system, T-2 toxin dissolved in olive oil was o.p. administered to rats, and the trichothecene compounds were analysed by GLC after clean-up with silicagel-florisil multicolumn. As shown in Fig. 2, HT-2 toxin was detected in the liver shortly after the intubation, and no other trichothecenes such as T-2 toxin, neosolaniol were detected. The kidneys also contained HT-2 toxin but ten times less than the liver. Since no detectable amount of T-2 toxin was found in the tissues, the authors concluded that T-2 toxin may be deacetylated before entrance into the blood circulation. Actually, several dermal anaerobic bacteria possess a potent activity which is capable to deacetylate T-2 toxin into HT-2 toxin. Furthermore, the dermal epithelium exhibited the esterase activity. In this regard, the author presumed that T-2 toxin administered orally to animals may be attacked by esterases of dermal microflora as well as dermal epitherium, and the resulting HT-2 toxin may transfer into the body circulation.

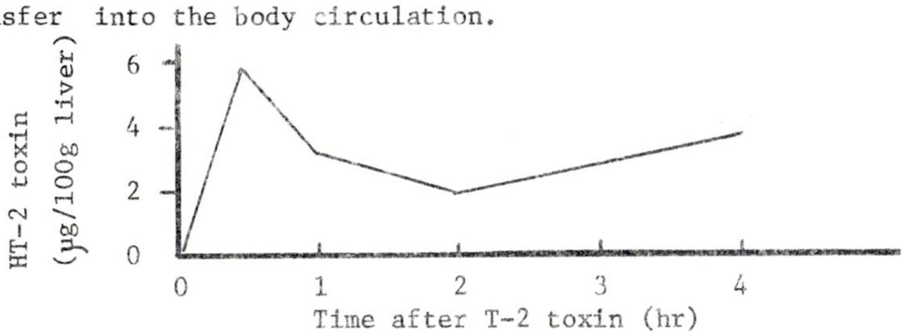

Fig. 3. HT-2 toxin content in the liver of rats.

EPOXIDE-SPECIFIC DETECTION METHOD OF TRICHOTHECENES

12,13-Epoxide of trichothecenes is reactive with 4-(*p*-nitrobenzyl)pyridine and the resulting blue-colored spots are estimated quantitatively by spectrodensitometry. This simplified TLC method is specific to the trichothecenes, since the 12,13-epoxide is a common functional group of trichothecene family (Takitani *et al.* 1979). The author adopted this technique for screening of trichothecene-producing fungi (Tanaka *et al.*, 1978) and survey of trichothecene metabolites in excreta. Actually, the author have detected HT-2 toxin and T-2 tetraol from the feces and HT-2 toxin from the urine of rats administered orally with T-2 toxin. This specific and simplified methodology is expected to give an information for toxicological evaluation of trichothecene mycotoxins.

REFERENCES

Bamburg, J. R., Riggs, N. V. and Strong, F. M. (1968). *Tetrahedron, 24,* 3329-3336.

Bamburg, J. R. and Strong, F. M. (1971). In S. Kadis, A. Ciegler and S. J. Ajl (Eds.), *Microbial Toxins*, Vol. 7, Academic Press, New York, pp. 207-292.

Eppley, R. M., Mazzola, E. P., Hight, R. J. and Bailey, W. J. (1977). *J.Org.Chem., 42,* 240-243.

Freeman, G. G., Gill, J. E. and Waring, W. S. (1959). *J.Chem.Soc.*, 1105-1132.

Ghosal, S., Chakrabarti, D. K. and Chaudhary, K. C. B. (1977). *Experientia, 33,* 574-575.

Greenway, J. A. and Puls, R. (1976). *Can.J.comp.Med., 40,* 12-19.

Hsu, I. H., Smalley, E. B., Strong, F. M. and Ribelin, W. E. (1972). *Appl.Microbiol. 24,* 684-690.

Ichinoe, M. (1978). *Proc.Jap.Assoc,Mycotoxicol., 8,* 1-5. (*in Japanese*)

Ishii, K., Ando, Y. and Ueno, Y. (1975). *Chem.Pharm.Bull.(Tokyo), 23,* 2162-2164.

Jemmali, M., Ueno, Y., Ishii, K., Frayssinet, C. and Etienne, M. (1978). *Experientia, 34,* 1333.

Kamimura, H., Nishijima, M., Saito, K., Takahashi, S., Ibe, A., Ochiai, S. and Naoi, Y. (1978). *Proc.Jap.Assoc.Mycotoxicol., 8,* 14-16. (*in Japanese*)

Masuko, H., Ueno, Y., Otokawa, M. and Yaginuma, K. (1977). *Jap.J.Med.Sci.Biol., 30,* 159-163.

Matsumoto, H., Ito, T. and Ueno, Y. (1978). *Jap.J.Exp.Med., 48,* 393-399.

Matsuoka, Y., Kubota, K. and Ueno, Y. (1979). *Toxicol.Appl.Pharmacol., in press.*

Mirocha, C. J., Pathre, S. V., Schauerhamer, B. and Christensen, C. M. (1976). *Appl.Environ.Microbiol., 32,* 553-556.

Ohta, M., Ishii, K. and Ueno, Y. (1977). *J.Biochem.(Tokyo), 82,* 1591-1598.

Ohta, M., Matsumoto, H., Ishii, K. and Ueno, Y. (1978). *J.Biochem. (Tokyo), 84,* 697-706.

Otokawa, M., Shibahara, Y. and Egashira, Y. (1979). *Jap.J.Med.Sci.Biol., 32,* 34-45.

Rosenstein, Y., Frayssinet, C. L., Lespinats, G., Lafont, P. and Frayssinet, C. (1979). *Immunology, 36,* 111-117.

Saito, M. and Tatsuno, T. (1971). In S. Kadis, A. Ciegler and S. J. Ajl (Eds.), *Microbial Toxins*, Vol. 7, Academic Press, New York, pp293-316.

Sato, N., Ueno, Y. and Enomoto, M. (1975). *Jap.J.Pharmacol., 25,* 263-270.

Sato, N., Ito, T., Kumada, H., Ueno, Y., Asano, K., Saito, M., Ohtsubo, K., Ueno, I. and Hatanaka, Y. (1978). *J.Toxicol.Sci., 3,* 335-356.

Tanaka, T., Ogata, K., Toyazakai, N., Matsuda, Y., Matsuki, Y. and Ueno, Y. (1978). *Proc.Jap.Assoc.Mycotoxicol., 8,* 16-19.

Takitani, S., Asabe, Y., Kato, T., Suzuki, M. and Ueno, Y. (1979). *J.Chromato., 172,* 335-342.

Tatsuno, T., Fugimoto, Y. and Morita, Y. (1969). *Tetrahedron Lett., 33,* 2823-2826.

Tsunoda, H., Toyazaki, M., Morooka, S., Nakano, N., Yoshiyama, H., Okubo, K. and Ishida, M. (1968). *Proc.Food Res.Inst., 23,* 89-116. (*in Japanese*).

Ueno, Y., Hosoya, M. and Ishikawa, Y. (1969a). *J.Biochem. (Tokyo), 66,* 419-422.

Ueno, Y., Ueno, I., Tatsuno, T., Ohtsubo, K. and Tsunoda, H. (1969b). *Experientia, 25, 1062.*

Ueno, Y., Ishikawa, Y., Amakai, K., Nakajima, M., Saito, M., Enomoto, M. and Ohtsubo, K. (1970). *Jap.J.Exp.Med., 40,* 33-38.

Ueno, Y., Ueno, I., Iitoi, Y., Tsunoda, H., Enomoto, M. and Ohtsubo, K. (1971). *Jap.J.Exp.Med., 41,* 521-539.

Ueno, Y., Ishii, K., Sakai, K., Kanaeda, S., Tsunoda, H., Tanaka, T. and Enomoto, M. (1972). *Jap.J.Exp.Med., 42,* 187-203.

Ueno, Y., Sato, N., Ishii, K., Sakai, K., Tsunoda, H. and Enomoto, M. (1973). *Appl.Microbiol., 25,* 699-704.

Ueno, Y., Ishii, K., Sato, N. and Ohtsubo, K. (1974). *Jap.J.Exp.Med., 44,* 123-127.

Ueno, Y., Nakajima, M., Sakai, K., Ishii, K., Sato, N. and Shimada, N. (1975). *J.Biochem. (Tokyo), 74,* 285-296.

Ueno, Y. (1977a). In J. V. Rodricks, C. W. Hesseltine and M. A. Mehlman (Eds.), *Mycotoxins in Human and Animal Health*, Pathotox Pub.Inc., Park Forest South, pp. 189-204.

Ueno, Y. (1977b). *Pure Appl.Chem., 49*, 1737-1745.

Ueno, Y. (1978). *Proc.Jap.Assoc.Mycotoxicol., 7*, 6-14.

Vesonder, R. F., Ciegler, A. and Jensen, A. H. (1973). *Appl.Microbiol., 26*, 1008-1010.

Vesonder, R. F., Ciegler, A., Rogers, R. F., Burbridge, K. A., Bothast, R. J. and Jensen, A. H. (1978). *Appl.Environ.Microbiol., 36*, 886-888.

Yoshizawa, T. and Morooka, N. (1973). *Agr.Biol.Chem., 37*, 2933-2934.

Yoshizawa, T. and Morooka, N. (1977). In J. V. Rodricks, C. W. Hesseltine and M. A. Mehlman (Eds.), *Mycotoxins in Human and Animal Health*, Pathotox Pub. Inc., Park Forest South, pp. 309-321.

Yoshizawa, T., Shirota, T. and Morooka, N. (1978). *J.Food Hygien.Soc.Jap., 19*, 178-184.

OCHRATOXINS: OCCURRENCE, BIOLOGICAL EFFECTS AND CAUSAL ROLE IN DISEASES

P. Krogh

Department of Veterinary Microbiology, Purdue University, West Lafayette, Indiana 47907, USA

ABSTRACT

Ochratoxin A is a fungal metabolite (mycotoxin) with pronounced nephrotoxic potency in all species of animals studied. It has shown teratogenic properties in three rodent species, and is a renal carcinogen in the mouse. Protein synthesis and RNA synthetase is competitively inhibited by the toxin. Ochratoxin A is a major disease determinant of mycotoxic porcine nephropathy, a disease occurring endemically in several countries. This disease resembles Balkan endemic nephropathy in man, suggesting a common causal relationship. Ochratoxin A has been found in foodstuffs in many countries, and the highest contamination frequency in foods has been encountered in an area of Yugoslavia, where Balkan endemic nephropathy is prevalent. As seven percent of the people in that area had ochratoxin A in the blood, compared to none in the controls, increasing evidence is provided supporting the suggestion, that ochratoxin A is a nephrotoxin in man.

KEYWORDS

Fungal toxin; nephrotoxin; foodstuff contaminant; protein synthesis inhibitor; porcine nephropathy; Balkan endemic nephropathy.

INTRODUCTION

Ochratoxin A, the leading member of the ochratoxin group, was discovered 15 years ago in South Africa during laboratory screening for toxicity of a number of molds isolated from cereal and legume crops (van der Merve and co-workers, 1965). The compound was encountered as a naturally occurring contaminant of foodstuffs (maize) four years later (Shotwell and co-workers, 1969), and has since been found in foodstuffs in many countries in Europe and North America. Ochratoxin A is a potent nephrotoxin, and has been observed as a major disease determinant of mycotoxic porcine nephropathy, a chronic renal disease in pigs endemic in Scandinavia and possibly also in other areas (Krogh, 1978). The toxin has been suggested as a disease determinant of Balkan endemic nephropathy (Krogh, 1974), a chronic renal disease in man occurring in certain areas of the Balkan peninsula. Lately increasing evidence for a causal role of ochratoxin A in this disease has been obtained, through the observation that locally grown foodstuffs in endemic areas are frequently contaminated with ochratoxin A (Krogh and co-workers, 1977), indicating pronounced human exposure. The observation that 7% of the population in an endemic area appears to have ochratoxin A in the blood (Hult and co-workers, 1979) is further documentation for a pronounced human exposure to this food contaminant.

FUNGAL FORMATION AND ENVIRONMENTAL OCCURRENCE OF OCHRATOXIN

The ochratoxins constitute a group of closely related derivatives of isocoumarin linked to L-β-phenylalanine (Fig. 1).

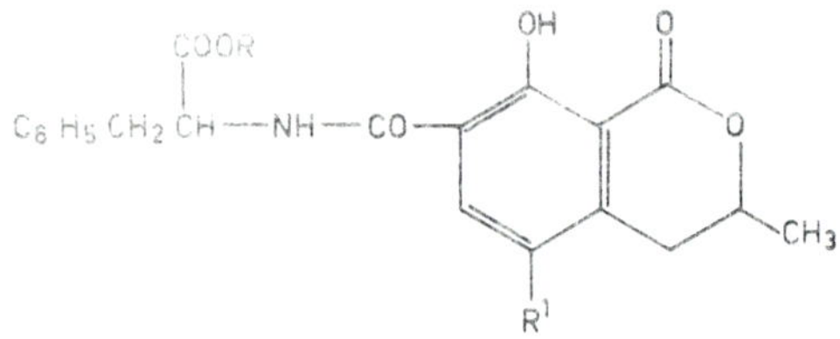

Fig. 1. The chemical structure of the ochratoxins; ochratoxin A: R=H, R_1=Cl; ochratoxin B: R=H, R_1=H; ochratoxin C: R=C_2H_5, R_1=Cl; methylester of ochratoxin A: R=CH_3, R_1=Cl; methyl and ethyl ester of ochratoxin B: R=CH_3 or C_2H_5, R_1=H.

The acids, the methyl and ethyl esters, and the isocoumarin part of ochratoxin B (ochratoxin β) have all been isolated from fungal cultures under experimental conditions (Review by Steyn, 1977; Scott, 1977). Ochratoxin α, the isocoumarin part of ochratoxin A, has been found in the intestine, urine, feces and liver of rodents (mouse, rat) experimentally fed ochratoxin A-containing feed, and is the cleavage product formed in the alimentary tract (Galtier and Alvinerie, 1976).

In contrast, only ochratoxin A and very rarely ochratoxin B are produced under natural conditions, in plant products. The ochratoxin-producing fungi are included in the genera Aspergillus and Penicillium. The toxins were first isolated from A. ochraceus (hence the name), but the main producers, at least under colder climatic conditions, are found among the Penicillia, with P. viridicatum being the leading producer (Krogh, 1978). Toxin production can occur in most plant products and is primarily governed by two factors: temperature and water, i.e. water activity (a_w) of the substrate (plant product). The temperature and a_w conditions for growth and ochratoxin A production have been determined for several fungal species (Northolt, van Egmond and Paulsch, 1979), and the conditions for P. viridicatum are illustrated in Fig. 2.

Although optimal conditions for ochratoxin production are found at a_w=0.95 and 24°C, the toxin is still being produced at a temperature as low as 4°C. The a_w values, determined under laboratory conditions, can be converted to the more practical parameter, water content (water %), specific for each commodity. Thus the lowest water % allowing ochratoxin A production by P. viridicatum is 18.5% in wheat and 21.6% in maize (at 24°C). Water content of cereals and other plant products is dependent on a number of factors, such as climatic conditions (precipitation) during growth and harvest period, and harvest and storage techniques. Thus submarginal agricultural techniques are conducive to high water content in plant products and subsequent ochratoxin A production by the ubiquitously occurring fungi.

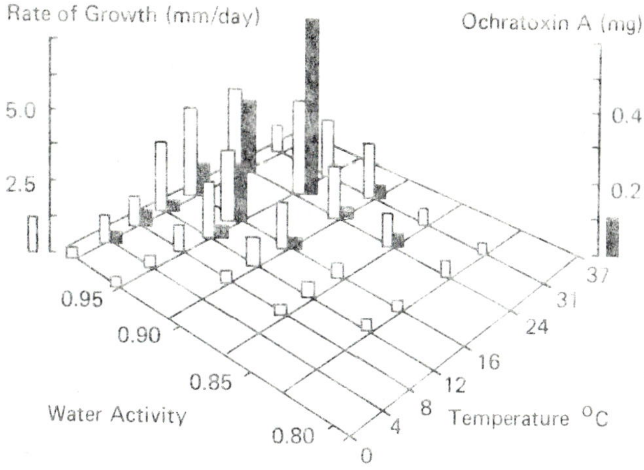

Fig. 2. Growth and ochratoxin A production by a strain of *P. viridicatum* on maize sucrose agar under various conditions of temperature and water activity.

Surveys of foodstuffs, mainly cereals, have revealed the presence of ochratoxin A in the following geographical areas: Europe: Czechoslovakia, Denmark, France, Hungary, Poland, Sweden, United Kingdom, Yugoslavia; North America: Canada, U.S.A. Actually, no survey for ochratoxin A appears to have been conducted with-

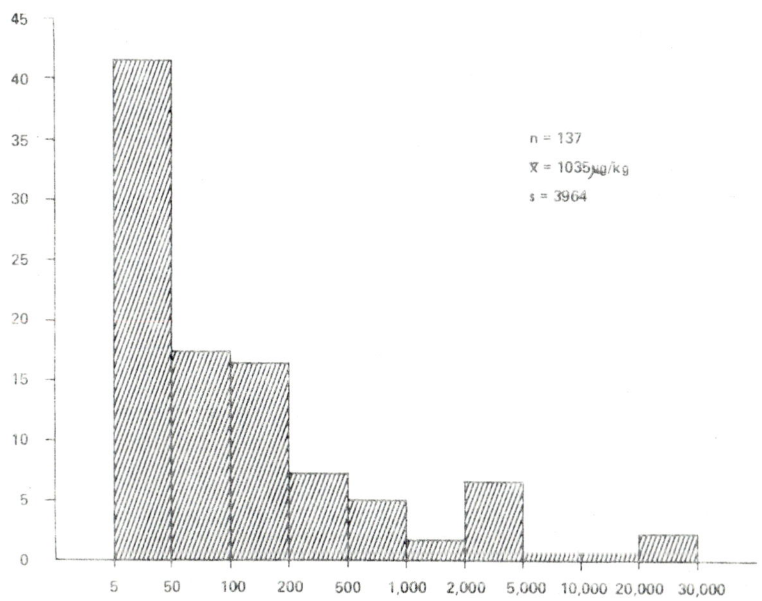

Fig. 3. Frequency of ochratoxin contamination levels, based

upon all reported surveys of foodstuffs. Abscissa: μg ochratoxin A/kg; ordinate: percentage of contaminated samples.

out finding the contaminant. In foods the frequency of contamination varies from 1% to 18.8% with levels in the range 5-360 μg/kg; in feeds up to 57.6% of samples have been found contaminated, with levels in the range 5-27,500 μg/kg (Review: Krogh, 1978). Although the mean level of ochratoxin A in all reported surveys is 1035 μg/kg (Fig. 3), 83% of the samples contains less than 200 μg/kg.

When food animals (pigs, poultry) are exposed to ochratoxin A-contaminated feed, a part of the ingested toxin will be retained, as residues, in the tissues. Thus carry-over of ochratoxin A from feed to food of animal origin is possible, and surveys at meat plants in Denmark and Sweden have revealed that 25-35% of pigs suffering from nephropathy contains residues of ochratoxin A (Krogh and co-workers, 1977; Rutqvist and co-workers, 1977).

BIOLOGICAL EFFECTS OF OCHRATOXIN A

Ochratoxin A is resorbed from the alimentary tract, starting already in the stomach and continuing in the small intestine (Galtier, 1979). By passing the intestine a part of ochratoxin A is cleaved forming ochratoxin α and phenylalanine, due to the hydrolytic activity of carboxypeptidase A and chymotrypsinogen (Suzuki, Satoh and Yamazaki, 1977) and of the intestinal bacteria and protozoa (in ruminants) (Galtier and Alvinerie, 1976). In the blood ochratoxin A is present as bound to serum albumin (Chu, 1971; Galtier, 1974a), and as free ochratoxin A; saturation in the rat occurs at 70 μg ochratoxin A/ml plasma.

TABLE 1 In Vitro Binding of Ochratoxin A to Serum Albumin of Several Species*

Animal Species	Number of Binding Sites	Intrinsic Association Constant (M^{-1})
Cattle	0.58	94,600
Pig	0.56	71,100
Man	0.58	63,500
Horse	0.57	57,400
Chicken	0.51	52,700
Rat	0.68	40,100
Sheep	0.88	22,600

*Adapted from Galtier (1979).

As indicated in Table 1 the binding of ochratoxin A to serum albumin is particularly strong in cattle, pig and man. Apart from the blood the highest tissue concentrations of ochratoxin A are found in the kidney and the liver in rats (Galtier, 1974b; Chang and Chu, 1977; Lillehoj and co-workers, 1979) and in pigs (Krogh, 1978; Rutqvist and co-workers, 1978), pointing to the target organs of this toxin.

Under experimental conditions ochratoxin A has revealed a pronounced acute toxic effect in a number of mammal, bird and fish species, with peroral LD_{50} in the range 3.4-62.4 mg/kg bw. The main pathologic changes observed during LD_{50} experiments are necrosis of the renal tubules and of periportal liver cells; additional findings (in the pig, rat and dog) are enteritis and necrosis of lymphoid tissue (Review: WHO, 1979). When lower doses of ochratoxin A have been employed, corresponding to feed levels below 5-10 mg/kg, the effect (in pigs) has been confined to the kidneys (Krogh, 1978). The effect of ochratoxin A above 5-10 mg/kg is only of marginal interest as such levels are rarely encountered in foodstuffs (See Fig. 3). The nephropathy induced in pigs during 4 months of exposure to ochratoxin A in the range 200-4000 μg/kg feed is characterized by impairment of proximal tubular function, indicated by a decrease of Tm_{PAH}/C_{In}, of the ability to concentrate urine, and by an increased urinary excretion of glucose, leucine aminopeptidase and protein. The changes of renal structure include atrophy of the proximal tubules, interstitial formation of connective tissue in the renal cortex, and in advanced cases sclerotized glomerular tufts (Krogh and co-workers, 1974). In a long term study in pigs fed 1 mg ochratoxin A/kg feed the renal impairment aggravated slightly during the two year period, without reaching a state of terminal renal failure (Krogh and co-workers, 1979).

Teratogenic effects of ochratoxin A have been demonstrated in the mouse (Hayes, Hood and Lee, 1974), the hamster (Hood, Naughton and Hayes, 1976) and the rat (Brown, Szczech and Purmalis, 1976). Renal carcinoma and liver tumors were induced in mice (Kanisawa and Suzuki, 1978).

Ochratoxin A is an inhibitor of tRNA synthetase and protein synthesis in several microorganisms (*Bacillus subtilis*, *B. stearothermophilus*, *Streptococcus faecalis*, yeasts) as well as in rat hepatoma cells (Konrad and Röschenthaler, 1977; Bunge, Dirheimer and Röschenthaler, 1978; Heller and Röschenthaler, 1978; Creppy and co-workers, 1979a; Creppy and co-workers, 1979b). The competitive inhibitory effect of ochratoxin A on tRNA synthetase and protein synthesis in rat hepatoma cells can be prevented by phenylalanine (Creppy and co-workers, 1979b), an observation suggesting the possibility of preventive measures in ochratoxin A-induced diseases. Thus the acute intraperitoneal effect of ochratoxin A (LD_{100}) in mice can be prevented by concomittant injection of phenylalanine (Creppy and co-workers, 1979c); it remains to be elucidated whether chronic effects (nephropathy) in animals also can be prevented by phenylalanine. Experiments in rats have shown, that ochratoxin A inhibits renal gluconeogenesis through an effect on renal phosphoenolpyruvate carboxykinase, whereas the corresponding hepatic enzyme is unaffected (Meisner and Selanik, 1979).

CAUSAL ROLE IN DISEASES

Mycotoxic porcine nephropathy is an endemically occurring disease in Denmark known for decades, and recently the disease has been observed in Sweden as well (Rutqvist and co-workers, 1978). At slaughter the kidneys appear pale and enlarged, with cortical fibrosis visible on the cut surface. Histologically atrophy of proximal tubules and interstitial cortical fibrosis is observed (Fig. 4).

Ochratoxin A is a major disease determinant of the disease (Krogh, 1978), but also other nephrotoxic mycotoxins, such as citrinin, might be involved. The prevalence rate of mycotoxic porcine nephropathy ranges from 10 to 70 cases per 10,000 pigs, heavily influenced by weather conditions (Krogh, 1976).

Balkan endemic nephropathy is a chronic renal disease in man, with unknown etiology so far. Because of the similarity of this disease with mycotoxic porcine nephropathy (with partly known etiology) attempts have been made to elucidate a possible causal role for ochratoxin A in this human condition. Surveys of locally grown foodstuffs in an endemic area of Yugoslavia, covering a 5-year period, have revealed that 8-12% of the cereals are contaminated with ochratoxin A, compared to an average of 3% for foods in all other European and North American countries (Krogh and co-workers, 1977; Pavlovic, Plestina and Krogh, 1979). These obervations indicate an increased exposure of the inhabitants in endemic areas to ochra-

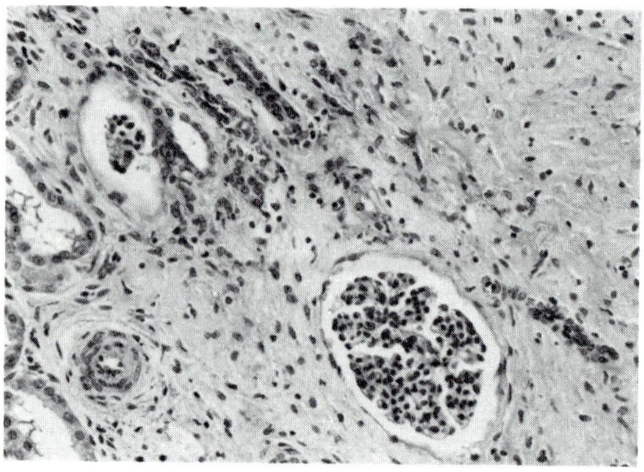

Fig. 4. Field case of mycotoxic porcine nephropathy causally associated with ochratoxin A; atrophic tubules, interstitial cortical fibrosis, a morphologically normal glomerulus; Ih-v.G. x 220.

toxin A, although the intake of this compound has not yet been measured in any part of the world. Indirect evidence for an increased exposure was recently provided by the observation that 7% of a fraction of the population (201 persons) in the endemic area of Yugoslavia mentioned above had ochratoxin A in the blood (maximal concentration: 1.8 μg/ml) compared to none in the control group (Hult and co-workers, 1979).

ACKNOWLEDGEMENTS

The use of Fig. 3, from Northolt and co-workers (1979), is gratefully acknowledged. Published as paper no 7855 of the Agricultural and Experiment Station, Purdue University, West Lafayette, Indiana, USA.

REFERENCES

Brown, M.H., G.M. Szczech, and B.P. Purmalis (1976). Teratogenic and toxic effects of ochratoxin A in rats. Toxicol. and App. Pharm. 37, 331-338.

Bunge, I., G. Dirheimer, and R. Roschenthaler (1978). In vivo and in vitro inhibition of protein synthesis in Bacillus stearothermophilus by ochratoxin A. Biochem. Biophys. Res. Comm. 83, 398-405.

Chang, F.C. and F.S. Chu (1977). The fate of ochratoxin A in rats. Fd. Cosmet. Toxicol. 15, 199-204.

Chu, F.S. (1971). Interaction of ochratoxin A with bovine serum albumin. Arch. Biochem. Biophys. 147(2), 359-366.

Creppy, E.-E., A.A.J. Lugnier, G. Beck, R. Röschenthaler and G. Dirheimer (1979b). Action of ochratoxin A on cultured hepatoma cells - reversion of inhibition by phenylalanine. FEBS Letters 104, 287-290.

Creppy, E.-E., A.A.J. Lugnier, F. Fasiolo, K. Heller, and R. Röschenthaler (1979a). In vitro inhibition of yeast phenylalanyl-tRNA synthetase by ochratoxin A. Chem.-Biol. Interact. 24, 257-261.

Creppy, E.-E., M. Schlegel, R. Röschenthaler, and G. Dirheimer (1979c). Action preventiv de la phenylalanine sur l'intoxication aigue par l'ochratoxine-A. Cont. R. Acad. Sci. (in Press).

Galtier, P. (1974a). Devenir de l'ochratoxine A dans l'organisme animal. I.

Transport sanguin de la toxine chez le rat. Ann. Rech. veter. 5, 311-318.

Galtier, P. (1974b). Devenir de l'ochratoxine A dans l'organisme animal. II. Distribution tissulaire et elimination chez le rat. Ann. Rech. veter. 5, 319-328.

Galtier, P. (1979). Etude toxicologique et pharmacocinetique d'une mycotoxine, l'ochratoxine A. These d'Etates Sciences pharmaceutiques. Toulouse, 1-50.

Galtier, P. and M. Alvinerie (1976). In vitro transformation of ochratoxin A by animal microbial floras. Ann. Rech. veter. 7, 91-98.

Hayes, A.W., R.D. Hood, H.L. Lee (1974). Teratogenic effects of ochratoxin A in mice. Teratology, 9, 93-97.

Heller, K. and R. Röschenthaler (1978). Inhibition of protein synthesis in Streptococcus faecalis by ochratoxin A. Can. J. Microbiol. 24, 466-472.

Hood, R.D., M.J. Naughton and A.W. Hayes (1976). Prenatal effects of ochratoxin A in hamsters. Teratology 13, 11-14.

Hult, K., E. Hökby, S. Gatenbeck, R. Plestina, and S. Ceovic (1979). Ochratoxin A and Balkan endemic nephropathy. IV. Occurrence of ochratoxin A in humans. Abstract:IV IUPAC Symposium on Mycotoxins and Phycotoxins, Lausanne.

Kanisawa, M. and S. Suzuki (1978). Induction of renal and hepatic tumors in mice by ochratoxin A, a mycotoxin. Gann. 69, 599-600.

Konrad, I. and R. Röschenthaler (1977). Inhibition of phenylalanine tRNA synthetase from Bacillus subtilis by ochratoxin A. FEBS Letters 83, 341-347.

Krogh, P. (1974). Mycotoxic porcine nephropathy - a possible model for Balkan (endemic) nephropathy. In: Endemic nephropathy (A. Puchlev), Bulgarian Academy of Sciences, Sofia, 266-270.

Krogh, P. (1976). Epidemiology of mycotoxic porcine nephropathy. Nord. Vet. -Med. 28, 452-458.

Krogh, P. (1978). Causal associations of mycotoxic nephropathy. Acta Path. microbiol. scand. Sect. A, Suppl. No. 269, 28.

Krogh, P., N.H. Axelsen, F. Elling, N. Gyrd-Hansen, B. Hald, J. Hyldgaard-Jensen, A.E. Larsen, A. Madsen, H.P. Mortensen, T. Møller, O.K. Petersen, U. Ravnskov, M. Rostgaard, and O. Aalund (1974). Experimental porcine nephropathy. Changes of renal function and structure induced by ochratoxin A-contaminated feed. Acta path. microbiol. scand., Section A, Supplementum No. 246, 21.

Krogh, P., F. Elling, Chr. Friis, B. Hald, A.E. Larsen, E.B. Lillehoj, A. Madsen, H.P. Mortensen, F. Rasmussen and U. Ravnskov (1979). Porcine nephropathy induced by long-term ingestion of ochratoxin A. Vet. Pathol. 16, 466-475.

Krogh, P., B. Hald, R. Plestina and S. Ceovic (1977). Balkan (endemic) nephropathy and foodborn ochratoxin A: Preliminary results of a survey of foodstuffs. Acta path. microbiol. scand. Sect. B, 85, 238-240.

Lillehoj, E.B., W.F. Kwolek, F. Elling and P. Krogh (1979). Tissue distribution of radioactivity from ochratoxin A - ^{14}C in rats. Mycopathol. Mycol. Applic. (in press).

Meisner, H. and P. Selanik (1979). Inhibition of renal gluconeogenesis in rats by ochratoxin. Biochem. J. 180, 681-684.

Van der Merwe, K.J., P.S. Steyn, L. Fourie, Scott De B, and J.J. Theron (1965). Ochratoxin A, a toxic metabolite produced by Aspergillus ochraceus Wilh. Nature 205, 1112-1113.

Northolt, M.D., H.P. Van Egmond, and W.E. Paulsch (1979). Ochratoxin A production by some fungal species in relation to water activity and temperature. J. Food Protect. 42, 485-490.

Pavlovic, M., R. Plestina and P. Krogh (1979). Ochratoxin A contamination of foodstuffs in an area with Balkan (endemic) nephropathy. Acta path. microbiol. scand. Sect. B 87, 243-246.

Rutqvist, L., N.-E. Björklund, K. Hult, E. Hökby, and B. Carlsson (1978). Ochratoxin A as the cause of spontaneous nephropathy in fattening pigs. Appl. Env. Microbiol. 36, 920-925.

Rutqvist, L., N.-E. Björklund, K. Hult, and S. Gatenbeck (1977). Spontaneous occurrence of ochratoxin residues in kidneys of fattening pigs. Zbl. Vet. Med. A 24, 402-408.

Scott, P.M. (1977). Penicillium mycotoxins. In T.D. Wyllie and L.G. Morehouse (Eds.), Mycotoxic Fungi, Mycotoxins, Mycotoxicoses, Vol. I, Marcel Dekker, New York, 283-356.

Shotwell, O.L., C.W. Hesseltine and M.L. Goulden (1969). Ochratoxin A: Occurrence as natural contaminant of a corn sample. Appl. Microbiol. 17, 765-766.

Steyn, P.S. (1977). Mycotoxins, excluding aflatoxin, zearalenone and the trichothecenes. In J.V. Rodricks, C.W. Hesseltine and M.A. Mehlman (Eds.), Mycotoxins in Human and Animal Health, Pathotox Publ., Illinois, 419-467.

Suzuki, S., T. Satoh and M. Yamazaki (1977). The pharmacokinetics of ochratoxin A in rats. Japan. J. Pharmacol. 27, 735-744.

World Health Organization (1979). Environmental Health Criteria 11, Mycotoxins, Geneva, 86-98.

METABOLISM AND MODE OF ACTION OF AFLATOXIN IN RELATION TO THE ETIOLOGY OF LIVER DISEASES IN MAN AND FARM ANIMALS

D. S. P. Patterson

Central Veterinary Laboratory, Weybridge, Surrey, KT15 3NB, UK

ABSTRACT

Aflatoxin B_1 and two of its metabolites (2,3 oxide and dihydrodiol) interact with the liver at several intracellular sites. There are also extrahepatic sites of action and this multi-locus reactivity may explain the potency of aflatoxin. Acute toxicity probably results from cumulative action in the short term. Chronic toxicity arises specifically from an interaction between the epoxide and hepatic DNA. With present day controls of aflatoxin-contaminated food and feedstuffs emphasis has been placed on a consideration of the possible toxic effects of low dietary concentrations of aflatoxin B_1.

KEYWORDS

Aflatoxin B_1; liver metabolism; multi-locus reactivity; cumulative action; low level dietary exposure.

INTRODUCTION

Although it was only discovered in 1961, more is probably known about the aflatoxins than any other group of mycotoxins or indeed other naturally occurring toxic substances (Heathcote and Hibbert, 1978; Uraguchi and Yamazaki, 1978; Wyllie and Morehouse, 1977). Aspergillus flavus and A. parasiticus are the two fungal species capable of producing aflatoxin and as they are virtually ubiquitous, the potential for contaminating food crops is considerable. Optimal conditions are generally encountered in tropical and sub-tropical latitudes however, and groundnut, cottonseed, and maize appear to be particularly susceptible to fungal attack and contamination with aflatoxin in the field or during storage.

Aflatoxin B_1 causes acute liver disease and has been found to be carcinogenic in all animal species so far tested (IARC, 1976; WHO, 1979). It is also the commonest and most potent of the four aflatoxins, B_1, B_2, G_1 and G_2 that occasionally contaminate human food and animal feeds in trace amounts (µg/kg range).

METABOLISM OF AFLATOXIN B_1

The liver is the major site of aflatoxin metabolism which is summarised in Fig. 1.

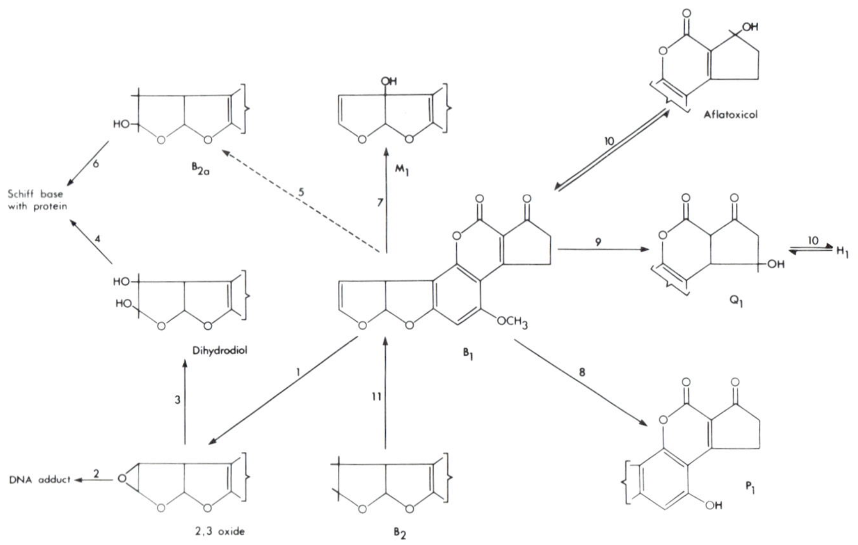

Fig. 1. Pathways for the metabolism of aflatoxin B_1 in the liver. Numbered reactions are referred to in the text.

Aflatoxin 2,3 oxide is formed by microsomal enzymes (1), alkylates DNA (2), may conjugate with glutathione, and is metabolised to the dihydrodiol (3). At physiological pH the dihydrodiol rearranges to form a dialdehydic phenolate ion which interacts with protein (Schiff base, 4). Aflatoxin B_{2a} which forms directly from B_1 under acidic conditions <u>in vitro</u> (5) reacts with protein similarly (6). Hydroxylated metabolites including M_1 are formed by microsomal mixed function oxidases (reactions 7, 8, 9). Other hydroxylation reactions (10) involve cytoplasmic NADP-linked steroid sensitive dehydrogenases. Aflatoxin B_2 may be converted to B_1 (11) but otherwise can be metabolised by pathways 7, 8, 9 and 10. Structures of aflatoxins G_1 and G_2 contain a δ-lactone ring in place of the cyclopentenone moiety of the B series and therefore cannot be metabolised by reactions 9 and 10. Conjugation of hydroxylated metabolites with glucuronic acid also occurs. Some metabolites may undergo further metabolism, e.g. aflatoxin M_1 in reaction 10.

Two pathways for aflatoxin B_1 are particularly important: (a) activation to form the mutagenic and carcinogenic metabolite, presumed to be the 2,3 oxide, which binds covalently to DNA, and (b) hydroxylation forming aflatoxin M_1 which is almost as toxic as the parent toxin and is excreted in cows' milk (see below). Both reactions appear to be common to livers of all animal species but in these and other pathways there are probably quantitative differences.

MODE OF ACTION OF AFLATOXIN B_1

Aflatoxin B_1 interacts with the liver cell at many sites (Table 1). At the molecular level, this probably results from specific interactions between activated forms of aflatoxin B_1 and enzymes, structural proteins, or DNA, but in some instances responses may be due to the action of the untransformed toxin.

TABLE 1 Interactions between Aflatoxin or its Metabolites and the Liver

Locus	Response or biochemical effect
Nucleus	mutagenic, carcinogenic: binds covalently to DNA inhibits DNA-dependent RNA polymerase stimulates DNA repair synthesis
Mitochondria	increases membrane permeability inhibits protein synthesis interrupts electron transport
Lysosomes	increases membrane permeability free acid hydrolases released
Endoplasmic reticulum	"degranulation" occurs mimics steroid sex hormones at polysome binding sites binds covalently to r-RNA inhibits mixed function oxidase activity inhibits protein (including blood clotting factor) synthesis, impairs enzyme induction inhibits glucose-6-phosphatase inhibits fatty acid and phospholipid synthesis feed-back control of cholesterol synthesis lost inhibits sialyl transferase activity inhibits lipid peroxidation
Cytoplasm	temporarily stimulates glycogenolysis/pentose shunt activity substrate/inhibitor for 17-hydroxysteroid dehydrogenase (NADP-linked)
General	aflatoxin dihydrodiol and hemiacetal (B_{2a}) form Schiff bases with free amino-groups of peptides and proteins with presumed inhibitory effect on many enzyme systems

For references to original data see reviews (Patterson, 1977 and 1979)

Interaction with Liver DNA

Covalent interaction between the presumed epoxide of aflatoxin B_1 and DNA is now generally believed to be fundamental to the carcinogenic and mutagenic action of aflatoxin but aflatoxin 2,3 oxide appears to be unstable and its formation by liver tissues in vitro has yet to be detected. However, several authors have reported the concentration dependent binding of radioactively labelled aflatoxin B_1 to DNA in the presence of liver microsomes and demonstrated the presence of the dihydrodiol which presumably is a metabolite of the epoxide.

Interactions with Liver Enzymes and Proteins

Both aflatoxin dihydrodiol and the hemiacetal B2a are capable of non-specific interaction with proteins to form Schiff bases and there are reports of the interaction between aflatoxin hemiacetal and enzymes, bovine serum albumin, and amino-acids. Either metabolite could therefore interact with key enzymes and membrane structures so as to disrupt metabolism and modify the permeability of cellular or intracellular organelle boundaries resulting in necrosis of the hepatic cell.

Species susceptibility to acute aflatoxin poisoning has been related to an animal's ability to metabolise aflatoxin rapidly to its hemiacetal, B_{2a} (Patterson, 1973) but in the light of recent experiments using improved analytical methodology (Neal and Patterson, unpublished observations) it is now almost certain that this metabolite should have been properly identified as the dihydrodiol. Consequently, while all animal species appear to be susceptible to chronic poisoning arising from interaction between the epoxide and DNA, an animal's susceptibility to acute aflatoxicosis probably depends upon the rate of aflatoxin dihydrodiol formation by epoxide hydrase (reaction 3, Fig. 1).

Hepatotoxicity of Untransformed Aflatoxin B_1

Even when not metabolically activated, aflatoxin B_1 may have considerable toxic potential. In impairing blood coagulation and interrupting mitochondrial electron transport it behaves like other coumarin derivatives not possessing the vinyl ether grouping, the bis-furan, or the cyclopentenone structures of aflatoxin. Aflatoxin B_1 may also be regarded as a pseudo-steroid since it can replace estrone and testosterone at their respective sex-determined binding sites on the hepatic endoplasmic reticulum and substitutes for these hormones at the active site of cytoplasmic NADP-dependent 17-hydroxysteroid dehydrogenase.

Extrahepatic Effects of Aflatoxin

Aflatoxin B_1 is capable of interacting with many body tissues, including the capillary wall, the skin, the immune system, phagocytic cells, and the developing foetus (see Table 2). The molecular basis of many of these interactions is uncertain, but the teratogenicity of aflatoxin B_1 probably involves DNA alkylation.

TABLE 2 Interactions between Aflatoxin or its Metabolites and Extra-Hepatic Sites

Site of interaction	Response
Capillaries	permeability increased intravascular blood coagulation occurs
Skin	toxin undergoes photochemical metabolism delayed hypersensitivity elicited
Immune system	antibody production depressed in response to bacterial and viral antigens cell-mediated immunity impaired
Phagocytosis	activity impaired
Conceptus	teratomas induced

For reference to original data see reviews (Patterson, 1977 and 1979)

Consequences of Multi-locus Reactivity

The ability of aflatoxin B_1 to interact with the liver and other tissues in a variety of ways (Tables 1 and 2) and in several different molecular forms probably explains its extreme potency but there may be other consequences.

Dietary levels of aflatoxin B_1 sufficient to cause death of farm livestock appear to be confined to a narrow range of about 0.7 to 1.8 mg/kg but of those animals considered in Table 3 only the duckling would ever be likely to ingest an LD_{50} dose of the toxin in a day's feed of rations containing, for example, 1 mg aflatoxin B_1/kg. Indeed for other stock, the quantity of a similar feed containing a single LD_{50} dose increases from 2.1 kg for the chicken up to highly improbable figures of around 1000 kg for large animals. Thus, experimentally determined LD_{50} values cannot be used to reliably predict acute toxicity arising from the ingestion of contaminated feeds and lethal effects on large animals like the pig, sheep, and cattle therefore appear to be due to the cumulative action of aflatoxin B_1.

TABLE 3 Acute Toxicity of Dietary Aflatoxin B_1 in Farm Animals

Species	Feed contamination[a] causing death (mg aflatoxin B_1/kg)	Estimated[a][b] LD_{50} dose (mg)	Calculated quantity of feed containing one LD_{50} dose (kg)
Duckling	0.7	0.017	0.02
Chicken	1.0	2.1 to 4.2	2.1 to 4.2
Pig	1.0 to 1.75	22.3	22.3 to 39
Sheep	more than 1.75	85.4	more than 149
Cattle	1.8	[800][c]	[1440]

(a) for references see Patterson (1979).
(b) estimated from LD_{50} values and body weight data tabulated by Patterson (1979) and Spector (1956) respectively.
(c) LD_{50} assumed to be 2 mg/kg body wt., as for sheep.

EXPOSURE TO LOW DIETARY LEVELS OF AFLATOXIN

Although crops like groundnut and maize are liable to be contaminated with aflatoxin they are such important sources of protein that it is difficult to avoid using them in the manufacture of human food and animal feeds. As a result, many countries have now introduced statutory control measures restricting the use of aflatoxin-containing commodities in such a way that the final concentration of aflatoxin B_1 in food and feeds is usually in the range 5-20 µg/kg.

No acute toxic or sub-clinical effects have been described at this level of contamination but it has been established that, at least in the rat and rainbow trout, chronic exposure will induce liver tumours (see review; WHO, 1979).

Effects on Farm Animals

As demonstrated above, LD_{50} values cannot be used to predict the acute effects produced by dietary levels of about 1 mg aflatoxin B_1/kg and at lower, µg/kg levels they have even less relevance. Many sub-clinical (i.e. biochemical and pathophysiological) responses by poultry to aflatoxin B_1 have been reported at experimental dietary concentrations of 0.63 to 10 mg/kg but this is 30 to 500 times higher than the maximum concentrations now included in poultry rations in EEC countries including the UK. Observations on aflatoxin metabolism by liver tissues *in vitro* are no more relevant. A survey of the literature shows that different investigators of rat liver metabolism used incubation media containing 1×10^{-5} to 5×10^{-4}M aflatoxin B_1 with the lowest figure close to that probably reached in the liver following the administration of a single LD_{50} dose of aflatoxin B_1.

Most of the known toxicological and physiological responses of experimental and farm animals and various metabolic interactions have therefore been produced by high doses and high *in vitro* concentrations of aflatoxin B_1 but assuming that all are dose-related, it is by no means certain that any one response would be physiologically significant at the very low concentrations likely to result from exposure to low dietary levels of aflatoxin B_1. Metabolic activation and alkylation of liver DNA can be singled out as the potentially most important interaction at μg/kg levels but in normal farming practice it is unlikely that any resulting hepatic tumours would be detected in livestock with their relatively short life spans. And when calves were recently fed rations containing only 10 μg aflatoxin B_1/kg for a period of 3 months regular weighing, clinical examination and standard methods of clinical pathology (including routine haematology, plasma and urine enzymes, blood clotting factors, serum proteins and urine analysis) failed to detect tissue damage or other abnormalities (unpublished data).

A few presumed cases of acute aflatoxicosis have been reported to this laboratory since the introduction of statutory control measures but all have involved cattle fed mixed rations containing groundnut meal with concentrations in the range 0.06 to 2 mg/kg (unpublished data). The response of calves was to grow at sub-optimal rates, dairy cattle produced less milk, and in some animals there was a tendency to resist gastro-intestinal and other infections less readily than usual (Patterson and others, 1977). Causal relationships were difficult to establish however.

Effects in Man

Occasional fatalities have been reported to be due to the ingestion of food contamination with aflatoxin B_1 and there have been various occupational incidents. There is possibly an association between dietary aflatoxin and Reye's syndrome in children, and aflatoxin B_1 and its metabolites have been detected in other liver specimens taken at autopsy (see review: WHO, 1979). Additionally, an outbreak of acute liver disease involving many deaths was reported in 1976 amongst the population of NW India and attributed to the ingestion of a diet contaminated with exceptionally high levels of aflatoxin B_1 (up to 6 mg per person were consumed).

Where man's diet is relatively unvaried and consistently contaminated with aflatoxin B_1, as it is in certain regions of Africa and SE Asia, it has been established that the crude incidence of primary liver cell cancer amongst the respective populations is directly related to the daily intake of aflatoxin B_1 (see reviews by Peers and Linsell, 1977; van Rensberg, 1977, and WHO, 1979). Daily amounts of up to 14 μg were found to be ingested but even in the Southeastern USA where daily intakes of aflatoxin B_1 are only about 0.2 μg it is considered that, statistically, it involves a small risk to human health (FDA, 1978).

Surveys carried out in many countries where the use of aflatoxin-contaminated dairy feedstuffs is carefully controlled show that milk is occasionally contaminated with trace amounts of aflatoxin M_1 and it has been demonstrated experimentally that following the ingestion of aflatoxin B_1, the toxic metabolite aflatoxin M_1 appears in cow's milk in dose-related concentrations (see reviews: Kiermeier, 1977; Patterson, 1977 and 1979). Recent improvements in analytical methods now make it possible to detect aflatoxin M_1 in milk at concentrations of 0.01 to 0.33 μg/litre when cattle are fed rations containing only 20 μg aflatoxin B_1/kg (Patterson Glancy and Roberts, 1979). Experimental "carry over" of aflatoxin has also been demonstrated in cattle and pig tissues and in eggs (see review: Rodricks and Stoloff, 1977) but natural contamination is uncommon and much less important than in the case of milk. While dietary habits vary from one population to another milk stands out as a food that, in one form or another, is ingested by man world wide perhaps at an average rate of about 0.5 litre daily. Of course, in infancy, the intake of milk relative to body weight is much greater. The risk to public health associated with continual low level exposure to dietary aflatoxin M_1 has yet to be satisfactorily assessed.

Liver Exposure to Aflatoxins B_1 and M_1 at Dietary Levels

As already discussed, there is little reference toxicological data with which to assess or predict the possible consequences of feeding diets contaminated with aflatoxin B_1 in the μg/kg range. However, following the approach of Claus, Krisko and Bolander (1974) it has proved instructive to calculate the approximate numbers of aflatoxin B_1 molecules that reach the average target cell under various experimental and field conditions using basic data from published reports (Table 4).

TABLE 4 Cellular Exposure and Responses to Aflatoxins B_1 and M_1

Cell type	Exposure (Reference) (a)	Calculated approx. no. molecules/ cell (b)	Response
Rat liver	Normal concentration of glutathione (1)	3×10^{12}	none
" "	" " " NADP (1)	1×10^{11}	none
" "	Oral LD_{50} dose of aflatoxin B_1 (2)	8 to 25 $\times 10^8$	acute lethal
Bacterium	microsomal metabolite of aflatoxin B_1 *in vitro* (3)	3×10^5 to 1×10^8	mutation
Rat liver	15 μg aflatoxin B_1/kg diet (4)	1×10^6	20% incidence of hepatomas
Bovine liver	daily ingestion of 200 μg aflatoxin B_1 (5)	1×10^5	none known
Human liver	8 μg aflatoxin B_1/kg diet) epidemiological	6×10^4	0.013% incidence of hepatomas
Human liver	0.1 μg aflatoxin B_1/kg) data (6) diet)	1×10^3	0.001% incidence of hepatomas
Human liver	50 g peanuts containing 2 μg aflatoxin B_1/kg (5)	3×10^2	none known
Human liver	0.4 litre milk containing 0.1 μg aflatoxin M_1 litre (5)	2×10^2	" "

(a) 1 = Long (1961); 2 = Butler (1974); 3 = Garner, Miller and Miller (1972); 4 = Wogan, Paglialunga and Newberne (1974); 5 = hypothetical but possible dietary exposure; 6 = Peers and Linsell, 1977.

(b) Calculated assuming that all the stated amounts of aflatoxin B_1 or its metabolite reached the relevant cells, that 1 gram molecule contains 6.02×10^{23} molecules, that a rat liver contained 1.4×10^9 cells, a human liver 5×10^{11} cells and a bovine liver 2.8×10^{12} cells (Claus, Krisko and Bolander, 1974 with arithmetic extrapolations). No allowance has been made for detoxification or possible differential accumulation by hepatocytes.

Calculated values for the levels of cellular exposure have been ranked in Table 4 and it will be seen that they range from about 10^8 molecules aflatoxin B_1/cell for acute liver damage in the rat and bacterial cell mutation down to 10^2 molecules/cell for a man eating peanuts or drinking milk contaminated with low levels of aflatoxin

B_1 or M_1. In this context, it is of interest that Claus, Krisko and Bolander (1974) concluded that a level of about 4 x 10^4 molecules/liver cell must be reached before the presence of a xenobiotic is even "registered" and it can be calculated that by comparison normal liver metabolites are in vast excess. Thus glutathione and the coenzyme NADP both of which play vital roles in normal intermediary metabolism and may be involved in detoxifying and other metabolic reactions of aflatoxin B_1 (see Fig. 1) appear to be present in the average liver cell at levels of 10^{11} or 10^{12} molecules/cell.

While this evaluation makes no allowance for metabolism and species differences and is generally insufficiently quantitative to permit a valid analysis of the risks to human and animal health, it does at least help to place into perspective contamination of food and feeds with aflatoxin in the µg/kg range.

REFERENCES

Butler, W. H. (1974). Aflatoxin. In I. F. H. Purchase (Ed.), Mycotoxins, Elsevier, Amsterdam, pp 1-28.

Claus, G., Krisko, I. and Bolander, K. (1974). Chemical carcinogens in the environment and in the human diet: can a threshold be established?. Fd Cosmet. Toxicol., 12, 737-746.

FDA, Food and Drug Administration (1978). Assessment of estimated risk resulting from aflatoxins in consumer peanut products and other food commodities, Bureau of Foods, US Food and Drug Administration, Washington DC.

Garner, R. C., Miller, E. C. and Miller, J. A. (1972). Liver microsomal metabolism of aflatoxin B_1 to a reactive derivative toxic to Salmonella typhimurium TA-1530. Cancer Res., 32, 2058-2066.

Heathcote, J. G. and Hibbert, J. R. (1978). Aflatoxins: Chemical and Biological Aspects, Developments in Food Science 1, Elsevier, Amsterdam.

IARC, International Agency for Research on Cancer (1976). Some naturally occurring substances, IARC Monograph on the Evaluation of Carcinogenic Risk of Chemicals to Man, Vol. 10, IARC, Lyon.

Kiermeier, F. (1977). The significance of aflatoxins in the dairy industry. Annu. Bull. Int. Dairy Fed. No. 98.

Long, C. (1961). Ed. Biochemists' Handbook, Spon Ltd, London.

Patterson, D. S. P. (1973). Metabolism as a factor determining the toxic action of aflatoxins in different animal species. Fd Cosmet. Toxicol., 11, 287-294.

Patterson, D. S. P. (1977). Aflatoxin and related compounds. Biochemistry and physiology. In T. D. Wyllie and L. G. Morehouse (Eds), Mycotoxic Fungi, Mycotoxins Mycotoxicoses: An Encyclopedic Handbook, Vol. 1, Marcel Dekker Inc., New York and Basel, pp 159-189.

Patterson, D. S. P. (1979). Foodborne diseases: Aflatoxicosis, In M. Rechcigl (Ed.), CRC Handbook of Nutrition and Food, CRC Press Inc., West Palm Beach, Fla., (in press).

Patterson, D. S. P., Glancy, E. M. and Roberts, B. A. (1979). The "carry-over" of aflatoxin M_1 into the milk of cows fed rations containing 10 µg aflatoxin B_1/kg. Fd Cosmet. Toxicol., (in press).

Patterson, D. S. P., Roberts, B. A., Shreeve, B. J., Wrathall, A. E. and Gitter, M. (1977). Aflatoxin, ochratoxin and zearalenone in animal feedstuffs: some clinical and experimental observations. Ann. Nutr. Aliment., 31, 643-650.

Peers, F. G. and Linsell, C. A. (1977). Dietary aflatoxins and human primary liver cancer. Ann. Nutr. Aliment., 31, 1005-1018.

Rodricks, J. V. and Stoloff, L. (1977). Aflatoxin residues in edible tissues of food producing animals. In J. V. Rodricks, C. W. Hesseltine and M. A. Mehlman (Eds), Mycotoxins in Human and Animal Health, Pathotox Publ. Inc., Park Forest South, Ill., pp 67-79.

Spector, W. S. (1956). Ed. Handbook of Biological Data, Wright Air Development Center, US Air Force, Wright-Patterson Air Force Base, Ohio.

Uraguchi, K. and Yamazaki, M. (1978). Toxicology, Biochemistry and Pathology of Mycotoxins, Kodansha, Tokyo, John Wiley & Son, New York.

Van Rensberg, S. J. (1977). Role of epidemiology in the elucidation of mycotoxin health risks. In J. V. Rodricks, C. W. Hesseltine and M. A. Mehlman (Eds), Mycotoxins in Human and Animal Health, Pathotox Publ. Inc., Park Forest South, Ill., pp 699-711.

WHO, World Health Organization (1979). Mycotoxins, WHO Environmental Health Criteria, No. 11, WHO, Geneva.

Wyllie, T. D. and Morehouse, L. G. (1977). Eds, Mycotoxic Fungi, Mycotoxins, Mycotoxicoses: an Encyclopedic Handbook, 3 vols., Marcel Dekker Inc., New York, and Basel.

Wogan, G. N., Paglialunga, S. and Newberne, P. M. (1974). Carcinogenic effects of low dietary levels of aflatoxin B_1 in rats. Fd Cosmet. Toxicol., 12, 681-685.

EFFECTS OF MYCOTOXINS ON IMMUNITY AND RESISTANCE OF ANIMALS

A. C. Pier, J. L. Richard and J. R. Thurston

National Animal Disease Center, U.S. Department of Agriculture, Science and Education Administration, Agricultural Research, Ames, Iowa, USA

ABSTRACT

Recognition of impaired immunogenesis among animals receiving dietary aflatoxin has added an important new parameter to the undesirable biological reactions caused by mycotoxin consumption. Experimental studies in laboratory animals, poultry, and swine have shown that moderate levels of aflatoxin (ca 0.25 ppm of feed or 0.07 mg/kg body weight B_1 activity) consumed during the period of immunization impaired the establishment of actively acquired immunity in some, but not all model systems. At these levels, thymic hypoplasia and defective cell mediated immune responses with normal antibody production were observed; clinical signs of intoxication other than reduced rate of gain were generally absent. At very high levels of aflatoxin intake, some investigators have reported alterations in the quality and quantity of antibody in addition to the effects on cell mediated immune mechanisms. In addition to aflatoxin, ochratoxin, stachybotryotoxin, diacetoxyscirpenol, and T-2 toxin have been found to adversely affect the thymus and cell mediated immune activity. Aflatoxin has also reduced the effectiveness of the mechanisms of resistance to infection; this effect has been related to a number of actions and has been reported as the basis of field outbreaks of naturally occurring animal disease. The minimal levels of aflatoxin or other mycotoxins affecting immune responses and native resistance remain to be determined.

KEYWORDS

Mycotoxin; aflatoxin; ochratoxin; T-2 toxin; diacetoxyscirpenol; stachybotryotoxin; sterigmatocystin; rubratoxin; immunosuppression; immunity; resistance; native defense mechanisms; cell mediated immunity; thymic involution; antibody; complement; interferon.

The major signs of clinically recognizable mycotoxicoses are usually dictated by the target organs affected by the specific toxin. Thus, acute mycotoxic diseases include the syndromes of aflatoxic hepatitis, ochratoxic nephritis and zearalenone induced estrogenism. However, other clinically important biological effects, apparently unrelated to target organ injury, result from consumption of several mycotoxins. Important among these latter reactions are the effects of aflatoxin, and apparently several other mycotoxins, on the lymphoreticular system which mediates the immune reactivity and native defense mechanisms of the affected consumer (Pier et al, 1979a). Because these latter effects may occur at toxin doses below those associated with clinically apparent mycotoxic disease, they are difficult to relate diagnostically with the causative mycotoxin. However, the medical and economic consequences of these effects may be of equal importance as the more clinically dramatic effects of acute intoxication.

The effects of aflatoxin and other mycotoxins on immunity and resistance have been reviewed extensively in several recent articles (Pier, 1973; Pier et al, 1977 ; Pier et al, 1979a; Pier et al, 1979b; Pier et al, 1979c; Richard et al, 1975; Richard et al, 1978). A brief review of the major known immunosuppressive effects as summarized in these articles will be presented here along with a review of recent scientific reports on this subject.

Aflatoxin has been shown to cause an immunosuppressive response in some model systems when animals were vaccinated while consuming experimentally contaminated rations. Turkey poults consuming 0.25 to 0.5 ppm aflatoxin (B_1 activity) did not develop a solid immunity when challenged 3 weeks after vaccination with virulent Pasteurella multocida (Pier & Heddleston, 1970). In a similar study, swine vaccinated against Erysipelothrix rhusiopathiae while receiving aflatoxin (0.065 mg B_1 activity/kg body wt) also failed to develop a solid protective immunity (Cysewski et al, 1978). Not all model systems have shown this immunosuppressive effect for turkeys receiving aflatoxin developed the same level of immunity as did vaccinated controls when the infectious model was Newcastle Disease Virus (Pier et al, 1971). Apparently the mechanisms of protective immunity for these models was different. The differences in the effects of aflatoxin on cell mediated immune responses and antibody formation have been explored by a number of investigators as recently reviewed by Pier et al, 1979a. Generally speaking, doses of aflatoxin sufficient to cause reduced rate of growth have been sufficient to cause thymic involution and a reduction in cell mediated immune activities as measured by several parameters (Giambrone et al, 1978; Pier et al, 1977). The minimal dose for this effect of aflatoxin has not been determined. A summary of the important effects of aflatoxin on cell mediated immune activities is presented in Table 1.

Aflatoxin has also been associated with impaired production of antibody and of certain nonspecific humoral substances (Giambrone et al, 1978; Pier et al, 1979a; Richard et al, 1978c). The suppression of antibody formation and hypoplasia of the related tissues of the Bursa of Fabricus in poultry is dose related and occurs at doses of toxin substantially above those that suppress cell mediated immune activity. At such levels aflatoxin has been shown to affect both the quantity and quality of antibody produced; the levels of IgG and IgA were reduced in broilers by rations containing 2.5 to 10 ppm total aflatoxin but IgM levels were not affected (Giambrone et al, 1978). At lower levels (0.25 to 0.5 ppm B_1 activity) neither qualitative or quantitative changes were seen in the levels of agglutinins, hemagglutination inhibition or serum neutralizing antibodies (Pier et al, 1979a). The production of complement (primarily C_4') is reduced by aflatoxin (Thurston et al, 1972; Thurston and Richard, 1979) and the toxin also causes a lag in interferon production (Pier, et al, 1971). The major reported effects of aflatoxin on the production of antibodies and nonspecific humoral substances are summarized in Table 2.

TABLE 1 Effects of Aflatoxin on Acquired Immunity and Cell Mediated Immune Responses

Effect	Model	Reference
Immunosuppression	Turkey, chicken (*P. multocida*)	Pier & Heddleston, 1970
Immunosuppression	Pig (*E. rhusiopathiae*)	Cysewski, et al, 1978
Normal immunogenesis	Turkey (Newcastle D.V.)	Pier et al, 1971
Thymic involution (bursa normal)	Turkey (*P. multocida*)	Pier et al, 1972
Thymic & bursal involution	Chicken (sheep rbc)	Thaxton et al, 1974
Phagocytosis impaired	Chicken (colloidal carbon)	Michael et al, 1973
Phagocytosis impaired	Rabbit macrophage (*A. fumigatus*)	Richard & Thurston, 1975
Phagocytosis impaired	Chicken monocyte (*E. cloacae*)	Chang & Hamilton, 1979
Lymphoblastogenesis suppression (*in vitro*)	Human lymphocytes (PHA)	Savel, et al, 1970
Cell mediated immune suppression (*in vivo*) (delayed hypersens.; MIF and lympholastogenesis)	Guinea pig (*N. asteroides*, PHA)	Pier et al, 1976
Lymphoblastogenesis suppression (*in vitro*)	Bovine lymphocytes (PHA, con A, PWM)	Paul et al, 1977
Cell mediated immune suppression (*in vivo*) (delayed hypersens., graft-host)	Chicken (allogeneic blood, tuberculin)	Giambrone et al, 1978

TABLE 2 Effects of Aflatoxin on Production of Antibody and Nonspecific Humoral Substances Related to Resistance and Immunity

Effect	Model	Reference
Antibody suppression (agglutinin)	Mice (*S. typhi*)	Galikeev et al, 1968
Antibody normal (agglut.)	Turkeys (*P. multocida*)	Pier & Heddleston, 1970
Antibody normal (HI & SN) Interferon lag	Turkeys (Newcastle D.V.)	Pier et al, 1971
Antibody normal (density grad. fractions, agglut., precipit.)	Turkeys (*P. multocida*)	Pier et al, 1972
Antibody normal (IHA)	Chicken (*S. pullorum*)	Adinarayanaiah et al, 1973
Antibody lag (HA)	Chicken (sheep rbc)	Thaxton et al, 1974
Complement reduction	Guinea Pig (sheep rbc lysis)	Thurston et al, 1972
Complement reduction Antibody normal (agglut., C.F.)	Guinea pig (*B. abortus*)	Thurston et al, 1974
Complement reduction Antibody normal (agglut., C.F.)	Guinea pig (*B. abortus*)	Richard et al, 1974a
IgG suppression (IgM normal)	Chicken	Tung et al, 1975
IgA and IgG suppression (IgM normal)	Chicken	Giambrone et al, 1978

In addition to the effects on acquired immune responses, aflatoxin consumption also has impaired native defense mechanisms associated with resistance to some infectious and parasitic diseases. Presumably these reactions are caused by the effects on phagocytosis, complement and interferon discussed above and perhaps by other mechanisms as well. Impaired resistance has not been manifest in all of the experimental models studied. The results of reported studies of the effects of aflatoxin on resistance as measured by incidence, severity or incubation period are summarized in Table 3.

TABLE 3 Effect of Aflatoxin on Resistance to Infection

Model	Enhanced susceptibility*	Reference
Chicken (*Salmonella gallinarum*)	-	Smith et al, 1969
Chicken (*Candida albicans*)	+	Hamilton & Harris, 1971
Turkey (*Aspergillus fumigatus*)	-	Richard et al, 1973
Chicken (*Eimeria tenella*)	+	Edds et al, 1973
Chicken (*Eimeria tenella*)	+	Wyatt et al, 1975
Hamster (*Mycobacterium paratuberculosis*)	-	Larsen et al, 1975
Chicken (Salmonella spp.: *S. worthington*, *S. derby*, & *S. thompson*)	+	Boonchuvit & Hamilton, 1975
Chicken (*S. typhimurium*)	+	Boonchuvit & Hamilton, 1975
Calf (*Fasciola hepatica*)	+	Edds & Osuna, 1976
Pigs (*Treponema hyodysenteriae*)	+	Joens & Pier, 1979**

*Increased incidence of infection, reduced incubation period, or increased severity of disease. **Unpublished data.

Certain other mycotoxins also appear capable of modifying the immune response. Rubratoxin and sterigmatocystin cause a reduction in complement activity; ochratoxin causes lymphoid necrosis and apparently impairs antibody formation indirectly. T-2 toxin and diacetoxyscirpenol cause thymic involution and reduce the clearance of inoculated bacteria and impair production of certain antibodies; a T-2 toxin-related enhancement in delayed hypersensitivity in mice has been ascribed to interference with suppressor cell activity. Stachybotryotoxin has been reported to impair both antibody production and delayed cutaneous hypersensitivity. These effects are summarized with appropriate references in Table 4.

DISCUSSION

Aflatoxin is established as an important modifier of the immune response. A number of its actions also impair the native defense mechanisms against infections. The primary effect of aflatoxin on immune reactivity appears to be some action on the thymus derived lymphocytes. The exact nature of that action is not known. In part, at least, there appears to be a selective lympholytic response in that

TABLE 4 Effects of Other Mycotoxins on Immunogenesis and Resistance

Toxin	Major Effects	Reference
T-2 toxin	Poult: thymic involution. No affect on P. multocida antibody.	Richard et al, 1978a
	Mice: thymic hypoplasia, reduced graft vs host & anti sheep rbc agglut.	Rosenstein et al, 1978
	Mice: reduced clearance Listeria + rise in antibody (tetanus antitox.).	Wiskott, 1978
	Mice: enhancement of delayed hypersensitivity (sheep rbc)	Masuko et al, 1977
DAS	Mice: thymic involution, depress sheep rbc agglut and graft vs host.	Rosenstein et al, 1978
	Mice: reduced tetanus antitox., reduced Listeria clearance, reduced immune response to Pasteurella.	Wiskott, 1978
Stachybotryotoxin	Mice: reduced sheep rbc agglutinins.	Danko & Krasznia, 1976
	Guinea pigs: reduced skin test reaction to BCG.	Danko & Krasznia, 1976
Ochratoxin	Dogs, Pigs: lymphoid necrosis (gut, spleen, et al.).	Szczech et al, 1973
	Mice: secondary reduction of antibody to B. abortus; lymphocytes normal.	Prior & Sisodia, 1979
Sterigmatocystin	Guinea pigs: reduced complement titer.	Richard et al, 1978b
Rubratoxin	Guinea pigs: reduced complement titer.	Richard et al, 1974b

cortical thymic regions are markedly depleted of lymphocytes by doses of aflatoxin that do not alter the architecture of the Bursa of Fabricius. At high levels of aflatoxin intake, the latter organ can also be affected with resultant impairment of antibody production. The thymus derived lymphocyte appears to have a similar order of sensitivity to aflatoxin as the hepatocyte. At least in turkey poults and guinea pigs impairment of immunogenesis and cell mediated immune responsiveness has been caused by levels of aflatoxin that cause little or no hepatic cell necrosis, albeit there may be some change in hepatic function. The first detectable sign of aflatoxicosis is generally considered to be a reduced growth response in young animals. Whether the impairment of cell mediated immune responsiveness can be induced by doses of aflatoxin lower than those affecting rate of gain remains to be determined.

Evidence is accumulating that other mycotoxins also influence the immune response; important among these appear to be ochratoxin, T-2 toxin, diacetoxyscirpenol and stachybotryotoxin. It seems likely that still other mycotoxins will be found to have activity on the immune system.

The immunosuppressive and resistance impairing aspects of mycotoxins presents some complex problems to the diagnostician. At least with aflatoxin, the impairment of immunogenesis and native defense mechanisms may occur in the absence of other clinical signs of intoxication except, perhaps, for a moderately depressed rate of gain by young animals. In such cases the clinical signs of disease are referable to the infectious agent rather than to the mycotoxin that predisposed the individual to infection.

The frequency with which these actions occur under field conditions is not known and will be very difficult to ascertain because the signs of disease are those associated with the infectious process rather than the mycotoxin. Some evidence that these effects do occur under field conditions is present in the literature. Both salmonellosis and candidosis were associated with early reports of Turkey X disease in 1960 (Siller et al). Following the appearance of aflatoxin in high levels in field corn grown in the Southeastern U.S. in 1977, a flurry of outbreaks of salmonellosis in swine were attributed to interaction with dietary aflatoxin (Miller et al, 1978). A high incidence of equine abortion caused by opportunistic bacterial infection was associated with T-2 toxin in feeds of southern Hokkaido (Tatsuno, 1979). Obviously, firm scientific proof of such field disease relationships is extremely difficult to establish. However, the experimental evidence indicates that it is a problem of substantial magnitude with significant importance to both veterinary and human medicine.

REFERENCES

Adinaryanaiah, G. L., R. D. Nanjiah, and B. S. Keshavamurthy (1973). Indian Vet. J. 50(4), 297-303.

Boonchuvit, B., and P. B. Hamilton (1975). Poult. Sci., 54, 1567-1573.

Chang, C. F., and P. B. Hamilton (1979). Poult. Sci., 562-566.

Cysewski, S. J., R. L. Wood, A. C. Pier, and A. L. Baetz (1978). Am. J. Vet. Res., 39(3), 445-448.

Danko, G., and G. Krasznia (1976). Magyar Allatorvosok Lapja, 31, 233-244.

Edds, G. T., K. P. C., Nair, and C. F. Simpson (1973). Am. J. Vet. Res., 34, 819-826.

Edds, G. T., and Osuna, O. (1976). Proc. 80th Ann. Meet. U.S. An. Hlth. Assoc., 434-441.

Galikeev, KH. L., O. R. Raipov, and R. A. Manyasheva (1968). Byul. Eksper. Biol. Med. (USSR), 65(5), 88-90.

Giambrone, J. J., D. L. Ewert, R. D. Wyatt, and C. S. Edison (1978). Am. J. Vet. Res., 39(2), 305-308.

Hamilton, P. B., and J. R. Harris (1971). Poult. Sci., 50, 906-912.

Larsen, A. B., S. J. Cysewski, and J. M. Miller (1975). Am. J. Vet. Res., 36, 1545-1547.

Masuko, H., Y. Ueno, M. Otokawa, and K. Yaginuma (1977). Jap. J. Med. Sci., 30, 159-163.

Michael, G. Y., P. Thaxton, and P. B. Hamilton (1973). Poult. Sci., 52(3), 1206-1207.
Miller, D. M., B. P. Stuart, W. A. Crowell, J. R. Cole, A. J. Goven, and J. Brown (1978). Proc. Am. Assoc. Vet. Lab. Diag., 135-146.
Paul, P. S., D. W. Johnson, C. J. Mirocha, F. F. Soper, C. O. Thoen, C. C. Mucoplat, and A. F. Weber (1977). Am. J. Vet. Res., 38(12), 2033-2035.
Pier, A. C. (1973). J. Am. Vet. Med. Assoc., 163(11), 1268-1269.
Pier, A. C., S. J. Cysewski, J. L. Richard, and J. R. Thurston (1977). Mycotoxins in Human and Animal Health (Pathotox), 745-750.
Pier, A. C., R. E. Fichtner, R. E, and S. J. Cysewski (1976). III. Intl. IUPAC Symp. Mycotoxins in Foodstuffs, Abstr. 61, 9.

Pier, A. C., and K. L. Heddleston (1970). Avian Dis., 14, 797-809.
Pier, A. C., K. L. Heddleston, W. A. Boney, and P. D. Lukert (1971). Proc. XIX Cong. Mundial de Med. Vet. Zootech., 1, 216-219.
Pier, A. C., K. L. Heddleston, S. J. Cysewski, and J. M. Patterson (1972). Avian Dis., 16, 381-387.
Pier, A. C., J. L. Richard, and J. R. Thurston (1979a). Proc. Symp. on the interactions of Mycotoxins in Animal Production, Nat'l. Acad. Sci., 56-66.
Pier, A. C., J. L. Richard, and J. R. Thurston (1979b). Proc. I.A.M.S. Congress, (in press).
Pier, A. C., J. L. Richard, and J. R. Thurston (1979c). Inadvertent Modifications of the Immune Response, FDA Science Symposium, (in press).

Prior, M. G., and C. S. Sisodia (1979). 6th Intl. Symp. on Animal, Plant, and Microbial Toxins, Toxicon, 17, 146.
Richard, J. L., A. C. Pier, S. J. Cysewski, and C. K. Graham (1973). Avian Dis., 17, 111-121.
Richard, J. L., and J. R. Thurston (1975). Appl. Microbiol., 30, 44-47.
Richard, J. L., J. R. Thurston, and A. C. Pier (1975). Microbiology - 1975, 388-396.
Richard, J. L., J. R. Thurston, B. L. Deyoe, and G. D. Booth (1974a). Appl. Microbiol., 29, 27-29.
Richard, J. L., J. R. Thurston, and C. K. Graham (1974b). Am. J. Vet. Res., 35, 957-959.
Richard, J. L., S. J. Cysewski, A. C. Pier, and G. D. Booth (1978a). Am. J. Vet. Res., 39, 1674-1679.
Richard, J. L., J. R. Thurston, E. B. Lillehoj, S. J. Cysewski, and G. D. Booth (1978b). Am. J. Vet. Res., 39, 163-166.
Richard, J. L., J. R. Thurston, and A. C. Pier (1978c). Proc. 5th Intl. Symp. Toxins: Animal, Plant, and Microbial, Pergamon, New York, 801-817.
Rosenstein, Y., C. Lafarge-Frayssinet, G. Lespinats, F. Loisillier, P. Lafont, and C. Frayssinet (1979). Immunology, 36, 111-117.
Savel, H., B. Forsyth, W. Schaeffer, and T. Cardella (1970) Proc. Soc. Exptl. Biol. Med..134(4), 1112-1115.
Siller, W. G., and D. C. Ostler (1961). Vet. Rec., 73(7), 134-138.
Smith, J. W., W. R. Prince, and P. B. Hamilton (1969). Appl. Microbiol., 18(5), 946-947.
Szczech, G. M., W. W. Carlton, J. Tuite, and R. Caldwell (1974). Vet. Path., 10, 347-364.
Tatsuno, T., H. Tsunoda, K. Ohkubo, K. Terao, K. Aibara, and T. Konishi (1979). Abstr. O(H)26 Am. Soc. Microbiol., 202.
Thaxton, J. P., H. T. Tung, and P. B. Hamilton (1974). Poult. Sci., 53, 721-725.

Thurston, J. R., J. L. Richard, S. J. Cysewski, A. C. Pier, and C. K. Graham (1972). Proc. Soc. Exp. Biol. Med., 138, 300-303.
Thurston, J. R., B. L. Deyoe, A. L. Baetz, J. L. Richard, and G. D. Booth (1974). Am. J. Vet. Res., 35, 1097-1110.
Thurston, J. R., and J. L. Richard (1979). Am. J. Vet. Res., 40, 1206-1208.
Tung, H. T., R. D. Wyatt, P. Thaxton, and P. B. Hamilton (1975). Tox. Appl. Pharmacol., 34, 320-326.
Wiskott, U. (1978). Doctoral dissertation, Ludwig-Maximilian, Univ. Munich.
Wyatt, R. D., M. D. Ruff, and R. K. Page (1975). Avian Dis., 19(4), 730-740.

Additional Paper

NEUROTOXINS AS TOOLS FOR BIOCHEMICAL CHARACTERIZATION OF ION CHANNELS

W. Schiebler, S. Stengelin and F. Hucho

Freie Universität Berlin, Fachbereich Chemie, Berlin, Federal Republic of Germany

ABSTRACT

Certain Neurotoxins may be used as tools for the characterization of molecular components involved in nerve impuls propagation. We intend to use them for the investigation of receptor-ion channel relationships in excitable membranes.

α-Neurotoxins from Cobra and Krait venom have been shown to block specifically nicotinic acetylcholine receptors. By hybridisation of toxin blocked receptor with receptor the ion translocation mechanism of which has been blocked by quinacrine mustard we have obtained evidence that receptor site and ion channel in the postsynaptic membrane of Torpedo electric tissue can be located on different molecules.

Anemone toxins have been shown to inhibit inactivation of voltage dependent sodium channels (Romey et al. PNAS 73, 4055-4059, 1976; Bergman et al., BBA 455, 173-184, 1976). From the three anemone toxins which have been purified and the aminoacid sequence of which has been elucidated we choose for our experiments ATX I, because this polypeptide can be labeled radioactively by gentle enzymatic methods. We iodinated ATX I by the lactoperoxidase method and we isolated monoiodo ATX I (^{125}I-ATX I) from the diiodo product and from unlabeled toxin by ion exchange chromatography. ^{125}I-ATX I was shown to bind specifically to the axonal membrane from Astacus leptodactylus main walking nerve. Astacus nerve bound 44 fmoles of ^{125}I-ATX I per mg nerve (wet weight). The axonal membrane surface of the nerve was determined to be 7 800 cm^2 per gram nerve. This amounts to a binding site density of around 35/μ^2 axonal surface. Binding was not inhibited by tetrodotoxin, the blocker of the selectivity filter of voltage dependent sodium channels.

^{125}I-ATX I therefore may bind to the sodium channel inactivating gate. The affinity of the nerve membrane receptors for ^{125}I-ATX I appears to be voltage dependent: K_D= 5 nM was found with whole crayfish nerves in the presence of tetrodotoxin, K_D= 40 nM in the absence of tetrodotoxin, and an even lower affinity was observed with axonal membrane fragments isolated from the nerve. Drugs destabilizing the membrane potential, e.g. veratridin, ouabain and sodium azide lowered the affinity or abolished binding completely.

The photoaffinity derivative NAP-^{125}I-ATX I (2-nitro-4-azidophenyl ^{125}I-ATX I) was synthesized, purified, and shown to have retained the toxicity of the native ATX I.

KEYWORDS

Acetylcholine receptor; reconstitution; receptor-ion channel-relationship; sodium channel; anemone toxin ATX I.

INTRODUCTION

Ion channels appear to be composed of two parts: A selectivity filter determining which ion may pass and which is excluded and a gate which determines in response to a signal when an ion may pass. The signal moving the gate may be a chemical one e.g. a transmitter substance or an electrical one, a change in membrane potential. This paper is dealing with one example of each type: The acetyl choline regulated ion channel of the postsynaptic membrane of nicotinic cholinergic synapses and the voltage dependent sodium channel of axonal membranes. Since both types are receptor sites for many neurotoxins both respond to chemical signals as well and might not be so principally different. Here we focus on the question as to how receptor site and ion channel are interrelated and we propose assay systems to solve this question.

THE NICOTINIC ACETYLCHOLINE RECEPTOR

Acetylcholine (ACh) regulates the ion permeability of the postsynaptic membrane of cholinergic synapses via a special membrane protein, the acetylcholine receptor (AChR). In the centre of the biochemists interest is the mechanism by which the receptor influences the membrane resistance: Does it interact with an ionophor, or represents it the ion channel itself? The receptor site for cholinergic effectors (Weill, McNamee, and Karlin, 1964; Hucho and co-workers, 1976) including the neurotoxins (Hucho and co-workers, 1976; Hucho, 1979) is located on a polypeptide of MW 40 000 dalton but at least in the electric tissue of <u>Torpedo californica</u> this receptor subunit appears to be part of a larger protein complex:

1. Four major and several minor protein components can be detected in receptor-rich membranes from <u>Torpedo</u>.
2. After solubilization of the membrane these four polipeptide chains remain associated and are co-purified by affinity chromatography.
3. The four chains can be cross-linked with diimidates. The cross-linked complex has a molecular weight of 270 000 (Hucho, Bandini, and Suárez-Isla, 1978).
4. Polypeptide chains of MW 68 000 and 55 000 are located within the membrane close to the receptor protein of MW 40 000, as evidenced by means of photoaffinity derivatives of α-bungarotoxin and α-Naja naja toxin (Hucho, 1979).
5. A protein kinase and a phosphatase appear to be endogenous to the receptor membrane. Polypeptide chains of MW 45 000 and 55 000 react with a photoaffinity derivative of ATP (Gordon and co-workers, 1979).

From structural investigations alone the relation between acetylcholine binding site (the receptor in the true sense of the word) and ion channel cannot be deduced. We therefore attempted to tackle the problem by reconstitution experiments. In this report we present evidence that in the case of the nicotinic acetylcholine receptor from the electric organ of <u>Torpedo californica</u> transmitter binding site and ion channel are not necessarily located on the same protein molecule. By hybridisation of receptor complexes in which the transmitter binding site is blocked with complexes in which the ion channel is irreversibly inhibited we were able to reconstitute active acetylcholine receptor complexes. The reconstitued system was similar to the native receptor in its ability to regulate the ion permeability of lipid vesicles in response to nicotinic cholinergic effectors.

The hybridisation experiment was performed with membrane fragments enriched in acetylcholine receptor prepared from the electric organs of Torpedo californica according to Duguid and Raftery,(1973) with the slight modifications described (Schiebler and Hucho, 1978). One sample of the receptor-enriched membranes was treated with α-bungarotoxin, a strong and virtually irreversible competitive inhibitor of the transmitter binding site in nicotinic acetylcholine receptors. Another sample of this preparation was treated with quinacrine mustard. Quinacrine has been shown to act upon the postsynaptic membrane of nicotinic cholinergic synapses as a local anaesthetic (Grünhagen, Ywatsubo, and Changeux, 1977), characterised by its blocking effect on the ion translocation through the membrane without competitively inhibiting transmitter binding. We have shown that the alkylating derivative quinacrine mustard irreversibly blocks the ion permeability response to agonists in receptor enriched membrane microsacs (Lauffer, Weber, and Hucho, 1979). These modified membranes still contained at least fifty percent of their high-affinity binding sites for ^{3}H-acetylcholine.

Both these modified samples were dissolved in detergent supplemented with lecithine, first separately, for the controls, later jointly, for the hybridisation experiment. Reconstitution of the detergent solubilised membranes to functional liposomal receptor-membrane systems was performed by column chromatograph with Sephadex G 50 as described before (Schiebler and Hucho, 1978). Receptor function was measured by determining the ^{22}Na efflux from reconstituted vesicles by the Millipore filtration assay developed by Popot, Sugijama, and Changeux,(1976). Maximum efflux was determined by adding gramicidin to the vesicles (open squares in figure 1). The first control experiment was aimed to show that under the conditions of the reconstitution experiment the bungarotoxin block is virtually irreversible (top frame of fig. 1, labeled "T", for toxin). The time dependent ^{22}Na efflux from vesicles reconstituted with toxin-blocked receptor could not be stimulated by 0.1 mM carbamoylcholine although considerable amounts of radioactivity could be released with gramicidin. A similar result was obtained in the second control experiment with quinacrine mustard blocked receptor (middle frame of the figure, labeled "Q"): the ^{22}Na efflux from vesicles reconstituted with mustard-blocked receptor could also not be stimulated by 0.1 mM carbamoyl choline. (In this experiment unstimulated "leakage" of ^{22}Na was higher as compared to the "T"-experiment. This increased leakage was consistently observed with quinacrine modified membranes (Lauffer, Weber, and Hucho, 1979) and may be due to the increase of lipid fluidity caused by the local anaesthetic).

Reconstitution of a one to one mixture of toxin-blocked and quinacrine mustard-blocked receptor-rich membranes resulted in vesicles in which the ^{22}Na efflux could be stimulated by 0.1 mM carbamoyl choline (bottom frame, labeled "TQ"). This stimulation (open circles) was prevented by preincubation of the reconstituted "TQ"-vesicles with Naja naja siamensis toxin, another competitive inhibitor of nicotinic acetylcholine receptors (closed squares).

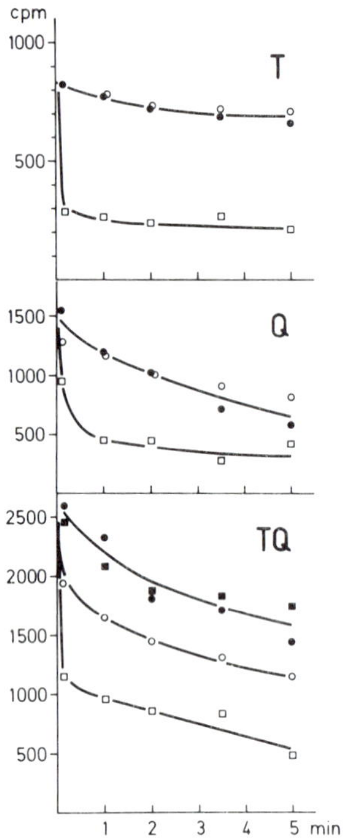

Fig.1: *Hybridisation of binding site-blocked (T) and ion channel blocked (Q) AChR yielding functionally active AChR (TQ).*

o-o-o ^{22}Na efflux in absence and presence ^{22}Na efflux from reconstituted AChR-lipid vesicles in the absence (●-●-●) and presence (o-o-o) of 10^{-4} M carbamoylcholine. Inhibition of carbamoylcholine stimulation by α-neurotoxin from Naja naja siamensis (■-■-■). ^{22}Na efflux in the presence of 0.1 mg/ml gramicidin A (□-□-□).

The simplest explanation of this result would be based on the following model: The nicotinic acetylcholine receptor of the Torpedo membrane is composed of two types of subunits, one carrying the transmitter binding site (being the receptor "sensu stricto"), the other translocating the cations (being the ion channel, ionophore).

Another possibility would be a complementation of two identical polypeptide chains forming together the active AChR complex, each containing both a ligand binding site and an ionophor. In our reconstitution experiment polypeptides with unblocked receptor sites would complement with chains containing unblocked ion channels. Both models, the first assuming distinct proteins for receptor and channel, the second postulating only one type of polypeptide chain, would imply that receptor and channel are not necessarily located on the same polypeptide chain and that in our reconstitution experiment exchange of chains, identical or not, took place. Several alternative explanations were investigated and ruled out by appropriate control experiments (not shown).

THE VOLTAGE DEPENDENT Na^+ CHANNEL OF THE AXON

Neither structural investigations nor reconstitution experiments with ion channels involved in action potential propagation are as advanced as with the AChR. We are attempting to obtain first biochemical informations by binding studies using radioactively labeled ATX I, a polypeptide neurotoxin from Anemonia sulcata. Anemone toxins have been shown to inhibit sodium conductance inactivation (Narahashi, Moore, and Shapiro, 1969; Bergman and co-workers; Romey and colleagues, 1976).

Its binding site in the axonal membrane might therefore be associated with the "gate" of the sodium channel (in analogy to the snake venom α-neurotoxins which bind to the gating mechanism of postsynaptic channels, the AChR). We labeled ATX I with ^{125}I and obtained pure monoiodo ATX I and a photoaffinity derivative (NAP-^{125}I-ATX I) was also prepared (Hucho, Béress, and Stengelin, 1979).

^{125}I-ATX I was shown to bind specifically to the axonal membrane from Astacus leptodactylus main walking nerve (Hucho, Stengelin, and Bandini, 1979). Specificity of binding was shown by saturability of the binding sites and by competitive binding of native and radioactive toxin. Astacus nerve bound 44 fmoles of ^{125}I-ATX I per mg nerve (wet weight). The axonal membrane surface of the nerve was determined to be 7 800 cm^2 per gram nerve. This amounts to a binding site density of around $35/\mu^2$ axonal surface. Binding was not inhibited by tetrodotoxin, the blocker of the selectivity filter of voltage dependent sodium channels. ^{125}I-ATX I therefore may bind to the sodium channel inactivating gate.

The affinity of the nerve membrane receptors for ^{125}I-ATX I appears to be voltage dependent: K_D= 5 μM was found with whole crayfish nerves in the presence of tetrodotoxin (fig. 2), K_D= 40 μM in the absence of tetrodotoxin (Hucho, Stengelin, and Bandini, 1979), and an even lower affinity was observed with axonal membrane fragments isolated from the nerve.

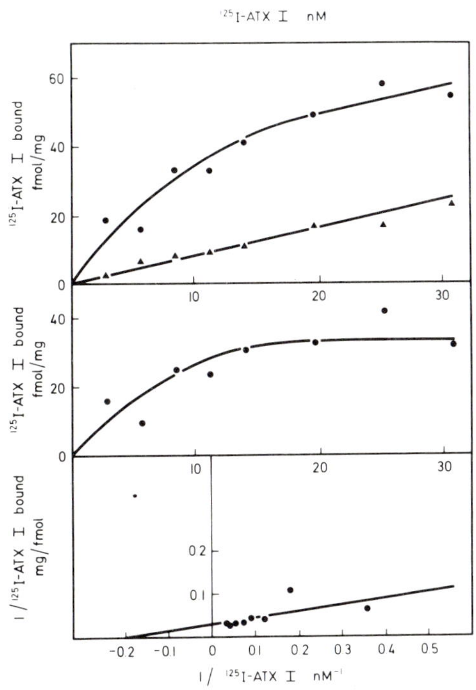

Fig.2: *Binding of ^{125}I-ATX I to crayfish nerves in the presence of TTX:*

Pieces from main walking nerves of Astacus leptodactylus (5 - 15 mg) were incubated in 0.27 ml buffer solutions containing ^{125}I-ATX I as indicated and 10 μM TTX. (a) o-o-o Total binding per mg nerve after 15 hours incubation. ▲-▲-▲ Binding in the presence of a 520 fold molar excess of ATX I. (b) Difference between the two curves, representing specific binding. (c) Double reciprocal plot of the data of (b). The plot extrapolates (regression analysis) to 35 fmol/mg bound ^{125}I-ATX I and to an apparent K_D= 5 nM.

Drugs destabilizing the membrane potential, e.g. veratridin, ouabain and sodium azide lowered the affinity or abolished binding completely (fig. 3a - d).

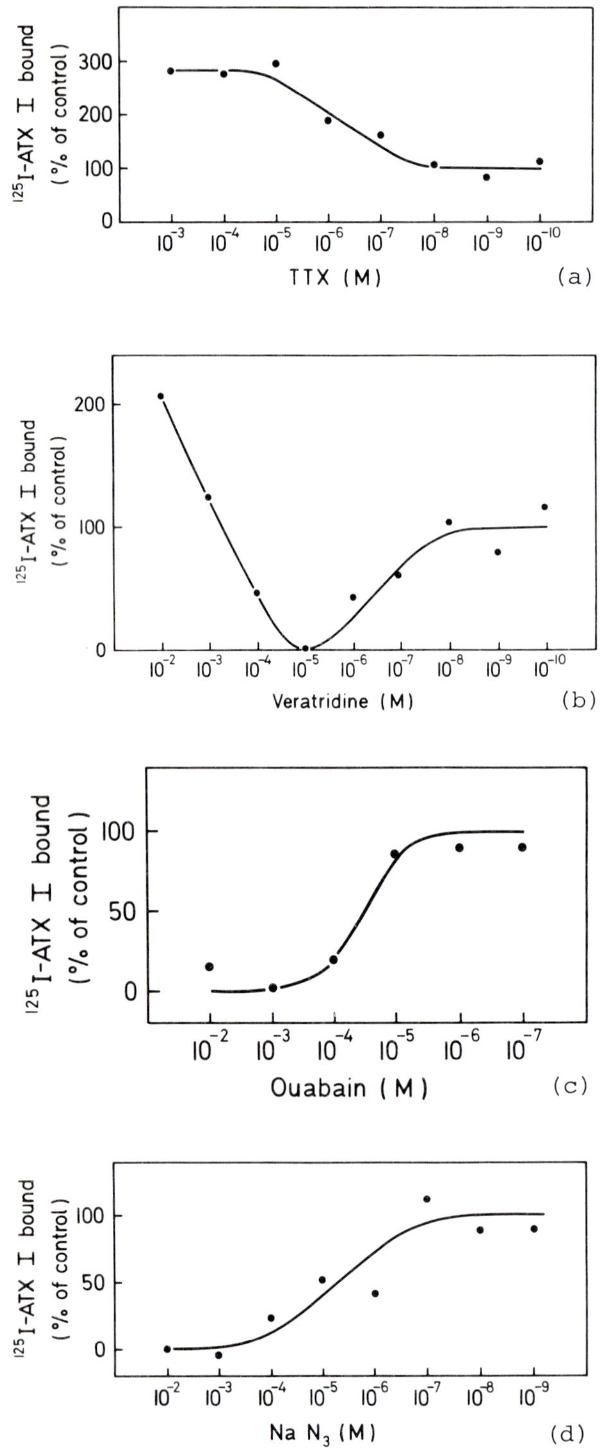

Fig.3: *Effect of various toxins on* ^{125}*I-ATX binding:*

Pieces from main walking nerves of Astacus leptodactylus (5 - 15 mg) were incubated in 0.26 ml buffer solution containing 25.3 nM ^{125}I-ATX I and the indicated concentrations of toxin. As a control (100 %) specific binding in the absence of effectors was determined by subtracting unspecific binding (obtained from samples containing 7.5 μM ATX I and 25.3 nM ^{125}I-ATX I) from total binding (obtained from samples containing only 25.3 nM ^{125}I-ATX I).

(a) About threefold enhancement of specific binding by TTX.

(b) Inhibition of ^{125}I-ATX I binding by veratridine.

(c) Inhibition of anemone toxin by ouabain.

(d) Inhibition of anemone toxin binding by sodium azide.

Binding in the presence of varying concentrations of veratridin appeared to be especially complex (fig. 3 b). Up to 10 μM veratridin inhibited ^{125}I-ATX binding, but a further increase stimulated it. We believe that the inhibition is due to the depolarizing effect of veratridin which is compensated at higher concentrations by the cooperativity of veratridin and ATX binding. This latter effect has been observed before with ^{22}Na flux experiments performed with neuroblastoma cells (Catterall and Béress, 1979).

ACKNOWLEDGEMENT

We would like to thank Dr. L. Béress and Mr. J. Zwick for generous gifts of ATX I. Also, the skilled technical assistance of Ms. Birsner is gratefully acknowledged. This work was supported by the Deutsche Forschungsgemeinschaft (SFB 138) and the Fonds der Chemischen Industrie.

REFERENCES

Bergmann, C., J.M. Dubois, E. Rojas, and W. Rathmayer (1976). Biochim. Biophys. Acta 455, 173-184.
Catterall, W.A., and L. Béress (1978). J. Biol. Chem. 253, 7793-7396.
Duguid, J.R., and M.A. Raftery (1973). Biochemistry 12, 3593-3597.
Gordon, A.S., R.J. Guillory, I. Diamond, and F. Hucho (1979). FEBS Letters, in press.
Grünhagen, H.-H., M. Iwatsubo, and J.P. Changeux (1977). Eur. J. Biochem. 80, 225-242.
Hucho, F., P. Layer, H.R. Kiefer, and G. Bandini (1976). Proc. Natl. Acad. Sci. USA, 73, 2624-2638.
Hucho, F., G. Bandini, und B. Suárez-Isla (1978). Eur. J. Biochem. 83, 334-340.
Hucho, F. (1979). FEBS Letters 103, 27-32.
Hucho, F. S. Stengelin, and G. Bandini (1979) Recent advances in receptor chemistry (Gualtieri, F., Gianella, M., Melchiorre, C., eds.) Elsevier/North-Holland, pp. 37-58.
Lauffer, L., K.-H. Weber, and F. Hucho (1979). Biochim. Biophys. Acta 587, 42-48.
Narahashi, T., J.W. Moore, and B.J. Shapiro (1969). Science 163, 680-681.
Popot, J.L., H. Sugijama, and J.P. Changeux (1976). J.Mol.Biol. 106, 469-483.
Romey, G., J.P. Abita, H. Schweitz, G. Wunderer, and M. Lazdunski (1976). Proc. Natl. Acad. Sci. USA, 73, 4055-4059.
Schiebler, W., and F. Hucho (1978). Eur. J. Biochem. 85, 55-63
Stengelin, S., L. Béress, and F. Hucho (1979). Function and molecular aspects of Biomembrane transport. (Quagliariello, E., Palmieri, F., Papa, S., Klingenberg, M., eds.) Elsevier/North-Holland, Amsterdam, New York, pp. 43-51.
Weill, C.L., M.G. McNamee, and A. Karlin (1974). Biochem.Biophys. Res. Commun. 61, 997-1003.

Author Index

Keyword Index

The page numbers in most cases refer to the first pages of the articles in which the keywords appear. T following a page number indicates a table.